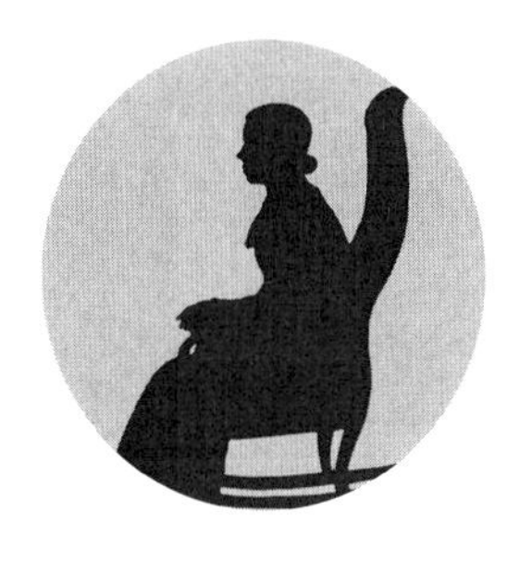

Aunt Minnie's Atlas
and
Imaging-Specific Diagnosis

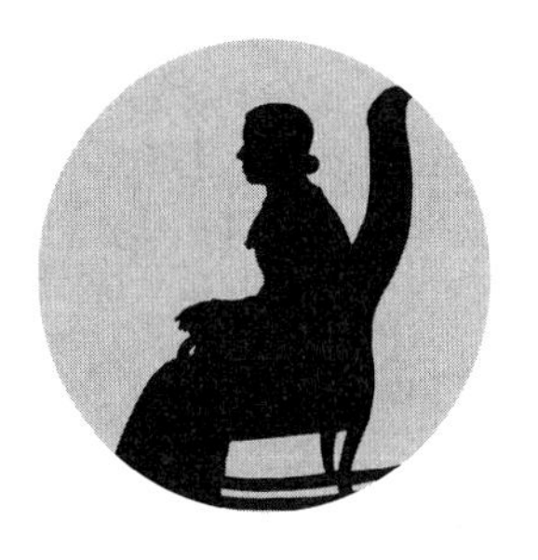

Aunt Minnie's Atlas and Imaging-Specific Diagnosis

KENNETH L. FORD III, MD

Staff Radiologist
Baylor University Medical Center
Dallas, Texas
Medical Director
Texas Diagnostic Imaging Center—Mesquite
Mesquite, Texas

THOMAS L. POPE Jr., MD

Professor and Section Head
Director of Education
Department of Radiology
Bowman Gray School of Medicine
Winston-Salem, North Carolina

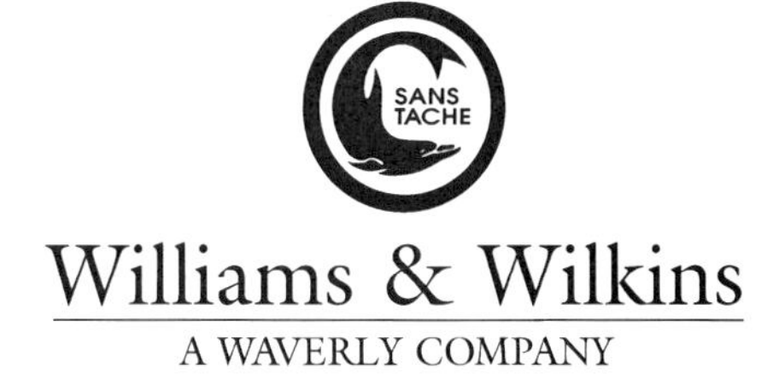

BALTIMORE • PHILADELPHIA • LONDON • PARIS • BANGKOK
BUENOS AIRES • HONG KONG • MUNICH • SYDNEY • TOKYO • WROCLAW

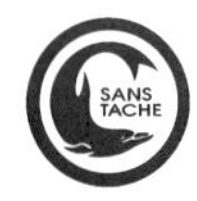

Editor: Charles W. Mitchell
Managing Editor: Grace E. Miller
Production Coordinator: Marette Magargle-Smith
Copy Editor: Therese Grundl
Designer: Dan Pfisterer
Illustration Planner: Lorraine Wrzosek
Composition: Mario Fernández
Digitized Illustrations: Publicity Engravers
Manufacturing: R.R. Donnelley & Sons

351 West Camden Street
Baltimore, Maryland 21201-2436 USA

Rose Tree Corporate Center
1400 North Providence Road
Building II, Suite 5025
Media, Pennsylvania 19063-2043 USA

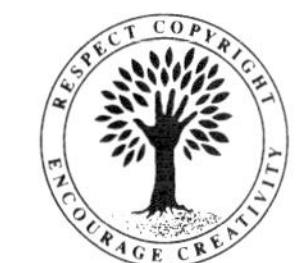

Printed in the United States of America

First Edition,

Library of Congress Cataloging-in-Publication Data

Aunt Minnie's atlas and imaging-specific diagnosis / [edited by] Kenneth L. Ford III, Thomas L. Pope, Jr.
p. cm.
Includes index.
ISBN 0-683-03309-3
1. Diagnostic imaging—Atlases. I. Ford, Kenneth L. II. Pope, Thomas Lee
[DNLM: 1. Diagnostic Imaging. 2. Radiography—methods. WN180 A926 1997]
RC78.7.D53A96 1997
616.07'54—dc20
DNLM/DLC
for Library of Congress 96-13796
CIP

To purchase additional copies of this book, call our customer service department at **(800) 638-0672** or fax **(800) 447-8438.** For other book services, including chapter reprints and large quantity sales, ask for the Special Sales department.

Canadian customers should call **(800) 268-4178** or fax **(905) 470-6780.** For all other calls originating outside of the United States, please call **(410) 528-4223** or fax us at **(410) 528-8550.**

Visit Williams & Wilkins on the Internet: **http://www.wwilkins.com** or contact our customer service department at **custserv@wwilkins.com**. Williams & Wilkins customer service representatives are available from 8:30 am to 6:00 pm, EST, Monday through Friday, for telephone access.

98 99 00 01
3 4 5 6 7 8 9 10

To my loving wife Holly and son Kenneth—their extraordinary support, encouragement, and sacrifice have allowed me to realize the dream of completing this text.

To the outstanding radiology residents at Bowman Gray, Mallinckrodt, and Baylor University Medical Center—their intellectual curiosity and eagerness to learn make this project worthwhile.

KENNETH L. FORD III

To my wife Lou, my boys David and Jason, my mom Florence, my brother Roger, and to Dad, whom I wish could have lived to see the book completed.

THOMAS L. POPE JR.

FOREWORD

As a child I dreaded summer vacations. All we ever did was visit relatives. One relative in particular was a mystery to me. You guessed it: my Aunt Minnie. I had heard about her and imagined how she might look, but my mental image of this grand lady was way off. When we finally met, I knew I would never forget her.

As radiologists we have our own "Aunt Minnies." They are diagnoses made on the basis of imaging features that are nearly specific or for which no significant differential diagnosis exists. Until we see these cases for the first time, we can feel frustrated when trying to define the condition. Once exposed to an "Aunt Minnie," however, we never forget her. Familiarity with these Aunt Minnies can bolster our confidence when reviewing cases with colleagues who have not seen them before. Conversely, like the aunt we have not met yet, the unfamiliar Aunt Minnie can produce anxiety when we attempt to generate a practical differential diagnosis.

Image interpretation requires radiologists to incorporate data from various imaging modalities and to evaluate the data with an essential understanding of pathology, laboratory results, and clinical information. This approach usually allows us to develop a lengthy differential diagnosis. Obviously, however, we would prefer to provide the referring clinician with a short list of possibilities or, better yet, a specific diagnosis. We are happiest when presented with Aunt Minnie images that allow us to be very specific in our suggested diagnosis.

The authors of this atlas present more than 250 Aunt Minnie cases covering virtually all imaging modalities and organ systems. Each case is presented in a concise format that includes a brief history, findings, diagnosis, discussion, and "Aunt Minnie's Pearls." Cases cover the subspecialties of pediatrics, musculoskeletal system, cardiovascular and interventional radiology, ultrasound, nuclear medicine, neuroradiology, thoracic radiology, mammography, and gastrointestinal and genitourinary radiology—the same familiar categories used in Louisville for the oral board examination.

The goal of this text is to present radiology residents and practicing radiologists with an extensive collection of practical Aunt Minnie cases; unfortunately for the older, more experienced radiologist, the authors succeed admirably in achieving their goal. This atlas may take away the edge we "seasoned" radiologists have gained by accumulating Aunt Minnies during the many years of radiology practice (a few years, at least). Our best defense is to make sure we include this atlas in our personal libraries.

THOMAS H. BERQUIST, MD, FACR
Chair, Department of Diagnostic Radiology
Mayo Clinic—Jacksonville
Jacksonville, Florida

PREFACE

The idea to create this atlas was formed during a noon conference that I (K.F.) attended during the spring of my third year of radiology residency at the Bowman Gray School of Medicine. A visiting professor was conducting a didactic teaching conference and called on one of our brightest seniors to "take a case," proclaiming that the diagnosis was "somewhat of an Aunt Minnie." An audible groan erupted in the audience because we all understood what that statement meant. The senior resident would either "hit a home run" or "strike out" miserably in his interpretation of the case. All the residents had been introduced to the term Aunt Minnie during their training and knew the unwritten definition: a disease or condition that cannot be correctly diagnosed unless you have seen the case before. The resident looked carefully at the case and said: "I've never seen anything like this before, so I might as well take my seat." All of us felt sorry for the senior, because the visiting professor had no idea that this particular fourth year resident was one of the best in our program and rarely missed a case. It was this experience that planted the seed that a collection of Aunt Minnie's could be put into an imaging atlas format so that residents and practicing radiologists could be exposed to these unique cases in one easily obtainable source *before* they are encountered in conference or daily practice (or worse, in a visiting professor's teaching session!).

The concept, Aunt Minnie, is well known in North America and is practiced in every radiology department to some degree. The term was popularized by Ben Felson in the introduction of the first edition of his book, *Fundamentals of Chest Roentgenology*: "As she enters the room you say, 'Hello, Aunt Minnie.' But how do you know it's Aunt Minnie? 'Well,' you shrug, 'well—look at her. It's Aunt Minnie all right!' "(Felson B. Fundamentals of chest roentgenology, Philadelphia: Saunders, 1960). Thus, just as one would easily recognize his or her favorite aunt, the term refers to diseases or conditions that are diagnosed because of the specificity of the imaging findings.

The editors encountered many personal and regional variations in the definition of Aunt Minnie in preparing this text. The conservative school of thought believes that this diagnostic process can be applied only to plain films. The more liberal definition of the Aunt Minnie approach also includes cases where the imaging findings are correlated in a multimodality manner and interpreted in the context of the patient's clinical presentation to reach a specific diagnosis. To broaden the educational message of this text, we have chosen the liberal interpretation of Aunt Minnie in preparing this atlas (and this does not necessarily reflect the political leanings of either editor!). The inclusion of some cases that require historical information to appreciate the specificity of the imaging findings closely reflects the clinical practice of radiology and in no way artificially enhances the specificity of the diagnosis. These cases also emphasize to radiology trainees the importance of obtaining clinical information before rendering a final interpretation. To underscore the educational message contained in this text, the editors have chosen the title, *Aunt Minnie's Atlas and Imaging-Specific Diagnosis,* to encompass both the conservative and liberal definitions of the term. Thus if a specific case does not fit the reader's personal definition of an Aunt Minnie, the editors hope that the case can still be enjoyed as a nice example of an imaging-specific diagnosis.

Generating a table of contents was a big challenge for the editors, and we purposely recruited experienced academic radiologists as senior authors for each chapter to ensure credibility in case selection. Newer imaging modalities have greatly increased the number of diseases that radiologists confidently diagnose, and every effort has been made to include contemporary imaging without excluding plain-film Aunt Minnies. The atlas also emphasizes diagnoses that are encountered in everyday clinical practice and attempts to exclude obscure or clinically impractical cases. The text and the references that accompany each case are intentionally concise and include the essential and distinguishing features of each disease or condition. Diagnostic pitfalls are also discussed when appropriate, so the reader might avoid Aunt Minnie impostors.

At the end of each case are "Aunt Minnie's Pearls." These short vignettes are intended to emphasize the key features and "take home messages" of each case and also provide a mechanism for quick review of the atlas. All images were reproduced from original x-rays by computer digitization, ensuring the best quality and resolution. No image is altered or computer enhanced.

Finally, the editors realize that nothing in medicine is absolute, and many instances exist where an apparent Aunt Minnie diagnosis is shown to be incorrect. The reader should therefore not assume that most cases in radiology are amenable to the Aunt Minnie approach to diagnosis. Each case that one encounters should be systematically analyzed for diagnostic possibilities and potential pitfalls, and only after this careful process can the radiologist render an imaging-specific diagnosis.

The major educational objective of this book is to introduce the reader to a compilation of diseases or conditions in which a confident diagnosis can be rendered based on the imaging findings and interpreted in the context of the patient's clinical presentation. *Aunt Minnie's Atlas and Imaging-Specific Diagnosis* is intended as a fun and informative educational tool that exposes readers to cases that would remain perplexing to all but the initiated. We hope you will enjoy the book and the experience.

Thanks to Sharon Meister, Nancy Ragland, and Donna Garrison at Bowman Gray for their excellent work editing the manuscript. Also, thanks to the numerous individuals at Bowman Gray and the Mallinckrodt Institute of Radiology who unselfishly donated their favorite cases and time, and, finally, thanks to the Mallinckrodt Abdominal Imaging Section for supporting me (K.F.) fully in the preparation of this text.

KENNETH L. FORD III
THOMAS L. POPE JR

CONTRIBUTORS

Sam T. Auringer, MD
Associate Professor
Department of Radiology
Bowman Gray School of Medicine
Winston-Salem, North Carolina

James D. Ball, MD
Associate Professor
Department of Radiology
Bowman Gray School of Medicine
Winston-Salem, North Carolina

Robert Bechtold, MD
Associate Professor
Department of Radiology
Bowman Gray School of Medicine
Winston-Salem, North Carolina

Caroline Chiles, MD
Associate Professor
Department of Radiology
Bowman Gray School of Medicine
Winston-Salem, North Carolina

Raymond B. Dyer, MD
Professor
Department of Radiology
Bowman Gray School of Medicine
Winston-Salem, North Carolina

Kenneth L. Ford III, MD
Staff Radiologist
Baylor University Medical Center
Dallas, Texas
Medical Director
Texas Diagnostic Imaging Center—Mesquite
Mesquite, Texas

Rita L. Freimanis, MD
Assistant Professor
Department of Radiology
Bowman Gray School of Medicine
Winston-Salem, North Carolina

David W. Gelfand, MD
Professor and Section Head
Department of Radiology
Bowman Gray School of Medicine
Winston-Salem, North Carolina

Edward K. Grishaw, MD
Fellow
Department of Nuclear Medicine
Mallinckrodt Institute of Radiology
Washington University
St. Louis, Missouri

Fernando Gutiérrez, MD
Associate Professor of Radiology
Mallinckrodt Institute of Radiology
St. Louis, Missouri

William D. Middleton, MD
Associate Professor of Radiology
Mallinckrodt Institute of Radiology
St. Louis, Missouri

Eric J. Pike, MD
Musculoskeletal Fellow
Department of Radiology
Bowman Gray School of Medicine
Winston-Salem, North Carolina

Thomas L. Pope Jr., MD
Professor and Section Head
Director of Education
Department of Radiology
Bowman Gray School of Medicine
Winston-Salem, North Carolina

William D. Routh, MD
Associate Professor and Section Head
Department of Radiology
Bowman Gray School of Medicine
Winston-Salem, North Carolina

H. Stuart Saunders, MD
Assistant Professor
Department of Radiology
Bowman Gray School of Medicine
Winston-Salem, North Carolina

Christopher A. Schlarb, MD
Staff Radiologist
Charleston Area Medical Center
Charleston, West Virginia

Roger Y. Shifrin, MD
Fellow
Department of Radiology
Stanford University
Palo Alto, California

Sharlene A. Teefey, MD
Assistant Professor of Radiology
Mallinckrodt Institute of Radiology
St. Louis, Missouri

Daniel W. Williams III, MD
Associate Professor
Department of Radiology
Bowman Gray School of Medicine
Winston-Salem, North Carolina

Thomas C. Winter III, MD
Associate Professor
Director of Ultrasound
Department of Radiology
University of Washington
Seattle, Washington

CONTENTS

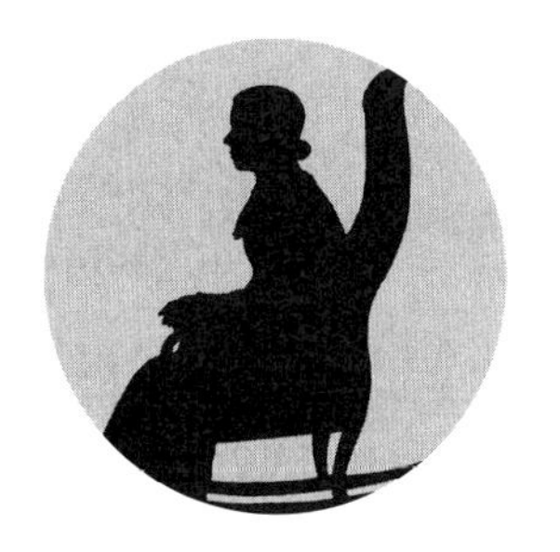

chapter 1

PEDIATRICS

SAM T. AURINGER

CASE 1

History. 3-day-old infant with acute onset of bilious vomiting

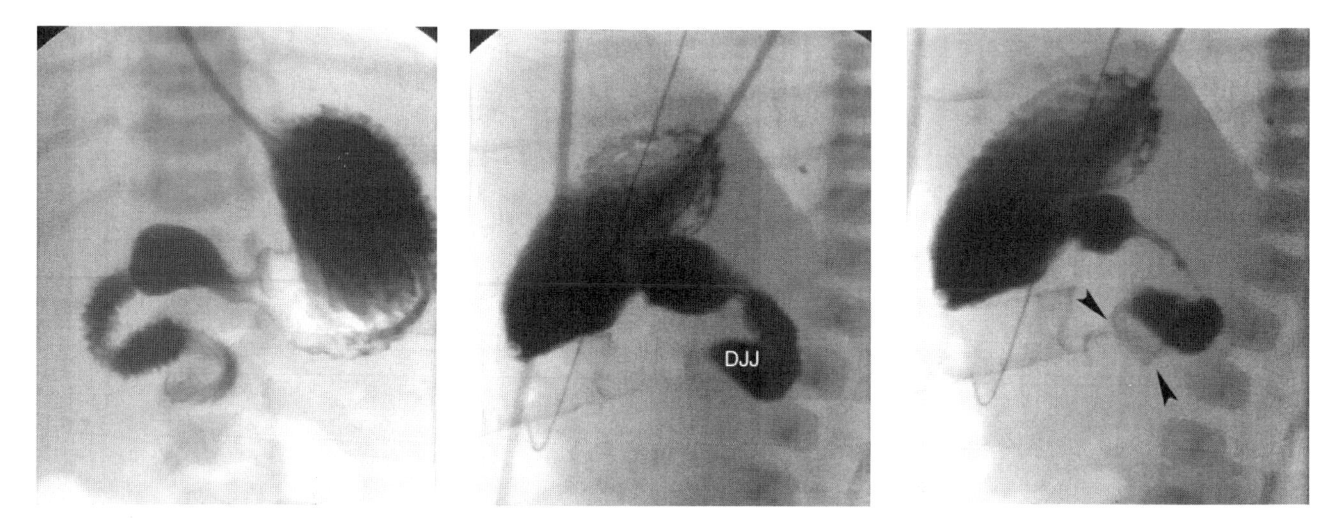

Figure 1.1.1. Figure 1.1.2. Figure 1.1.3.

Findings. Anteroposterior (Fig. 1.1.1) and lateral (Fig. 1.1.2) upper gastrointestinal series reveal partial duodenal obstruction, abnormal position of duodenal-jejunal junction (DJJ), and proximal small bowel in the right abdomen. A spiral or corkscrew configuration of the distal duodenum and proximal jejunum is also seen (Fig. 1.1.3, *arrowheads*).

Diagnosis. Malrotation with midgut volvulus

Discussion. Midgut malrotation complicated by midgut volvulus presents most frequently in the first month of life and is a true pediatric surgical emergency because of potential bowel ischemia. Because plain films are unreliable for diagnosis or exclusion of midgut volvulus, an emergent upper gastrointestinal series with barium or nonionic water-soluble contrast medium is indicated to diagnose the duodenal obstruction and the abnormally positioned duodenal-jejunal junction (i.e., duodenal-jejunal junction is *not* to the left of the spine and at the level of the bulb). A Ladd's operation is performed to diagnose and reduce the volvulus, resect any dead bowel, and lyse dense, aberrant peritoneal bands, also known as Ladd's bands (1).

Aunt Minnie's Pearls

- *Bilious vomiting in a newborn is malrotation with midgut volvulus until proven otherwise.*
- *Check for abnormal position and appearance of the duodenal-jejunal junction and proximal small bowel on upper gastrointestinal series.*

CASE 2

History. Newborn with bilious vomiting, Down's syndrome, and maternal polyhydramnios

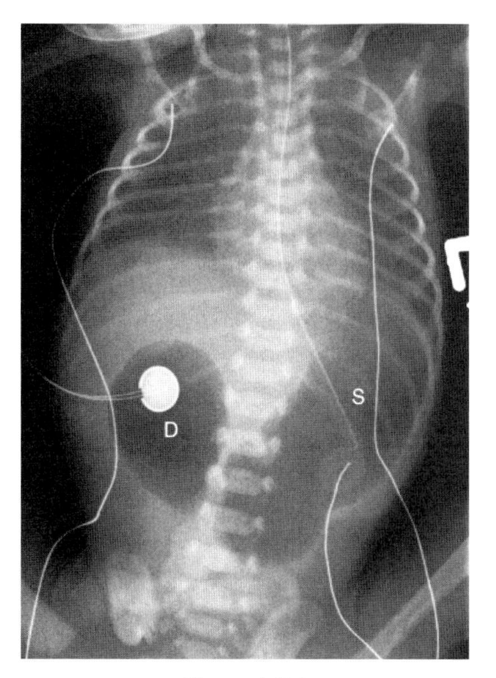

Figure 1.2.1.

Findings. Anteroposterior supine view of the chest and abdomen (Fig. 1.2.1) demonstrates a classic "double-bubble" sign—gaseous distention of the stomach (S) and an enlarged duodenal bulb or "mega bulb" (D). No intestinal gas is seen distal to the duodenum.

Diagnosis. Duodenal atresia

Discussion. Duodenal atresia is complete congenital intrinsic obstruction of the duodenum and is thought to be secondary to failed recanalization. Approximately 30% of affected infants have Down's syndrome (trisomy 21), 40% have maternal polyhydramnios, and 50% have some type of associated anomaly. Plain film demonstration of the double-bubble sign is diagnostic and may be aided by injection of air through a nasogastric tube, as in the case presented. Upper gastrointestinal series is not indicated unless distal gas is present (i.e., partial duodenal obstruction exists). Distal gas requires further investigation for other etiologies of neonatal duodenal obstruction (e.g., duodenal stenosis or web, malrotation with Ladd's bands or volvulus, annular pancreas, or duplication cyst) (2).

Aunt Minnie's Pearls

- *A double-bubble sign without distal bowel gas is diagnostic of duodenal atresia.*

CASE 3

History. 3-month-old infant with lethargy and an interhemispheric subdural hematoma on a head CT

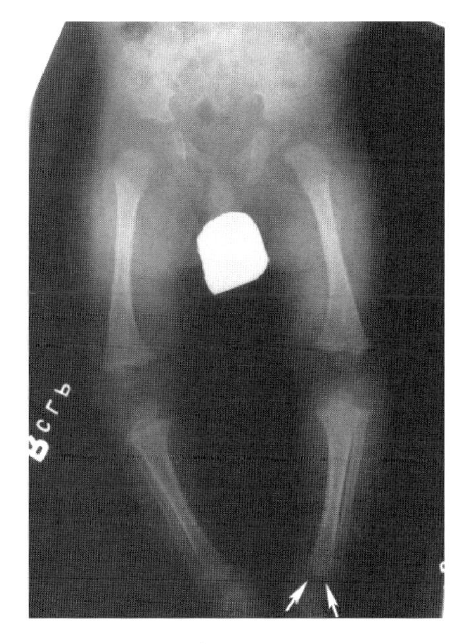

Figure 1.3.1.

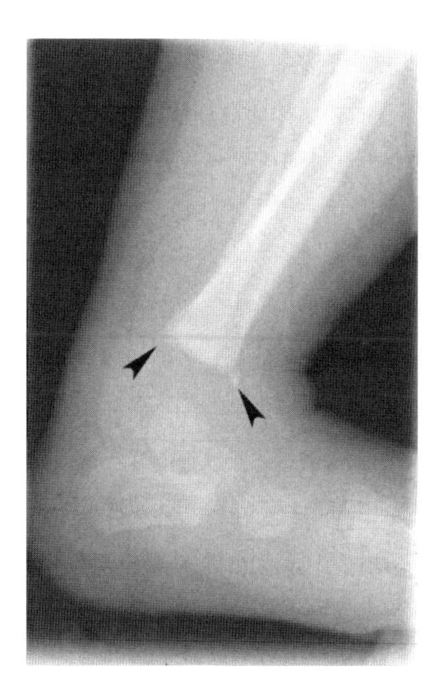

Figure 1.3.2.

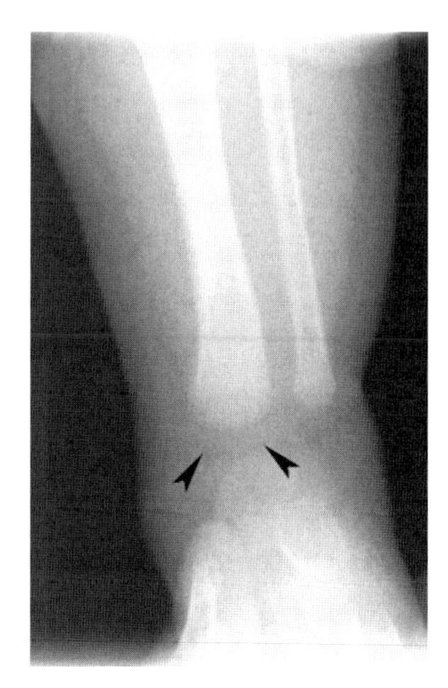

Figure 1.3.3.

Findings. Anteroposterior view of the lower extremities (Fig. 1.3.1) from a skeletal survey reveals subtle irregularity of the distal left tibia (*arrowheads*). Dedicated views of the left ankle reveal the classic metaphyseal "corner" (Fig. 1.3.2, *arrowheads*) and "bucket handle" (Fig. 1.3.3, *arrowheads*) fractures of the distal left tibia.

Diagnosis. Battered child syndrome

Discussion. The classic metaphyseal "corner" and "bucket handle" fractures are considered virtually pathognomonic of battered child syndrome and result from indirectly applied shearing forces during shaking (3). These fractures are often subtle, and the case presented reinforces the importance of following suspicious areas on skeletal surveys with dedicated high-quality radiographs. Shaken infants commonly present with seizures, lethargy, coma, retinal hemorrhages on funduscopic examination, and interhemispheric subdural hematomas caused by rupture of bridging veins from the cerebral cortex to the superior sagittal sinus (4).

Aunt Minnie's Pearls

- *Metaphyseal "corner" and "bucket handle" fractures are virtually pathognomonic of the battered child syndrome.*

CASE 4

History. Newborn male infant with bilateral hydronephrosis detected in utero

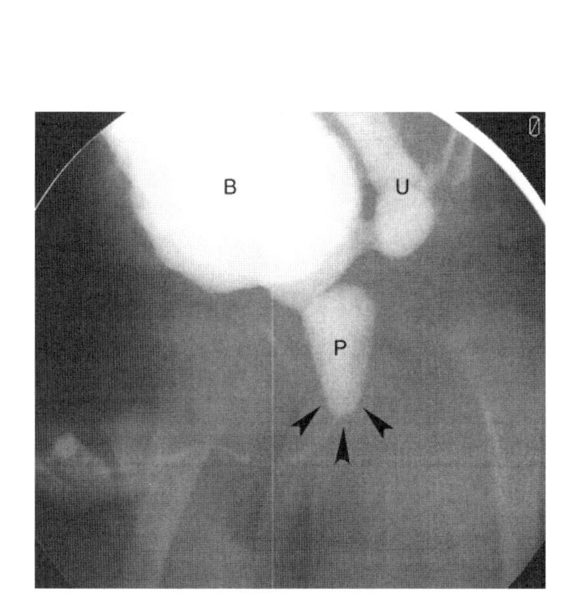

Figure 1.4.1.

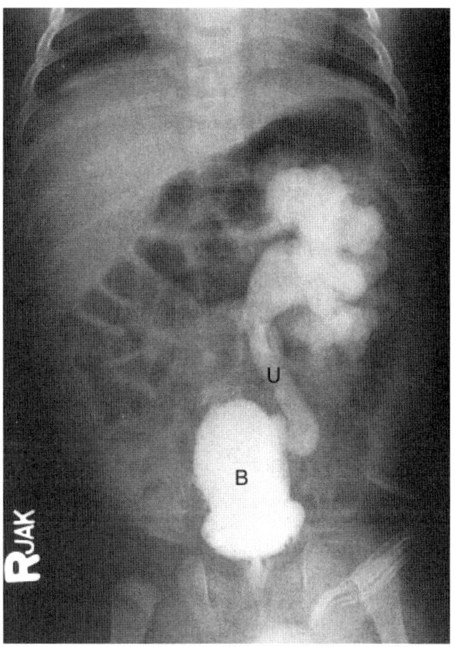

Figure 1.4.2.

Findings. Voiding cystourethrogram (Fig. 1.4.1) and postvoid KUB (Fig. 1.4.2) demonstrate "bullet nosed" dilatation (*arrowheads*) of the posterior urethra (P), a thick-walled trabeculated bladder (B), and severe vesicoureteral reflux on the left (U).

Diagnosis. Posterior urethral valves

Discussion. Posterior urethral valves are the most common cause of bilateral hydronephrosis in a male infant. Affected infants may present with maternal oligohydramnios, pulmonary hypoplasia, and cystic renal dysplasia. Vesicoureteral reflux tends to be unilateral and may lead to forniceal rupture and urinary ascites. Older children or adolescents may present with urinary tract infections, voiding difficulty, or end-stage renal disease. Type I valves are the most common and extend from the verumontanum distally, leaving a small opening posteriorly for the passage of urine. Voiding cystourethrogram is the test of choice for diagnosis. Treatment frequently involves early urinary diversion and subsequent valve ablation (5).

Aunt Minnie's Pearls

- *"Bullet nosed" dilatation of the posterior urethra resulting in bilateral hydronephrosis in a male infant = posterior urethral valves.*

CASE 5

History. 2-year-old child with an abdominal mass, proptosis, anemia, and elevated urinary catecholamines

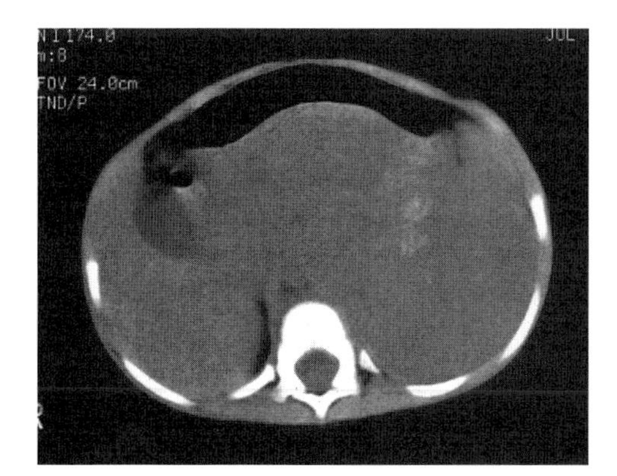

Figure 1.5.1.

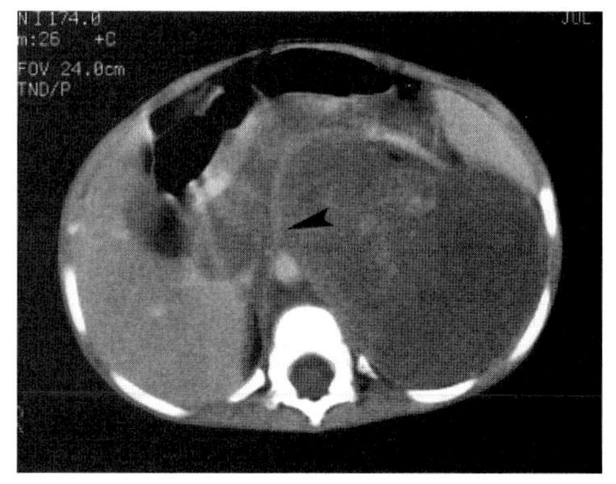

Figure 1.5.2.

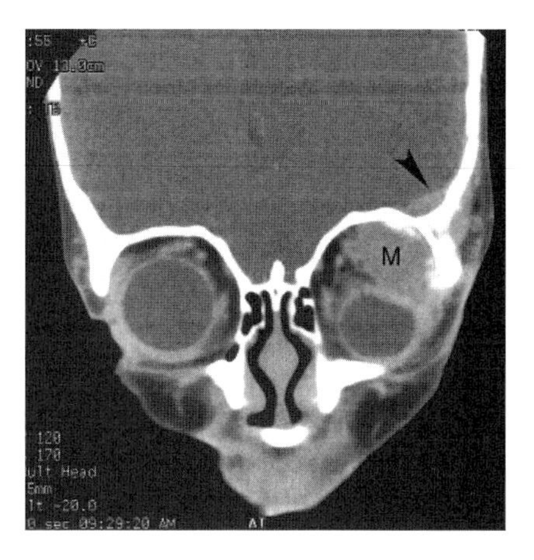

Figure 1.5.3.

Findings. Unenhanced (Fig. 1.5.1) and contrast-enhanced (Fig. 1.5.2) CT images through the abdomen demonstrate an inhomogeneous mass in the left upper quadrant that contains calcifications, crosses the midline, and encases the celiac axis (*arrowhead*). Orbital CT with contrast (Fig. 1.5.3) reveals a soft tissue mass in the superolateral left orbit (M) that displaces the globe inferiorly and is associated with bone destruction and extradural extension of tumor (*arrowhead*). Other images not shown reveal a normal left kidney that is displaced inferiorly by the mass.

Diagnosis. Neuroblastoma with orbital metastasis

Discussion. Neuroblastoma is a common malignancy of childhood that originates in the sympathetic chain ganglia and adrenal medulla. Two-thirds of cases arise in the abdomen, and two-thirds of abdominal tumors arise in the adrenal medulla. Peak age of presentation is 2 years; 70% of patients present with metastatic disease to cortical bone (especially skull), bone marrow, liver, and lymph nodes.

The main challenge in imaging these tumors is differentiating neuroblastoma from Wilms tumor. Calcification, suprarenal location with a displaced but normal ipsilateral kidney, vessel encasement, retrocrural adenopathy, and extension across the midline are features that allow a confident diagnosis of neuroblastoma. Paraspinal tumor may invade the spinal canal and is best evaluated with MRI. Initial diagnosis is often based on plain films and ultrasonography; CT, MRI, bone scans, and MIBG scans are required for complete staging. Age, stage, N-myc oncogene amplification, and Shimada histology are important prognostically. Overall, the prognosis remains poor (6).

Aunt Minnie's Pearls

- *A childhood suprarenal mass with calcification that crosses the midline and encases the celiac axis is almost certainly a neuroblastoma.*

CASE 6

History. Newborn with respiratory distress during feedings, failure to pass a nasogastric tube, and limb anomalies

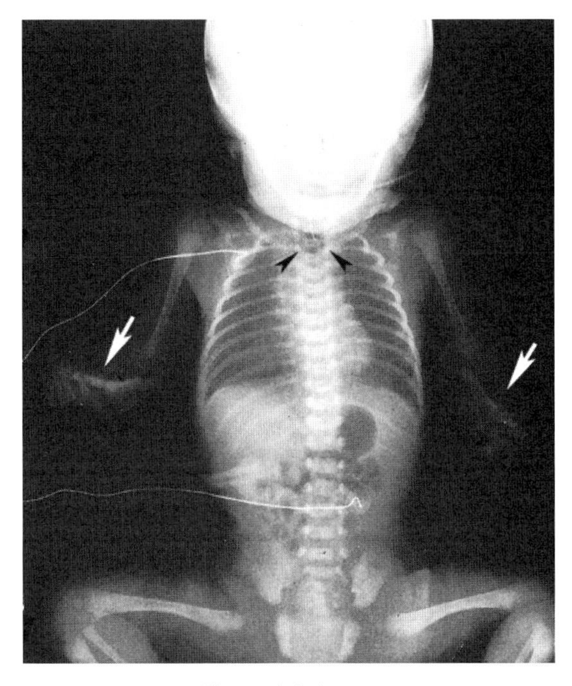

Figure 1.6.1.

Findings. Anteroposterior supine "babygram" (Fig. 1.6.1) shows that the nasogastric tube terminates in a gas-filled proximal esophageal pouch (*arrowheads*). Bowel gas is present. The radii are absent (*arrows*).

Diagnosis. Esophageal atresia with tracheoesophageal fistula and radial ray anomalies (VATER association)

Discussion. The VATER association includes vertebral and cardiovascular anomalies, anorectal malformations, tracheoesophageal fistula, and renal and radial ray anomalies. The most common type of tracheoesophageal fistula is proximal esophageal atresia with a distal tracheoesophageal fistula, which is diagnosed on the basis of plain films demonstrating a feeding tube coiled in the proximal pouch with gas present distally. A barium "pouchogram" is not indicated, but the esophageal pouch can be made more conspicuous by injecting air through the nasogastric tube. Echocardiography and renal sonography are indicated to screen for congenital heart disease and renal anomalies, most commonly patent ductus arteriosus, ventricular septal defect, and renal agenesis. Complications of esophageal atresia with tracheoesophageal fistula include aspiration pneumonia, postoperative leak and stricture, recurrent fistula, disordered esophageal motility, gastroesophageal reflux, congenital esophageal stenosis, and tracheomalacia (7).

Aunt Minnie's Pearls

- *In the proper clinical setting, esophageal atresia is diagnosed by failure to pass an nasogastric tube and visualization of an air containing esophageal pouch.*
- *Always look for the VATER association in patients with esophageal atresia.*

CASE 7

History. 3-year-old child with a lap belt ecchymosis after a motor vehicle accident

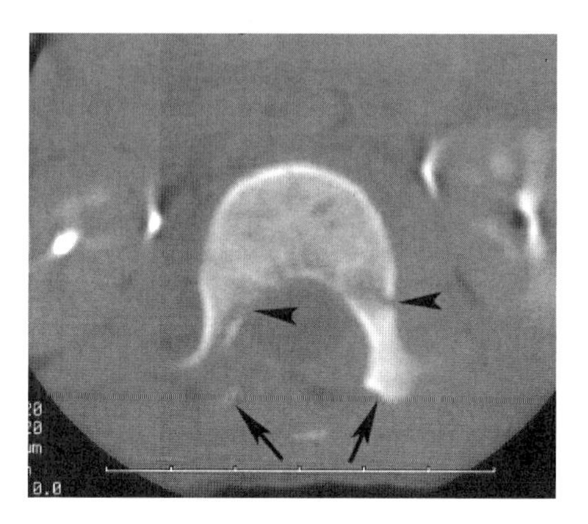

Figure 1.7.2.

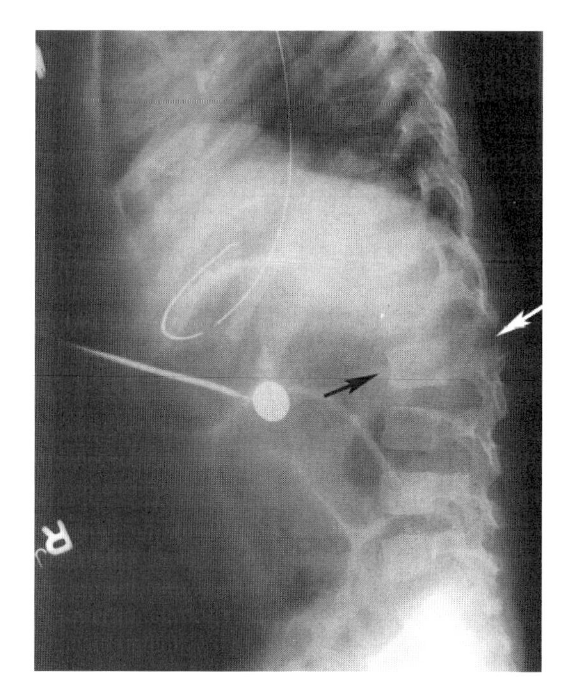

Figure 1.7.1.

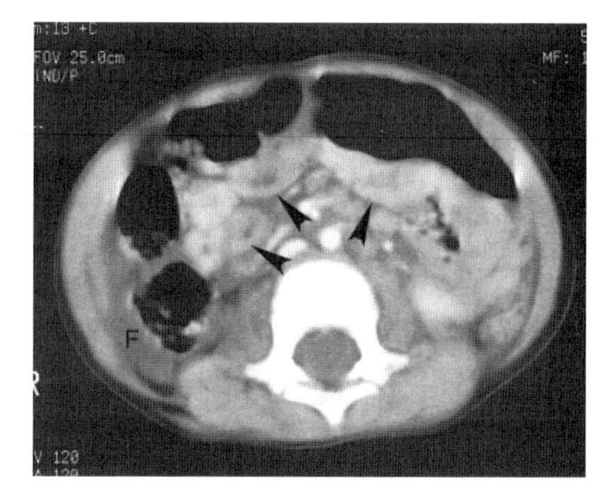

Figure 1.7.3.

Findings. Distraction and separation of the posterior elements of L1 and L2 vertebrae without anterior compression are seen on a lateral view of the thoracolumbar spine (Fig. 1.7.1, *arrows*). Axial CT of L2 (Fig. 1.7.2) demonstrates the "naked facet" sign or lack of opposing facets at L2 (*arrows*) and bilateral pedicle fractures (*arrowheads*). Contrast-enhanced abdominal CT (Fig. 1.7.3) reveals bowel-wall thickening and bowel-wall enhancement (*arrowheads*) as well as free intraperitoneal fluid (F).

Diagnosis. Lap belt injury complex (lap belt ecchymosis, distraction fracture of the lumbar spine, and bowel injury)

Discussion. In a sudden deceleration accident, hyperflexion around the axis of a lap belt disrupts the posterior spinal ligaments and distracts the posterior elements, resulting in the "naked facet" sign. The anterior vertebral body is not compressed, but a horizontal fracture through the vertebral body (i.e., "Chance" fracture) may also occur. Injuries to bowel and abdominal viscera may dominate the clinical picture, and the unstable spine injury may be overlooked without lateral radiography. Manifestations of bowel injury on CT scans include bowel-wall enhancement, bowel-wall thickening, free fluid, free air, and extraluminal oral contrast. In this clinical setting, unexplained intraperitoneal fluid on CT is a bowel injury until proven otherwise (8).

Aunt Minnie's Pearls

- *Lap belt injury complex = lap belt ecchymosis, distraction fracture of the lumbar spine, and bowel injury.*

CASE 8

History. 1-year-old child with abdominal pain, fever, and reluctance to sit up

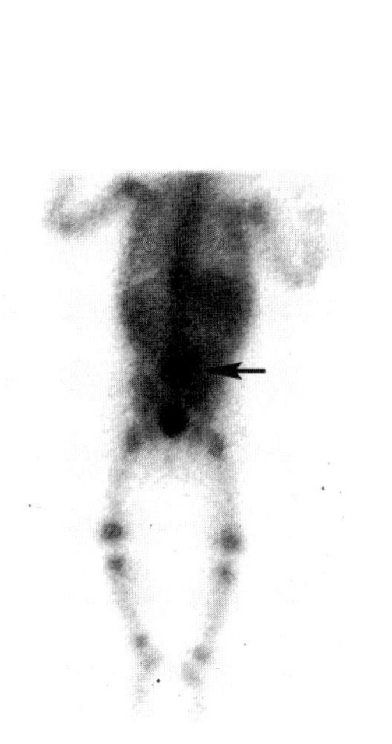

Figure 1.8.1. Posterior gallium scan.

Figure 1.8.2.

Findings. Initial plain films and a bone scan were interpreted as normal. A subsequent gallium scan (Fig. 1.8.1) shows increased activity in the lower lumbar spine (*arrow*). A follow-up lateral lumbar radiograph obtained 3 months later reveals narrowing of the L4–L5 intervertebral disc space and erosive irregularity and sclerosis of adjacent end plates (Fig. 1.8.2, *arrow*).

Diagnosis. Discitis

Discussion. Discitis is an inflammatory process that usually involves the lumbar intervertebral disc spaces. Variable symptoms include fever, abdominal pain, limp, refusal to walk or sit up, and pain in the back, hip, or knee. Children aged 6 months to 4 years are the most commonly affected age group. A second peak is seen at 10–14 years. *Staphylococcus aureus* is recovered in one-third to one-half of patients. Plain film results are negative early, but bone-scan results are generally positive. Gallium scans and MR imaging are useful in equivocal cases. MR imaging also allows delineation of paraspinal or epidural abscesses and disc herniation in complicated cases (9).

Aunt Minnie's Pearls

- *Discitis is an inflammatory process centered on a lumbar intervertebral disc.*
- *Children aged 6 months to 4 years are most frequently affected.*

CASE 9

History. 32-week, 1500-gram premature infant with abdominal distention, increased gastric residuals, and thrombocytopenia on day 6 of life

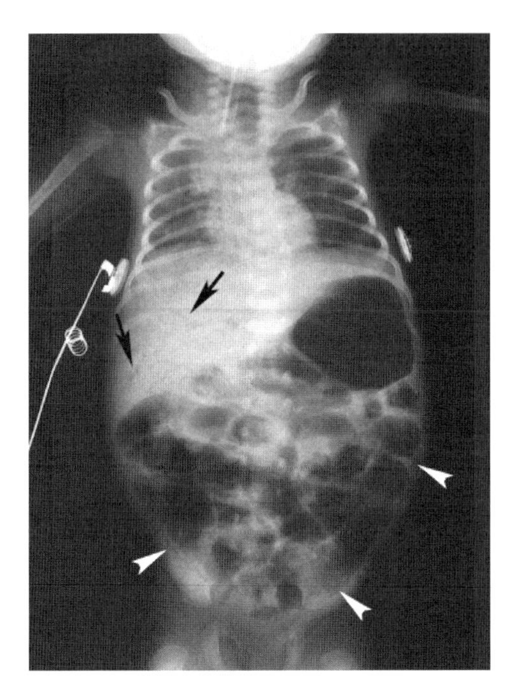

Figure 1.9.1.

Findings. Anteroposterior supine film of chest and abdomen (Fig. 1.9.1) demonstrates diffuse gaseous distention of bowel, linear and crescentic areas of pneumatosis intestinalis (*arrowheads*), and portal venous gas (*arrows*).

Diagnosis. Necrotizing enterocolitis

Discussion. Necrotizing enterocolitis most frequently affects premature infants or full-term infants with congenital heart disease. The underlying pathophysiology is multifactorial, but the mucosal injury is probably due to ischemia compounded by hyperosmolar feedings and infection. The earliest roentgen signs are nonspecific dilatation and separation of loops. Pneumatosis and portal venous gas indicating severe disease appear subsequently. Pneumoperitoneum, ascites, or both signal perforation and the need for surgical intervention. The mortality rate in children with necrotizing enterocolitis approaches 40%. Colonic strictures are a common late complication in survivors (10).

Aunt Minnie's Pearls

- *Necrotizing enterocolitis occurs in premature infants or full-term infants with congenital heart disease.*
- *Look for dilated bowel loops, pneumatosis, and portal venous gas.*
- *Pneumoperitoneum, ascites, or both indicate bowel perforation and the need for immediate surgery.*

CASE 10

History. Full-term infant with progressive respiratory distress

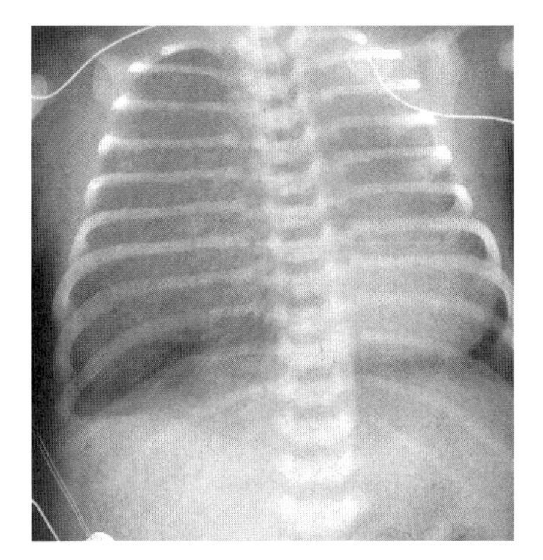

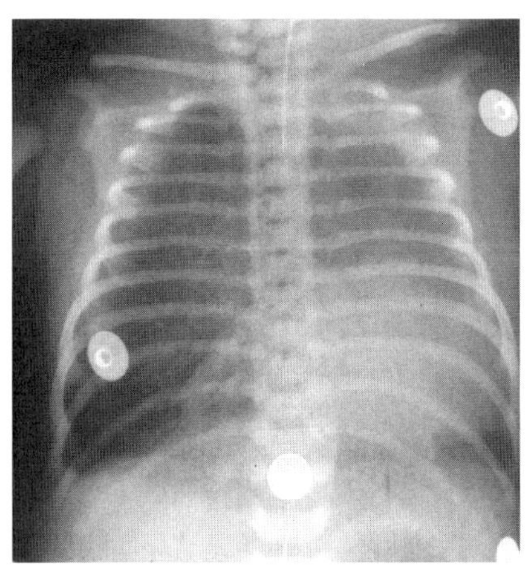

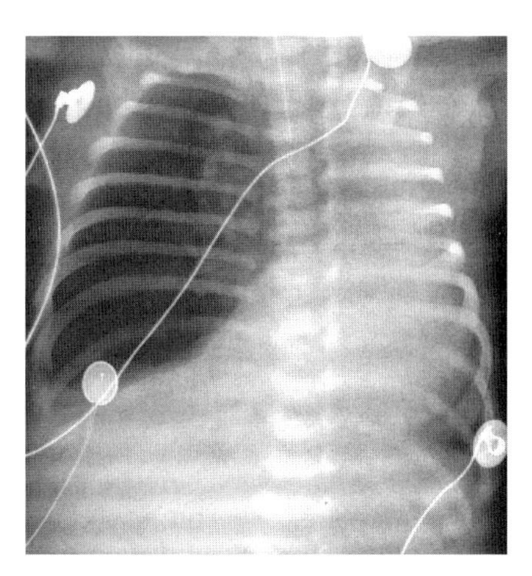

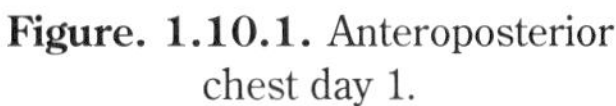

Figure. 1.10.1. Anteroposterior chest day 1.

Figure 1.10.2. Anteroposterior chest day 2.

Figure 1.10.3. Anteroposterior chest day 3.

Findings. A series of chest films obtained from day 1 to day 4 of life demonstrates initial opacification of the right upper lobe (Fig. 1.10.1), which subsequently becomes interstitial or reticular (Fig. 1.10.2) and finally hyperlucent (Fig. 1.10.3). Right-to-left mediastinal shift and progressive right middle and lower lobe collapse are also identified.

Diagnosis. Congenital lobar emphysema of right upper lobe

Discussion. Mediastinal shift is the hallmark of "surgical" causes of neonatal respiratory distress. The etiology of congenital lobar emphysema remains unclear. In most cases, congenital lobar emphysema is congenital in origin and is associated with an intrinsic ball-valve obstruction in the affected bronchus. The result is progressive air trapping with mediastinal shift and compressive atelectasis of adjacent lobes. The initial opacification of the affected lobe is due to impaired drainage of fetal lung fluid. The upper lobes and the right middle lobe are most frequently affected. Differentiation of congenital lobar emphysema from other surgical lesions of the lung in newborns (sequestration and cystic adenomatoid malformation) requires recognition of the characteristic location and temporal evolution of this abnormality. Infants with severe respiratory distress are treated by lobectomy, whereas functional assessment with ventilation-perfusion scanning and nonsurgical management may be indicated in less severely affected infants (11).

Aunt Minnie's Pearls

- *Progressive air trapping in the middle or either upper lobe in a newborn = congenital lobar emphysema.*

CASE 11

History. Full-term neonate with the classic obstructive triad of bilious vomiting, abdominal distention, and failure to pass meconium

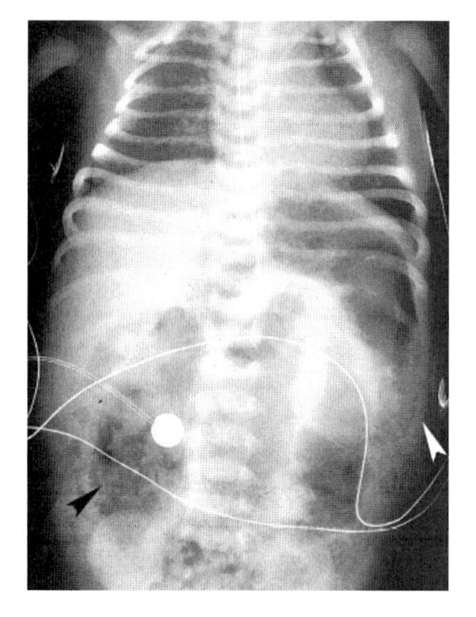

Figure. 1.11.1.

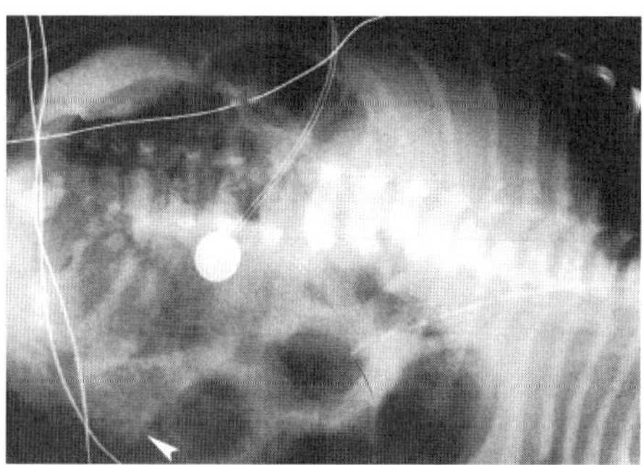

Figure 1.11.2.

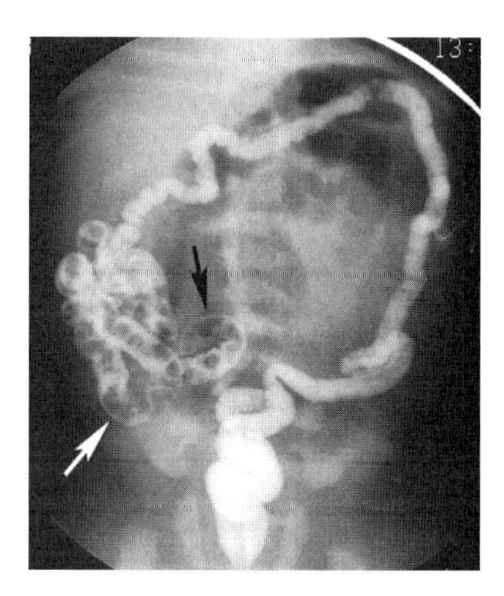

Figure 1.11.3.

Findings. Anteroposterior supine (Fig. 1.11.1) and left lateral decubitus (Fig. 1.11.2) views of the abdomen demonstrate dilated loops of small bowel containing stool with a "soap bubble" appearance (*arrowheads*). No air-fluid levels are seen on the lateral view. A contrast enema (Fig. 1.11.3) reveals a microcolon with "rabbit pellet" filling defects in the ileum (*arrows*).

Diagnosis. Meconium ileus

Discussion. Meconium ileus is the neonatal presentation of cystic fibrosis. Hydramnios and a family history of cystic fibrosis may be present. With simple meconium ileus, abnormally viscid meconium obstructs the ileum, and a water-soluble contrast enema with ileal reflux to the level of the dilated loops may relieve the impaction. This disorder is said to produce the smallest of all microcolons because the obstructing meconium causes the colon to be completely unused. In nearly half of cases, meconium ileus may be complicated by volvulus, atresia, stenosis, perforation, peritonitis, or pseudocyst formation. Complicated meconium ileus may present early, and severe abdominal distention and respiratory distress may require corrective surgery (12).

A similar diagnosis may be made in older children with cystic fibrosis in whom viscid stool obstructs the ileum and cecum. This disorder is known as meconium ileus equivalent.

Aunt Minnie's Pearls

- *Meconium ileus is diagnostic of cystic fibrosis.*
- *A water-soluble contrast enema is diagnostic and therapeutic in uncomplicated cases.*
- *Meconium ileus produces the smallest of all microcolons.*

CASE 12

History. 1-year-old immigrant child with growth failure

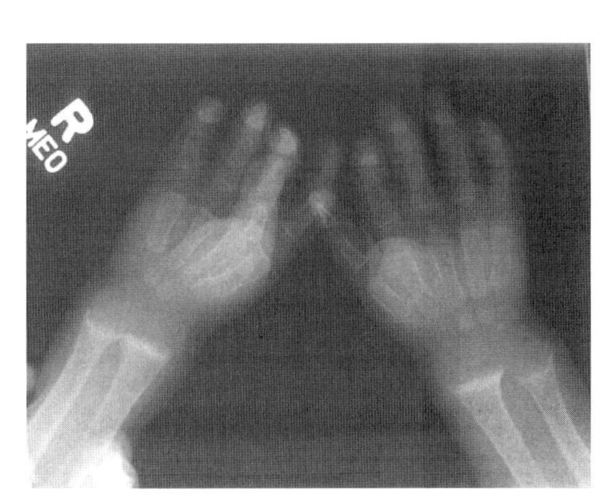

Figure 1.12.1.

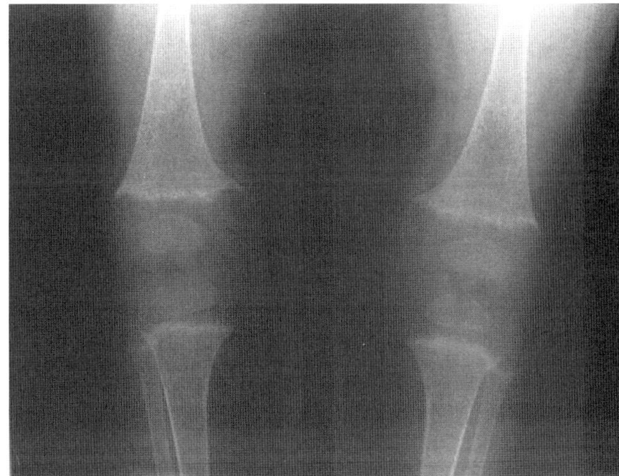

Figure 1.12.2.

Findings. Metaphyseal cupping, fraying, and splaying are demonstrated on anteroposterior views of the wrists (Fig. 1.12.1) and knees (Fig. 1.12.2). Also apparent is loss of the zone of provisional calcification, which is seen radiographically as widening of the physes and loss of the epiphyseal and metaphyseal margins. The visualized skeleton shows diffuse coarse demineralization.

Diagnosis. Rickets

Discussion. Deficient mineralization of osteoid in children is known as rickets, whereas in adults the same pathologic process is osteomalacia. Many types and causes of rickets result in this classic Aunt Minnie appearance. Rachitic changes on radiographs reflect a relative or absolute deficiency of vitamin D or its hormonally active derivative 1,25-dihydroxycholecalciferol. Remembering that the biosynthetic pathway of vitamin D involves skin, gut, liver, and kidney assists formulation of a basic differential diagnosis. Other pathologic processes in the gut or kidneys that result in calcium or phosphorus wasting can also result in rickets.

Because rachitic changes are best visualized at the ends of the most rapidly growing bones, a rickets survey routinely includes views of the wrists and knees. Rickets is rarely encountered before 6 months of age in full-term infants, and most cases are diagnosed before the patient is 2 years old (13).

Aunt Minnie's Pearls

- *In rickets, the metaphyses are cupped, frayed, and splayed.*
- *Vitamin D deficiency causes poor osteoid mineralization.*

CASE 13

History. Obese black male adolescent with pain in the left hip

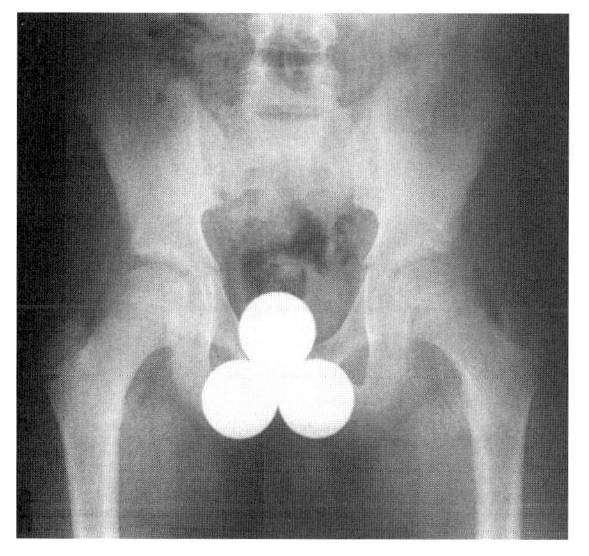

Figure 1.13.1.

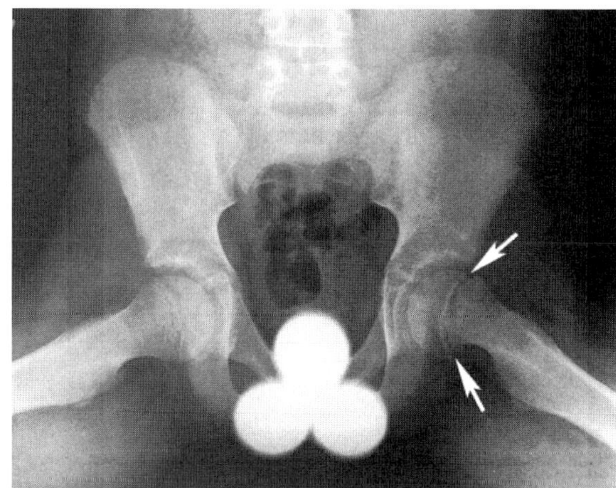

Figure 1.13.2.

Findings. Anteroposterior view of the pelvis (Fig. 1.13.1) shows widening of the left proximal femoral physis, metaphyseal irregularity, and regional osteopenia. Lines drawn along the lateral femoral necks would intersect less femoral epiphysis on the left. The frog-leg lateral view (Fig. 1.13.2) reveals posterior displacement of the epiphysis relative to the metaphysis (*arrows*), producing the classic "ice cream falling off the cone" appearance.

Diagnosis. Slipped capital femoral epiphysis (SCFE)

Discussion. SCFE, which is a Salter-Harris type I fracture of the proximal growth plate of the femur, is usually encountered during the adolescent growth spurt. Black (male or female) and male (of any race) patients are most commonly affected. Children with SCFE are usually overweight and present with hip pain, limp, or referred knee pain. Younger and older presentations suggest hypothyroidism, hypopituitarism, and prior radiation therapy. Both hips are affected in approximately 25% of patients.

Anteroposterior and frog-leg lateral radiographs of the hips should be obtained in suspected cases of SCFE. A line, also known as Klein's line, drawn along the lateral edge of the femoral neck should bisect at least one-sixth of the femoral epiphysis on an anteroposterior view. If the line intersects less than this amount, SCFE should be suspected. Because the primary direction of slippage is posterior and medial, the frog-leg lateral view may show the epiphyseal displacement to best advantage.

SCFE is a true orthopedic emergency, and the goal of treatment is to prevent further slippage by internal fixation. Complications of SCFE include avascular necrosis, chondrolysis, varus deformity with femoral neck shortening, and early degenerative osteoarthritis. The epiphysis is fixated in the position in which it is found because attempts to reduce the epiphysis increase the risk of avascular necrosis (14).

Aunt Minnie's Pearls

- *SCFE occurs most frequently in adolescent males.*
- *25% of cases are bilateral.*
- *SCFE is an orthopedic emergency, and the epiphysis is pinned "as is" to prevent further slippage.*

CASE 14

History. 1-year-old girl with acute onset of wheezing

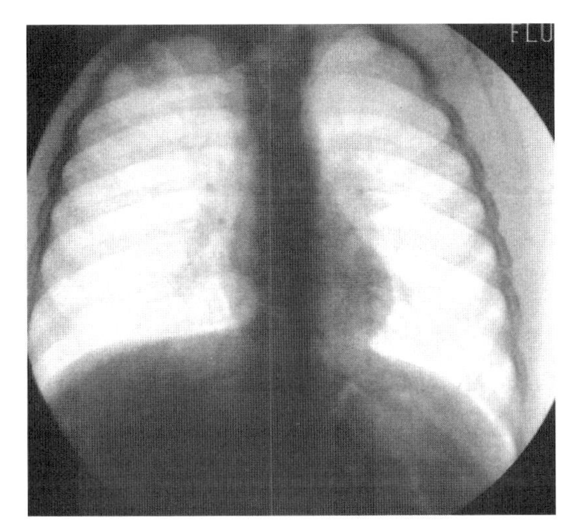

Figure 1.14.1.

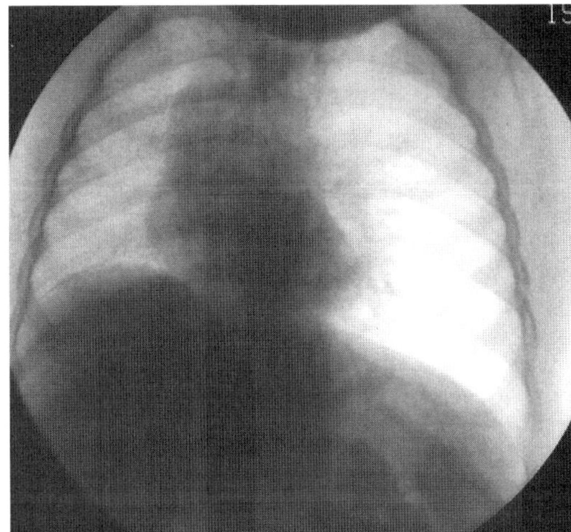

Figure 1.14.2.

Findings. Anteroposterior spot film (Fig. 1.14.1) obtained during fluoroscopy appears normal. A film obtained during expiration (Fig. 1.14.2) shows impressive left-to-right mediastinal shift and unilateral left-sided air trapping.

Diagnosis. Foreign body (peanut) in the left main stem bronchus

Discussion. Foreign bodies in the lower airway are a commonly encountered pediatric problem, especially in children younger than age 3. The child may present either acutely with cough, respiratory distress, and wheezing or more insidiously with fever, cough, recurrent pneumonia, pneumomediastinum, or pneumothorax. Peanuts are the most common foreign body to be aspirated, and bronchial impaction occurs more frequently on the right than on the left. The affected lung may be collapsed, normally aerated, or emphysematous. Inspiratory views alone have a normal appearance in 20% of patients, necessitating an expiratory view of the chest or chest fluoroscopy. Decubitus views are also helpful, because when an obstructing foreign body is present, the dependent lung is hyperinflated. Radiologic evaluation may still be normal in up to 30% of children with proven lower-airway foreign bodies, hence the need for bronchoscopy in any child with strong clinical suspicion and negative films (15).

Aunt Minnie's Pearls

- *Foreign body aspiration is most common in children younger than age 3.*
- *Unilateral air trapping during expiration is diagnostic in the appropriate clinical setting.*

CASE 15

History. Previously well 2-year-old in acute respiratory distress after playing "in the shed"

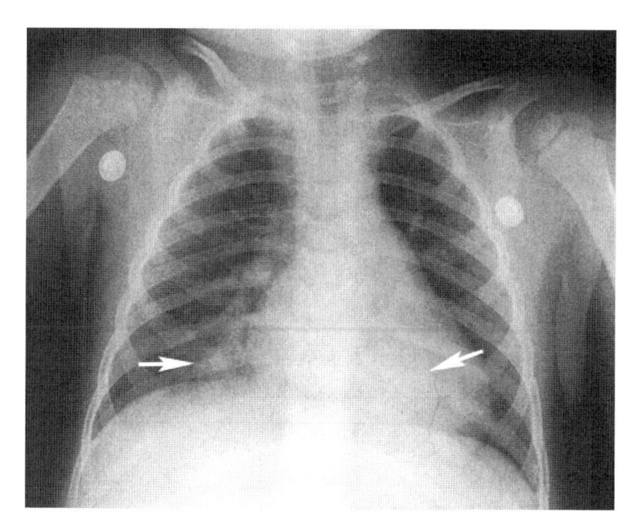

Figure 1.15.1.

Findings. Anteroposterior portable chest film demonstrates medial bibasilar infiltrates (Fig. 1.15.1, *arrows*).

Diagnosis. Hydrocarbon aspiration

Discussion. Children may ingest and readily aspirate hydrocarbons (e.g., gasoline, kerosene, furniture polish, lighter fluid) commonly available around the house. Because hydrocarbons possess low viscosity and surface tension, they are easily aspirated during swallowing. The aspirated fluid induces a chemical pneumonitis that destroys surfactant and produces local edema and atelectasis. Because of aspiration in the erect position, the patchy air-space opacities are classically in the medial lower lobes. Radiographic changes may not develop until 6–12 hours after hydrocarbon aspiration. Hence it is clinically important to assess gas exchange with pulse oximetry and blood gases. If these parameters and a 12-hour radiograph are normal, it is unlikely that significant aspiration has occurred. A normal radiograph 24 hours after ingestion excludes significant aspiration. Once present, radiographic findings are slow to clear. Pneumatocele development is a classic late complication (16).

Aunt Minnie's Pearls

- *Medial lower lobe patchy opacities in a child with a history of caustic ingestion = hydrocarbon aspiration until proven otherwise.*
- *Radiographic changes may not develop for 6–12 hours after aspiration, so one normal chest film during this period does not exclude the diagnosis.*

CASE 16

History. Newborn with severe respiratory distress

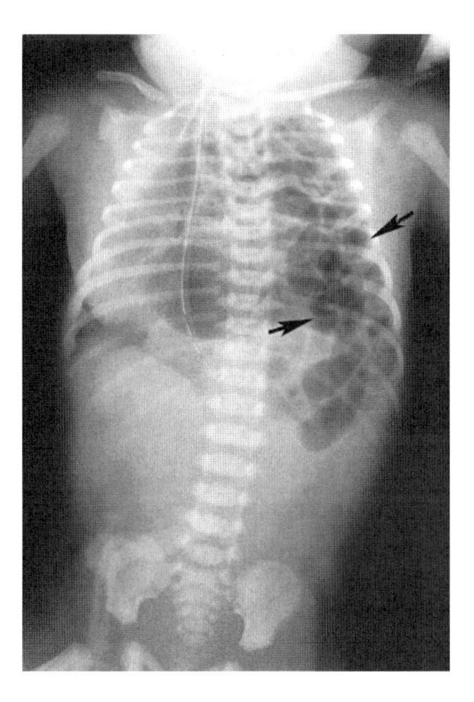

Figure 1.16.1.

Findings. Anteroposterior chest and abdomen film (Fig. 1.16.1) shows marked left-to-right shift of the heart, mediastinum, and support apparatus. The left side of the chest contains multiple tubular radiolucencies (*arrows*), and the abdomen is gasless.

Diagnosis. Congenital diaphragmatic hernia, Bochdalek type

Discussion. Congenital Bochdalek-type diaphragmatic hernia is a common "surgical" cause of neonatal respiratory distress. Herniation of abdominal contents occurs through a posterolateral diaphragmatic defect or persistent pleuroperitoneal canal. It is convenient to remember that Bochdalek hernias occur in the back, are more common on the left than right, and are associated with a scaphoid, gasless abdomen. Intestinal malrotation is present in all cases. The degree of associated pulmonary hypoplasia and persistent fetal circulation from pulmonary hypertension determines prognosis and management. Delayed appearance of diaphragmatic hernias is often right-sided and may be idiopathic or may be associated with previous group B streptococcal pneumonia. Sonography is useful for both prenatal and postnatal diagnosis of diaphragmatic hernia. On prenatal sonograms, the presence of the stomach bubble adjacent to the heart on a true transverse image should alert the radiologist to this diagnosis (17).

Aunt Minnie's Pearls

- *The presence of bowel in the left chest in a newborn is diagnostic of a congenital diaphragmatic hernia.*
- *Older infants with right-sided hernias often have a history of previous group B streptococcal pneumonia.*
- *On a transverse obstetrical ultrasound image, look for the stomach bubble adjacent to the heart to suggest this diagnosis.*

CASE 17

History. Full-term infant with abdominal distention and failure to pass meconium

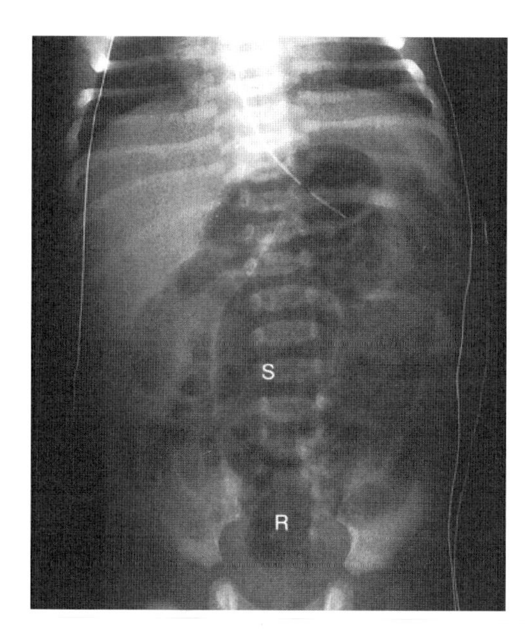

Figure 1.17.1.

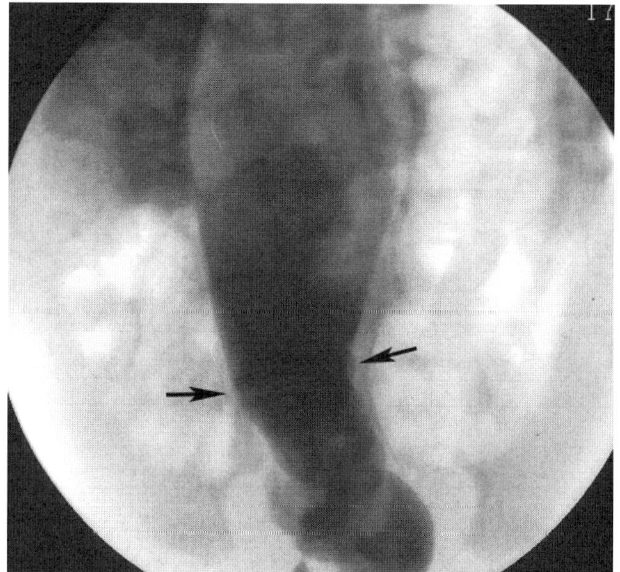

Figure 1.17.2.

Findings. Anteroposterior supine abdominal film (Fig. 1.17.1) demonstrates dilated large and small bowel. The distal sigmoid colon (S) is more dilated than the rectum (R). Anteroposterior view from a contrast enema (Fig. 1.17.2) confirms the rectosigmoid transition zone (*arrows*).

Diagnosis. Short-segment Hirschsprung disease

Discussion. Hirschsprung disease is a functional colonic obstruction characterized by an aganglionic hypertonic distal segment of bowel with associated proximal dilatation. Radiographic demonstration of the transition zone between the dilated proximal ganglionic bowel and the nondilated distal aganglionic bowel is the most reliable diagnostic finding of Hirschsprung disease. Other roentgen findings include an abnormal rectosigmoid index (a fancy term to signify that the sigmoid should not be bigger than the rectum), a corrugated or saw-toothed rectosigmoid, and delayed evacuation of contrast medium. Enemas in these patients should be performed with no bowel preparation to prevent false-negative studies.

Eighty percent of patients with Hirschsprung disease present during the first 6 weeks of life, and these patients account for 20% of all cases of neonatal bowel obstruction. Short-segment disease accounts for 80% of cases, has a rectosigmoid transition zone, and exhibits a male predominance. Long-segment disease accounts for 15% of cases and mimics small left colon meconium plug syndrome (therefore this variant is not an Aunt Minnie). Total colonic aganglionosis accounts for 5% of cases, may be familial, and has no sex predilection. Uncommon but severe complications of Hirschsprung disease include fulminant enterocolitis and bowel perforation (18).

Aunt Minnie's Pearls

- *80% of patients with Hirschsprung disease present in the first 6 weeks of life.*
- *Contrast enemas reveal the transition point between the aganglionic distal segment and the dilated proximal bowel.*
- *Perform enemas without bowel preparation to diagnose this disorder.*

CASE 18

History. 4-month-old boy evaluated in the emergency room for abdominal distention and bilious vomiting

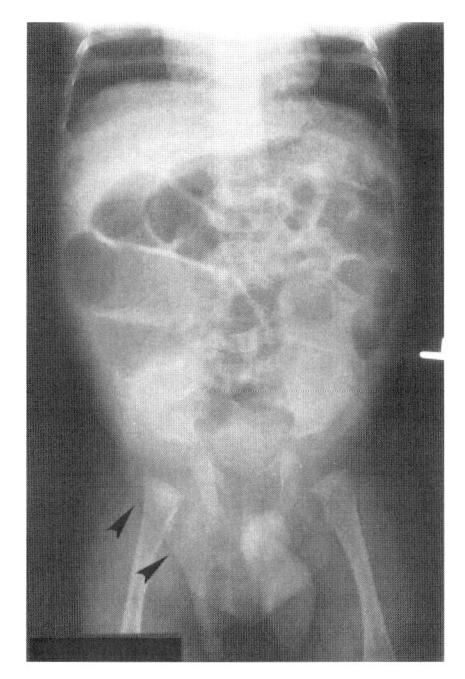

Figure 1.18.1.

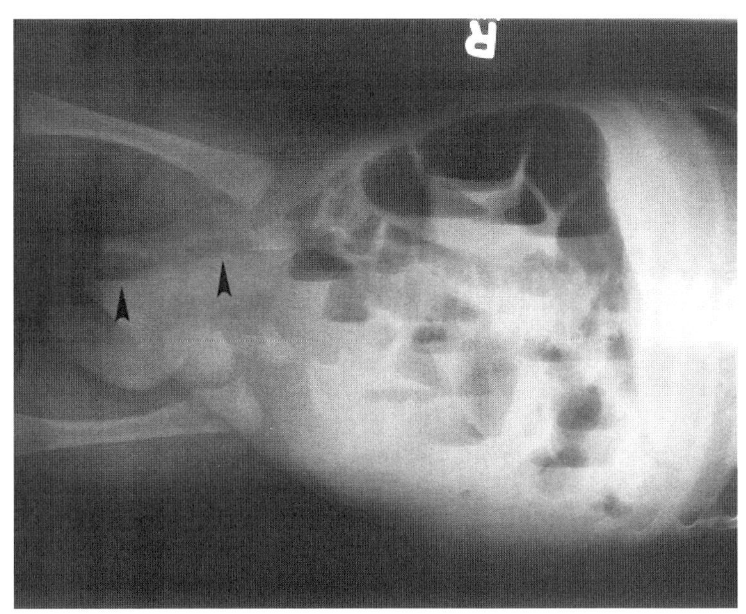

Figure 1.18.2.

Findings. Important findings on the supine anteroposterior view of the abdomen (Fig. 1.18.1) include distended bowel loops with no visible rectal gas, a widened right inguinoscrotal fold (*arrowheads*), and tubular gas in the right scrotum. The left lateral decubitus view (Fig. 1.18.2) demonstrates multiple air-fluid levels in the abdomen, right inguinal region, and right scrotum (*arrowheads*).

Diagnosis. Small-bowel obstruction resulting from an incarcerated right inguinal hernia

Discussion. The embryologic connection between the celomic cavity and the scrotum is known as the processus vaginalis. When the processus remains patent during the first year of life, small bowel may descend into the inguinal canal and scrotum, resulting in the indirect inguinal hernia of childhood. Inguinal hernias are more common in infant boys and more frequently right-sided. After the immediate newborn period and until the fourth month of life, incarcerated inguinal hernia is the most common cause of small-bowel obstruction. Besides small-bowel obstruction, plain films may show gas in the scrotum or inguinal canal, but more often a widened inguinoscrotal fold is the only clue to the diagnosis. Both plain films and sonography may be used to diagnose inguinal hernias, but physical examination is usually sufficient for diagnosis (19).

Aunt Minnie's Pearls

- *Look for a small-bowel dilatation with a thickened inguinoscrotal fold or inguinal bowel gas to diagnose an incarcerated inguinal hernia in children.*

CASE 19

History. 15-year-old African-American boy with fever and chest pain

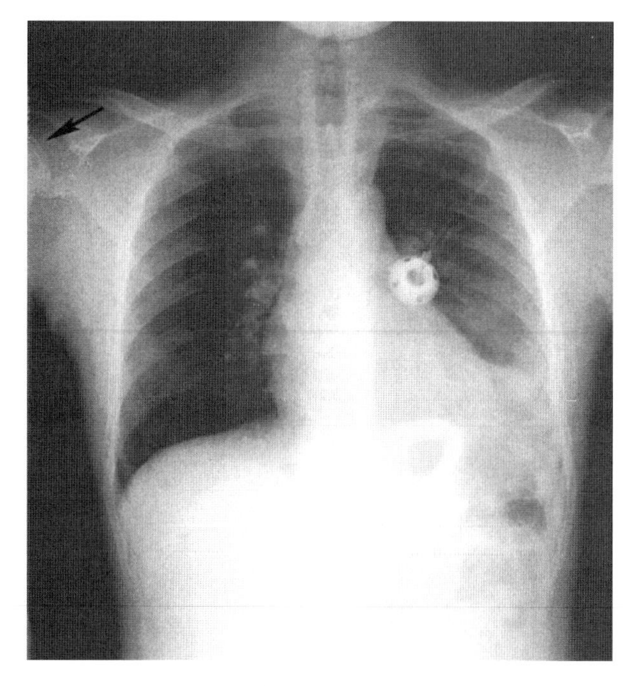

Figure 1.19.1.

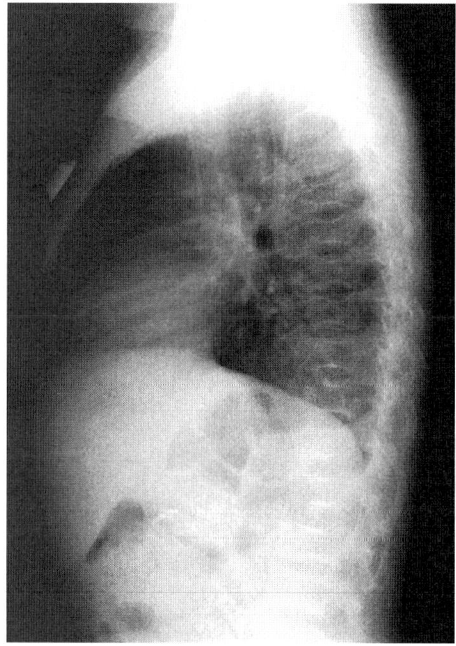

Figure 1.19.2.

Findings. Posteroanterior (Fig. 1.19.1) and lateral (Fig. 1.19.2) views of the chest reveal multiple findings, including a left lower lobe infiltrate, H-shaped or "Lincoln log" vertebrae with central endplate depressions, cholecystectomy clips, mild cardiomegaly, absent splenic shadow, and avascular necrosis of the right humeral head (*arrow*).

Diagnosis. Sickle cell disease

Discussion. Children homozygous for hemoglobin S have the classic severe chronic hemolytic anemia known as sickle cell anemia or sickle cell disease. Sickle cell disease exhibits many abnormalities on chest films, including a small, absent, or calcified splenic shadow resulting from progressive splenic infarction, pulmonary opacities caused by pneumonia or infarction, pigment gallstones from hemolysis, and cardiomegaly from the high-output state induced by anemia. Sludging of sickled erythrocytes in bone leads to infarction or avascular necrosis involving the central vertebral body end plates and the humeral heads. Bone infarction may be complicated by or difficult to differentiate from *Salmonella* osteomyelitis in patients with sickle cell disease (20).

Aunt Minnie's Pearls

- *To diagnose sickle cell disease on the basis of a chest film, look for H-shaped vertebral bodies, avascular necrosis of the humeral heads, cardiomegaly, cholecystectomy clips, and infiltrates.*

CASE 20

History. Neonate with imperforate anus and a family history of sacral and pelvic anomalies

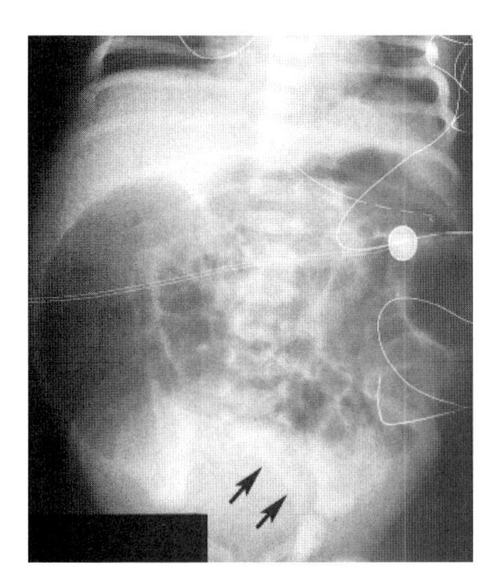

Figure. 1.20.1.

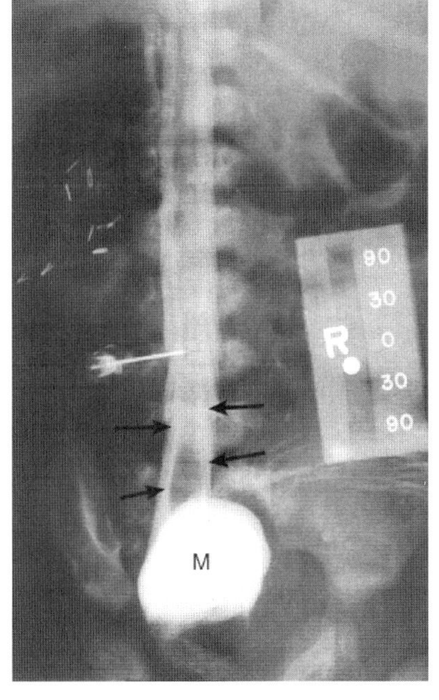

Figure 1.20.2.

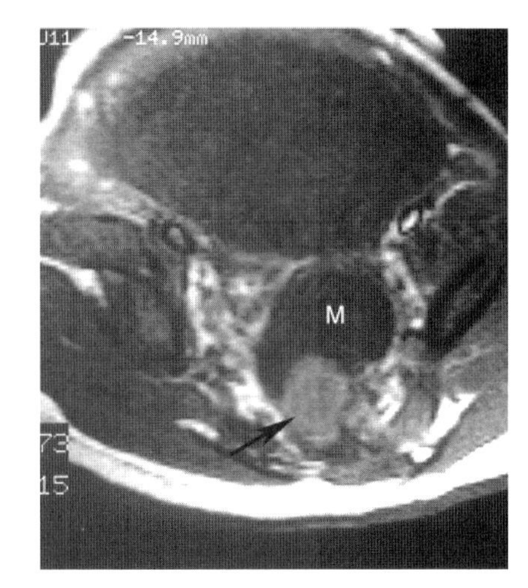

Figure 1.20.3. SE 750/20 without gadolinium.

Findings. Anteroposterior abdominal film demonstrates dilated bowel loops and the classic "scimitar" sacrum (Fig. 1.20.1, *arrows*). A myelogram (Fig. 1.20.2) shows a presacral meningocele (M) with an enlarged and tethered distal spinal cord (*arrows*). An axial T1-weighted MR image through the low pelvis reveals a soft-tissue mass (Fig. 1.20.3, *arrow*) within the meningocele (M).

Diagnosis. The Currarino triad: anorectal malformation, presacral mass, and sacral abnormality

Discussion. The Currarino triad is a hereditary complex of congenital caudal anomalies. Included in the triad are an anorectal malformation and a sacral bony defect such as malsegmentation or crescentic partial agenesis (i.e., "scimitar" sacrum). The presacral mass may be a teratoma, enteric cyst, anterior meningocele, or a combination of the three. This patient had a presacral meningocele that contained an enteric duplication cyst. The patient's mother was born with a "scimitar" sacrum, a presacral teratoma, and an imperforate anus (21).

Aunt Minnie's Pearls

- *The Currarino triad consists of anorectal malformation, presacral mass, and sacral anomaly.*

CASE 21

History. Hypotonic short-limbed infant with a rapidly increasing head circumference

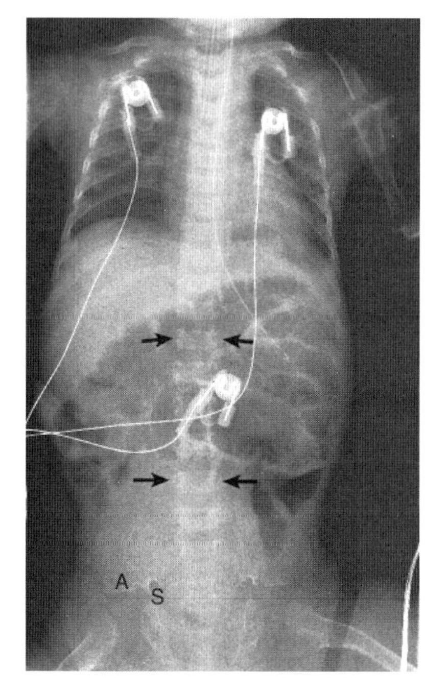

Figure 1.21.1.

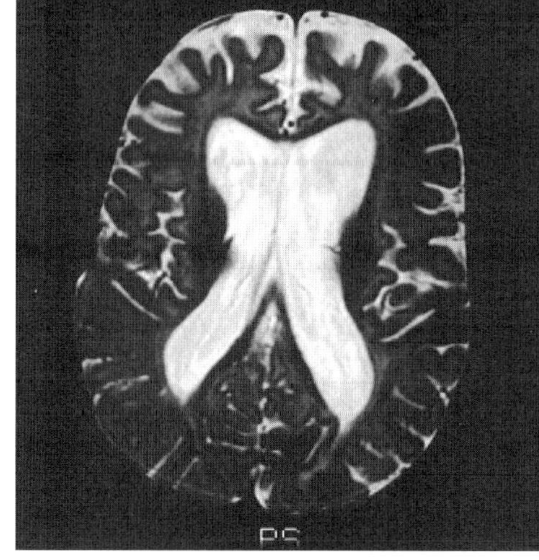

Figure 1.21.2. Axial SE 4000/90.

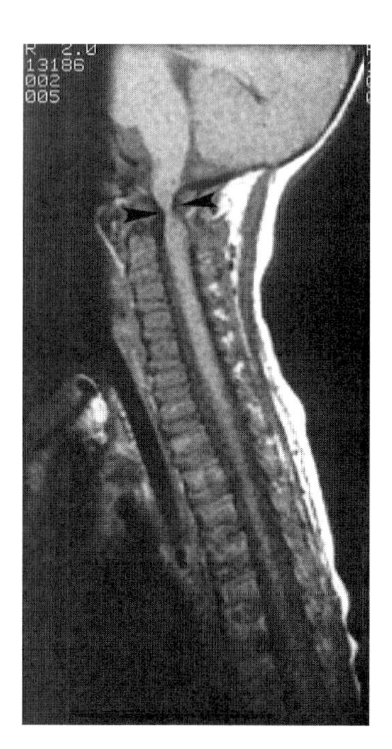

Figure 1.21.3. Sagittal SE 600/23.

Findings. Anteroposterior chest/abdomen film (Fig. 1.21.1) demonstrates narrow lumbar interpediculate distances (*arrows*), short and squared ilia, narrowed sacrosciatic notches (S), horizontal acetabular roofs (A), and a short humerus. MR images of the brain and cervical spinal cord show hydrocephalus (Fig. 1.21.2), caused by stenosis at the foramen magnum, constricting the spinal canal and spinal cord (Fig. 1.21.3, *arrowheads*).

Diagnosis. Achondroplasia

Discussion. Achondroplasia, the most common type of short-limbed dwarfism, results from a defect in endochondral bone formation. Rhizomelia or proximal-limb shortening and craniofacial involvement are the dominant clinical features. Classic plain film findings of achondroplasia not illustrated include short and thick tubular bones, which may have a ball-and-socket epiphyseal-metaphyseal configuration. Vertebral changes are characteristic and include decreased vertebral body height, short pedicles, posterior vertebral body scalloping, and progressively decreasing interpediculate distances down the lumbar spine. Because the membranous bone of the calvarium develops normally, these patients have a relatively large calvarium. However, the skull base, which is formed from endochondral bone, is underdeveloped. This underdevelopment leads to constriction of the foramen magnum that may result in disabling obstructive hydrocephalus, paraplegia, and infant mortality. Tibial bowing, spinal stenosis with thoracolumbar kyphosis, and hydrocephalus may cause complications later in childhood and adulthood (22).

Aunt Minnie's Pearls

- *Achondroplasia is the most common rhizomelic dwarfism.*
- *The basic defect is abnormal endochondral bone formation.*
- *One serious complication is narrowing of the foramen magnum, which causes hydrocephalus and cord compression.*

CASE 22

History. 2-year-old with bowed lower extremities

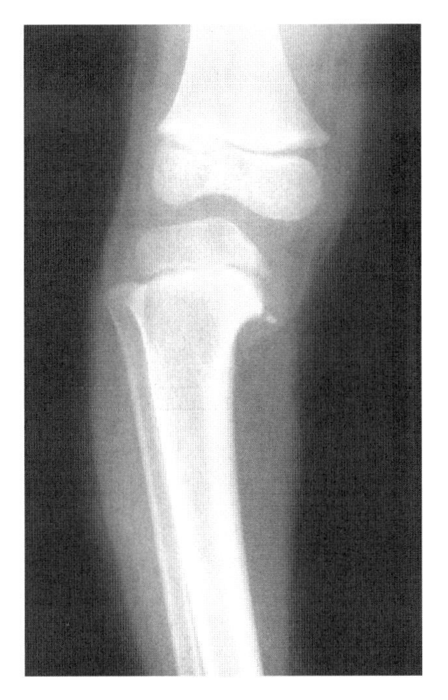

Figure 1.22.1.

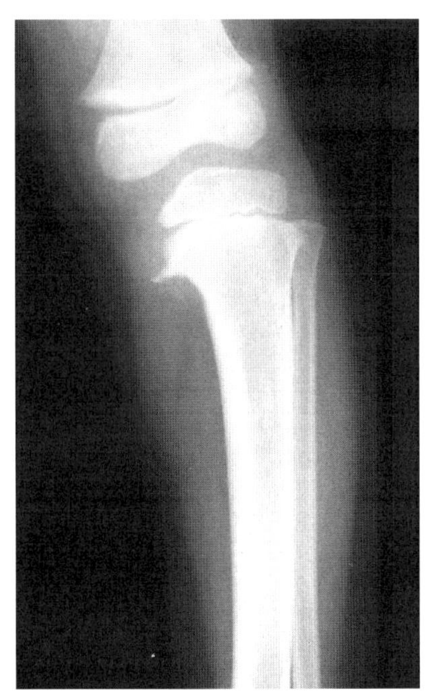

Figure 1.22.2.

Findings. Anteroposterior views of the right (Fig. 1.22.1) and left (Fig. 1.22.2) tibia show beaking, fragmentation, and depression of the medial tibial metaphyses. Hypoplasia and medial sloping of the proximal tibial epiphyses are also evident.

Diagnosis. Blount disease (infantile tibia vara)

Discussion. The underlying abnormality in Blount disease is faulty endochondral bone formation in the medial proximal tibia, which results from abnormal mechanical stresses on the physis. Blount disease may present in infants or adolescents. Infantile Blount disease, or tibia vara, represents persistent physiologic bowing or genu varum that fails to regress as the child begins to walk. Radiographs are useful to differentiate the various causes of bowed legs, such as physiologic bowing, rickets, Blount disease, posttraumatic physeal arrest, and focal fibrocartilaginous dysplasia. Infantile Blount disease may be unilateral or bilateral and asymmetric. Adolescent Blount disease occurs in older children who are overweight. This form of the disease is usually milder, is often unilateral, and is posttraumatic. Either form may resolve spontaneously, but tibial osteotomies are frequently required (23, 24).

Aunt Minnie's Pearls

- *Blount disease is due to abnormal stresses on the medial proximal tibial physis.*
- *Beaking, fragmentation, and sloping characterize the medial proximal tibia.*
- *Infantile and adolescent varieties occur.*

CASE 23

History. 4-month-old with a large anterior fontanelle and widened calvarial sutures

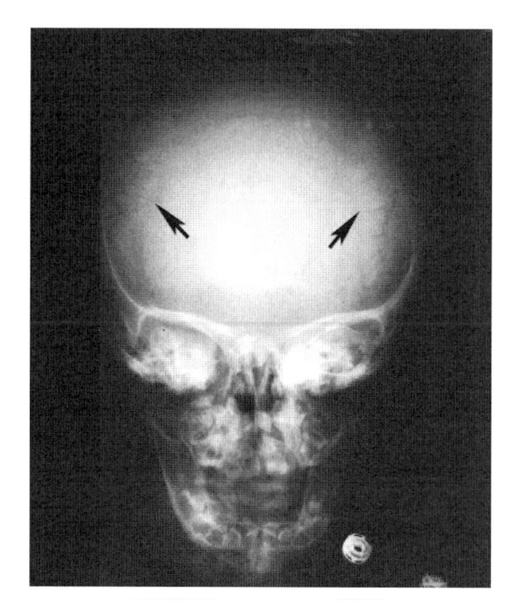

Figure 1.23.1.

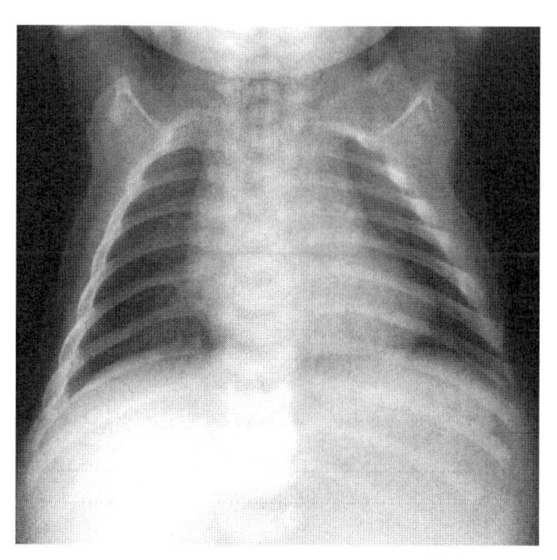

Figure 1.23.2.

Findings. Anteroposterior view of the skull (Fig. 1.23.1) reveals wormian bones (intrasutural bone, *arrows*). Frontal view of the chest (Fig. 1.23.2) shows a hypoplastic left clavicle and absence of the right clavicle.

Diagnosis. Cleidocranial dysplasia

Discussion. Cleidocranial dysplasia is an autosomal dominant disorder that affects membranous bone formation. Patients are characterized clinically by an enlarged head with wide fontanelles and sutures, drooping shoulders, and joint hypermobility. Plain film skull findings include retarded membranous ossification with wormian bones and delayed closure of sutures and fontanelles. Because the clavicles and parasymphyseal bone of the pubis are formed from membranous bone, total or partial aplasia of one or both clavicles and abnormal pelvic ossification with a widened symphysis pubis are also seen. Finally, large pseudoepiphyses of the metacarpals and metatarsal bones are characteristic of this disorder (24).

Aunt Minnie's Pearls

- *Hypoplastic or absent clavicles, wormian bones, and a wide symphysis pubis = cleidocranial dysplasia.*

REFERENCES

1. Kirks DR, Caron KH. Gastrointestinal tract. In: Kirks DR, ed. Practical pediatric imaging: diagnostic radiology of infants and children, 2nd ed. Boston: Little, Brown, 1991:775–782.
2. Auringer ST, Sumner TE. Congenital anomalies of the small bowel. In: Chen MYM, Zagoria RJ, Ott DJ, Gelfand DW, eds. Radiology of the small bowel. New York: Igaku-Shoin, 1992:107–110.
3. Kleinman PK. Diagnostic imaging of child abuse. Baltimore: Williams & Wilkins, 1987:10–20.
4. Kleinman PK. Diagnostic imaging in infant abuse. AJR 1990;155:703–712.
5. Slovis TL, Sty JR, Haller JO. Imaging of the pediatric urinary tract. Philadelphia: Saunders, 1989:87–89.
6. Cohen MD. Imaging of children with cancer. St. Louis: Mosby-Year Book, 1992:134–169.
7. Barnes JC, Smith WL. The VATER association. Radiology 1978;126:445–449.
8. Taylor GA, Eggli KD. Lap belt injuries of the lumbar spine in children: a pitfall in CT diagnosis. AJR 1988;150:1355–1358.
9. Afshani E, Kuhn JP. Common causes of low back pain in children. RadioGraphics 1991;11:269–291.
10. Stringer DA. Pediatric gastrointestinal imaging. Philadelphia: Decker, 1989:394–403.
11. Kennedy CD, Habibi P, Matthew DJ, Gordon I. Lobar emphysema: long-term imaging follow-up. Radiology 1991;180:189–193.
12. Auringer ST, Sumner TE. Congenital anomalies of the small bowel. In: Chen MYM, Zagoria RJ, Ott DJ, Gelfand DW, eds. Radiology of the small bowel. New York: Igaku-Shoin, 1992:115–120.
13. Oestreich AE. Skeletal system. In: Kirks DR, ed. Practical pediatric imaging: diagnostic radiology of infants and children, 2nd ed. Boston: Little, Brown, 1991:397–403.
14. Staheli LT. Fundamentals of pediatric orthopedics. New York: Raven, 1992:7.1–7.20.
15. Hedlund GL, Kirks DR. Respiratory system. In: Kirks DR, ed. Practical pediatric imaging: diagnostic radiology of infants and children, 2nd ed. Boston: Little, Brown, 1991:683.
16. Harris VJ, Brown R. Pneumatoceles as a complication of chemical pneumonia after hydrocarbon ingestion. AJR 1975;125:531–537.
17. Leonidas JC, Berdon W. The neonate and young infant. In: Silverman FN, Kuhn JP, eds. Caffey's pediatric x-ray diagnosis: an integrated imaging approach, 9th ed. St. Louis: Mosby-Year Book, 1993;2:2002–2006.
18. Kirks DR, Caron KH. Gastrointestinal tract. In: Kirks DR, ed. Practical pediatric imaging: diagnostic radiology of infants and children, 2nd ed. Boston: Little, Brown, 1991:861–866.
19. Currarino G. Incarcerated inguinal hernia in infants: plain films and barium enema. Pediatr Radiol 1974;2:247–251.
20. Bohrer SP. Bone changes in the extremities in sickle cell anemia. Semin Roentgenol 1987;22:160–167.
21. Currarino G, Coln D, Votteler T. Triad of anorectal, sacral, and presacral anomalies. AJR 1981;137:395–398.
22. Kao SCS, Waziri MH, Smith WL, Sato Y, Yuh WTC, Franken EA Jr. MR imaging of the craniovertebral junction, cranium, and brain in children with achondroplasia. AJR 1989;153:565–569.
23. Langenskiold A. Tibia vara: a critical review. Clin Orthop 1989;246:195–207.
24. Oestreich AE. Skeletal system. In: Kirks DR, ed. Practical pediatric imaging: diagnostic radiology of infants and children, 2nd ed. Boston: Little, Brown, 1991:380–381.
25. Taybi H, Lachman RS. Radiology of syndromes, metabolic disorders, and skeletal dysplasias, 3rd ed. Chicago: Year Book, 1990:703–704.

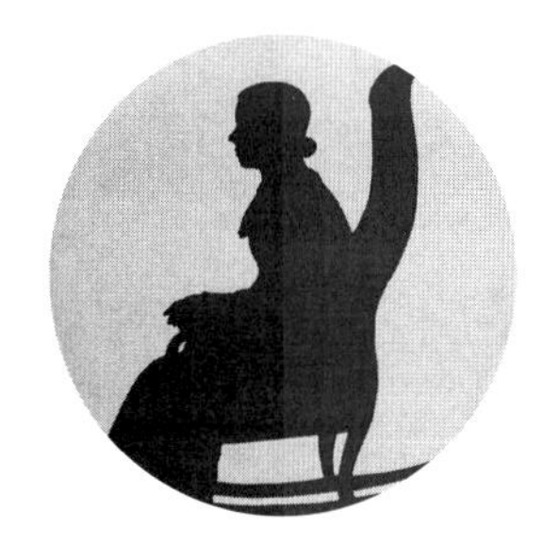

chapter 2

MUSCULOSKELETAL SYSTEM

ERIC J. PIKE AND THOMAS L. POPE JR.

CASE 1

History. Chronic foot pain

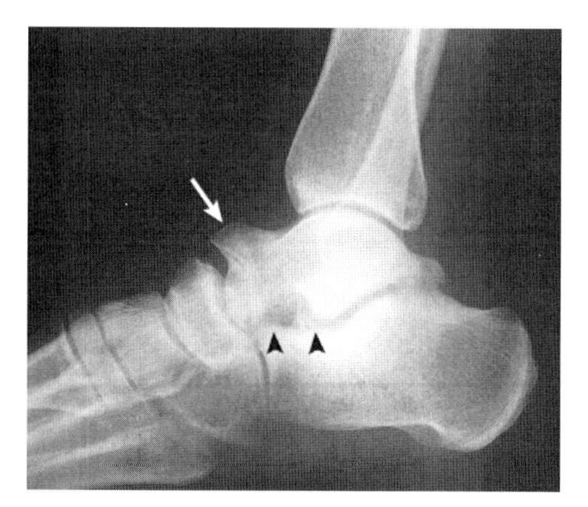

Figure 2.1.1.

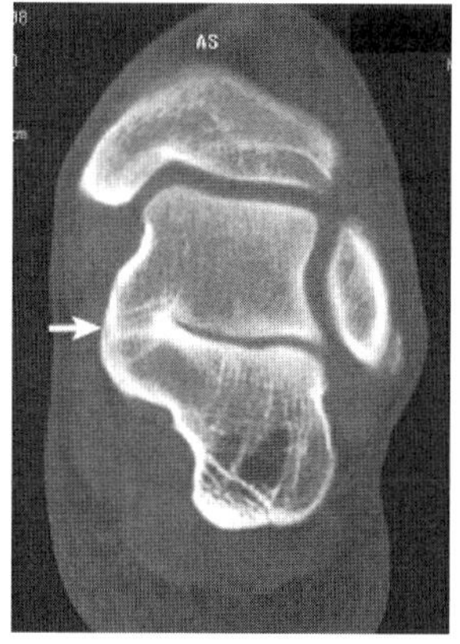

Figure 2.1.2.

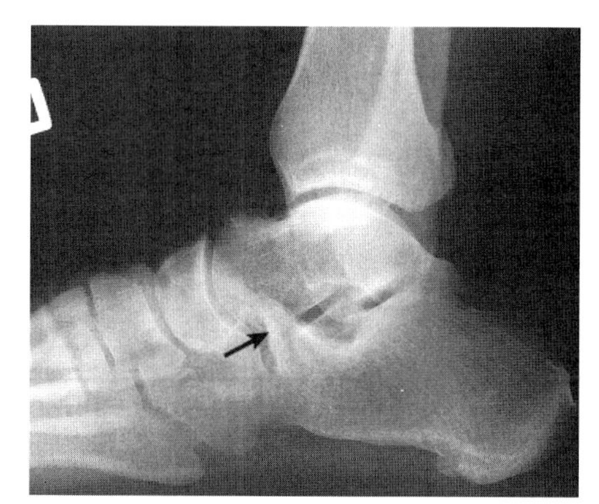

Figure 2.1.3.

Findings. A lateral view of the left foot (Fig. 2.1.1) demonstrates a prominent talar beak (*arrow*) and bony sclerosis overlying the middle facet (*arrowheads*). A coronal CT image in this patient through the middle facet shows talocalcaneal fusion, with bony bridging between the talus and the sustentaculum tali of the calcaneus (Fig. 2.1.2, *arrow*).

Diagnosis. Tarsal coalition

Discussion. Tarsal coalition, an abnormal fusion of one or more of the tarsal bones, may be fibrous, cartilaginous, or osseous and can be congenital (developmental) or acquired secondary to trauma, articular diseases, infection, or surgery. The most common tarsal coalitions are calcaneonavicular and talocalcaneal (1). Almost all talocalcaneal coalitions occur between the sustentaculum tali of the calcaneus and the middle facet of the talus. Tarsal coalition is more common in male patients, is bilateral in up to 25% of patients, and is most commonly discovered during the second and third decades of life. The peroneal spastic flatfoot deformity may be the initial clinical manifestation in many of these patients because of decreased subtalar motion.

Radiographically, the calcaneonavicular coalition may be suspected because of elongation of the anterior facet of the calcaneus (anteater sign) on plain films (Fig. 2.1.3, *arrow*). The 45° medial oblique view is the best diagnostic plain-film projection to demonstrate this coalition. Talocalcaneal coalition can result in dorsal beaking of the talar head, a ball-and-socket ankle mortise, asymmetry of the inferior talar necks, widening of the lateral talar process, and close approximation between the talus and calcaneus. For definitive diagnosis, CT is the investigation of choice (2).

Aunt Minnie's Pearls

- *The most common types of tarsal coalition are talocalcaneal and calcaneonavicular.*
- *The condition is bilateral in up to 25% of patients.*

CASE 2

History. 23-year-old man with pain in the right hip

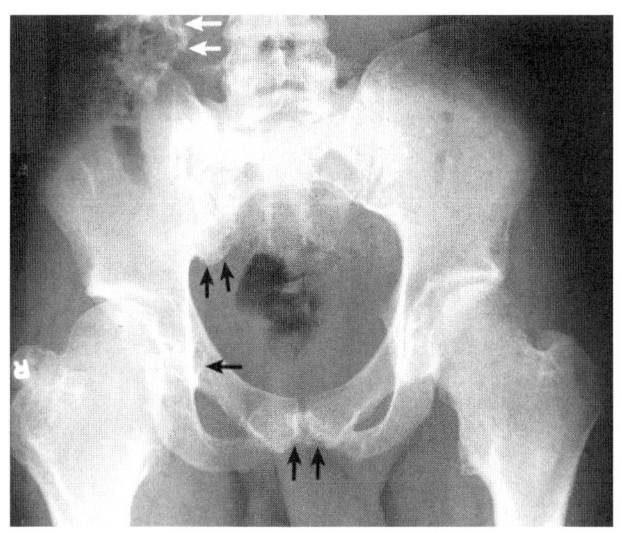

Figure 2.2.1.

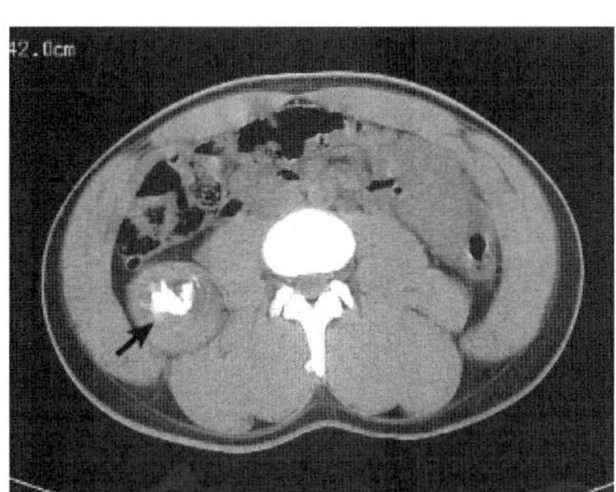

Figure 2.2.2.

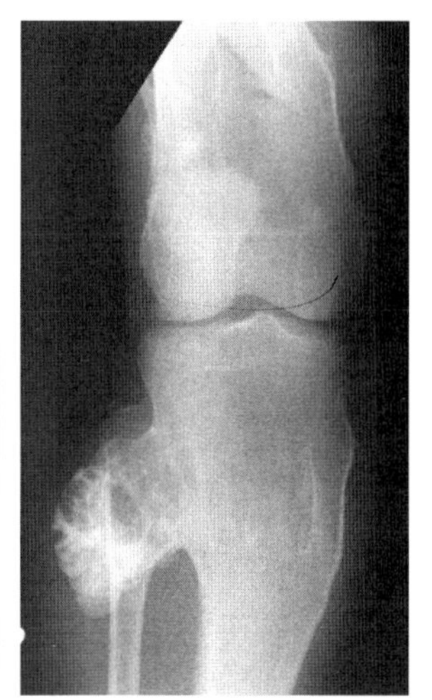

Figure 2.2.3.

Findings. Anteroposterior view of the pelvis (Fig. 2.2.1) shows flaring of the metaphyseal regions of the proximal femurs and numerous osteochondromas arising from the right iliac crest, pubic bones, and proximal right femur (*arrows*). An axial CT image through the upper pelvis demonstrates a large right exostosis with an associated soft tissue mass (Fig. 2.2.2, *arrow*). Anteroposterior view of the knee shows multiple osteochondromas arising from the femur and the fibula (Fig. 2.2.3).

Diagnosis. Multiple hereditary exostosis (diaphyseal aclasia)

Discussion. Multiple hereditary exostosis is an autosomal dominant disorder that usually becomes manifest in the first or second decade of life. Initial symptoms include palpable masses adjacent to joints, compression of neurovascular structures, decreased range of motion, and deformities caused by bowing or shortening of bones. The osteochondromas are generally bilateral and most commonly involve the distal and proximal portions of the femur, tibia, fibula, and humerus. The scapula, innominate bone, ribs, radius, and ulna may also be affected.

The complications occurring in multiple hereditary exostosis are the same as those in a solitary exostosis: fracture, vascular injury, bursa formation, neurological compromise, osseous deformity, and malignant transformation. The risk of malignant transformation in multiple hereditary exostosis is 5%, whereas in the solitary exostosis it is <1%. Clinical features of pain, swelling, and a mass and imaging changes showing growth of a previously stable exostosis, bony erosion, or development of calcifications are warning signs of malignant transformation. The most frequent malignant tumor is chondrosarcoma, which generally occurs in the femur, tibia, humerus, or innominate bone (Fig. 2.2.2, *arrow*) (3). The definitive diagnosis of a developing malignancy is determined by open biopsy and pathological examination.

Aunt Minnie's Pearls

- *Abnormal modeling of bone and osseous deformity are characteristic of multiple hereditary exostosis.*
- *New pain, mass, bony erosion, or calcifications may indicate malignant transformation.*

CASE 3

History. Withheld

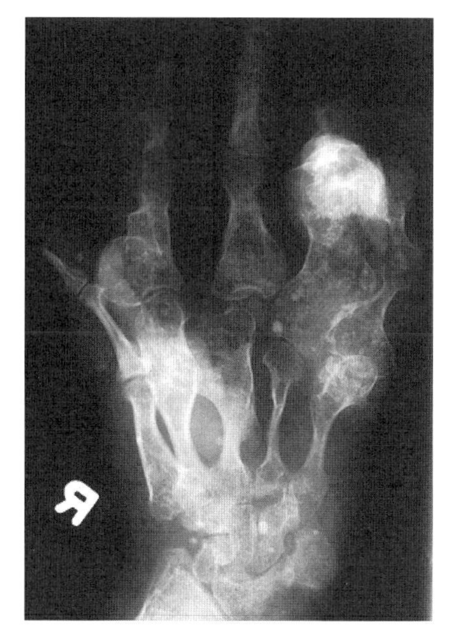

Figure 2.3.1.

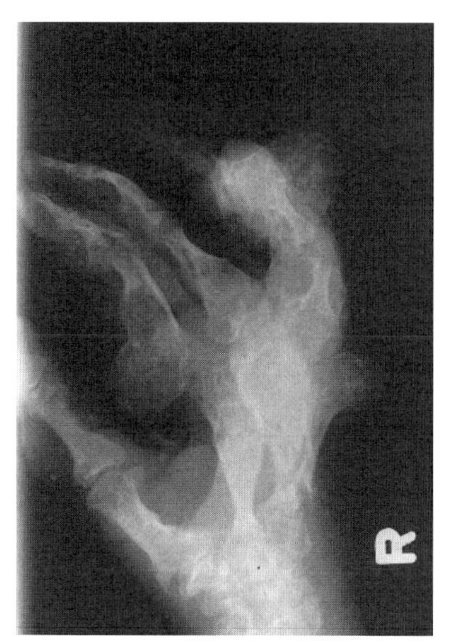

Figure 2.3.2.

Findings. Anteroposterior and oblique views of the right hand (Figs. 2.3.1 and 2.3.2) show multiple metacarpal and phalangeal chondroid lesions representing enchondromas. Numerous hand and finger soft tissue masses containing phleboliths are identified.

Diagnosis. Maffucci's syndrome (multiple enchondromatosis with soft tissue hemangiomas)

Discussion. The diagnosis of Maffucci's syndrome is made on the basis of a combination of multiple nonhereditary enchondromatosis and soft tissue hemangiomas. The hemangiomas, usually detected at birth or shortly after, are variable in size and number and can become quite large, resulting in growth disturbance. Their distribution does not correlate with that of the enchondromas. Hemangiomas that occur in the head, neck, or gastrointestinal tract can lead to stridor, epistaxis, and dysphagia (4). There is also a higher rate of malignant transformation of the enchondromas to chondrosarcoma in Maffucci's syndrome (18–27%). Other malignancies, including hemangiosarcomas, lymphangiosarcomas, and fibrosarcomas, have been described (5).

The imaging appearance of Maffucci's syndrome is similar to that of Ollier's disease, except that these patients also have soft tissue masses and phleboliths. Involvement of the hands and feet is usually severe, and CT scanning or MR imaging is useful to evaluate the extent of the soft tissue and bony lesions.

Aunt Minnie's Pearls

- *Multiple enchondromas + soft tissue hemangiomas = Maffucci's syndrome.*
- *Involvement of the hands and feet is frequent and severe.*

CASE 4

History. Three patients with "dense bones"

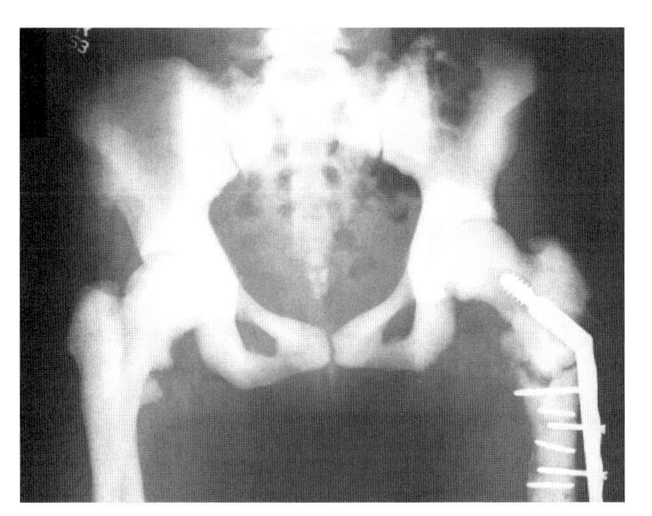

Figure 2.4.1.

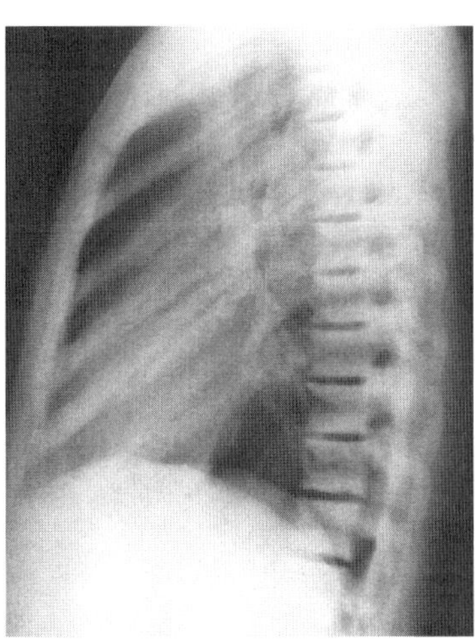

Figure 2.4.2.

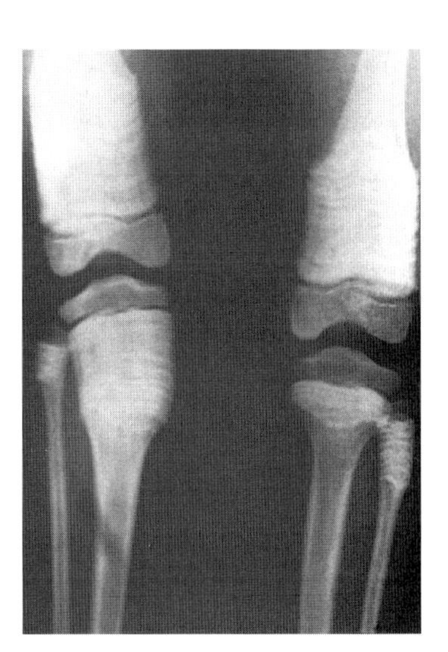

Figure 2.4.3.

Findings. Anteroposterior view of the pelvis (Fig. 2.4.1) in a 22-year-old woman shows diffuse uniform bony sclerosis and a pathologic subtrochanteric fracture of the proximal left femur. A lateral chest radiograph in another patient (Fig. 2.4.2) shows a sandwich appearance involving the vertebral bodies, with sclerosis of the superior and inferior endplates. Plain radiographs of the knees in a younger patient (Fig. 2.4.3) show splaying of the metaphyses and alternating radiolucent bands in the distal femora and proximal tibia and fibula bilaterally.

Diagnosis. Osteopetrosis

Discussion. Osteopetrosis is a complex hereditary disorder that is characterized by a defect in osteoclastic resorption. Four different subtypes with distinct clinical and radiographic features are recognized, but the two most common are the precocious and delayed types. Patients affected with the autosomal recessive, precocious, or lethal form usually die shortly after birth or survive for only a few years. Clinically they are characterized by hepatosplenomegaly, failure to thrive, and blindness. Patients with the autosomal dominant, delayed form are generally asymptomatic but may have mild anemia, cranial nerve deficits, pathologic fracture, or bleeding problems after tooth extraction (6).

Osteopetrosis is characterized by generalized osteosclerosis and diffuse cortical thickening with narrowing of the medullary cavity. The typical plain-film features include a bone-within-bone appearance, metaphyseal undermodeling and widening (Erlenmeyer flask deformity), radiolucent and radiodense bands near the ends of long bones, and obliteration of mastoid air cells and paranasal sinuses. The potential complications of osteopetrosis include fractures (bones are weaker than normal), crowding of normal bone marrow space, pancytopenia and extramedullary hematopoiesis, and osteosclerosis of the basal foramina of the skull with resultant cranial nerve deficits (7).

Aunt Minnie's Pearls

- *Osteosclerosis + alternating radiolucent bands + metaphyseal widening = osteopetrosis.*
- *Complications include pathologic fractures, pancytopenia, and cranial nerve defects.*

CASE 5

History. 74-year-old woman with knee pain and a palpable mass

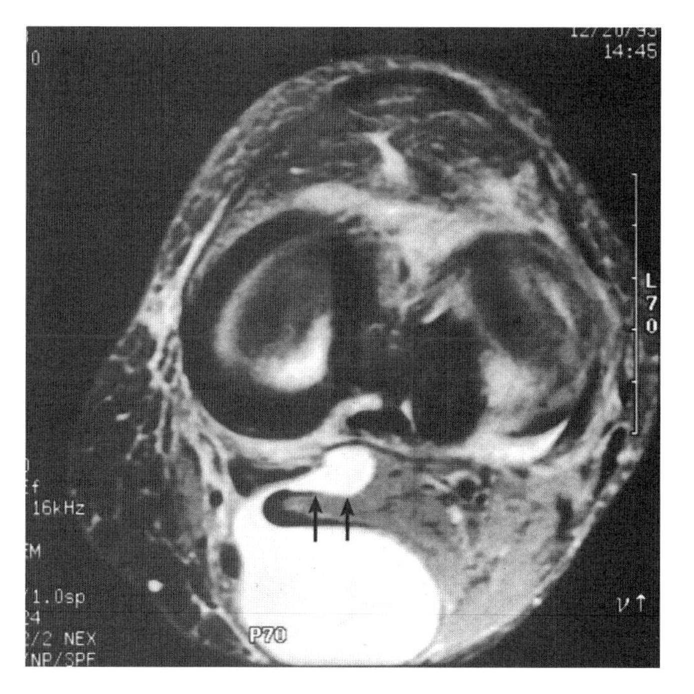

Figure 2.5.1. FSE 4000/18, ET = 8.

Findings. T2-weighted axial MR image (Fig. 2.5.1) demonstrates a moderate-sized, well-defined, cystic mass in the popliteal region. A channel between the semimembranosus and medial gastrocnemius muscles connects the cyst to the joint (*arrows*).

Diagnosis. Popliteal (Baker's) cyst

Discussion. Although various potential bursae are located around the knee joint, most synovial cysts develop in the popliteal region. The semimembranosus-gastrocnemius bursa, located between the tendons of the medial gastrocnemius and semimembranosus muscles posterior to the medial femoral condyle, is the most commonly encountered synovial cyst in the knee. Normally, a communication may be present between the posterior joint capsule and the anterior limit of the bursa, but when the bursa distends, it is called a popliteal or Baker's cyst. These cysts are often large enough to cause pain and to be palpable but are often discovered as incidental findings on MR imaging of the knee performed for other reasons. Any traumatic, inflammatory, neoplastic, or degenerative condition producing a joint effusion can lead to the formation of these cysts (8).

MR imaging provides the most accurate information regarding the extent of the cyst and the amount of synovial inflammation (9). However, ultrasonography is a less expensive test that can be used to confirm the presence and characteristic location of a popliteal cyst (10).

Aunt Minnie's Pearls

- Baker's cyst is the most common popliteal fossa cyst.
- Connection to joint is between the tendons of the semimembranosus and the medial gastrocnemius muscles.

CASE 6

History. 11-year-old boy with right arm pain after a fall

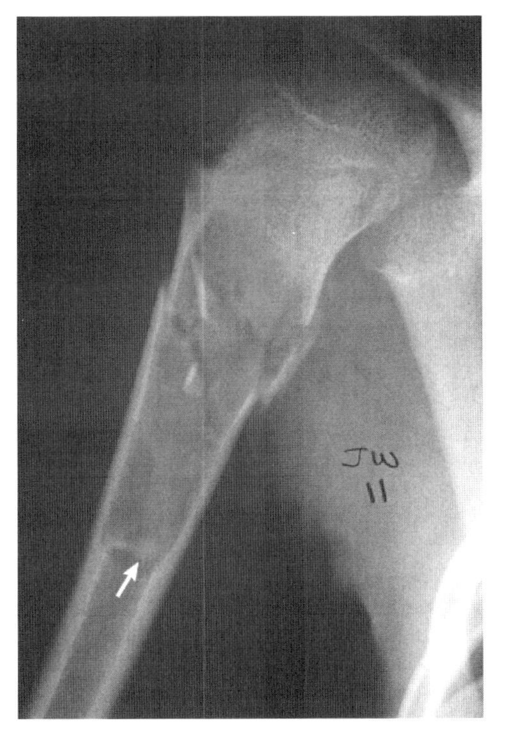

Figure 2.6.1.

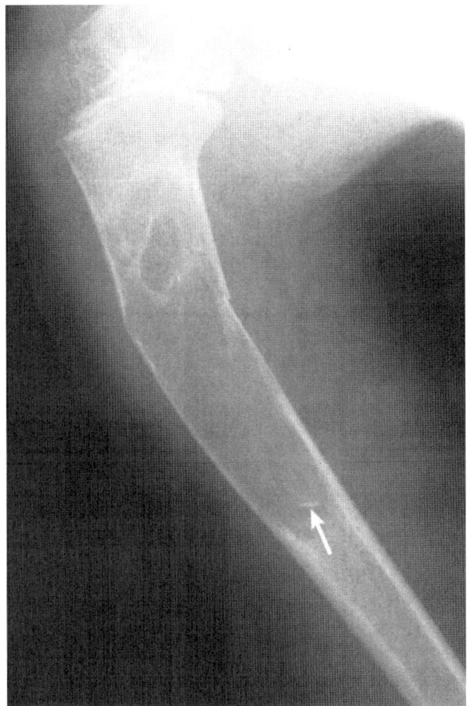

Figure 2.6.2.

Findings. Anteroposterior and lateral views of the proximal right humerus (Figs. 2.6.1 and 2.6.2) demonstrate a well circumscribed, geographic lytic abnormality in the metaphysis. The margins of the lesion are well defined, and no matrix is present. A pathologic, comminuted fracture is associated with the lesion, and fragments of cortex have fallen to its dependent portion (*arrows*). This latter finding is the distinguishing feature in this case, as the fragments reach this position because of the lesion's cystic nature.

Diagnosis. Unicameral bone cyst with fallen fragment sign (11)

Discussion. Unicameral or simple bone cysts are benign lesions of unknown pathogenesis that are often discovered clinically because of pathologic fracture. They involve the proximal humerus, femur, tibia, or fibula most commonly. Most lesions are identified in the second decade, with a 2:1 male predominance. Lesions near the metaphysis are active, whereas those that have migrated toward the diaphysis because of bone growth are inactive. Treatment includes curettage and packing with bone chips or steroid injection. Some lesions spontaneously resolve (12).

Aunt Minnie's Pearls

- *Unicameral bone cysts are most common in the proximal humerus and femur.*
- *The fallen fragment confirms the cystic nature of the lesion.*

CASE 7

History. 55-year-old woman with foot pain

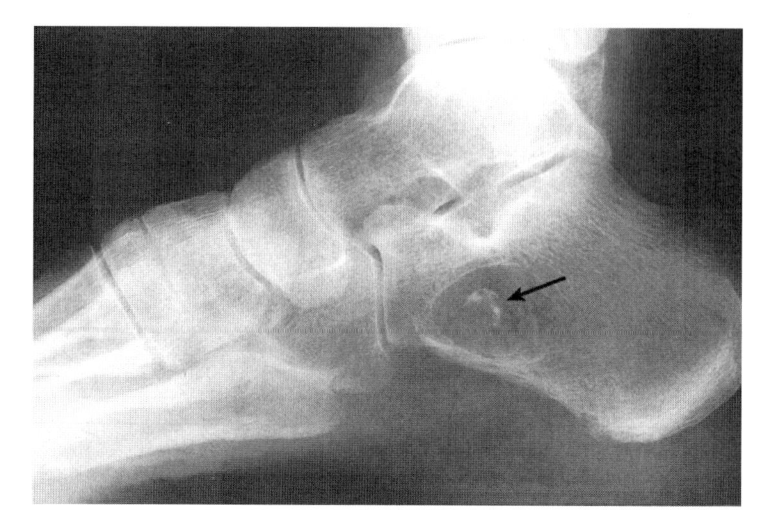

Figure 2.7.1.

Findings. A lateral view of the left foot (Fig. 2.7.1) shows a well-defined lytic lesion in the anterior aspect of the calcaneus with a thin sclerotic border and central calcification (*arrow*). No soft tissue mass or other aggressive features are present.

Diagnosis. Intraosseous lipoma

Discussion. Intraosseous lipomas are most commonly diagnosed in the fourth to sixth decades of life, although they have been reported to occur in patients aged 5–75 years. Male and female patients are equally affected, and the lesion is usually found within the metaphyses of the long tubular bones of the femur, tibia, and fibula or within the calcaneus (13, 14). Multiple intraosseous lipomas are exceedingly rare.

The intraosseous lipoma is characterized by radiolucency with a thin sclerotic margin, which sometimes contains lobulation or intraosseous ridges. Bony expansion, when it occurs, is usually within the small tubular bones. In the calcaneus, this lesion occurs in the relatively lucent triangle between the trabecular groups and may show a central calcified or ossified nidus, whereas lipomas arising in the proximal femur cause ossification along the margin of the intertrochanteric line. Histologically, intraosseous and extraosseous lipomas are identical (15). Either CT or MR imaging can be used as adjunct imaging tests to confirm the diagnosis of lesions suspected to be lipomas. Treatment is usually not necessary when characteristic lesions are seen in asymptomatic patients. If the patient complains of pain, a biopsy followed by bone grafting may be required.

Aunt Minnie's Pearls

- *Lytic lesion with thin sclerotic border and central calcification (especially within the calcaneus) = intraosseous lipoma until proven otherwise.*
- *Average size of intraosseous lipoma is 5–6 cm.*

CASE 8

History. Adolescent child with pain in the leg.

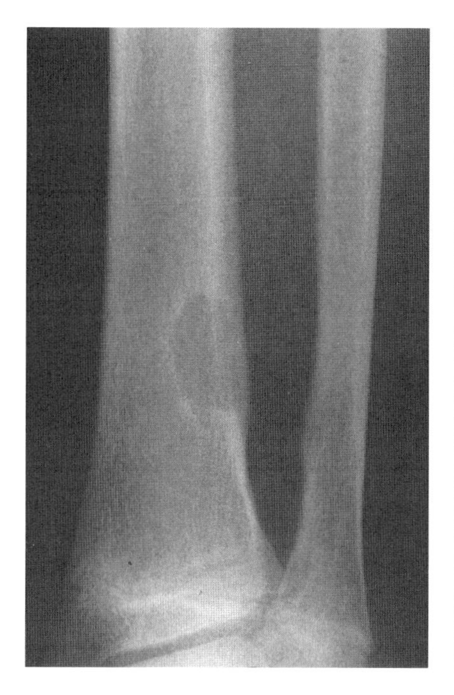

Figure 2.8.1.

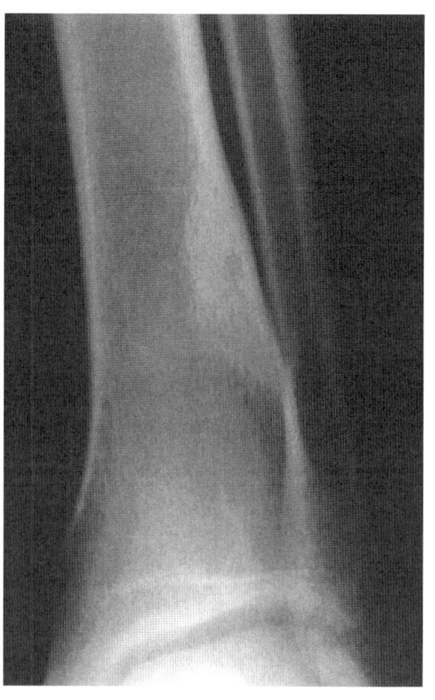

Figure 2.8.2.

Findings. There is a well-defined eccentric radiolucent lesion with a thin sclerotic border adjacent to the cortex of the distal tibia (Fig. 2.8.1). A film 7 years later shows a well-defined sclerotic lesion in the same location (Fig. 2.8.2).

Diagnosis. Fibrous cortical defect or nonossifying fibroma of bone

Discussion. Fibrous cortical defect (FCD), the common designation for this entity, is used synonymously with nonossifying fibroma (NOF). Although the lesions are identical histologically, some authorities call lesions 2 cm and larger NOF, whereas those smaller than this are called FCD. The FCD/NOF is usually discovered as an incidental finding on films done for other reasons and rarely cause symptoms (16).

FCD/NOFs occur in up to 40% of children older than 2 years; 95% of the lesions occur in patients younger than 20 years. Eighty percent of the lesions occur in the lower extremity, and about 25% of lesions are polyostotic. Lesions arise adjacent to the physis, and as limb lengthening occurs, they migrate away from the joint. Typically, FCD/NOF is radiolucent, has a thin sclerotic margin, and shows no periosteal reaction; rarely, it may be expansile. The natural history of FCD/NOF is to involute during adolescence and to become sclerotic, as in this example. When the characteristic imaging features are encountered on plain film, no further imaging and no treatment are necessary ("don't touch lesion") (17).

Aunt Minnie's Pearls

- *Eccentric, well-defined lucent lesion in a young asymptomatic patient is most likely an FCD/NOF.*
- *When classic plain-film findings are present, no treatment or further imaging is necessary.*

CASE 9

History. 12-year-old boy with pain in the lower leg and 10-year-old boy with pain in the foot

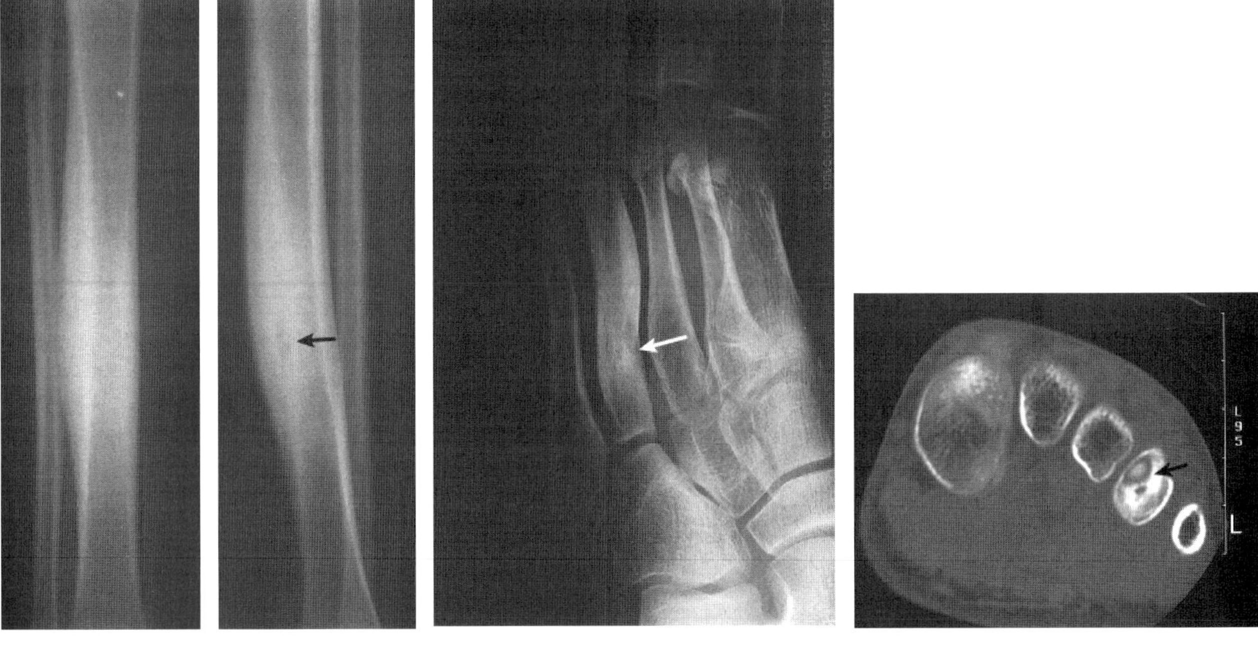

Figure 2.9.1. **Figure 2.9.2.** **Figure 2.9.3.** **Figure 2.9.4.**

Findings. Anteroposterior (Fig. 2.9.1) and lateral (Fig. 2.9.2) views of the lower leg in the first patient show a focal area of sclerosis in the midshaft of the tibia with a central area of radiolucency (*arrow*). In the second patient, an oblique view of the left foot (Fig. 2.9.3) shows sclerosis of the shaft of the fourth metatarsal with an associated central radiolucency (*arrow*). A corresponding axial CT image (Fig. 2.9.4) demonstrates the region of sclerosis and confirms the central radiolucency (*arrow*).

Diagnosis. Osteoid osteoma

Discussion. Osteoid osteoma is a benign osteoblastic neoplasm composed of a central core of vascular osteoid tissue and a peripheral zone of sclerotic bone. The etiology is unknown. Most osteoid osteomas occur in patients between 5 and 25 years old. The male-to-female prevalence is 3:1. With rare exceptions, pain is a hallmark of osteoid osteoma, and if pain is absent, the diagnosis should be questioned. The characteristic history is pain, worse at night, relieved by small doses of aspirin (salicylates). Symptoms and signs of a systemic illness are generally absent, and results of laboratory tests are usually normal.

Osteoid osteoma has a predilection for the diaphysis of the long bones of the lower extremity; about 60% of the lesions occur in the femur and tibia. Other common sites are the humerus, bones of the hands and feet, and posterior elements of the spine, where they are usually located at the base of the transverse process, pedicle, or lamina (18). The classic radiographic appearance, virtually diagnostic of osteoid osteoma, is demonstrated in these two examples: a centrally located ovoid radiolucent area (nidus), measuring <1 cm in diameter, surrounded by a zone of uniform bone sclerosis. Other useful imaging modalities in this setting are bone scintigraphy and CT scanning. The double-density sign on bone scans, with intense accumulation centrally and less marked uptake in the periphery, is characteristic of osteoid osteoma. CT is particularly useful for evaluating lesions in the spine, pelvis, or femoral neck. Complete excision of the nidus with an open or percutaneous approach is necessary to ensure a good clinical outcome (19).

Aunt Minnie's Pearls

- *Pain that is worse at night and relieved by salicylates is characteristic of osteoid osteoma.*
- *Excision of the nidus is usually curative; recurrence is rare.*

CASE 10

History. 35-year-old woman with pain in the right knee

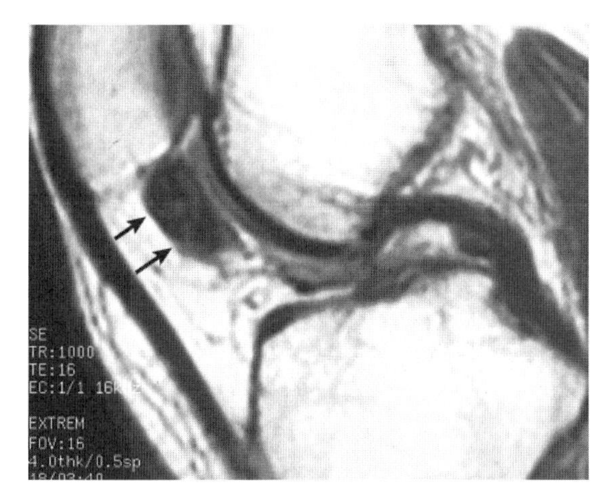

Figure 2.10.1. SE 1000/16

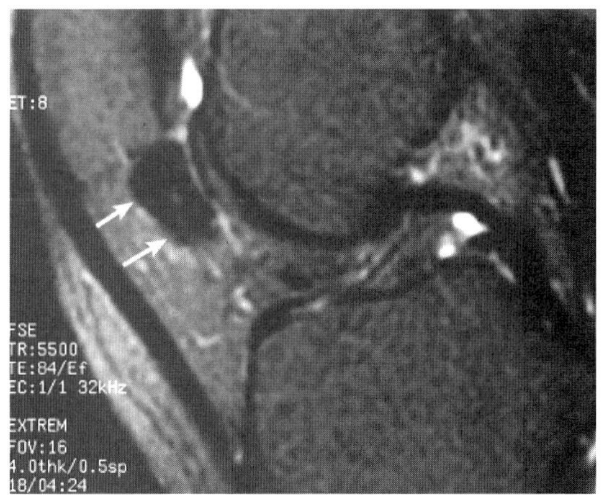

Figure 2.10.2. FSE 5500/84, ET = 8.

Findings. Sagittal proton-density (Fig. 2.10.1) and T2-weighted (Fig. 2.10.2) MR images of the right knee joint demonstrate a low-signal-intensity mass in the upper aspect of the infrapatellar fat pad on both imaging sequences (*arrows*).

Diagnosis. Pigmented villonodular synovitis

Discussion. Pigmented villonodular synovitis (PVS), a proliferative disorder of the synovium, usually affects adults in the third and fourth decades of life. The exact etiology is unknown, but it is likely related to an inflammatory process. The knee is the most commonly involved joint, followed in frequency by the hip, elbow, and ankle, although any joint may be affected. Generally, the involvement is monarticular. The male population is affected slightly more often than the female population. A history of trauma is present in about 50% of cases.

Symptoms depend on whether the disease is focal or diffuse and include pain, swelling, and diminished range of motion. Aspiration of the joint may show the hemorrhagic and characteristic "chocolate" effusion.

Classic radiographic features of PVS include soft tissue swelling, joint effusion, preservation of joint space, absence of osteoporosis, and bony erosions or cysts. Evidence of calcification or metaplastic cartilage in essence excludes PVS as the diagnosis. The MR imaging features of low-signal-intensity synovial masses on T1-weighted, T2-weighted, or gradient-echo sequences from the deposition of hemosiderin are typical of PVS. However, deposition of hemosiderin with low signal intensity can be seen in other conditions, such as hemophilia, synovial hemangioma, or neuropathic osteoarthropathy, all of which are associated with a chronic hemarthrosis (20–22). Treatment of PVS is arthroscopic or surgical excision of the lesions with synovectomy.

Aunt Minnie's Pearls

- *Lesions of PVS are generally low in signal intensity on T1- and T2-weighted MR images.*
- *Aspiration of hemorrhagic or "chocolate" effusion is typical of PVS.*

CASE 11

History. 52-year-old man with a prior shoulder injury

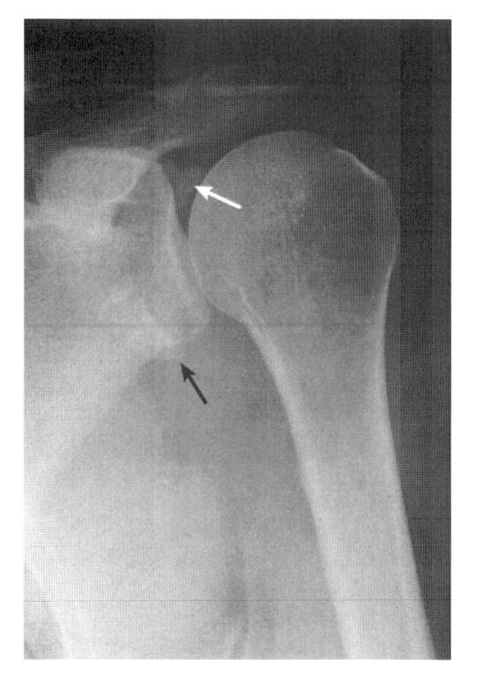

Figure. 211.1.

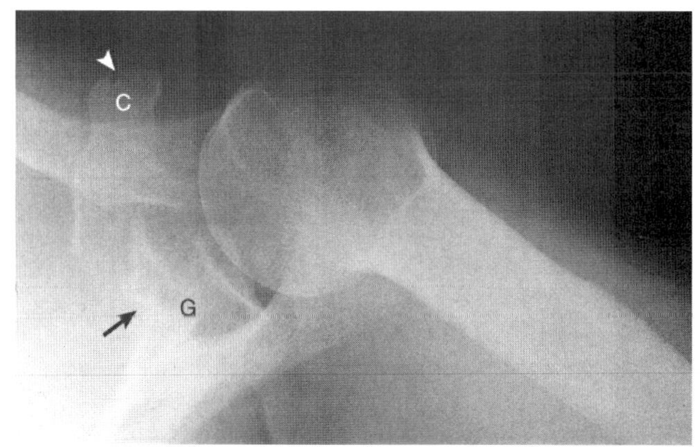

Figure 2.11.2.

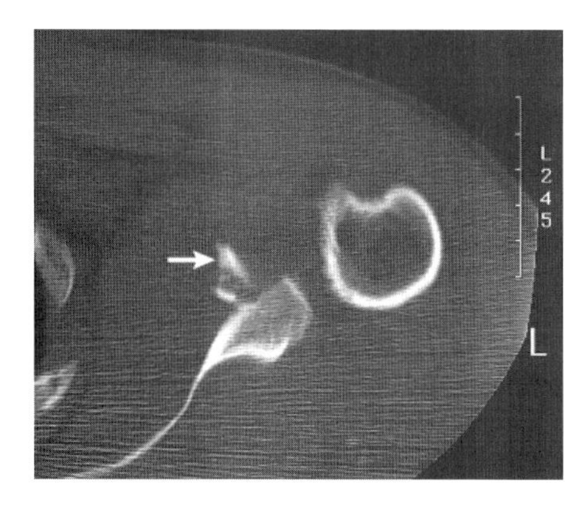

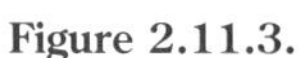

Figure 2.11.3.

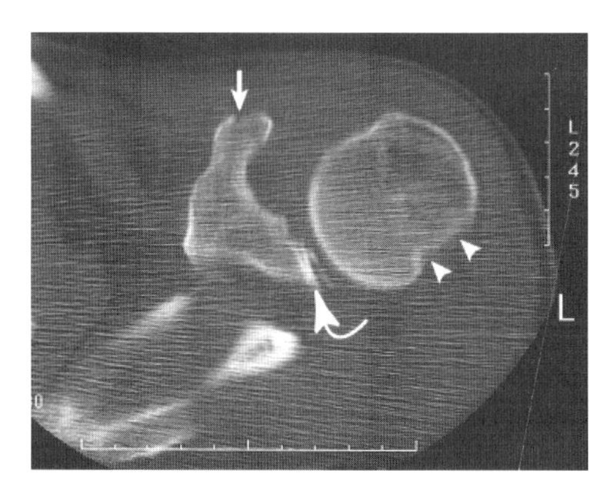

Figure 2.11.4.

Findings. Anteroposterior (Fig. 2.11.1) and axillary (Fig. 2.11.2) views show small fragments of bone (*arrows*) adjacent to the superior and inferior aspect of the glenoid (G) and a nondisplaced coracoid (C) fracture (*arrowhead*). Axial CT images through the shoulder joint show a fracture of the anteroinferior aspect of the glenoid (Bankart lesion) (Fig. 2.11.3, *arrow*). Another CT image (Fig. 2.11.4) reveals fractures of the superior glenoid (*curved arrow*), coracoid process (*arrow*), and a compression fracture of the posterolateral aspect of the humeral head (Hill-Sachs lesion) (*arrowheads*).

Diagnosis. Bony Bankart lesion of the shoulder with an associated Hill-Sachs deformity of the humeral head

Discussion. The Bankart lesion or deformity is an avulsion or compression defect of the anterior and inferior rim of the glenoid. The injury may be purely cartilaginous or osseous and is virtually always the result of an anterior dislocation of the shoulder. When the humeral head dislocates anteriorly and inferiorly, it impinges on the anterior and inferior glenoid labrum. This mechanism may result in a compression fracture of the superoposterolateral humeral head (Hill-Sachs lesion), stripping of the anterior capsule of the joint, and fractures of the cartilaginous labrum or of the osseous rim of the glenoid (Bankart lesion). Large osseous glenoid fractures can be seen on standard anteroposterior or axillary shoulder views, but smaller bony injuries require specialized plain-film views (West Point and Didiee projections). Demonstration of the fibrocartilaginous Bankart lesion requires CT arthrography or MR imaging (23, 24).

Aunt Minnie's Pearls

- *The Bankart lesion is due to traumatic anterior dislocation of the shoulder.*
- *Compression fracture of the posterolateral humeral head (Hill-Sachs deformity) is often an associated finding.*
- *CT or MR is required to diagnose the purely fibrocartilaginous Bankart lesions.*

CASE 12

History. 16-year-old basketball player with pain in his left knee

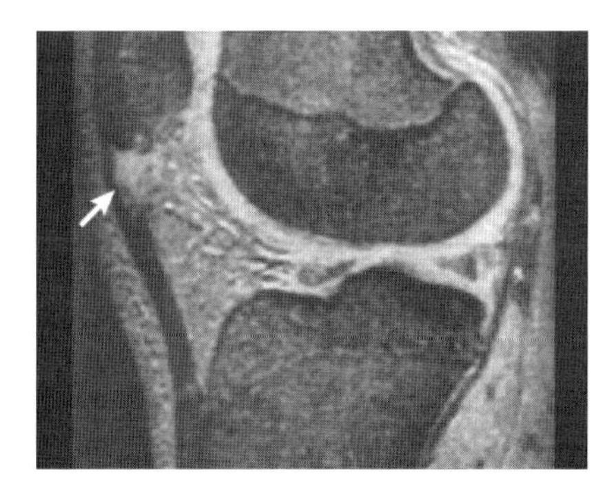

Figure 2.12.1. FSE 4000/84, ET = 8.

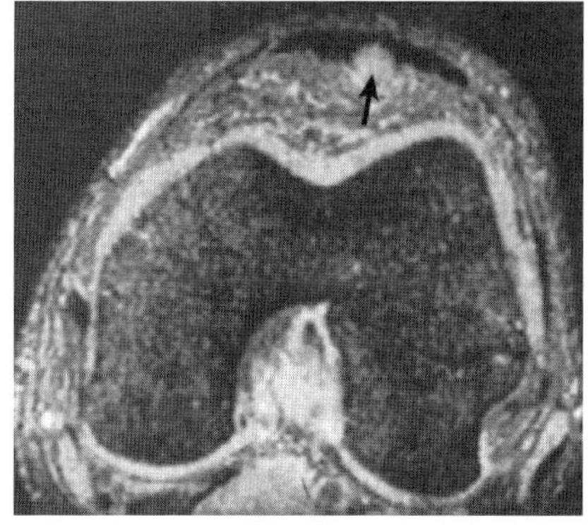

Figure 2.12.2. FSE 4000/84, ET = 8.

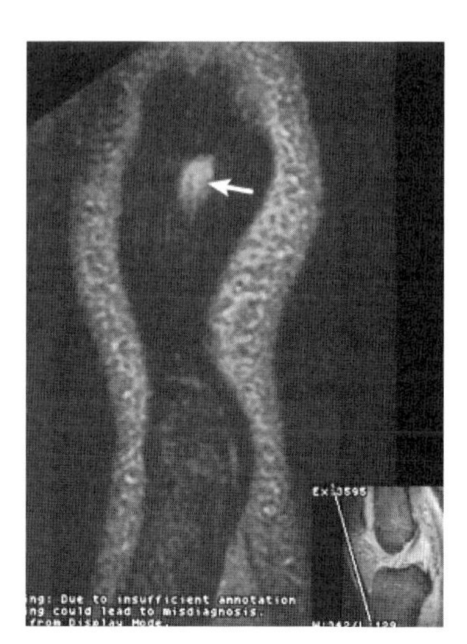

Figure 2.12.3. FSE 4000/84, ET = 8.

Findings. Sagittal (Fig. 2.12.1), axial (Fig. 2.12.2), and coronal (Fig. 2.12.3) fat saturated T2-weighted MR images of the left knee show a focal area of high signal intensity within the patellar tendon just below the lower aspect of the patella (*arrows*).

Diagnosis. Patellar tendinitis (jumper's knee)

Discussion. Jumper's knee is an overuse syndrome occurring in athletes involved in sports that require kicking, jumping, and running—activities that place tremendous stress on the knee in general and the patellofemoral joint in particular. Over time, if the athlete does not rest, necrosis, fibrosis, and degeneration within the tendon may occur and may lead to patellar tendon rupture. This sequence of events results in pain, swelling, and tenderness in the patella-patellar tendon junction. A similar clinical presentation can occur in adolescents with an associated bony fragmentation of the lower pole of the patella. This syndrome is referred to as Sinding-Larsen-Johansson disease, one of the many osteochondroses thought to be caused by chronic repetitive stress (25, 26).

MR imaging is the diagnostic investigation of choice to confirm the clinical suspicion of patellar tendinitis. The MR features, as shown in this example, are an enlarged proximal patellar tendon with areas of increased signal intensity on T1- and T2-weighted images. The areas of abnormal, increased signal intensity may be more evident on inversion-recovery sequences, which are more sensitive for areas of edema. If a patellar disruption is encountered, axial images must be obtained so that the degree of tendon injury can be estimated (27).

Aunt Minnie's Pearls

- *Patellar tendinitis (jumper's knee) is common in sports requiring jumping and abrupt quadriceps contraction.*
- *T2-weighted or inversion-recovery sequences are preferred to identify the extent of the tendon injury.*

CASE 13

History. 21-year-old man with worsening pain in the left wrist after an injury to the wrist 6 months ago (Fig. 2.13.1)

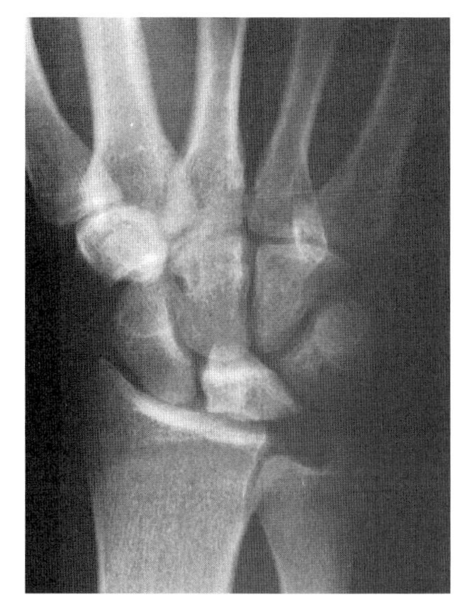

Figure 2.13.1.

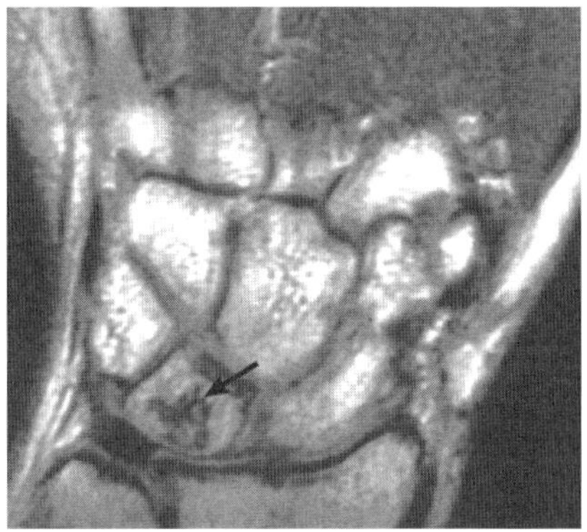

Figure 2.13.2. SE 600/30.

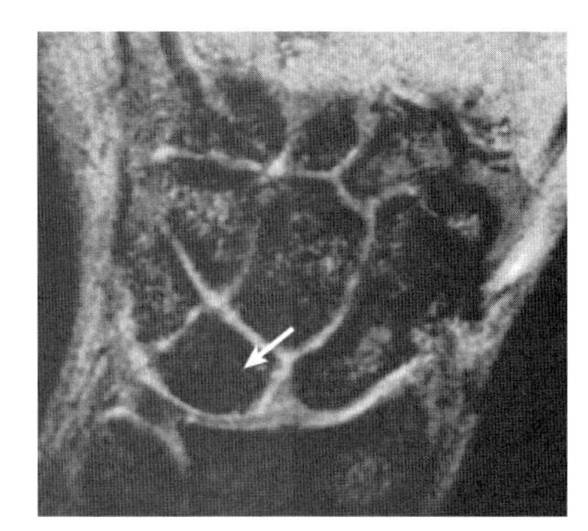

Figure 2.13.3. GRE 500/15/30.

Findings. Anteroposterior view of the left wrist (Fig. 2.13.1) shows a shortened ulna in relation to the radius (negative ulnar variance) and sclerosis with loss of height of the lunate bone. See discussion for findings of Figures 2.13.2 and 2.13.3.

Diagnosis. Kienböck's disease or lunatomalacia

Discussion. Kienböck's disease is by definition osteonecrosis of the lunate bone. It is most common in patients 20–40 years old and has a predilection for the dominant hand in individuals involved in manual labor. The exact cause is not known, but trauma, either single or repetitive, is thought to be a prominent predisposing factor in most cases. The lunate is considered vulnerable to injury from trauma because of its precarious blood supply and its fixed position in the wrist (28, 29). A shortened ulna in relation to the radius, or negative ulnar variance, increases the force on the lunate and is seen in about 75% of patients with Kienböck's disease (30).

The imaging findings, which do not always correlate with the patient's symptoms, include plain-film features of increased density or sclerosis of the lunate and, eventually, alteration in the normal bony shape with collapse. MR imaging may show abnormalities in the lunate when plain films are normal. For example, in a 46-year-old man with wrist pain, a coronal T1-weighted image (Fig. 2.13.2) demonstrates low signal intensity in the lunate (*arrow*) and negative ulnar variance. The gradient-recalled-echo MR image (Fig. 2.13.3) shows the signal intensity within the lunate to remain low (*arrow*). These features are diagnostic of Kienböck's disease.

Aunt Minnie's Pearls

- *On plain films, sclerosis of the lunate and negative ulnar variance are suggestive of Kienböck's disease.*
- *MR imaging is indicated in symptomatic patients with negative ulnar variance and a normal lunate on plain films.*

CASE 14

History. 18-year-old man with acute injury of the right knee

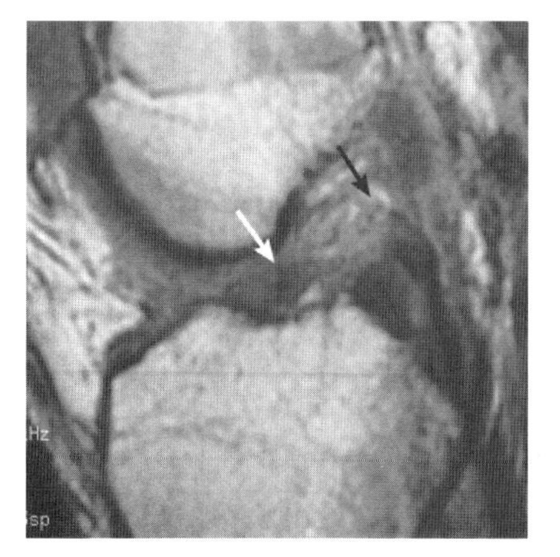

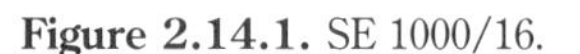

Figure 2.14.1. SE 1000/16.

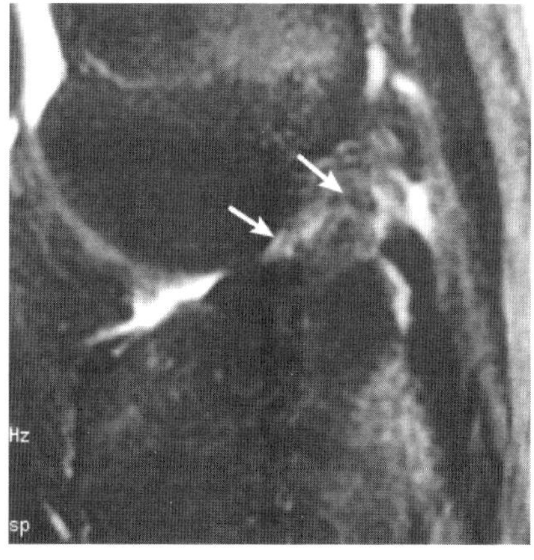

Figure 2.14.2. FSE 5500/84, ET = 8.

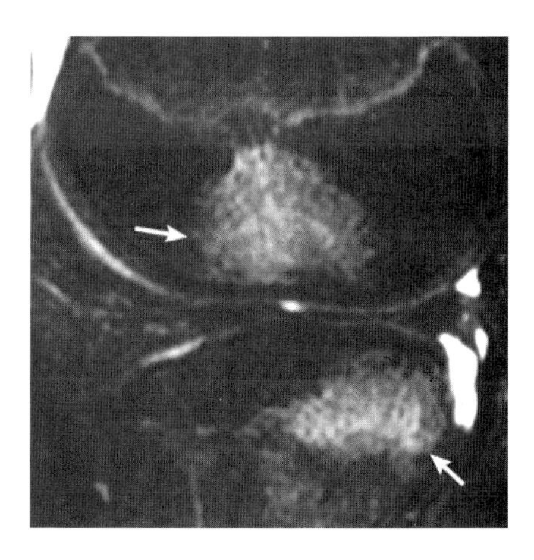

Figure 2.14.3. FSE 5500/84, ET = 8.

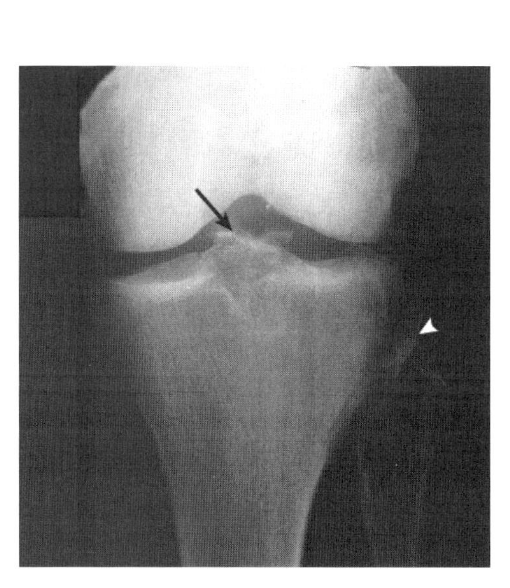

Figure 2.14.4.

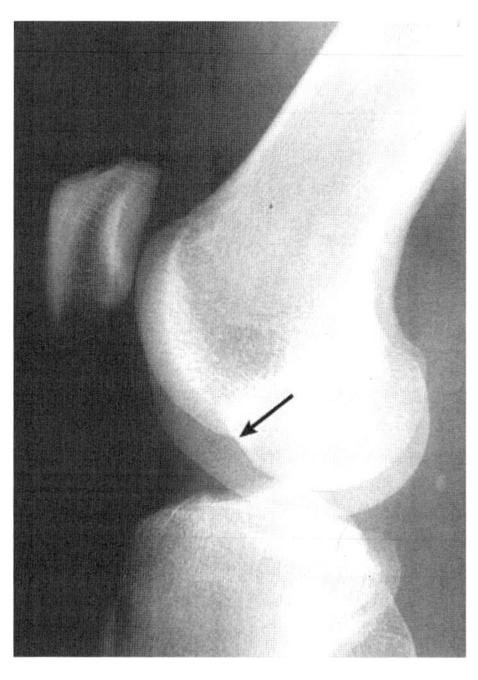

Figure 2.14.5.

Findings. Sagittal proton-density (Fig. 2.14.1) and fast spin-echo T2-weighted (Fig. 2.14.2) MR images show an area of increased signal intensity within the anterior cruciate ligament (ACL) [so-called pseudomass (*arrows*)], nonvisualization of the normal ACL fibers, and joint effusion. A sagittal T2-weighted MR image through the lateral joint compartment (Fig. 2.14.3) shows subchondral high signal intensity areas in the midportion of the lateral femoral condyle and in the posterolateral tibial plateau [so-called kissing contusions (*arrows*)]. Figures 2.14.4 and 2.14.5 are explained under "Discussion."

Diagnosis. Complete tear of the anterior cruciate ligament

Discussion. ACL injury is a frequent sequela of knee trauma and is seen in up to 70% of patients with acute traumatic hemarthroses. The classic mechanism of injury is indirect trauma from deceleration, hyperextension, or twisting forces, often accompanied by an audible pop and the rapid onset of pain, swelling, and disability. About one-third of patients with an ACL injury have other associated ligamentous disruptions.

Plain-film findings of ACL tear include avulsion fractures off either the femoral or tibial attachment of the ACL (Fig. 2.14.4, *arrow*), a Segond fracture (Fig. 2.14.4, *arrowhead*), or a deep lateral sulcus sign (Fig. 2.14.5, *arrow*). On the lateral plain film, a sulcus deeper than 1.5 mm has a high association with ACL injury (31). MR imaging features of the torn ACL are an irregular or wavy contour and a decreased slope on the sagittal images ("laying down"), increased signal intensity on proton-density and T2-weighted spin-echo sequences in the region of the ACL (pseudomass), posterior displacement of the lateral meniscus (uncovered meniscus sign), loss of the normal obtuse curvature with increased angulation of the posterior cruciate ligament, and undulation of the patellar tendon. Bone impaction forces result in medullary contusions of the posterolateral tibial plateau and midportion of the lateral femoral condyle in about 70–80% of patients up to 9 weeks after injury (32–34).

Various ACL reconstruction procedures are available, and most operations can be performed arthroscopically.

Aunt Minnie's Pearls

- *70% of acute traumatic hemarthroses have ACL injury.*
- *On plain films, a lateral femoral condyle sulcus of >1.5 mm (deep sulcus sign) is highly suggestive of ACL tear.*
- *Increased signal within the ligament, loss of slope of the ligament, and associated bone contusions are important features of ACL tears on MRI.*

CASE 15

History. 19-year-old man with worsening pain in the right knee after a recent injury

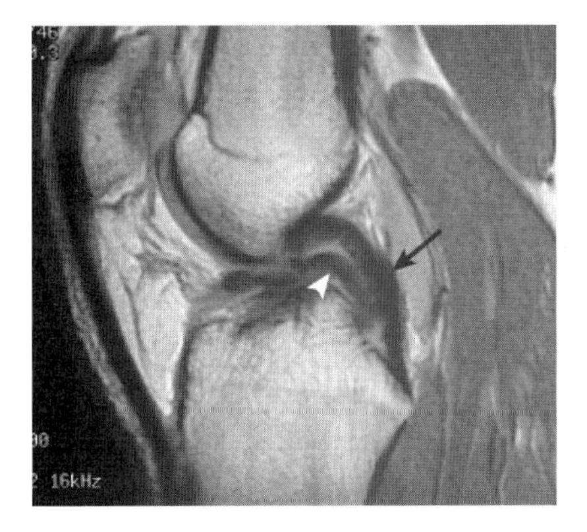

Figure 2.15.1. SE 2500/20

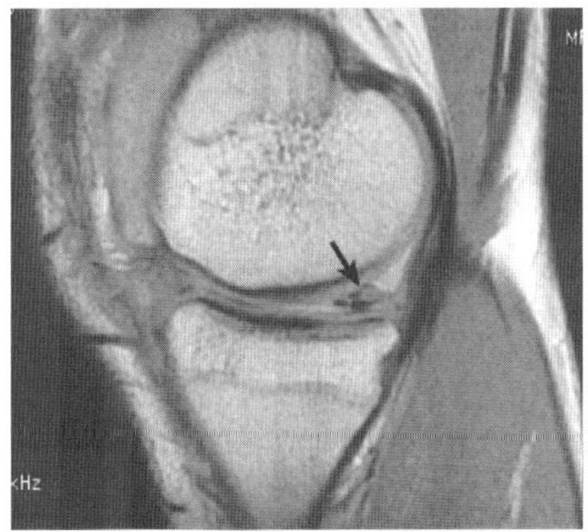

Figure 2.15.2. SE 2500/20.

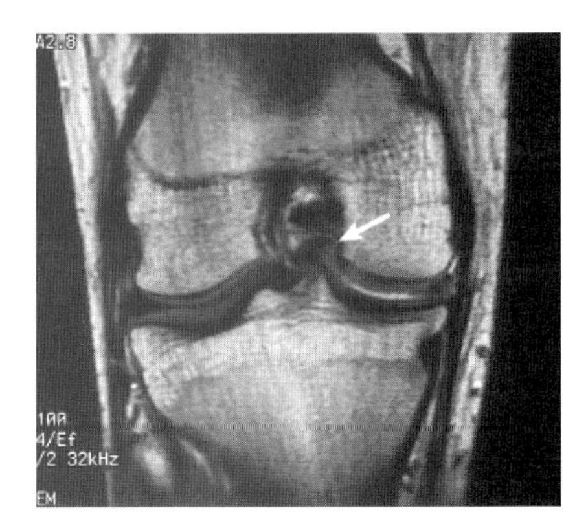

Figure 2.15.3. FSE 4100/14, ET = 8.

Findings. A sagittal proton-density MR image of the right knee (Fig. 2.15.1) shows a normal posterior cruciate ligament (PCL)[3] (*arrow*) with an apparent second PCL underneath (double PCL sign, *arrowhead*). A sagittal proton-density image through the medial meniscus (Fig. 2.15.2) shows increased signal in its posterior horn (*arrow*) and diminished visualization of the anterior horn. A corresponding coronal proton-density weighted image reveals the displaced meniscal fragment in the intercondylar notch (Fig. 2.15.3, *arrow*).

Diagnosis. Displaced bucket handle tear of the medial meniscus

Discussion. The bucket handle tear, usually caused by acute trauma, is a longitudinal meniscal rent in which the central, unstable fragment migrates into the intercondylar notch. The migrated fragment represents the handle of the bucket, and the remainder of the meniscus remains in situ and represents the bucket (35).

Many MR imaging features suggest a bucket handle tear. On 4-mm sagittal images, the medial meniscus should be seen on three consecutive MR slices. If the meniscus is not seen on all these slices, one must prove by using other imaging planes that a portion of it is not missing. The double PCL sign is produced by displacement of the meniscal fragment into the intercondylar notch and its coming to rest inferior to and in front of the PCL. Another useful sign of a bucket handle tear is the flipped meniscus sign, which is a shortened posterior horn and an abnormally tall anterior horn (≥6 mm) on sagittal images or a meniscus-shaped area of low signal just posterior to the normally shaped anterior horn (36, 37).

Aunt Minnie's Pearls

- *The double PCL sign and flipped meniscus sign on sagittal MR images are highly characteristic of a bucket handle tear*
- *The fragment seen within the intracondylar notch on coronal MR images is also typical of a bucket handle tear.*

CASE 16

History. 19-year-old man with pain in the left knee

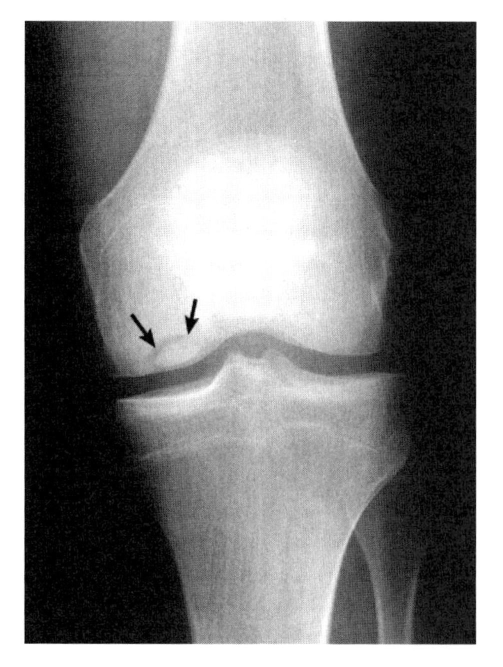

Figure 2.16.1.

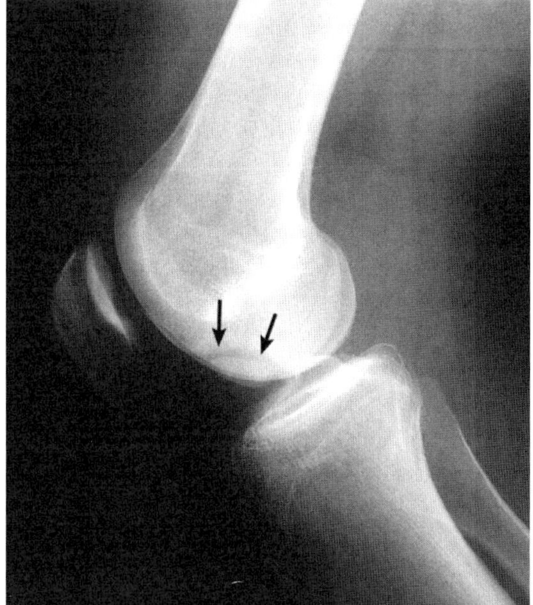

Figure 2.16.2.

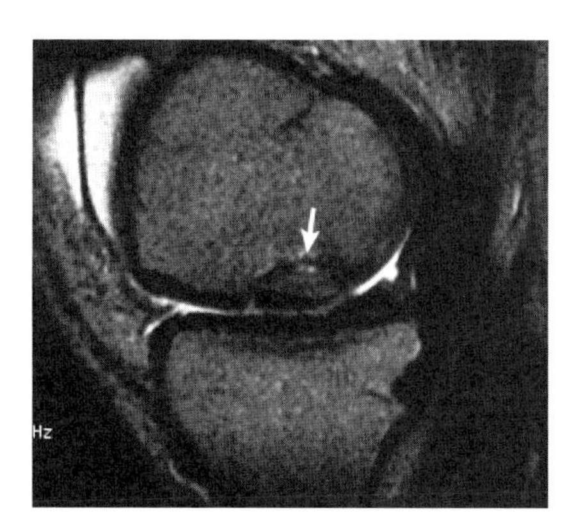

Figure 2.16.3. SE 2250/80.

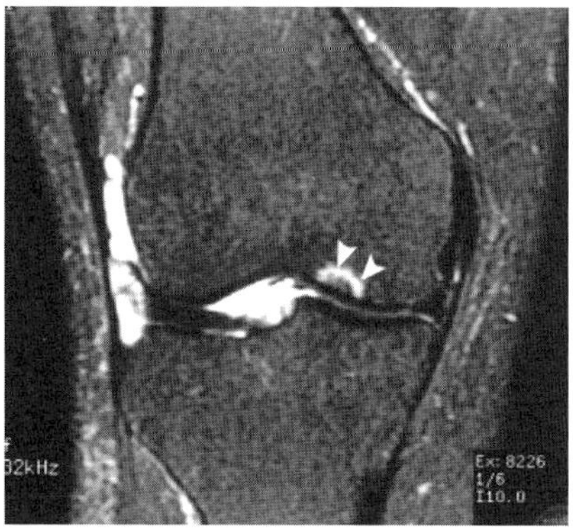

Figure 2.16.4. FSE 5500/90, ET = 8.

Findings. Anteroposterior (Fig. 2.16.1) and lateral (Fig. 2.16.2) plain films of the left knee show a semicircular region of subchondral lucency with a bony fragment adjacent to the inner aspect of the medial femoral condyle (*arrows*). An accompanying T2-weighted coronal MR image in this patient demonstrates the semicircular region with minimal increased signal between the subchondral bone and the fragment (Fig. 2.16.3, *arrow*). The fragment is low signal intensity and is not completely surrounded by cartilage.

Diagnosis. Osteochondritis (osteochondrosis) dissecans of the medial femoral condyle with a loose in situ fragment

Discussion. Osteochondritis dissecans occurs most commonly during adolescence and is believed to be a sequelae of an osteochondral fracture that was initially caused by shearing, rotatory, or tangentially aligned impaction forces. Common locations for osteochondritis dissecans include the knee (inner aspect of the medial femoral condyle), humeral head, capitellum of elbow, and talus (38). Clinically, patients may complain of pain, swelling, locking, and decreased range of motion.

MR imaging is valuable in determining the stability of fragments. The presence of high signal intensity on T2-weighted images, indicative of fluid or granulation tissue between the fragment and donor site, is strong evidence of potential instability (Fig. 2.16.4, *arrowheads*). Focal cystic areas beneath the fragment, or denuding of articular cartilage, are also strong evidence for an unstable fragment. All patients with plain-film evidence of osteochondritis dissecans should probably undergo MR imaging before surgical intervention to assess the integrity of the donor fragment (39).

Aunt Minnie's Pearls

- *The medial femoral condyle, talus, and capitellum are common sites for osteochondritis dissecans.*
- *Encircling fluid or focal cystic areas beneath the fragment on MR images usually indicate a potentially loose or unstable fragment.*

CASE 17

History. 39-year-old man with an acute knee injury

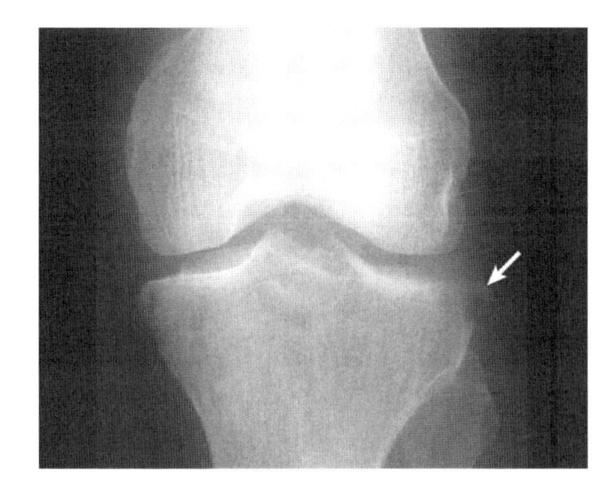

Figure 2.17.1.

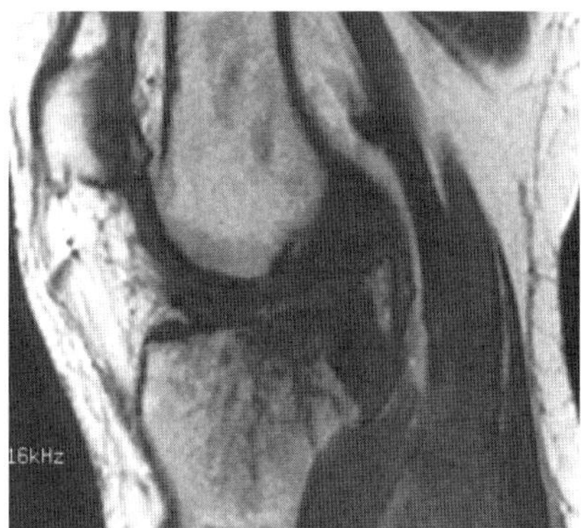

Figure 2.17.2. SE 1000/16.

Findings. Anteroposterior view of the left knee shows a corticated sliver of bone (Fig. 2.17.1, *arrow*) adjacent to the lateral aspect of the lateral tibial plateau. A nondisplaced fracture of the medial tibial plateau is also seen. A sagittal proton-density MR image of the knee in the same patient (Fig. 2.17.2) exhibits an anterior cruciate ligament tear, a nondisplaced tibial plateau fracture, and a large contusion in the tibia.

Diagnosis. Segond fracture

Discussion. The Segond fracture, an avulsion fracture of the lateral capsular ligament from its insertion site on the lateral tibial plateau, is usually caused by internal rotatory and varus forces. The avulsion occurs posteriorly and proximally to the insertion site of the iliotibial band and is therefore felt to represent an avulsion fracture of the lateral capsular ligament. The presence of a Segond fracture fragment should alert the physician to underlying anteroposterior instability of the knee because 90% of these patients have anterior cruciate ligament tears, and of these, 60% have associated meniscal tears (40). On MR images, the Segond fracture fragment itself often is not seen. However, a trabecular microfracture or bone marrow edema is seen adjacent to the avulsion fracture site in most cases (41).

Aunt Minnie's Pearls

- *An avulsion fracture of the lateral capsular ligament from the lateral tibial plateau = Segond fracture.*
- *A Segond fracture is almost always accompanied by an ACL tear.*

CASE 18

History. 80-year-old woman with back pain

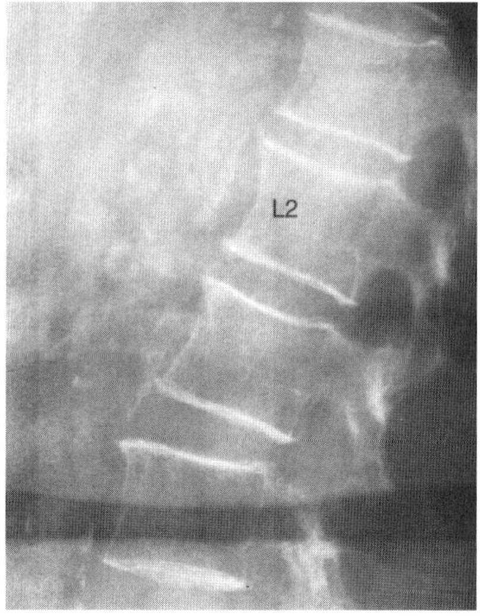

Figure 2.18.1. One year before presentation.

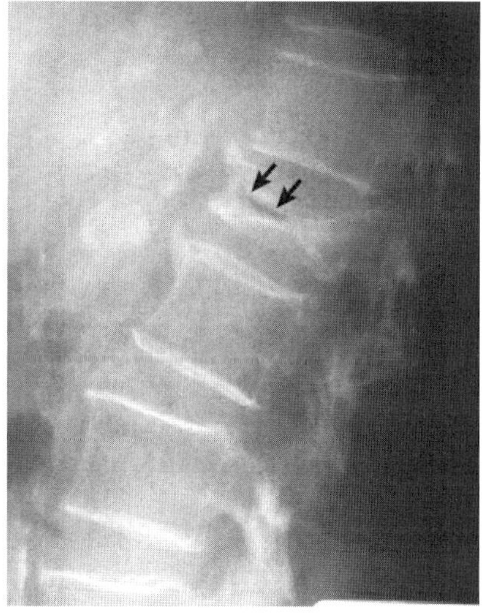

Figure 2.18.2. Presentation.

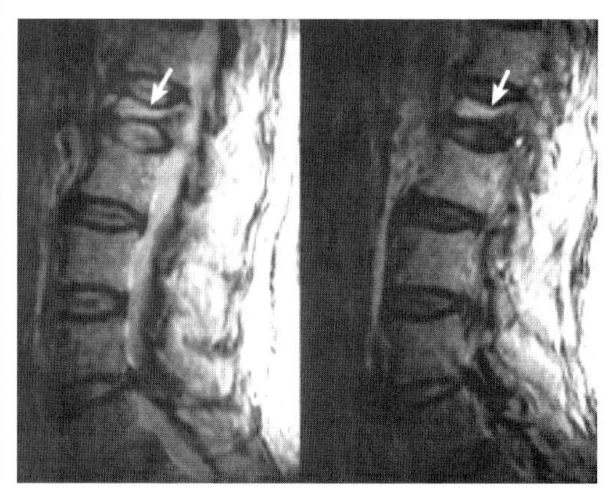

Figure 2.18.3. SE 2000/60.

Findings. A lateral view of the lumbar spine 1 year before her acute presentation shows a normal L2 vertebral body (Fig. 2.18.1). At presentation, the lateral view of the lumbar spine (Fig. 2.18.2) demonstrates marked collapse and sclerosis of the L2 vertebral body and a cleft of air (*arrows*) within the center of the vertebral body.

Diagnosis. Vertebral osteonecrosis (Calvé-Kümmel disease)

Discussion. Calvé-Kümmel's disease is a form of delayed, posttraumatic collapse of a vertebral body occurring weeks or months after an injury. The most widely accepted etiology is osteonecrosis, although traumatic, neurologic, vasomotor, or nutritional factors are other potential causes.

An association between vertebral body ischemia and the presence of gas within the vertebral body, also known as the intravertebral vacuum cleft, is characteristic. Theoretically, an episode of trauma leads to ischemia and delayed vertebral collapse. It is important to recognize the intravertebral gas because this finding effectively excludes neoplastic or infectious involvement of the vertebral body (42). Radiographically, the cleft appears as a radiolucent transverse band in the centrum of the collapsed vertebra or adjacent to one of its end plates. The cleft may increase in size with spinal extension and be inhomogeneous on CT scans. On MR images, vertebral osteonecrosis typically appears as fluid within the cleft, with high signal intensity on T2-weighted sequences (Fig. 2.18.3, *arrows*). Prolonged positioning of the patient in supine position may lead to displacement of the air cleft by fluid. When seen centrally in the vertebrae, this change appears to also be specific for osteonecrosis (43).

Aunt Minnie's Pearls

- *A cleft of air seen in the centrum of a collapsed vertebral body is diagnostic of vertebral osteonecrosis.*
- *This cleft of air effectively excludes neoplasm or infection.*

CASE 19

History. 49-year-old man and 35-year-old man with previous knee injuries

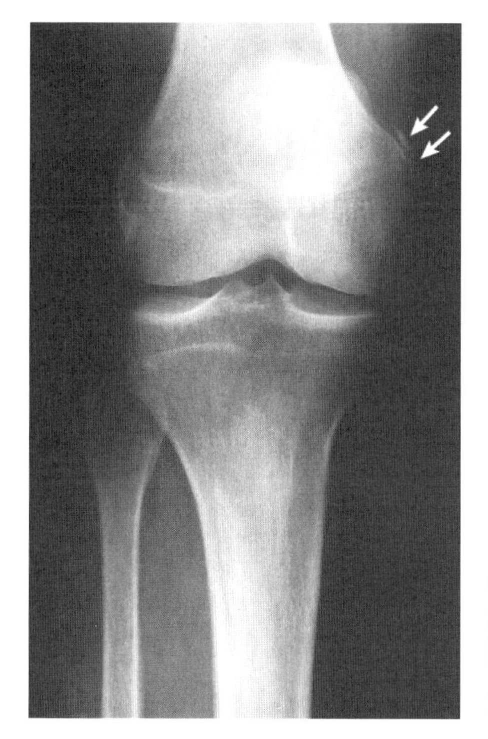

Figure 2.19.1.

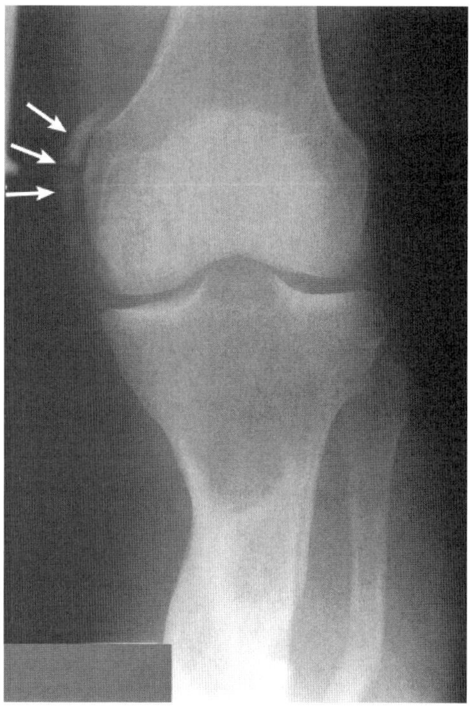

Figure 2.19.2.

Findings. In the 49-year-old, an anteroposterior view of the right knee (Fig. 2.19.1) shows an arcuate area of calcification along the superior aspect of the medial femoral condyle (*arrows*). In the 35-year-old, an anteroposterior view of the left knee shows a more prominent area of curvilinear calcification or ossification along the superior and medial aspect of the medial femoral condyle (*arrows*). Incidentally noted are healing fractures of the proximal tibia and fibula at the inferior aspect (Fig. 2.19.2).

Diagnosis. Pellegrini-Stieda disease or posttraumatic calcification of the medial collateral ligament

Discussion. Posttraumatic calcification or ossification of tendons or ligaments may be seen at various sites. When it occurs in the medial collateral ligament of the knee, this process is called Pellegrini-Stieda disease for the two individuals who first described it (44). The condition, actually a form of localized myositis ossificans, consists of deposition of heterotopic bone adjacent to the adductor tubercle of the femur but not connected to it except by fibrous tissue (i.e., it is not a chip or avulsion fracture). Patients frequently have a history of trauma or surgery in this region. Degrees of ossification or calcification vary, probably according to the severity of the original injury. Significant new local symptoms and signs may indicate a fracture of the ossified deposit (45).

Aunt Minnie's Pearls

- *Curvilinear calcification or ossification in the location of the medial collateral ligament = Pellegrini-Stieda disease.*
- *Most patients have a history of trauma or surgery to the knee.*

CASE 20

History. 54-year-old man with pain in the left shoulder

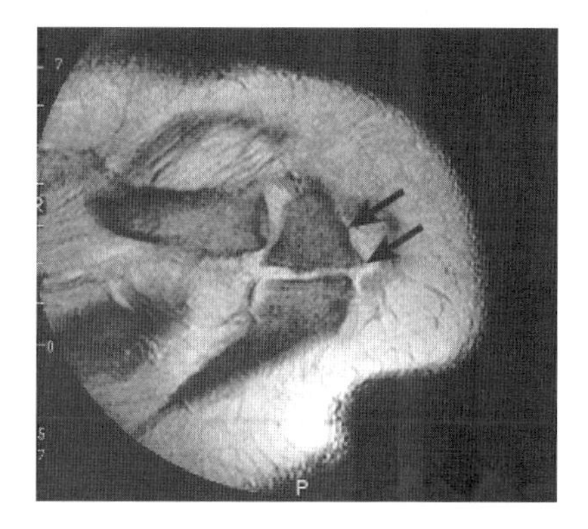

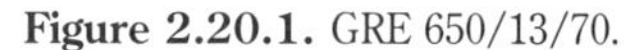

Figure 2.20.1. GRE 650/13/70.

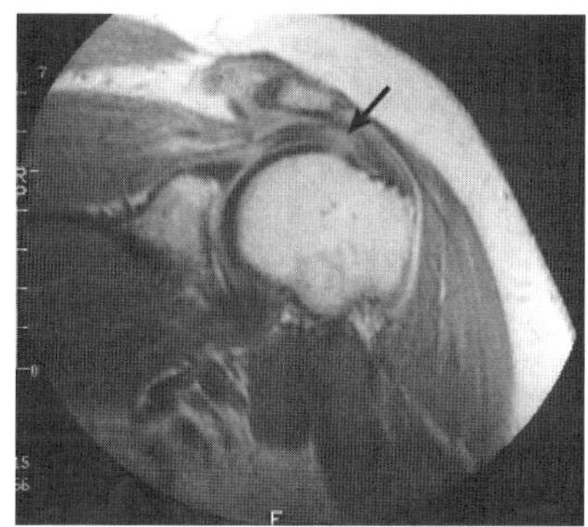

Figure 2.20.2. SE 2000/20.

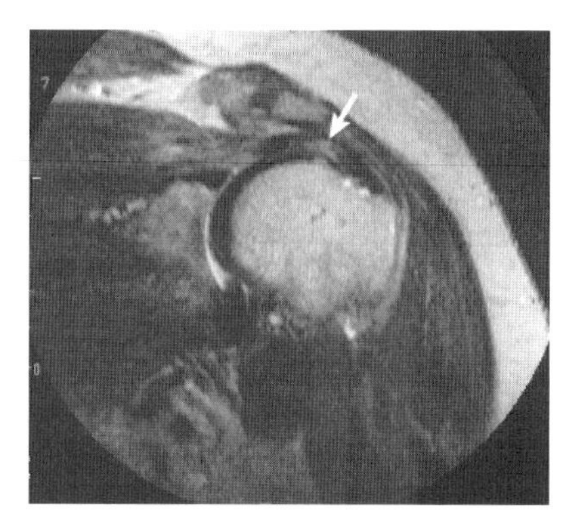

Figure 2.20.3. SE 2000/80.

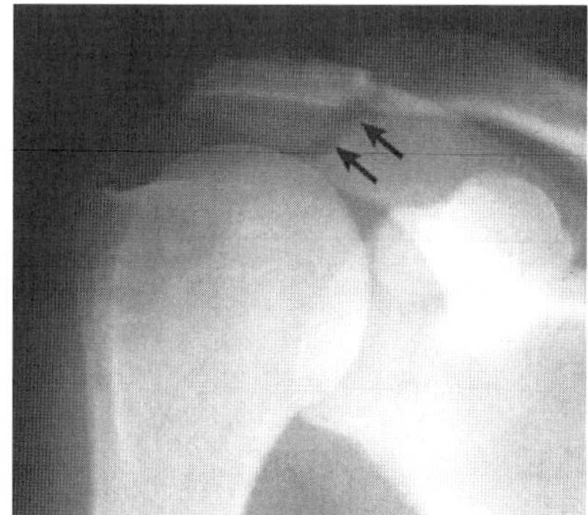

Figure 2.20.4.

Findings. An axial gradient-recalled echo image of the left shoulder (Fig. 2.20.1) shows a well-corticated triangular bony structure adjacent to the acromion (*arrows*). Proton density and T2-weighted coronal oblique images of the shoulder (Figs. 2.20.2 and 2.20.3) show hypertrophic changes that involve the acromioclavicular joint and cause impingement as well as increased signal intensity within the distal aspect of the supraspinatus tendon, indicative of tendinosis (*arrows*).

Diagnosis. Os acromiale or persistent separate ossification center for the acromion with associated supraspiratus tendon pathology

Discussion. Persistent ossification centers are normal skeletal variants that are commonly encountered. A separate site of ossification occurring at the free end of the acromion is termed an os acromiale and may normally occur in up to 15% of individuals. The os acromiale, triangular and variable in size, generally forms a synchondrosis with the acromion but may also articulate with the clavicle. This variation is important because it can cause pain, and patients with the anomaly have an increased association of impingement and rotator cuff tears (46).

The os acromiale, with its sclerotic margins, can usually be distinguished easily from an acute acromial fracture, which has no sclerosis around the fragment (Fig. 2.20.4, *arrows*).

Aunt Minnie's Pearls

- *Patients with an os acromiale are predisposed to impingement and rotator cuff tear.*
- *An os acromiale can occur in up to 15% of individuals.*

CASE 21

History. 59-year-old patient with a history of acute knee injury after falling down

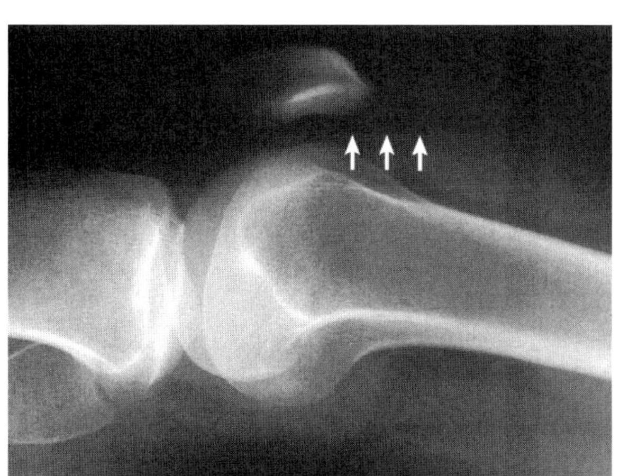

Figure 2.21.1.

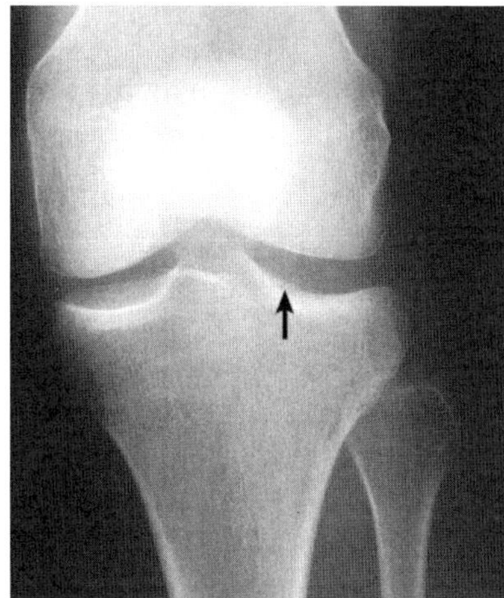

Figure 2.21.2.

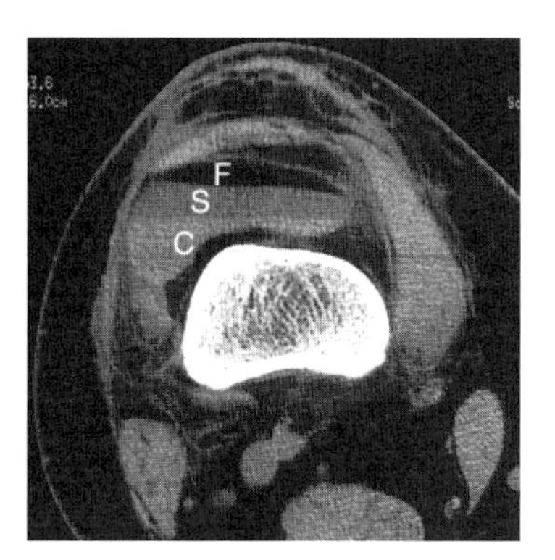

Figure 2.21.3.

Findings. A cross-table lateral view of the left knee demonstrates a fat-fluid level (Fig. 2.21.1, *arrows*) composed of radiolucent fat superiorly and comparatively radiodense blood inferiorly. Anteroposterior view of the knee joint in the same patient shows a fracture involving the lateral tibial plateau (Fig. 2.21.2, *arrow*).

Diagnosis. Lipohemarthrosis

Discussion. Lipohemarthrosis, a combination of bloody synovial effusion and fat globules, is most commonly seen after trauma to a joint and usually indicates a fracture that communicates with the joint. In the absence of fracture, hemarthrosis is likely related to significant soft tissue injury. The most common sites for lipohemarthrosis are the knee and shoulder, although other joints may be involved (47).

On plain films, the lipohemarthrosis is best demonstrated on the cross-table lateral view as a radiopaque straight line at the interface of lower density fat superiorly and the higher density fat inferiorly. On CT or MR images, three distinct layers (fat, serum, and layered red cells) may be seen (48). An axial CT image through the left knee joint (Fig. 2.21.3) demonstrates a lipohemarthrosis with multiple layers. The fat (F) lies most anteriorly, and cellular material (C) is seen posteriorly. The intermediate zone is serum (S).

Aunt Minnie's Pearls

- *Lipohemarthrosis is best demonstrated on the cross-table lateral view.*
- *Lipohemarthrosis usually indicates an intraarticular communication of an acute fracture.*

CASE 22

History. 81-year-old man who fell and injured his right shoulder and presented in the emergency room with his arm locked in an abducted position

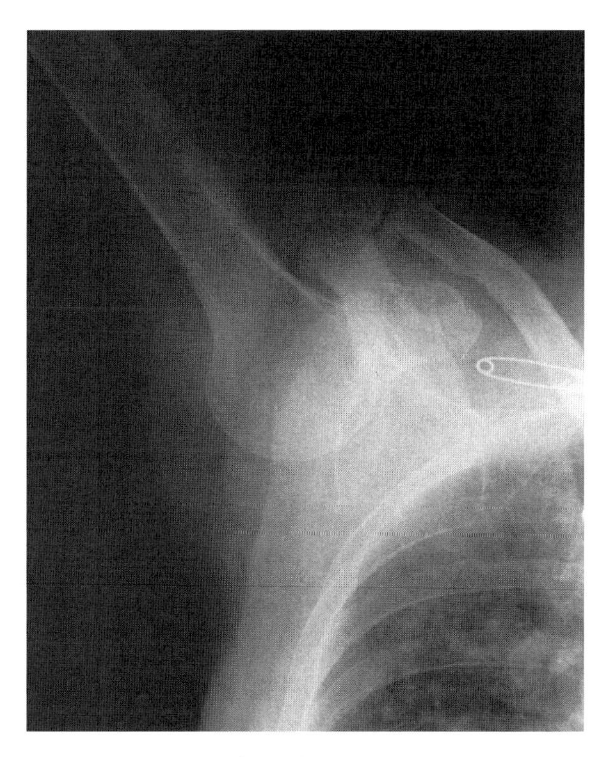

Figure 2.22.1.

Findings. The right humeral head is dislocated inferiorly at the glenohumeral joint. The superior aspect of the humeral head does not contact the inferior aspect of the glenoid rim, and the arm is held over the patient's head in a "fixed" position (Fig. 2.22.1).

Diagnosis. Luxatio erecta

Discussion. Luxatio erecta is an uncommonly encountered clinical scenario. It usually occurs when a direct, axial force is applied to a fully abducted arm or when a hyperabduction force leads to leverage of the humeral head across the acromion, resulting in inferior dislocation of the humerus. Clinically, the patient holds the arm in an elevated, immobile position over the head because the humeral head is fixed below the inferior aspect of the glenoid. With luxatio erecta, the inferior capsule is almost always torn, and fractures of the greater tuberosity, acromion, clavicle, coracoid process, and glenoid may be associated bony injuries. The most serious complications are injuries to the brachial plexus and axillary artery. Long-term sequelae of luxatio erecta include adhesive capsulitis and recurrent subluxations or dislocations (49, 50). The treatment of luxatio erecta is reduction (usually under general anesthesia) and evaluation for the associated injuries.

Aunt Minnie's Pearls

- *The patient who holds an arm in a fixed, elevated position over the head probably has luxatio erecta.*
- *Serious potential complications of luxatio erecta include injuries to the brachial plexus and axillary artery.*

Case 23

History. 65-year-old woman with insulin-dependent diabetes and recent swelling of the left foot (Fig. 2.23.1)

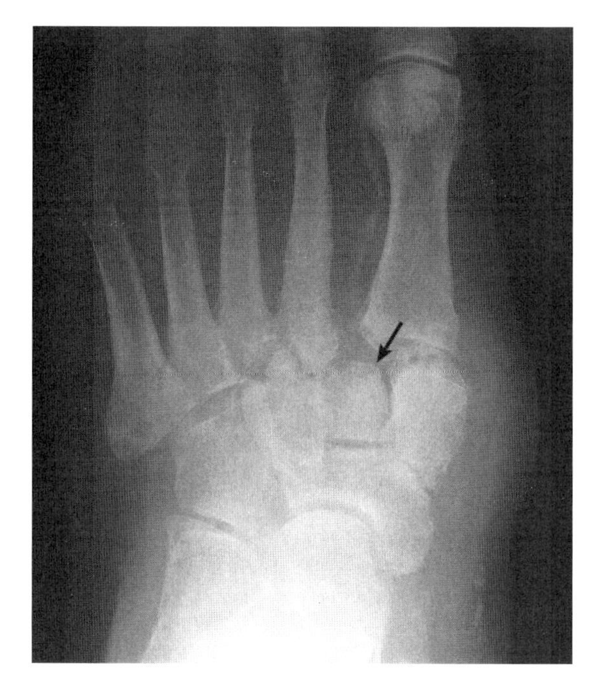

Figure 2.23.1.

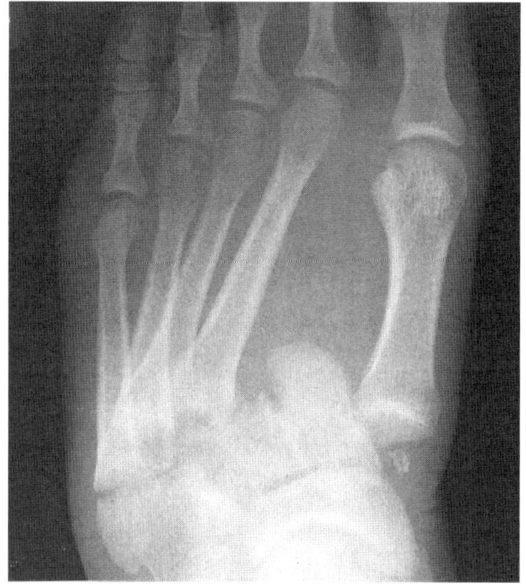

Figure 2.23.2.

Findings. Anteroposterior (Fig. 2.23.1) view of the left foot demonstrates vascular calcification, soft tissue swelling, lateral subluxation of the second through the fifth metatarsals in relation to the cuneiforms, and early destructive changes at the tarsal-metatarsal joints. Note that the medial aspect of the second cuneiform does not align with the medial aspect of the second metatarsal as it normally should (*arrow*).

Diagnosis. Diabetic with Charcot changes and homolateral type of Lisfranc fracture-dislocation of the foot

Discussion. The Lisfranc fracture-dislocation is named for Napoleon's surgeon, Lisfranc, who described an amputation procedure at the tarsometatarsal joint that now bears his name. The Lisfranc injury refers to a dorsal and lateral dislocation of the metatarsals in relation to the cuneiforms and is the most common dislocation in the foot. The injury may result from various acute traumatic mechanisms or can develop as a result of Charcot changes. There are two distinct forms of the Lisfranc complex: homolateral and divergent. In the homolateral type all metatarsals are dislocated laterally in relation to the cuneiforms (Fig. 2.23.1). In the divergent type, there is lateral displacement of the second through the fifth metatarsals and medial or dorsal shift of the first metatarsal (Fig. 2.23.2).

Diabetics develop neuropathic changes because of the peripheral loss of pain and proprioceptive sensations. The arthropathy primarily involves the tarsometatarsal (Lisfranc), intertarsal, and metatarsal-phalangeal joints of the foot. The characteristic radiographic changes include soft tissue swelling, vascular calcification, bone destruction and fragmentation, multiple fractures, and soft tissue ossific debris from the destructive changes (51, 52). Soft tissue infection also occurs, and distinguishing noninfected neuropathic changes from osteomyelitis is difficult preoperatively.

Aunt Minnie's Pearls

- *Lisfranc fracture/dislocation is commonly seen in diabetic neuropathy.*
- *Malalignment of the second cuneiform-second metatarsal relationship is the most important finding in making this diagnosis.*

CASE 24

History. 32-year-old man with sudden onset of calf pain during a tennis match

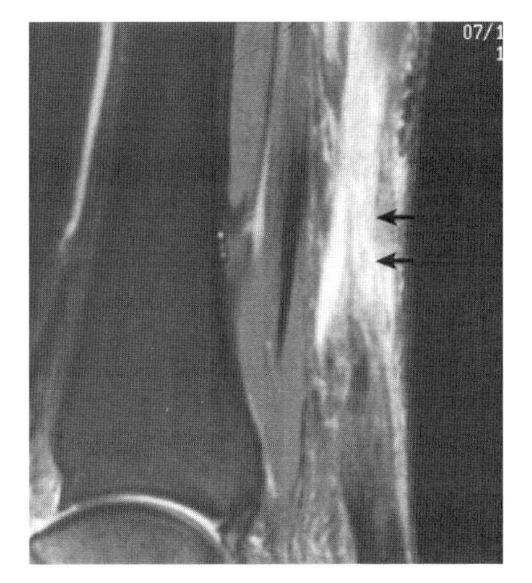

Figure 2.24.1. FSE 4100/20, ET = 8.

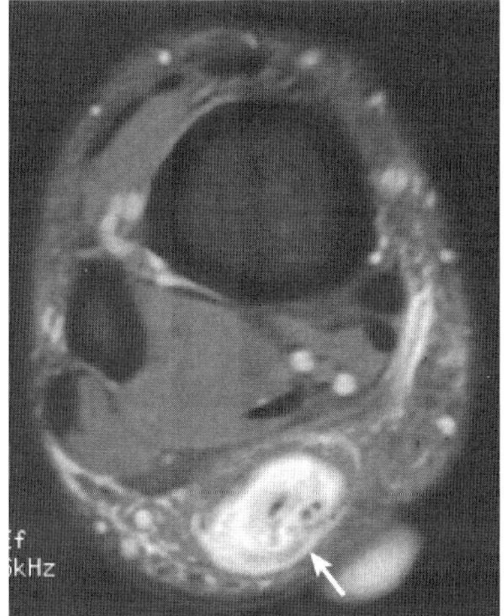

Figure 2.24.2. FSE 4100/19, ET = 8.

Findings. A sagittal proton-density MR image of the lower calf (Fig. 2.24.1) demonstrates increased signal intensity at the musculotendinous junction of an apparently disrupted Achilles tendon (*arrows*). An axial proton-density image through this area reveals a mass of increased signal intensity in the expected location of the Achilles tendon (Fig. 2.24.2, *arrow*).

Diagnosis. Complete tear of the Achilles tendon

Discussion. The Achilles tendon, formed by the confluence of the gastrocnemius and soleus tendons, is the strongest and longest tendon of the lower leg. The critical zone, the site of most acute tears, is 2–6 cm proximal to its calcaneal insertion site in an area of relative hypovascularity. The typical clinical scenario is that of a middle-aged, sedentary man who engages in strenuous activity requiring sudden or forceful dorsiflexion or push off the foot.

Plain films may support the clinical diagnosis by showing marked soft tissue swelling behind the distal tibia and ankle and obliteration of the pre-Achilles fat pad. Ultrasonography can reliably show the degree of tendon injury and has the advantage of enabling evaluation of the patient in a real-time format; however, the technique is highly observer dependent (53). MR imaging features of a partial tear of the Achilles tendon include tendon enlargement and edema, discontinuity of some of the tendon's fibers, intratendinous areas of increased signal intensity on T2-weighted or inversion recovery sequences, and surrounding soft tissue edema. Axial sections are important for estimating the degree of tendon disruption. In a complete rupture, a tendinous gap is present and is filled with high signal blood and edema (as shown in this case) (54).

Aunt Minnie's Pearls

- *Most Achilles tendon tears occur 2–6 cm proximal to its calcaneal insertion site.*
- *MR imaging and ultrasonography help assess severity of the tear.*

Case 25

History. 24-year-old woman with neck pain

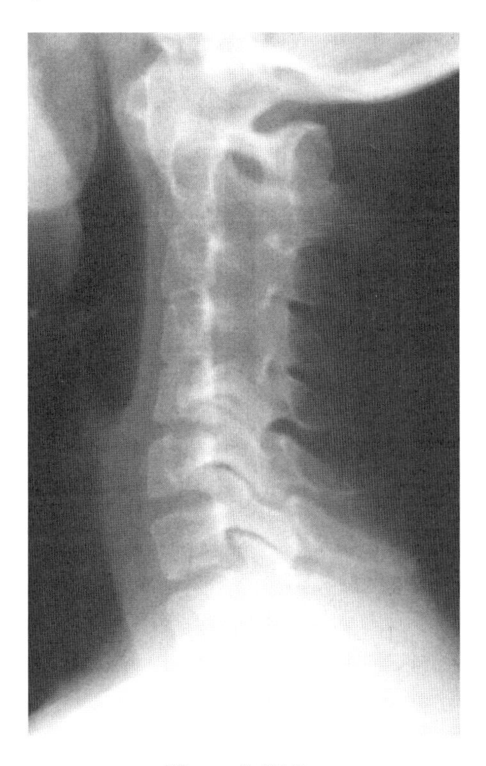

Figure 2.25.1.

Findings. Lateral view of the cervical spine (Fig. 2.25.1) shows ankylosis of the apophyseal joints of the second through fifth cervical vertebral bodies. The vertebral bodies are hypoplastic, and there is erosion of the dens, with atlantoaxial subluxation.

Diagnosis. Juvenile chronic arthritis

Discussion. Juvenile rheumatoid arthritis is best termed juvenile chronic arthritis (JCA). JCA has numerous subgroups, each with distinct clinical, laboratory, and radiographic findings. Subgroups include juvenile-onset adult type (seropositive) rheumatoid arthritis, Still's disease (systemic, polyarticular, and monarticular types), and juvenile-onset ankylosing spondylitis. Still's disease, the largest of these groups, comprises 70% of the cases. It results in systemic or articular symptoms and signs in the absence of positive serological tests for rheumatoid factor. Patients with Still's disease are usually younger than those with other types of JCA. Because articular changes in JCA occur in rapidly growing bones, the radiographic changes are quite different from those in older children.

The radiographic changes that may be seen in Still's disease include periarticular soft tissue swelling, osteopenia, which may be diffuse or juxta-articular, periostitis, overgrown epiphyses (knee, ankle, wrist), and advanced skeletal maturation leading to decreased bone length from premature fusion. Loss of articular space and erosive changes occur late in the disease. Ankylosis can also affect the small joints of the hands and spine, and when it occurs in the apophyseal joints of the cervical spine as illustrated, it is almost pathognomonic of JCA (55, 56).

Aunt Minnie's Pearls

- *Hypoplastic vertebral bodies with fusion of the apophyseal joints are characteristic of JCA.*
- *Still's disease is the largest subgroup of JCA.*

CASE 26

History. 21-year-old man with prior puncture wound to the leg

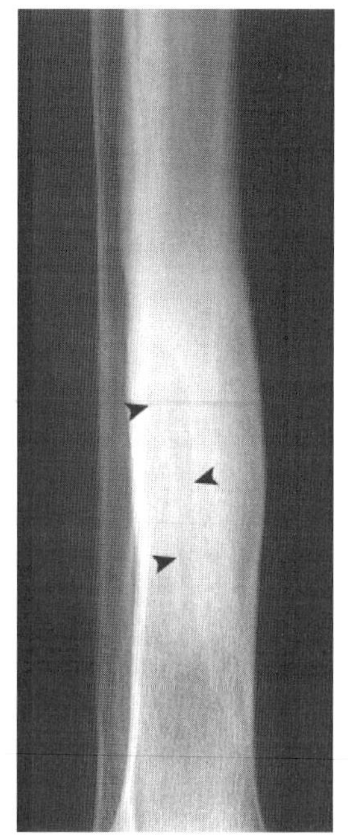

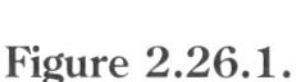

Figure 2.26.1.

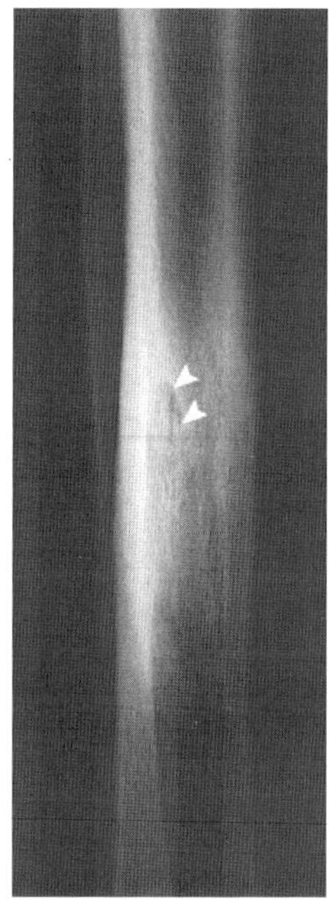

Figure 2.26.2.

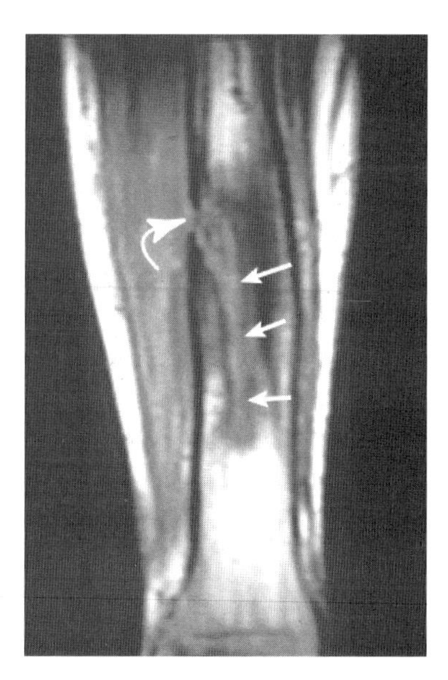

Figure 2.26.3. SE 500/20.

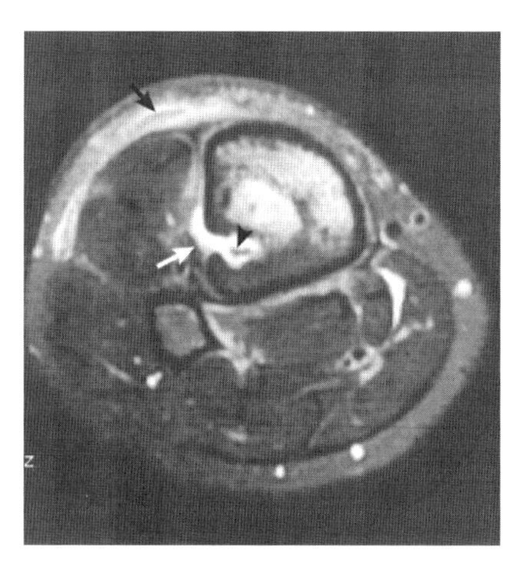

Figure 2.26.4. FSE 4000/84, ET= 8.

Findings. Plain radiographs of the right tibia (Figs. 2.26.1 and 2.26.2) show a vague linear radiolucency (*arrowheads*) within an area of sclerosis in the distal third of the tibia. A coronal T1-weighted MR image of the tibia reveals a serpiginous region of decreased marrow signal extending over several centimeters (Fig. 2.26.3, *arrows*) and a defect in the lateral tibial cortex (*curved arrow*). An axial T2-weighted MR image through the same region demonstrates a bony sequestrum (Fig. 2.26.4, *arrowhead*) and increased signal intensity (marrow edema) within the tibia. A sinus tract (cloaca) extends through the lateral aspect of the posterior tibia (*white arrow*), with edematous changes in the subcutaneous tissues, which extend to the skin surface anteriorly (*black arrow*).

Diagnosis. Chronic osteomyelitis with draining sinus tract

Discussion. Osteomyelitis may be classified as acute, subacute, or chronic. The three basic mechanisms responsible for dissemination of osteomyelitis and septic arthritis are hematogenous seeding, spread of infection from adjacent structures, and penetrating injury or surgery. *Staphylococcus aureus* is the most common organism in musculoskeletal infections. *Salmonella* is common in patients with sickle cell disease, whereas the *Serratia* and *Pseudomonas* species are associated with intravenous drug abusers.

The imaging workup of the patient with suspected osteomyelitis includes plain films, nuclear imaging, ultrasonography, or MR imaging. In acute osteomyelitis, the earliest plain-film radiographic change is obscuration of the normal fat planes as a result of soft tissue swelling. Bony changes usually do not appear until 1–2 weeks after onset of infection. The MR features of acute osteomyelitis include areas of diminished signal intensity on T1-weighted images compared with the normal high signal intensity of bone marrow. T2-weighted images usually show areas of increased signal in muscle, cortical bone, and periosteum that are not well demonstrated on the T1-weighted sequences. T1-weighted fat-suppressed gadolinium-enhanced images increase sensitivity and specificity in the diagnosis of infection (57).

Chronic osteomyelitis results from inadequately treated or untreated acute osteomyelitis. The plain-film findings of chronic osteomyelitis include prominent cortical thickening and a mixed pattern of osteosclerosis and osteolysis. Signs suggesting reactivation of infection include the development of new, ill-defined areas of osteolysis, thin, linear periostitis, or the presence of a sequestrum and draining sinus tract (58).

Nuclear medicine scanning with technetium methylene diphosphonate, gallium, and indium is used in the investigation of chronic osteomyelitis. However, MR imaging is the best imaging study to define the overall extent of the process (59). Squamous cell carcinomas may rarely form inside a longstanding sinus tract.

Aunt Minnie's Pearls

- *Chronic osteomyelitis is characterized by sequestra, a draining sinus tract, and mixed osteosclerosis and osteolysis.*
- *Staphylococcus aureus is the most common organism in this disease.*

CASE 27

History. Two 50-year-old patients who complain of joint pain

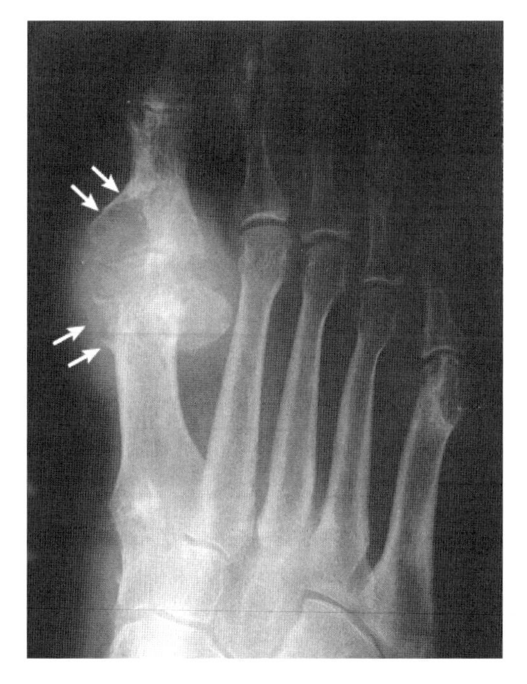

Figure 2.27.1.

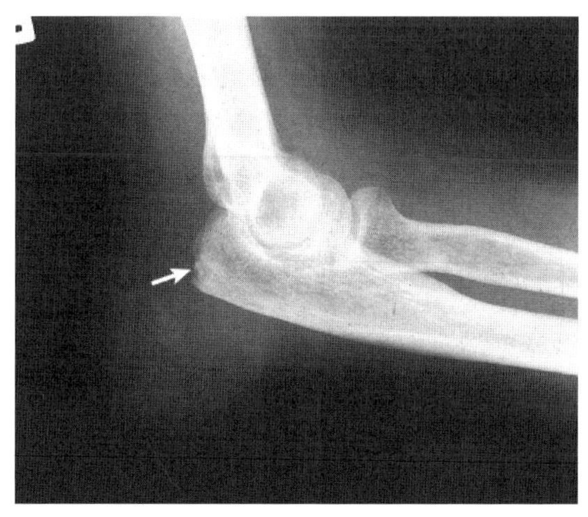

Figure 2.27.2.

Findings. Anteroposterior view of the right foot of the first patient shows soft tissue swelling, extensive periarticular erosions with sclerotic borders, and overhanging edges in the first metatarsophalangeal joint (Fig. 2.27.1, *arrows*) with preservation of the articular space. A lateral view of the right elbow in a different patient reveals marked soft tissue swelling and faint radiopacity in the region of the olecranon bursa. Minimal erosive changes are noted in the posterior surface of the olecranon (Fig. 2.27.2, *arrow*).

Diagnosis. Gouty arthritis

Discussion. Gout is the result of deposition of negatively birefringent monosodium urate crystals into synovial fluid. It has been divided into idiopathic and secondary causes. Idiopathic gout, with a male-to-female ratio of 20:1, is typically encountered in men in their fifth decade and in postmenopausal women. Gout has a predilection for joints of the lower extremities, particularly the first metatarsophalangeal joint, the intertarsal joints, the ankle, and the knee. The first metatarsal phalangeal joint is a frequent site of the initial attack and becomes involved in up to 75–90% of patients.

The radiographic changes of gout occur in about 50% of patients and develop over 6–12 years. The most common findings are punched-out erosions with sclerotic borders and overhanging cortical margins. The erosions may be intraarticular or periarticular, or they may be located some distance from the joint. Soft tissue tophi may be identified as masses (which may calcify) adjacent to the areas of bony erosion. Generally, the articular space is preserved, and periarticular osteopenia is minimal. When bursal swelling occurs, it usually affects the elbow at the olecranon (60–62).

Aunt Minnie's Pearls

- *Erosions with sclerotic borders and overhanging margins with preservation of the articular space are typical of gout.*
- *Bilateral olecranon bursitis almost always indicates gout.*

Case 28

History. 23-year-old patient with a chronic disease

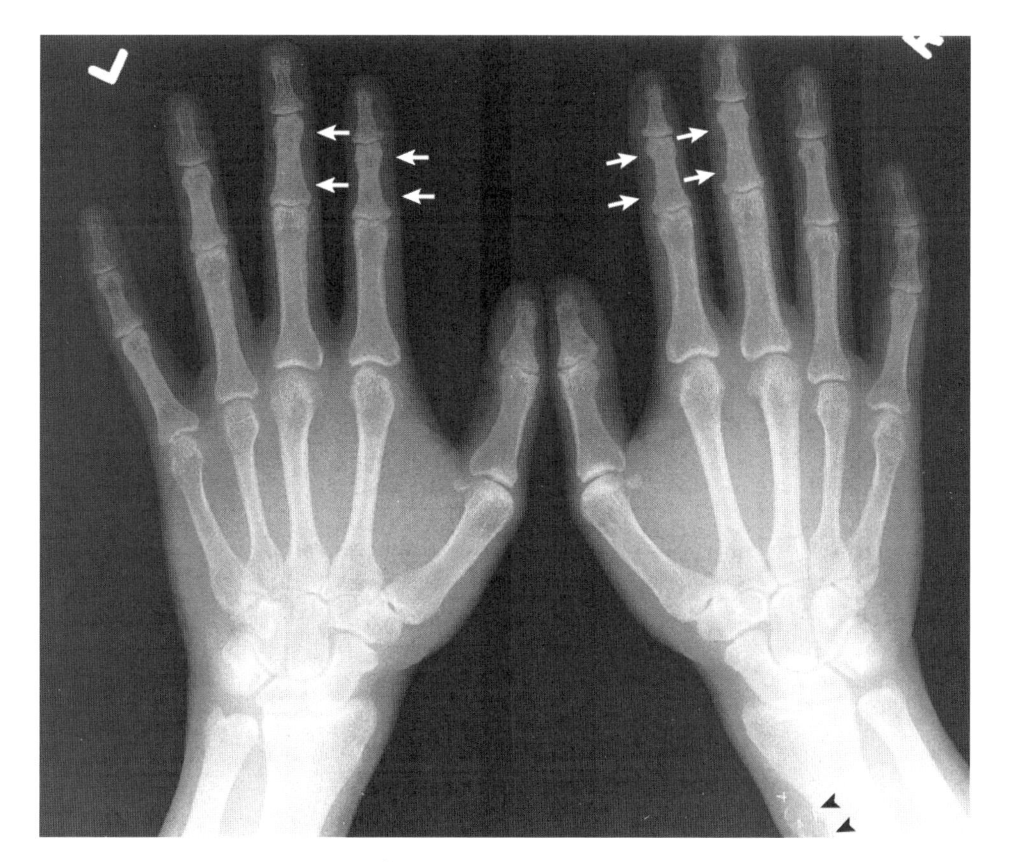

Figure 2.28.1.

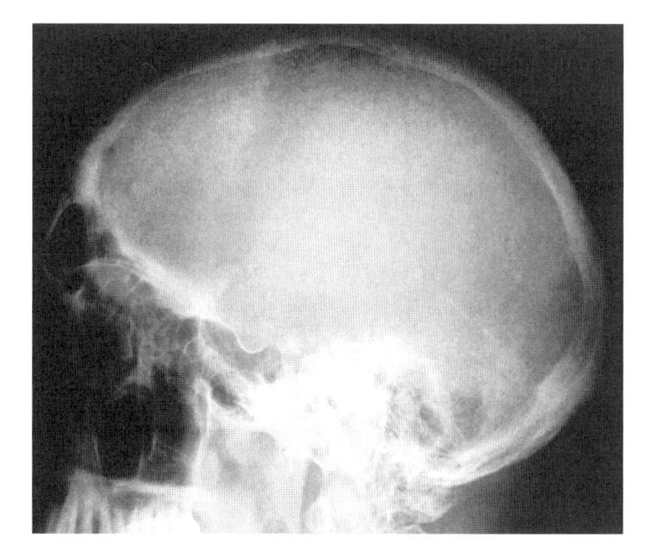

Figure 2.28.2.

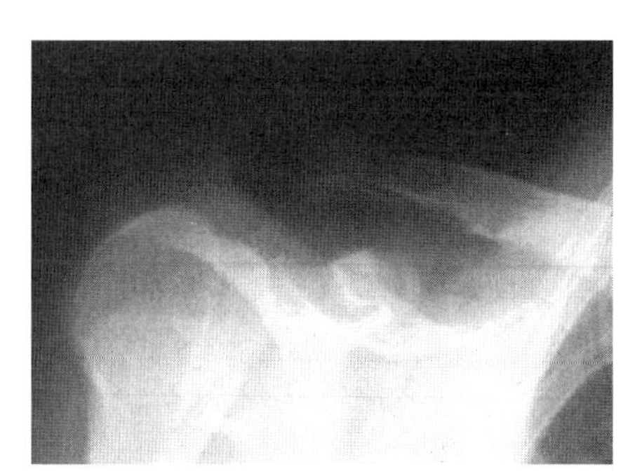

Figure 2.28.3.

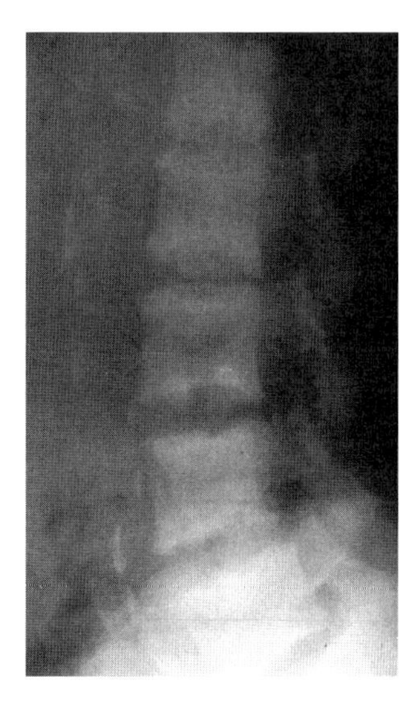

Figure 2.28.4.

Findings. Anteroposterior view of the hands of a patient with chronic renal failure shows subperiosteal resorption along the radial aspect of the middle phalanges of the index and middle fingers (Fig. 2.28.1, *arrows*). There are vascular clips from a graft at the radial aspect of the right wrist (*arrowheads*). A lateral view of the skull in the same patient (Fig. 2.28.2) shows a salt-and-pepper appearance.

Diagnosis. Secondary hyperparathyroidism

Discussion. Hyperparathyroidism is a general term referring to an increased serum level of parathyroid hormone. Primary hyperparathyroidism results from an intrinsic abnormality in the parathyroid gland (e.g., an adenoma, hyperplasia, or carcinoma). Secondary hyperparathyroidism is caused by a diffuse, adenomatous hyperplasia, whereas tertiary hyperparathyroidism develops from an autonomous parathyroid adenoma caused by the chronic overstimulation of hyperplastic glands in renal insufficiency. Hyperparathyroidism is most common in middle-aged women, and the clinical findings are generally attributable to renal, skeletal, and gastrointestinal changes (63).

There are many distinct radiographic changes of hyperparathyroidism. Bone resorption along the radial aspect of the middle phalanges is considered diagnostic of hyperparathyroidism. Although less specific for hyperparathyroidism, other sites of bone resorption include the sacroiliac joints, symphysis pubis, and distal end of the clavicle (Fig. 2.28.3). Bone softening may lead to basilar invagination, wedged vertebrae, bowing of long bones, and slipped capital femoral epiphyses. Brown tumors, lytic expansile lesions that may mimic metastases or myeloma, occur in the jaw, rib, and pelvis and are most commonly seen in primary hyperparathyroidism. Osteosclerosis, most commonly seen in secondary hyperparathyroidism, is characterized by bandlike sclerosis on the superior and inferior surfaces of the vertebral body ("rugger-jersey" spine, Fig. 2.28.4). Soft tissue calcifications can occur in the viscera, cornea, periarticular regions, and hyaline or fibrocartilage, causing chondrocalcinosis. Erosive arthritis simulating rheumatoid arthritis does rarely occur. The major complications of hyperparathyroidism include renal stones, fractures, peptic ulcers, and pancreatitis (64–66).

Aunt Minnie's Pearls

- *Subperiosteal resorption along the radial aspect of the second and third middle phalanges of the hand is diagnostic of hyperparathyroidism.*
- *Chondrocalcinosis and brown tumors are more commonly seen in primary hyperparathyroidism.*
- *Soft tissue calcifications and osteosclerosis are more commonly seen in secondary hyperparathyroidism.*

Case 29

History. 35-year-old woman with a history of a chronic disease and pain in her right thigh

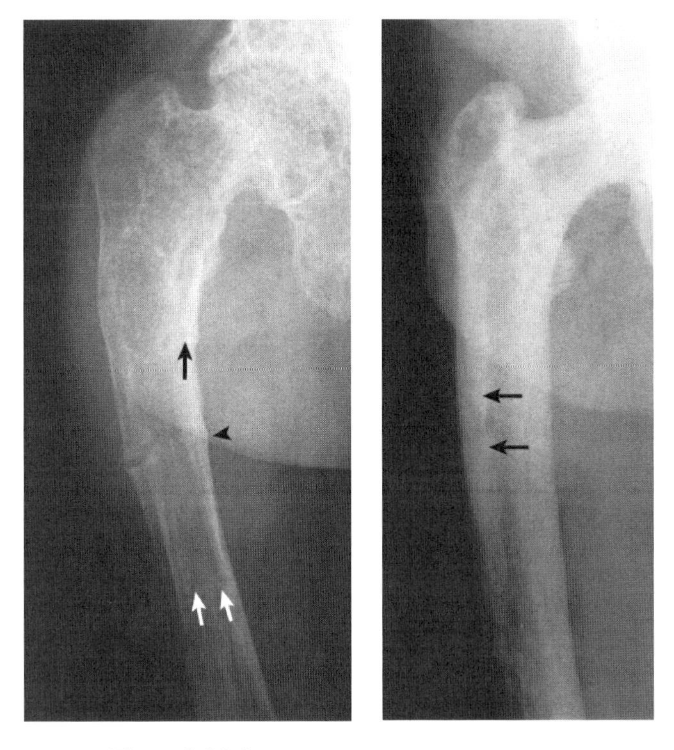

Figure 2.29.1. **Figure 2.29.2.**

Findings. Anteroposterior view of the proximal right femur demonstrates multiple lucent bands (Fig. 2.29.1, *arrows*) on the medial side oriented at right angles to the cortex. One lucency traverses the entire bone width (Fig. 2.29.1, *arrowhead*).

Diagnosis. Looser's zones (pseudofractures) of osteomalacia with a pathologic fracture

Discussion. Looser's (pronounced "Lowzer") zones, or pseudofractures, are considered to be insufficiency stress fractures occurring at sites of increased stress and are most commonly secondary to vitamin D deficiency. They are usually symmetric and bilateral, occur on the compressive (concave) surface, and are seen at characteristic sites such as the medial aspects of the proximal femora, axillary margins of the scapulae, superior and inferior pubic rami, ribs, and posterior margins of the proximal ulnae. They also may remain unchanged for long periods, and most patients have no history of trauma.

Radiographically, Looser's zones are wide, often incomplete radiolucent bands with well-defined parallel margins oriented at right angles to the cortex. The radiolucent appearance is due to the presence of unmineralized osteoid seams. Similar-appearing radiolucent bands may also be seen in bones affected by other conditions such as Paget's disease or fibrous dysplasia. However, the radiolucencies in these diseases are typically seen on the tensile (convex) surface of the bone in contrast to the compressive surface in osteomalacia. Also, Paget's disease often manifests other specific imaging features of its own (Fig. 2.29.2, *arrows*) (see Case 31).

Aunt Minnie's Pearls

- *Looser's zones are insufficiency fractures that occur on the concave (compressive) side in osteomalacia and as a lucent band perpendicular to the cortex at sites of increased stress.*
- *They tend to be bilateral and symmetric and commonly occur in the proximal femora, scapulae, and ulnae.*

CASE 30

History. Elderly man with back pain

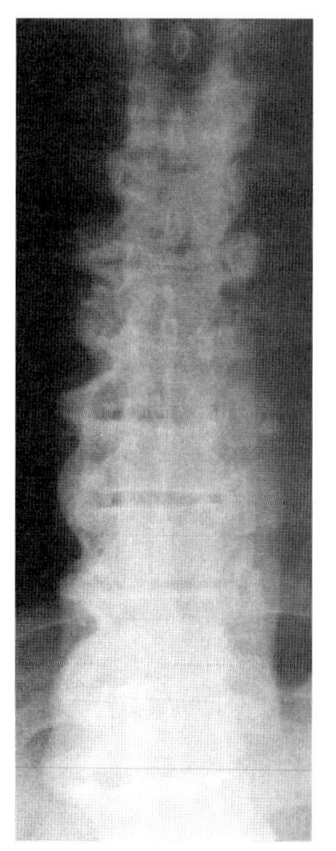

Figure 2.30.1.

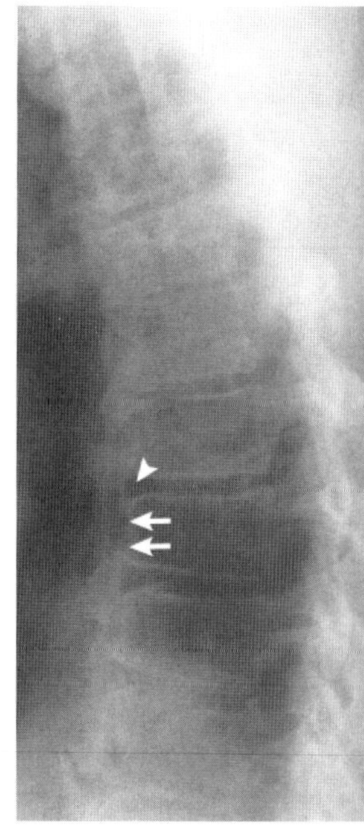

Figure 2.30.2.

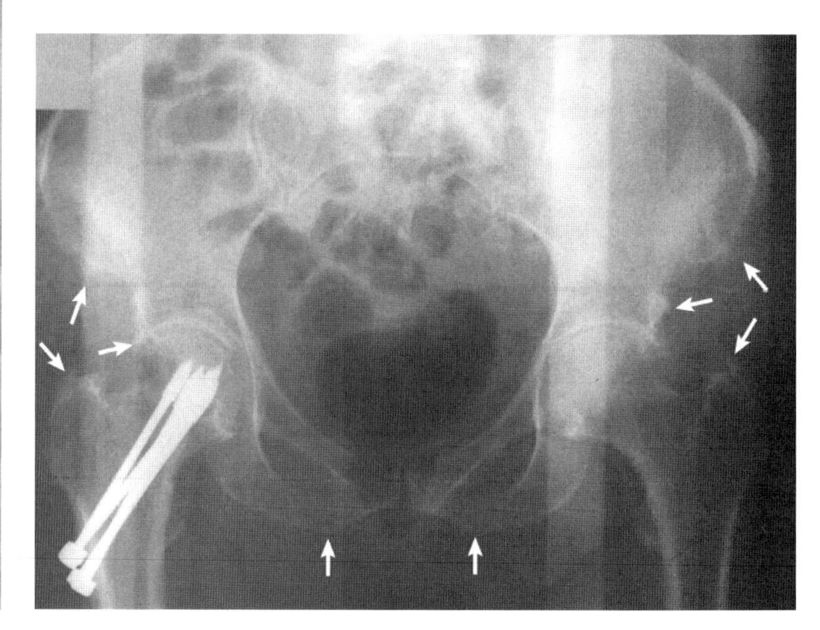

Figure 2.30.3.

Findings. Anteroposterior (Fig. 2.30.1) and lateral (Fig. 2.30.2) views of the thoracic spine show "flowing" ossification along the anterior and right lateral aspect of the thoracic spine, bridging more than four consecutive levels. The intervertebral disc spaces are reasonably well preserved, and no bony ankylosis is present. On Figure 2.30.2, lucency separates the flowing ossification from the adjacent vertebral body (*arrows*). Also, radiolucency extends from the disc space under the ossification (*arrowhead*), creating a Y-shaped lucency and a bumpy bony excrescence at the disc level.

Diagnosis. Diffuse idiopathic skeletal hyperostosis

Discussion. Diffuse idiopathic skeletal hyperostosis (DISH), or Forestier's disease, is a bone forming diathesis (enthesopathy) affecting up to 10% of the elderly population. It is not considered an arthropathy because the articular cartilage, adjacent bone marrow, and synovium are not affected. Although DISH has been called senile ankylosing spondylitis, it has no association with HLA-B27 antigen and is easily differentiated from ankylosing spondylitis radiographically by thicker, more disorganized paravertebral excrescences, lucency between the excrescences and the vertebral bodies, and no involvement of the posterior elements (67, 68).

The spine-related findings of DISH are normal mineralization, flowing ossification of at least four contiguous vertebral bodies, and preservation of disc or joint space. The most prominent features are seen in the mid-to-lower thoracic spine, although the lumbar and cervical spine may also manifest changes. Other prominent findings of DISH are ossification at tendinous and ligamentous insertions without intrinsic joint abnormalities, absence of apophyseal joint ankylosis, and sacroiliac joint erosion, sclerosis, or intraarticular osseous fusion. These latter changes are illustrated in an anteroposterior view of the pelvis in an elderly woman (Fig. 2.30.3, *arrows*). The extensive paravertebral ossification is usually seen primarily on the right side because, it is believed, pulsations of the descending aorta limit the ossification on the left.

Aunt Minnie's Pearls

- *Ossification at four contiguous vertebral body levels + preservation of the disc space + no ankylosis in an elderly patient = DISH.*
- *Paravertebral ossification is most marked on the right side.*

Case 31

History. Three elderly patients with pain

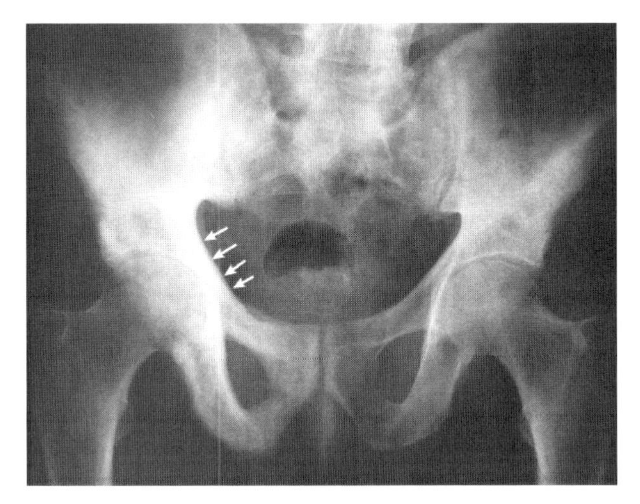

Figure 2.31.1.

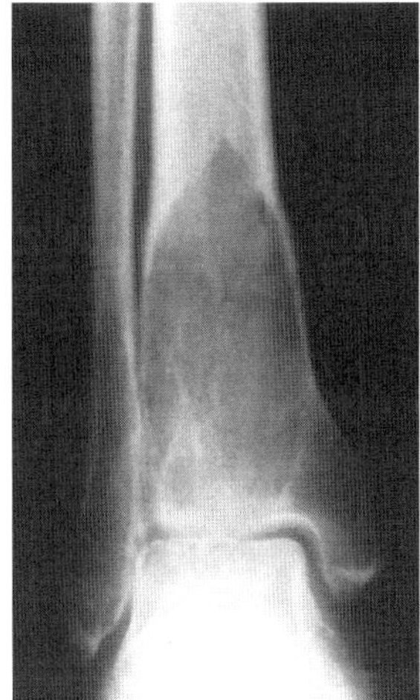

Figure 2.31.2.

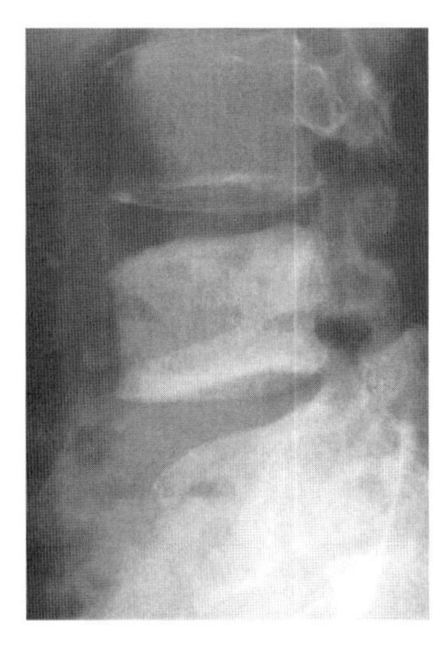

Figure 2.31.3.

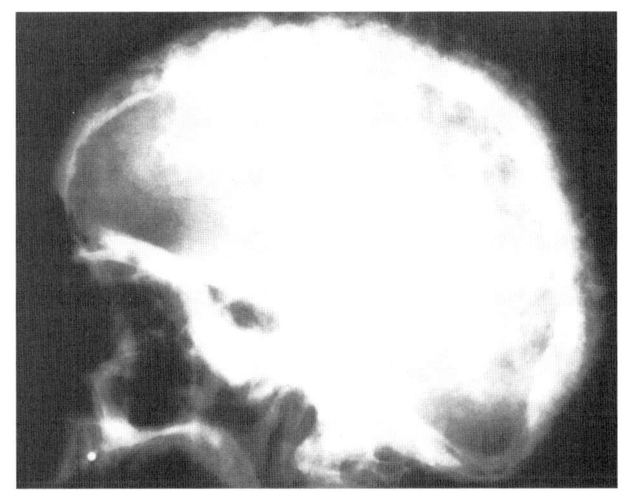

Figure 2.31.4.

Findings. Anteroposterior view of the pelvis (Fig. 2.31.1) in an elderly man shows extensive thickening of the iliopectineal line on the right (*arrows*) with coarsening of the trabecular pattern and increased sclerosis throughout the entire right hemipelvis.

Diagnosis. Paget's disease (osteitis deformans)

Discussion. Paget's disease, a condition of unknown etiology, occurs more commonly in men older than 40 years and has a higher incidence rate in temperate climates. The essential pathologic abnormality is disordered bone remodeling affecting osteoblastic and osteoclastic activity. Osseous involvement may be monostotic or polyostotic, and 80% of patients are asymptomatic. Levels of serum alkaline phosphatase and serum and urinary hydroxyproline are usually elevated. Paget's disease maybe divided into acute, intermediate, and late phases. In the acute phase, active and unbalanced osteoclastic bone resorption usually causes areas of lytic bone destruction. In the intermediate stage, increased osteoblastic activity results in thickening of the cortex, coarsening of the trabecular pattern, generalized bone overgrowth, and loss of corticomedullary differentiation. In the late, or inactive, phase there is a diffuse increase in the density of involved bone.

The characteristic, but not pathognomonic, plain-film findings in the acute phase are osteoporosis circumscripta, in which an advancing lytic area is seen in the frontal or occipital regions of the skull, and subarticular osteolysis of the skull in the diaphyses of the tubular bones, especially the tibia, yielding a flame or "blade of grass" shape (Fig. 2.31.2). In the intermediate stage there may be bowing of long bones, an "ivory" or "picture frame" vertebral body (Fig. 2.31.3), and more extensive calvarial osteosclerosis superimposed on a background of osteolysis, resulting in the "cotton wool" appearance of the skull (Fig. 2.31.4).

Potential complications of Paget's disease include spinal cord compression secondary to basilar invagination or compression fracture, cranial nerve involvement, high output cardiac failure caused by A-V shunting within pagetoid bone, protrusio acetabula, pathologic fractures of tubular bones, and premature degenerative arthritis. The most serious complication, however, is sarcomatous degeneration, usually to an osteosarcoma, in 10% of the patients. Giant cell tumor is also a well-recognized secondary lesion and has a predilection for the skull and facial bones (69, 70).

Aunt Minnie's Pearls

- *Elevated serum alkaline phosphatase and urine hydroxyproline are characteristic of Paget's disease.*
- *Characteristic, but nonspecific, plain-film patterns of Paget's disease include "blade of grass" appearance in long bones, "ivory" vertebral body, and the cotton wool or osteoporosis circumscripta appearance in the skull.*
- *Sarcomatous degeneration, usually to an osteosarcoma, can occur in up to 10% of patients.*

Case 32

History. 20-year-old woman with generalized bone pain

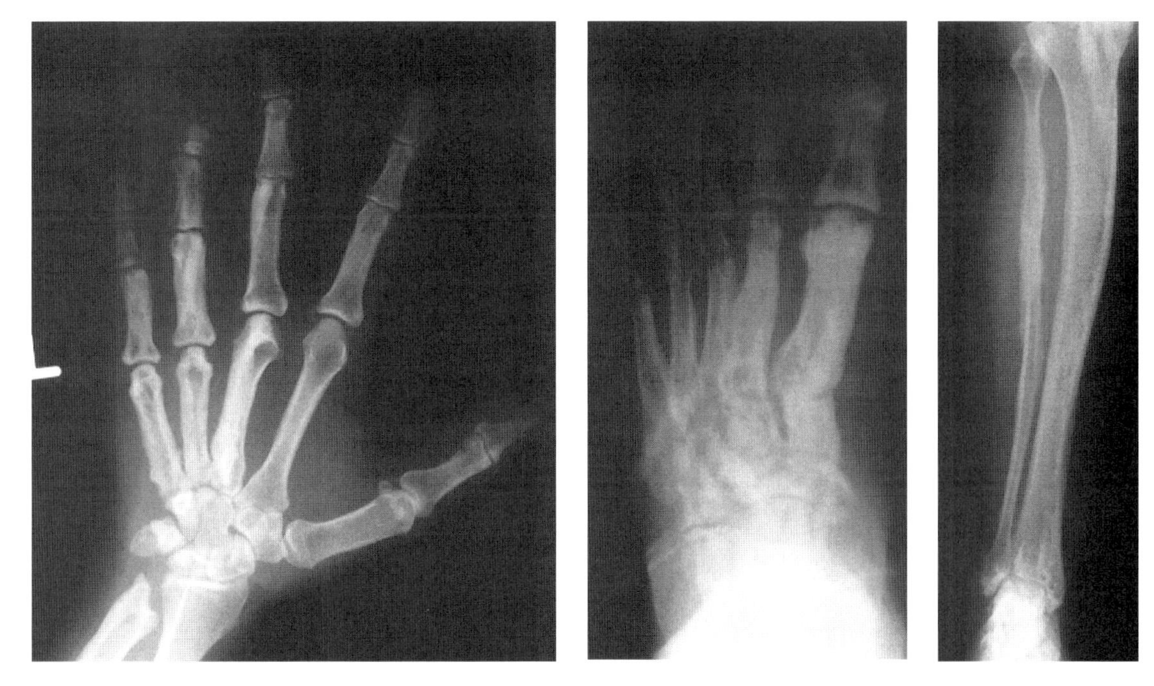

Figure 2.32.1. **Figure 2.32.2.** **Figure 2.32.3.**

Findings. Anteroposterior view of the left hand (Fig. 2.32.1) demonstrates wavy hyperostosis involving the periosteal and endosteal surfaces of the middle, ring, and little finger metacarpals as well as the phalanges in each of these fingers (along the sensory distribution of the ulnar nerve). Shortening of the ulna is also noted. Anteroposterior views of the left foot (Fig. 2.32.2) and of the right tibia and fibula (Fig. 2.32.3) demonstrate similar involvement of the bony structures of the lower extremity. Hyperostosis, deformity, and enlargement of the tarsal and metatarsal bones are most marked in the medial ray.

Diagnosis. Melorheostosis

Discussion. Melorheostosis is a rare disorder of unknown etiology that becomes apparent in early childhood. No hereditary features have been established, and men and women are equally affected. Clinical findings include pain, swelling, decreased range of motion, stiffness, and soft tissue contractures, which may become quite profound as the severity of the disease process increases. Bones of the lower extremities are most commonly involved, and the condition usually involves multiple bones in the same extremity or ray. Patterns may be monostotic, monomelic, or polyostotic, and the distribution usually corresponds to dermal sclerotomes (71).

The highly characteristic radiographic changes of melorheostosis include peripherally located (cortical) hyperostosis with osseous excrescences extending along the length of a bone that resemble wax dripping from a burning candle (Fig. 2.32.1).The wavy and sclerotic bony contour may involve only one side of the tubular bones in the upper or lower extremity and may extend distally to involve the carpus and tarsus as well as the metacarpals, metatarsals, and phalanges. The endosteal hyperostosis may obliterate the medullary cavity. Soft tissue ossification and calcification may be seen in periarticular regions (71, 72).

Aunt Minnie's Pearls

- *Wavy hyperostosis resembling candle wax drippings is characteristic of melorheostosis.*
- *The involvement is typically along spinal sensory nerve dermatomal distributions.*

REFERENCES

1. Stormont DM, Peterson HA. The relative incidence of tarsal coalition. Clin Orthop 1983;181:28–36.
2. Wechsler RJ, Karasick D, Schweitzer ME. Computed tomography of talocalcaneal coalition: imaging techniques. Skeletal Radiol 1992;21:353–358.
3. Shapiro F, Simon S, Glimcher MJ. Hereditary multiple exostosis: anthropometric, roentgenographic, and clinical aspects. J Bone Joint Surg 1979;61:815–824.
4. McAlister WH. Enchondromatosis with hemangioma. Semin Roentgenol 1973;8:230.
5. Lewis RJ, Ketcham AS. Maffucci's syndrome: functional and neoplastic significance. J Bone Joint Surg 1973;55:1465–1479.
6. McAlister WH, Herman TE. Osteochondrodysplasias, dysostoses, chromosomal aberrations, mucopolysaccharidoses, and mucolipidoses. In: Resnick D, ed. Diagnosis of bone and joint disorders, 3rd ed. Philadelphia: Saunders, 1995;6:4163–4244.
7. Hinkel CL, Beiler DD. Osteopetrosis in adults. AJR 1955;74:46–64.
8. Gristing AG, Wilson PD. Popliteal cysts in adults and children: review of 90 cases. Arch Surg 1964;88:357–363.
9. Fielding JR, Franklin PD, Kustan J. Popliteal cysts: a reassessment using magnetic resonance imaging. Skeletal Radiol 1991;20:433–435.
10. Pathria MN, Zlatkin M, Sartoris DJ, Scheible W, Resnick D. Ultrasonography of the popliteal fossa and lower extremities. Radiol Clin North Am 1988;26:77–78.
11. Reynolds J. The "fallen fragment sign" in the diagnosis of unicameral bone cysts. Radiology 1969;92:949–953.
12. Kricun ME. Imaging of bone tumors. Philadelphia: Saunders, 1993:47–188.
13. Leeson MC, Kay D, Smith BS. Intraosseous lipoma. Clin Orthop 1983;181:186–190.
14. Mohan V, Gupta SK, Cherian J, Lal S. Intraosseous lipoma of the calcaneum. J Postgrad Med 1981;27:127–128.
15. Resnick D, Kyriakos M, Greenway GD. Tumors and tumor-like lesions of bone: radiographic principles. In: Resnick D, ed. Diagnosis of bone and joint disorders, 3rd ed. Philadelphia: Saunders, 1995;6:3628–3938.
16. Caffey J. On fibrous defects in cortical walls of growing tubular bones: their radiologic appearance, structure, prevalence, natural course, and diagnostic significance. Adv Pediatr 1955;7:13–51.
17. Helms SC. Fundamentals of skeletal radiology, 2nd ed. Philadelphia: Saunders, 1995;7–33.
18. Klein MH, Shenkman S. Osteoid osteoma: radiologic and pathologic correlation. Skeletal Radiol 1992;21:23–31.
19. Kransdorf MJ, Stull MA, Gilkey FW, Moser RP Jr. Osteoid osteoma. RadioGraphics 1991;11:671–696.
20. Kindblom LG, Gunterburg B. Pigmented villonodular synovitis involving bone. J Bone Joint Surg 1978;60:830–832.
21. Breimer CW, Freiberger RH. Bone lesions associated with villonodular synovitis. AJR 1958;79:618–629.
22. Scott PM. Bone lesions in pigmented villonodular synovitis. J Bone Joint Surg 1968;50:306–311.
23. Bankart ASB. The pathology and treatment of recurrent dislocation of the shoulder joint. Br J Surg 1938;26:23–29.
24. Shuman WP, Kilcoyne RF, Matsen FA, Rogers JV, Mack LA. Double contrast computed tomography of the glenoid labrum. AJR 1983;141:581–584.
25. Roels J, Martens M, Muller JC, Barssens A. Patellar tendinitis (jumper's knee). Am J Sports Med 1978;6:362–368.
26. Blazina ME, Kerlan RK, Jobe FW, Carter VS, Carlson GJ. Jumper's knee. Orthop Clin North Am 1973;4:665–675.
27. El-Khoury GY, Wira RL, Berbaum KS, Pope TL Jr, Monu JU. MR imaging of patellar tendinitis. Radiology 1992;184:849–854.
28. Cave EF. Kienböck's disease of the lunate. J Bone Joint Surg 1939;21:858.
29. Simmons EH, Dommisse I. The pathogenesis and treatment of Kienböck's disease. Clin Orthop 1974;105:300 (abstract).
30. Gelberman RH, Salamon PB, Jurist JM, Posh JL. Ulnar variance in Kienböck's disease. J Bone Joint Surg Am 1975;57:674–676.
31. Cobby MJ, Schweitzer ME, Resnick D. The deep lateral femoral notch sign: an indirect sign of a torn anterior cruciate ligament. Radiology 1992;184:855–858.
32. Tung GA, Davis LM, Wiggins ME, Fadale PD. Tears of the anterior cruciate ligament; primary and secondary signs at MR imaging. Radiology 1993;188:661–667.
33. Remer EM, Fitzgerald SW, Friedman H, Rogers LF, Hendrix RW, Shafer MF. Anterior cruciate ligament injury: MR imaging diagnosis and patterns of injury. RadioGraphics 1992;12:901–915.
34. Chan WP, Peterfy C, Fritz RC, Genant HK. MR diagnosis of complete tears of the anterior cruciate ligament of the knee: importance of anterior subluxation of the tibia. AJR 1994;162:355–360.
35. De Smet AA, Tuite MJ, Norris MA, Swan JS. MR diagnosis of meniscal tears: analysis of causes of errors. AJR 1994;163:1419–1423.
36. Wright DH, De Smet AA, Norris M. Bucket-handle tears of the medial and lateral menisci of the knee: value of MR imaging in detecting displaced fragments. AJR 1995;165:621–625.
37. Haramati N, Staron RB, Rubin S, Shreck EH, Feldman F, Kiesman H. The flipped meniscus sign. Skeletal Radiol 1993;22:600–601.
38. Clanton TO, DeLee JC. Osteochondritis dissecans. History, pathophysiology and current treatment concepts. Clin Orthop 1982;167:50–64.
39. De Smet AA, Fisher DR, Graf BK, Lange RH. Osteochondritis dissecans of the knee: value of MR imaging in determining lesion stability and the presence of articular cartilage defects. AJR 1990;155:549–553.
40. Resnick D. Internal derangements of joints. In: Resnick D, ed. Diagnosis of bone and joint disorders, 3rd ed. Philadelphia: Saunders, 1995;5:2899–3228.

41. Weber WN, Neumann CH, Barakos JA, Steinbach LS, Genant HK. Lateral tibial rim (Segond) fractures: MR imaging characteristics. Radiology 1991;180:731–734.
42. Brower AC, Downey EF Jr. Kümmell disease: report of a case with serial radiographs. Radiology 1981;141:363–364.
43. Malghem J, Maldague B, Labaisse MA, et al. Intravertebral vacuum cleft: changes in content after supine positioning. Radiology 1993;187:483–487.
44. Nachlas IW, Olpp JL. Paraarticular calcification (Pellegrini-Stieda) in afflictions of the knee. Surg Gynecol Obstet 1945;81:206.
45. Norman A, Dorfman HA. Juxtacortical circumscribed myositis ossificans: evolution and radiographic features. AJR 1970;96:301–306.
46. Edelson JG, Zuckerman J, Hershkovitz I. Os acromiale: anatomy and surgical implications. J Bone Joint Surg Br 1993;75:551–555.
47. Arger PH, Oberkircher PE, Miller WT. Lipohemarthrosis. AJR 1974;121:97–100.
48. Kier R, McCarthy SM. Lipohemarthrosis of the knee: MR imaging. J Comput Assist Tomogr 1990;14:395–396.
49. Zimmers T. Luxatio erecta: an uncommon shoulder dislocation. Ann Emerg Med 1983;12:716–717.
50. Freundlich BD. Luxatio erecta. J Trauma 1983;12:434–436.
51. El-Khoury GY, Kathol MH. Neuropathic fractures in patients with diabetes mellitus. Radiology 1980;134:313–316.
52. Lesko P, Maurer RC. Talonavicular dislocations and midfoot arthropathy in neuropathic diabetic feet. Natural course and principles of treatment. Clin Orthop 1989;240:226–231.
53. Martinoli C, Derchi LE, Patroino C, Bertolotto M, Silvestri E. Analysis of echotexture of tendons with US. Radiology 1993;186:839–843.
54. Keene JS, Lash EG, Fisher DR, DeSmet AA. Magnetic resonance imaging of Achilles tendon ruptures. Am J Sports Med 1989;17:333–337.
55. Brower AC. Arthritis in black and white. Philadelphia: Saunders, 1988:317–329.
56. Forrester DM, Brown JC. The radiology of joint disease, 3rd ed. Philadelphia: Saunders, 1987;407–506.
57. Resnick D, Niwayama G. Osteomyelitis, septic arthritis and soft tissue infection: mechanisms and situations. In: Resnick D, ed. Diagnosis of bone and joint disorders, 3rd ed. Philadelphia: Saunders, 1995:2325–2418.
58. Mason MD, Zlatkin MB, Esterhai JL, et al. Chronic complicated osteomyelitis of the lower extremity: evaluation with MR imaging. Radiology 1989;173:355–359.
59. Morrison WD, Schweitzer ME, Bock GW, Mitchell DG, Hume EL, Pathria MN, Resnick D. Diagnosis of osteomyelitis. Utility of fat-suppressed contrast-enhanced MR imaging. Radiology 1993;189:251–257.
60. Rodman GP. Early theories concerning etiology and pathogenesis of the gout. Arthritis Rheum 1965;8:599–609.
61. Martel W. The overhanging margin of bone: a roentgenologic manifestation of gout. Radiology 1968;91:755–756.
62. Brower AC. Arthritis in black and white. Philadelphia: Saunders, 1988;257–270.
63. Gleason DC, Potchen EJ. The diagnosis of hyperparathyroidism. Radiol Clin North Am 1967;5:277–287.
64. Resnick DL. Erosive arthritis of the hand and wrist in hyperparathyroidism. Radiology 1974;110:263–269.
65. Parfitt AM. Renal osteodystrophy. Orthop Clin North Am 1972;3:681–698.
66. Murphey MD, Sartoris DJ, Quale JL, Patria MN, Martin NL. Musculoskeletal manifestations of chronic renal insufficiency. RadioGraphics 1993;13:357–379.
67. Brower AC. Arthritis in black and white. Philadelphia: Saunders, 1988:243–256.
68. Sartoris DJ. Musculoskeletal imaging: the requisites. St. Louis: Mosby, 1996:121.
69. Edeiken J, DePalma AF, Hodes PJ. Paget's disease: osteitis deformans. Clin Orthop 1966;46:141–153.
70. Resnick D, Niwayama G. Paget's disease. In: Resnick D, ed. Diagnosis of bone and joint disorders, 3rd ed. Philadelphia: Saunders, 1995;4:1923–1968.
71. Campbell CJ, Papademetriou T, Bonfiglio M. Melorheostosis: a report of the clinical, roentgenographic, and pathological findings in 14 cases. J Bone Joint Surg Am 1968;50:1281–1304.
72. Taybi H, Lachman RS. Radiology of syndromes, metabolic disorders and skeletal dysplasias, 3rd ed. Chicago: Year Book, 1990.

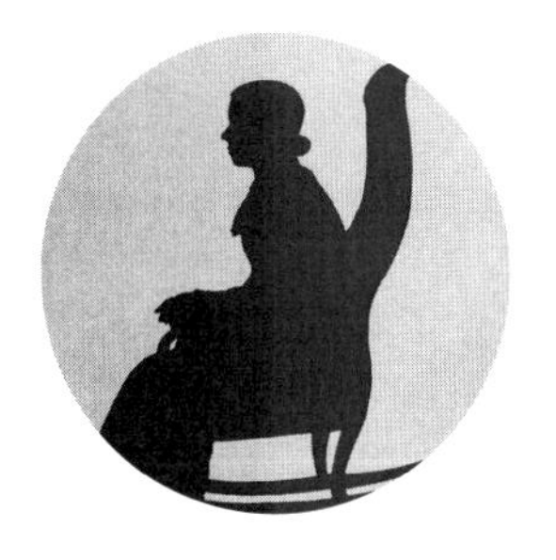

chapter 3

CARDIOVASCULAR AND INTERVENTIONAL RADIOLOGY

WILLIAM D. ROUTH, KENNETH L. FORD III,
AND FERNANDO GUTIERREZ

CASE 1

History. Sudden onset of pain radiating to the back

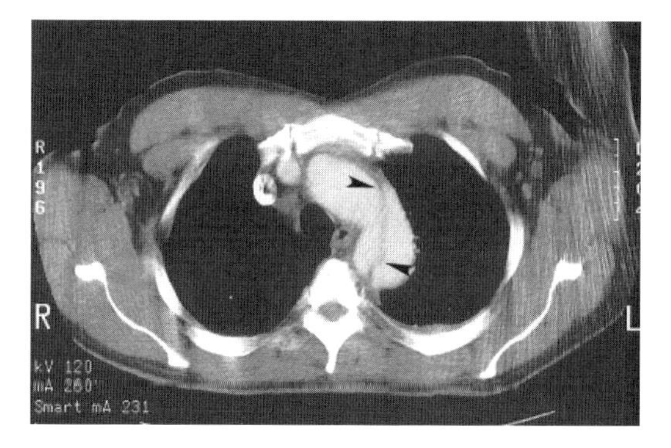

Figure 3.1.1.

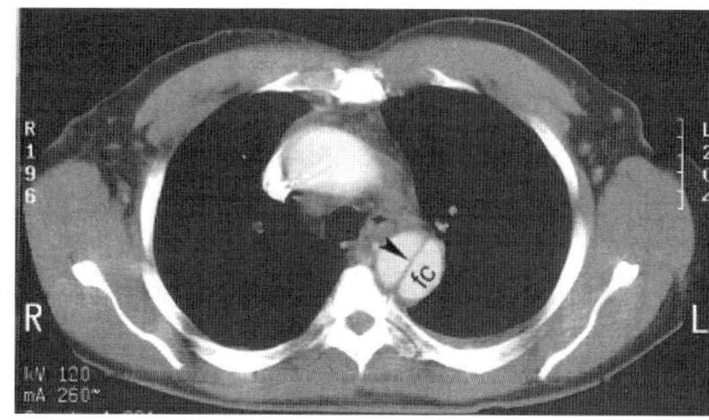

Figure 3.1.2.

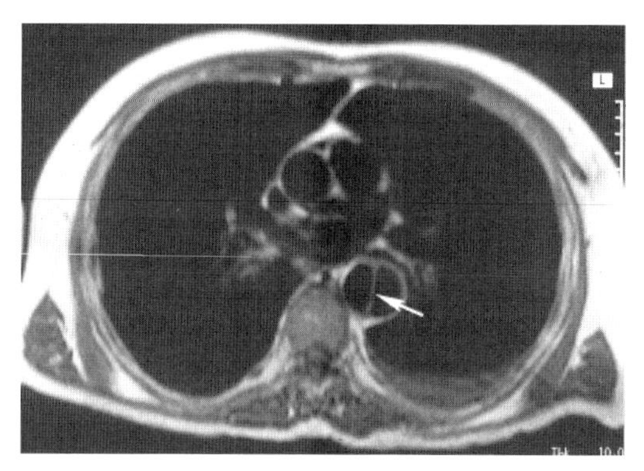

Figure 3.1.3. SE 537/30.

Findings. Axial contrast-enhanced CT images through the chest reveal an intimal flap within the aortic lumen that originates near the left subclavian artery (Fig. 3.1.1, *arrowheads*) and extends inferiorly down the thoracic aorta (Fig. 3.1.2, *arrowhead*). The larger, false channel (fc) is located in the posterolateral descending aorta. The ascending aorta is normal. No active extravasation of contrast material from the aorta is identified. In a different patient with the same abnormality, an axial ECG-gated T1-weighted MR image also demonstrates an intimal flap (Fig. 3.1.3, *arrow*).

Diagnosis. Aortic dissection (DeBakey type III or Stanford type B)

Discussion. Dissection of the aorta occurs when a pathologic communication develops between the true aortic lumen and the aortic wall. The most common predisposing factor to the development of aortic dissection is hypertension (1). Other predisposing factors include Marfan and Ehlers-Danlos syndromes, pregnancy, trauma, aortic valve disease, and coronary artery bypass surgery (2). Dissections that involve the ascending aorta (DeBakey types I and II and Stanford type A) may lead to rapid death because of rupture into the pericardium, acute valvular insufficiency, or coronary artery occlusion (3). Therefore, these types of dissections are managed with emergent surgery (4). Dissections that involve only the descending aorta distal to the left subclavian artery (DeBakey type III or Stanford type B) are usually managed medically by control of the patient's hypertension.

Aunt Minnie's Pearls

- *Emergent surgery is required for Stanford type A dissections.*
- *Always check for aortic rupture and branch vessel involvement.*
- *If dissection involves the ascending aorta, look for pericardial hematoma.*

CASE 2

History. Cyanosis

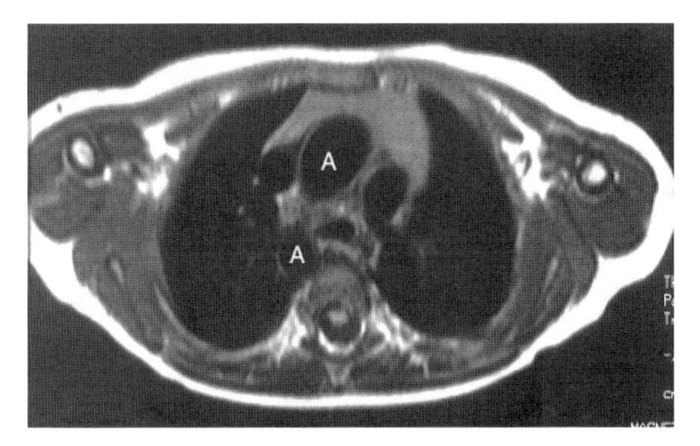

Figure 3.2.1. SE 515/30.

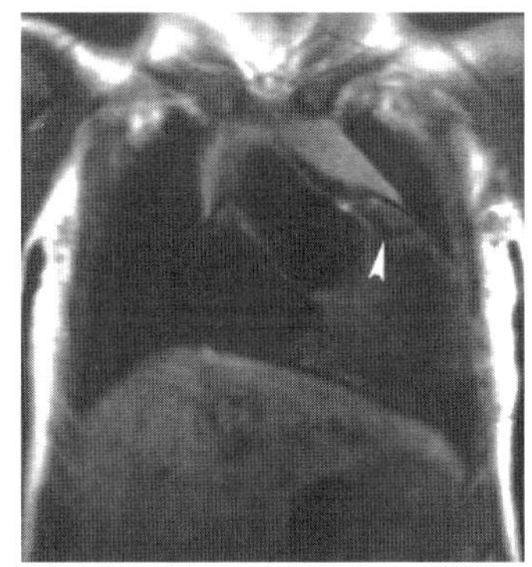

Figure 3.2.2.

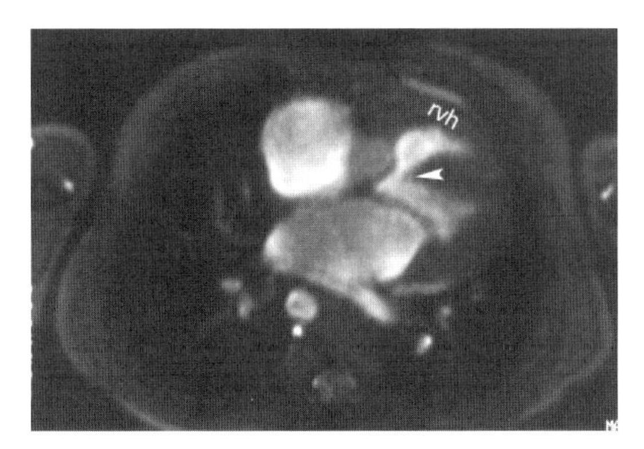

Figure 3.2.3. Flash 40/10/50°.

Findings. Axial ECG-gated T1-weighted MR images at the level of the great vessels demonstrate a right aortic arch (A) (Fig. 3.2.1). Coronal T1-weighted MR image demonstrates hypoplasia of the pulmonary infundibulum (Fig. 3.2.2, *arrowhead*). Axial gradient-recalled-echo MR images through the heart (Fig. 3.2.3) reveal right ventricular hypertrophy (rvh) and a high membranous ventricular septal defect (*arrowhead*).

Diagnosis. Tetralogy of Fallot

Discussion. Tetralogy of Fallot is characterized by a combination of (*a*) infundibular pulmonic hypoplasia, (*b*) ventricular septal defect, (*c*) right ventricular hypertrophy, and (*d*) overriding of the aortic root above the ventricular septal defect (5). The pulmonic infundibular stenosis and overriding of the aorta facilitate shunting of deoxygenated blood from the right ventricle to the aorta, thereby producing cyanosis. Approximately one-fourth of patients with tetralogy of Fallot also have a right aortic arch, usually with mirror-image branching. In fact, the plain-film findings of right aortic arch with decreased pulmonary vasculature should strongly suggest this diagnosis. Cardiomegaly usually is not present in these patients.

In planning surgery for tetralogy of Fallot, it is important to assess the degree of hypoplasia of the pulmonary arteries and the development of collateral vessels from the systemic to pulmonary arteries. Surgical correction varies from palliative shunt procedures (Blalock-Taussig) to complete repair of the infundibular outflow obstruction and patching of the ventricular septal defect (Lillehei procedure).

Aunt Minnie's Pearls

- *Infundibular stenosis + ventricular septal defect + overriding aorta + right ventricular hypertrophy = tetralogy of Fallot.*
- *Right arch + decreased pulmonary flow + no cardiomegaly on plain films = think tetralogy of Fallot.*

CASE 3

History. Newborn with cyanosis

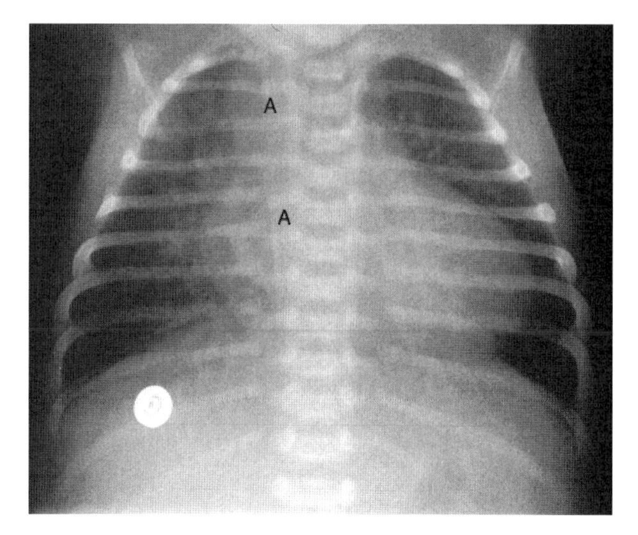

Figure 3.3.1.

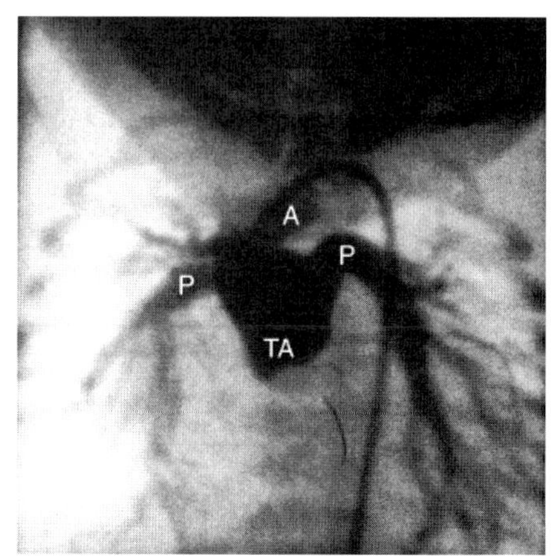

Figure 3.3.2.

Findings. A frontal chest x-ray demonstrates a right-sided aortic arch (A), cardiomegaly, and increased pulmonary blood flow (Fig. 3.3.1). An angiogram on another patient obtained by injection of contrast material into the aortic root (Fig. 3.3.2) reveals a single vascular trunk (TA), which gives rise to both the aorta (A) and the pulmonary arteries (P).

Diagnosis. Persistent truncus arteriosus

Discussion. Between the 5th and 7th weeks of embryologic development, the aorta, pulmonary artery, and high ventricular septum are formed by fusion of the truncoconal ridges, which divide the truncus arteriosus into the aorta and pulmonary artery (6). Failure of the ridges to fuse causes a persistent truncus arteriosus and a defect in the ventricular septum.

Radiographically, this diagnosis is strongly suggested when a right aortic arch (35% of cases), cardiomegaly, and increased pulmonary vascularity are present. Angiography or MR imaging can confirm the diagnosis by visualization of the persistent truncus. The truncal valve has two to five leaflets but is most commonly tricuspid (7). The most familiar classification scheme for persistent truncus arteriosus is the Collett and Edwards system (8), which is based on the variable origin of the pulmonary arteries from the truncus. A main pulmonary artery arising from the left posterolateral aspect of the truncus (type I) is the most common type. Surgical correction involves creating a new pulmonary outflow tract with synthetic graft material, while the truncal vessel becomes the aortic root. Before surgery, it is important to assess the position and origins of the coronary arteries on the imaging studies so that they are not inadvertently injured during the surgical procedure.

Aunt Minnie's Pearls

- *Embryologic separation of the aorta from the pulmonary artery fails to occur in persistent truncus arteriosus.*
- *Right arch + increased pulmonary flow + cyanosis = think persistent truncus arteriosus.*

CASE 4

History. 18-year-old woman with cyanosis as a newborn

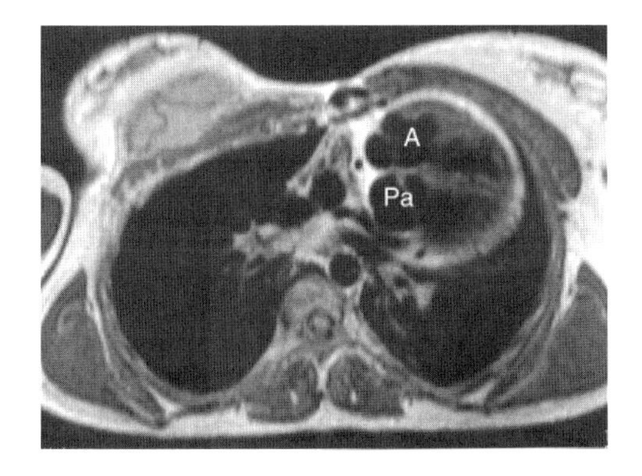

Figure 3.4.1. SE 1019/30.

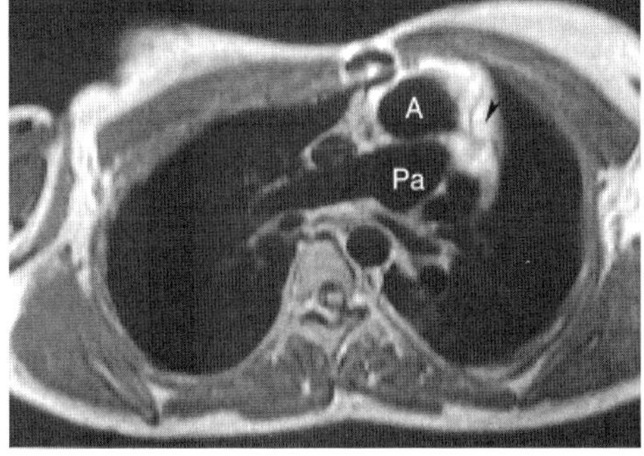

Figure 3.4.2. SE 1022/30.

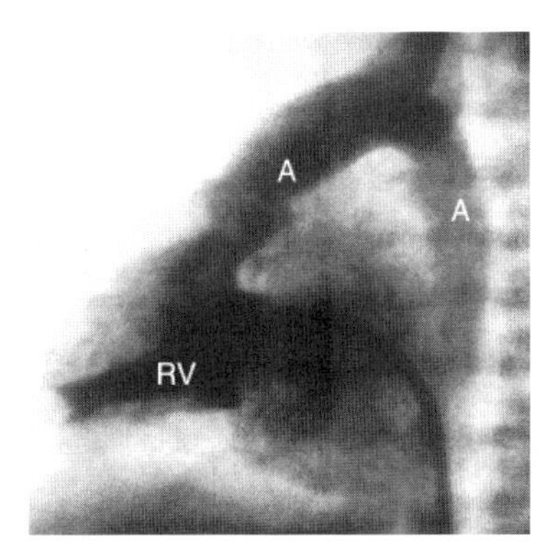

Figure 3.4.3.

Findings. Axial ECG-gated spin-echo T1-weighted MR images of the heart are presented. The abnormal position of the aortic valve and aorta (A) anterior to the pulmonic valve and pulmonary artery (Pa) (Figs. 3.4.1 and 3.4.2) defines D-transposition. A coronary artery is seen originating from the aortic root (Fig. 3.4.2, *arrowhead*). In a different patient, a lateral view from an angiogram obtained with injection of contrast material into the right ventricle (RV) (Fig. 3.4.3) shows contrast opacifying the anteriorly displaced aorta (A).

Diagnosis. D-Transposition of the great vessels

Discussion. Transposition of the great arteries is the most common congenital cyanotic heart lesion in the newborn. MR imaging allows a specific diagnosis of this lesion if the segmental method of cardiac analysis described by Van Praagh (9) is followed. In normal cardiac development, the inferior vena cava empties into a right-sided atrium, and the aortic valve is located posterior to and to the right of the pulmonic valve. This arrangement describes situs solitus, normal aortic position, and a normal D-bulboventricular loop, respectively. The aorticopulmonary septum, which is responsible for dividing the truncus arteriosus into the two great vessels, normally undergoes a clockwise spiral. If this fails to occur, the aortic valve will lie anteriorly to the pulmonic valve, thereby defining transposition (10).

Aortic transposition results in ventriculoarterial discordance (the right ventricle empties into the aorta). Atrioventricular concordance still exists in D-transposition; therefore, venous blood will travel from the right atrium to the right ventricle and out the aorta. An atrial septal defect, ventricular septal defect, or patent ductus arteriosus is necessary to allow blood to mix between the systemic and pulmonary circulations.

Aunt Minnie's Pearls

- *If the aortic valve is anterior to the pulmonic valve, transposition is present.*
- *D indicates that the aortic valve is to the right of the pulmonic valve.*

CASE 5

History. Murmur identified on physical examination

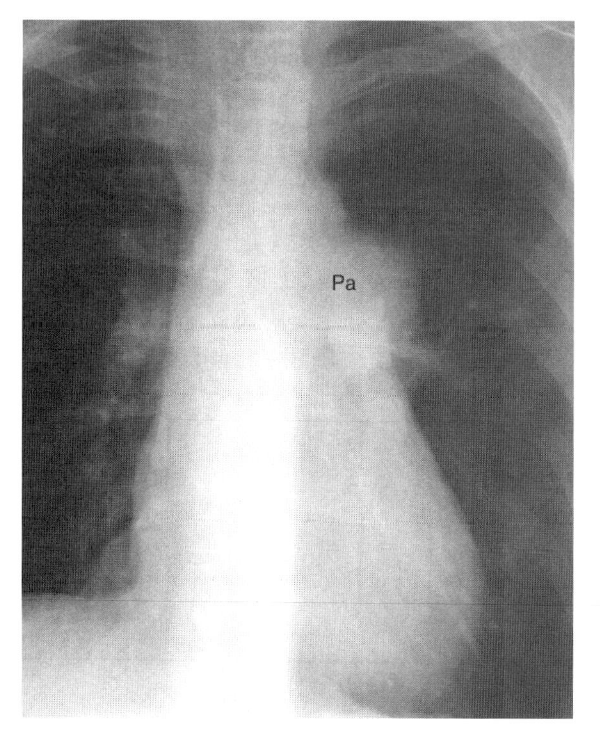

Figure 3.5.1.

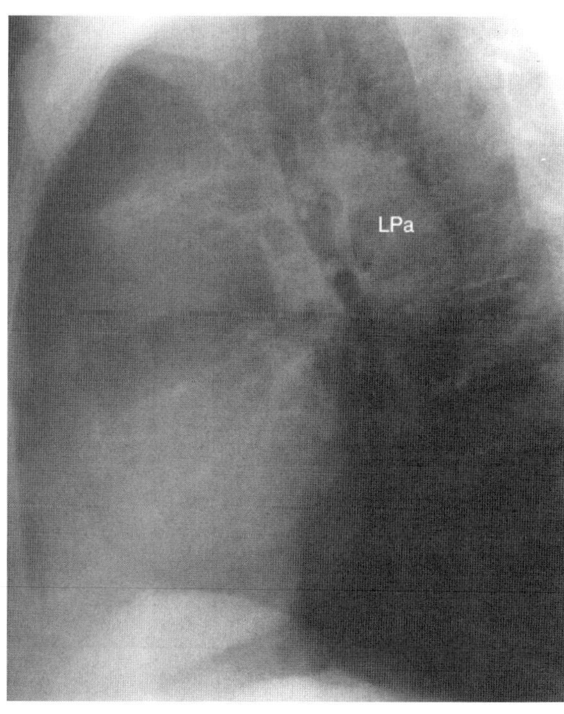

Figure 3.5.2.

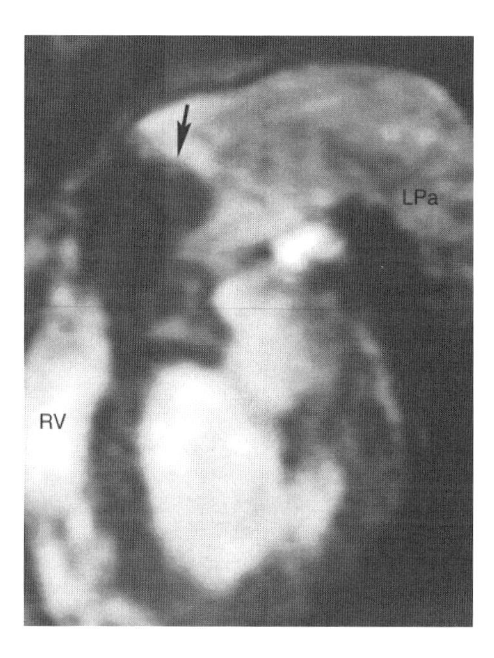

Figure 3.5.3. Flash 40/10/50°.

CASE 5 *(continued)*

Findings. Enlargement of the main and left pulmonary artery (Pa) is seen on the posteroanterior and lateral film of the chest (Figs. 3.5.1 and 3.5.2). Gradient-recalled-echo MR image (Fig. 3.5.3) reveals a signal void distal to the pulmonic valve (*arrow*) and entering the left pulmonary artery (LPa). This signal void signifies a systolic jet of blood passing the stenotic pulmonary valve. RV, right ventricle.

Diagnosis. Valvular pulmonic stenosis

Discussion. Congenital commissural fusion of the pulmonic valve leaflets results in valvular stenosis. The clinical presentation of valvular pulmonic stenosis depends on the severity of the abnormality. Mild stenosis may result in few clinical findings. If the stenosis is severe enough that right-sided heart failure and shunting across an atrial septal defect ensue, then the stenosis is labeled "critical" (11). Plain radiographs demonstrate hypertrophy of the right ventricle and enlargement of the main and left pulmonary arteries. This occurs because the stenotic jet of contrast preferentially enters the left pulmonary artery, which is in more direct alignment with the valvular apparatus. In severe cases, atresia of the main pulmonary artery occurs.

Aunt Minnie's Pearls

- *Hypertrophy of the right ventricle + enlargement of main and left pulmonary artery and left pulmonary artery on chest film = valvular pulmonic stenosis.*

CASE 6

History. Young woman with severe cyanosis as a newborn

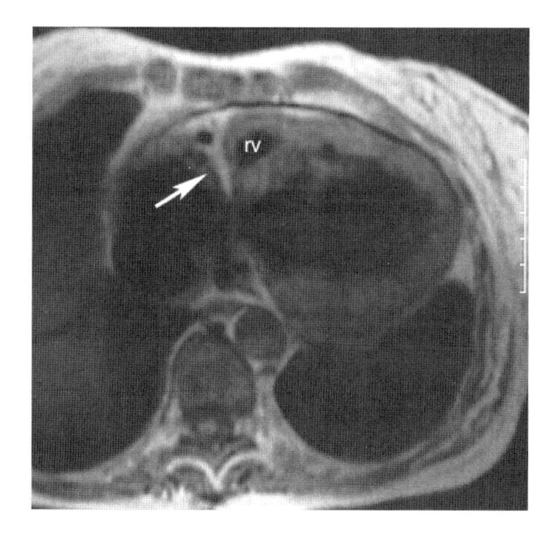

Figure 3.6.1. SE 618/17.

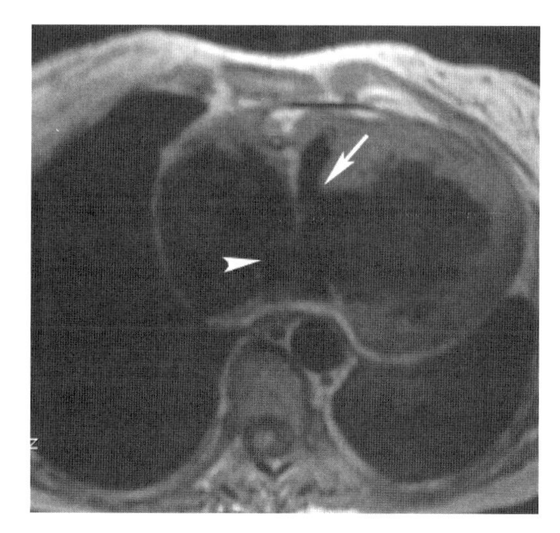

Figure 3.6.2. SE 618/17.

Findings. ECG-gated T1-weighted spin-echo MR images reveal a linear bar of high signal intensity in the expected location of the tricuspid valve (Fig. 3.6.1, *arrow*). A large atrial septal defect (Fig. 3.6.2, *arrowhead*) and a large ventricular septal defect (Fig.3.6.2, *arrow*) are present, as is an extremely hypoplastic right ventricle (rv) (Fig. 3.6.1).

Diagnosis. Tricuspid atresia

Discussion. When the tricuspid atrioventricular valve fails to develop normally, tricuspid atresia is present. The newborn presents with cyanosis, and plain-film evaluation classically demonstrates decreased pulmonary vascularity. MR imaging reveals a muscular and fatty ridge of tissue that separates a large right atrium from the hypoplastic right ventricle. A patent foramen ovale or atrial septal defect is necessary for blood to bypass the atretic valve and flow into the left atrium. Also present is a ventricular septal defect, which allows a small amount of blood to pass into the pulmonary circulation via the hypoplastic right ventricle. Approximately 30% of patients with tricuspid atresia also have transposition of the great vessels (12), and pulmonic stenosis is also a common coexistent lesion. The presence of these associated lesions can have a great impact on the associated plain-film findings. Surgical correction involves palliative shunts to the pulmonary artery from the superior vena cava (Glenn) or right atrium (Fontan) and correction of the accompanying intracardiac shunts or transposition.

Aunt Minnie's Pearls

- *Chest x-ray shows decreased pulmonary vascularity.*
- *MR imaging demonstrates muscular and fatty ridge in location of tricuspid valve and a hypoplastic right ventricle.*
- *Tricuspid atresia is associated with an atrial septal defect and a ventricular septal defect in all cases and transposition of the great vessels in 30%.*

CASE 7

History. Mild cyanosis and a long systolic murmur identified on physical examination

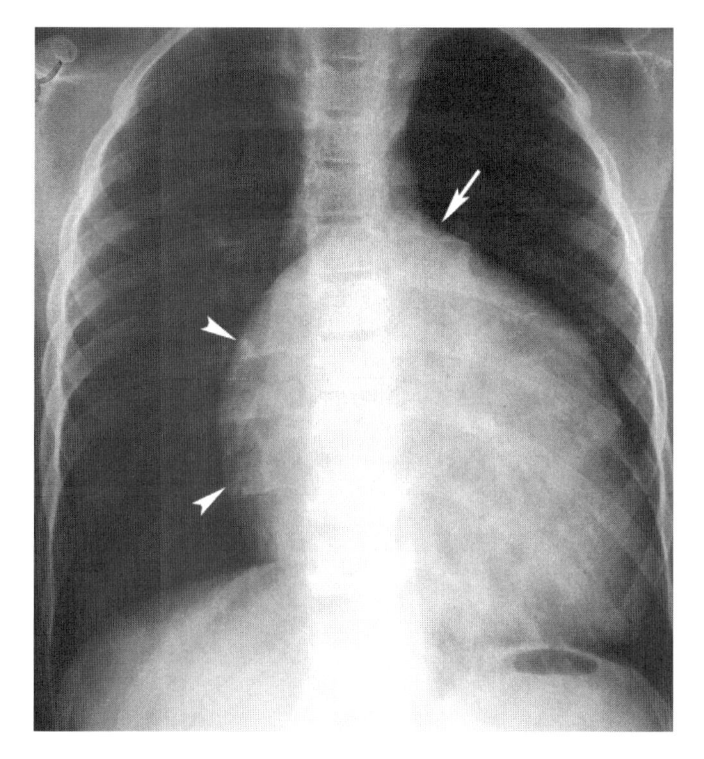

Figure 3.7.1.

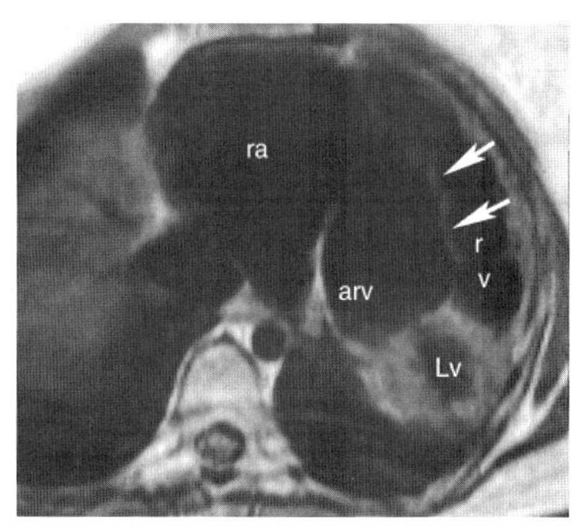

Figure 3.7.2.

Findings. Frontal view of the chest demonstrates an elongated and enlarged right atrium, which results in a box-shaped contour (Fig. 3.7.1, *arrowheads*). The pulmonary vascularity is decreased, and the area of the main pulmonary artery is concave on the frontal view (Fig. 3.7.1, *arrows*). In a different patient, an axial ECG-gated T1-weighted MR image of the heart reveals downward displacement and tethering of the tricuspid valve into the right ventricle (Fig. 3.7.2, *arrows*). This image also shows that a portion (arv) of the right ventricle (rv) is incorporated into the right atrium (ra). The left ventricle is also seen (Lv).

Diagnosis. Ebstein anomaly

Discussion. The Ebstein anomaly is abnormal downward displacement of the septal and posterior leaflets of the tricuspid valve into the right ventricle. As a result of this displacement, much of the right ventricle is anatomically incorporated into the right atrium, i.e., "atrialized" (arv) (Fig. 3.7.2). This portion of the ventricle has an abnormally thin wall, and tricuspid regurgitation occurs. An associated patent foramen ovale or secundum atrial septal defect is present in most cases. Plain films may demonstrate a nearly pathognomonic appearance of an elongated and enlarged right atrium with a box-shaped contour, as seen in the example case. Echocardiography, MR imaging, or angiography can confirm the diagnosis by demonstrating the displaced tricuspid leaflets and associated abnormalities. ECG abnormalities are frequently found and include right bundle branch block, prolonged P-R intervals, and Wolff-Parkinson-White syndrome (13). Interestingly, an association has been described between this anomaly and the use of lithium in early pregnancy (14).

Aunt Minnie's Pearls

- *Downward displacement of the septal and posterior leaflets of the tricuspid valve into the right ventricle indicates the Ebstein anomaly.*
- *Ebstein anomaly is associated with ECG conduction abnormalities and in utero lithium exposure.*

CASE 8

History. Acyanotic 11-year-old girl with upper extremity hypertension

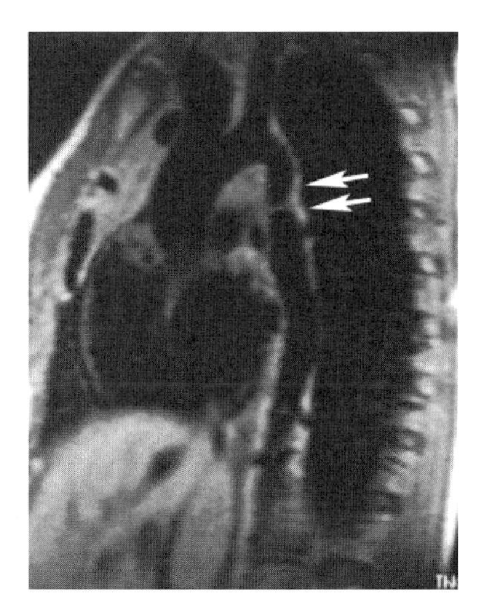

Figure 3.8.1. SE 813/20.

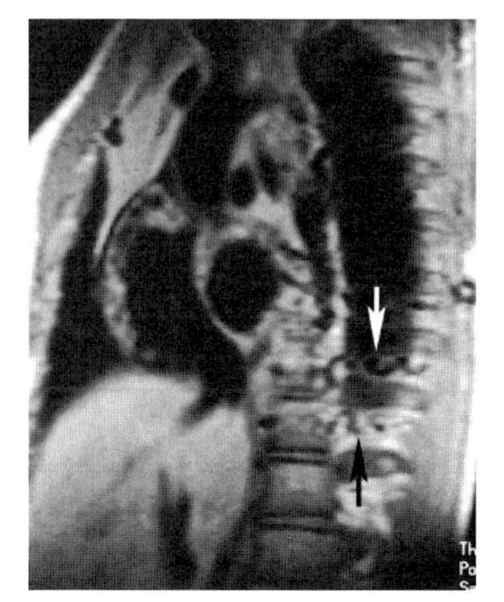

Figure 3.8.2. SE 813/20.

Findings. Oblique sagittal ECG-gated T1-weighted MR image of the aorta demonstrates an area of abnormal narrowing in the region of the aortic isthmus (Fig. 3.8.1, *arrows*). Another image obtained off the midline reveals dilated, tortuous intercostal arterial collaterals (Fig. 3.8.2, *arrows*).

Diagnosis. Coarctation of the aorta

Discussion. The juxtaductal portion of the aorta is congenitally narrowed in coarctation of the aorta. If the narrowing occurs proximal to the ductus, blood is shunted to the descending thoracic aorta via the patent ductus. Once the ductus closes, clinical symptoms may quickly develop with congestive heart failure and left to right shunting across a ventricular septal defect. Postductal coarctations produce the more familiar presentation in which the plain radiographs demonstrate left ventricular hypertrophy, an indistinct aortic knob with a "three" contour, and bilateral rib notching. Coarctation of the aorta is associated with bicuspid aortic valve, ventricular septal defect, patent ductus arteriosus, Berry aneurysms, and Turner's syndrome. Pseudocoarctation refers to elongation of the thoracic aorta with kinking in the juxtaductal region, but no significant pressure gradient exists across the narrowing and no collateral vessels are present (15).

Surgical correction in patients younger than 10 years usually involves placement of a patch across the posterior aorta. Older patients, who are less subject to physical growth, are treated with a subclavian artery patch. Postsurgical restenosis is often treated with balloon dilatation.

Aunt Minnie's Pearls

- *Coarctation = juxtaductal narrowing of aortic arch with pressure gradient across lesion (vs. pseudocoarctation = no pressure gradient).*
- *This anomaly is frequently associated with bicuspid aortic valve, ventricular septal defect, and patent ductus arteriosus.*

CASE 9

History. Systolic murmur

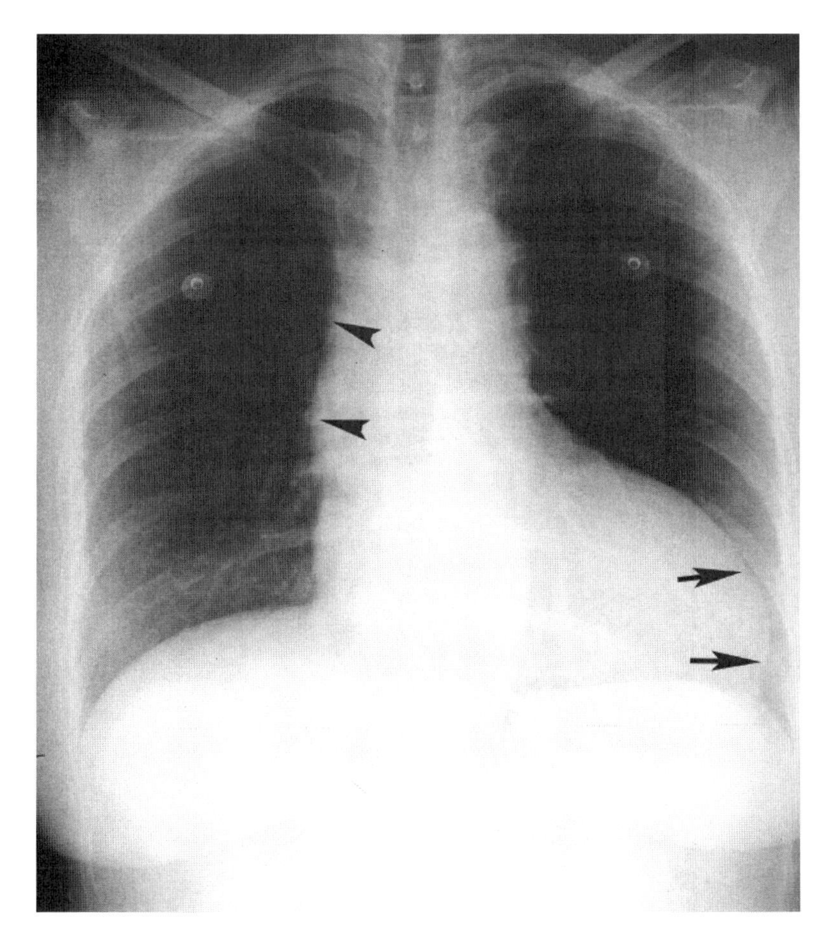

Figure 3.9.1.

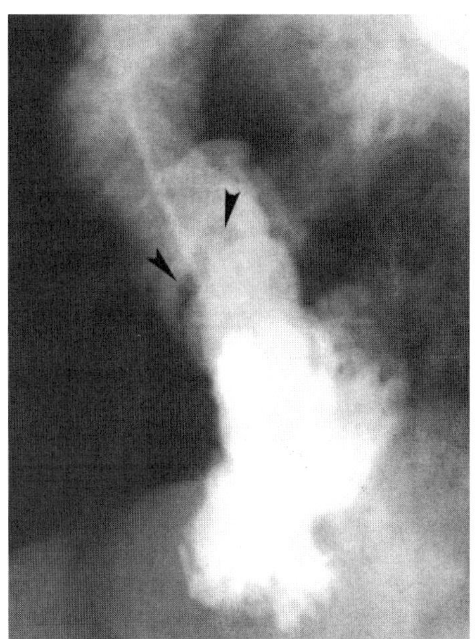

Figure 3.9.2.

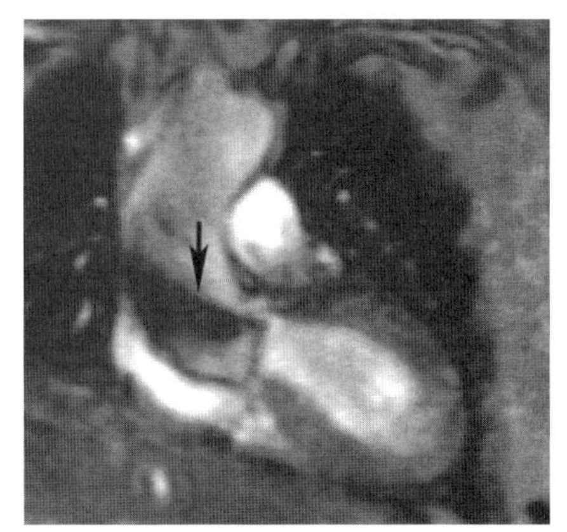

Figure 3.9.3. Flash 40/10/50°.

Findings. Ectasia of the ascending aorta (Fig. 3.9.1, *arrowheads*) and left ventricular enlargement (Fig. 3.9.1, *arrows*) are identified on the frontal view of the chest. Cardiac catheterization with injection of the left ventricle demonstrates a domed and thickened aortic valve (Fig. 3.9.2, *arrowheads*), which spans the entire chamber of the aortic root. A coronal gradient-recalled-echo MR image reveals a signal void across the aortic valve in systole (Fig. 3.9.3, *arrow*), consistent with a poststenotic jet of turbulent blood flow.

Diagnosis. Bicuspid aortic valvular stenosis

Discussion. Congenital fusion of the commissures of the aortic valve cusps results in a bicuspid aortic valve. This anomaly occurs in 1–2% of the general population and more frequently in patients with coarctation of the aorta. Degeneration of the bicuspid valve leads to a hemodynamically significant pressure gradient (≥25 mmHg) when the patient is middle-aged or younger. Calcification of the aortic valve on plain film is diagnostic of aortic stenosis and also signifies a significant pressure gradient. Other common causes of aortic valvular stenosis are rheumatic fever and degeneration of a tricuspid valve.

Radiographs demonstrate enlargement of the ascending aorta with sparing of the aortic knob and descending thoracic aorta. Hypertrophy and eventual enlargement of the left ventricle are also seen. MR imaging, echocardiography, and angiography allow for direct visualization of the thickened and domed bicuspid valve, which spans the entire aortic root, producing the characteristic “fish mouth” appearance (16). Surgical valve replacement and balloon commissurotomy are the current treatment options.

Aunt Minnie’s Pearls

- Enlargement of ascending aorta in young person = think bicuspid aortic valve.
- Calcification of aortic valve on lateral chest film = hemodynamically significant aortic stenosis.

CASE 10

History. 65-year-old man with intermittent hematochezia

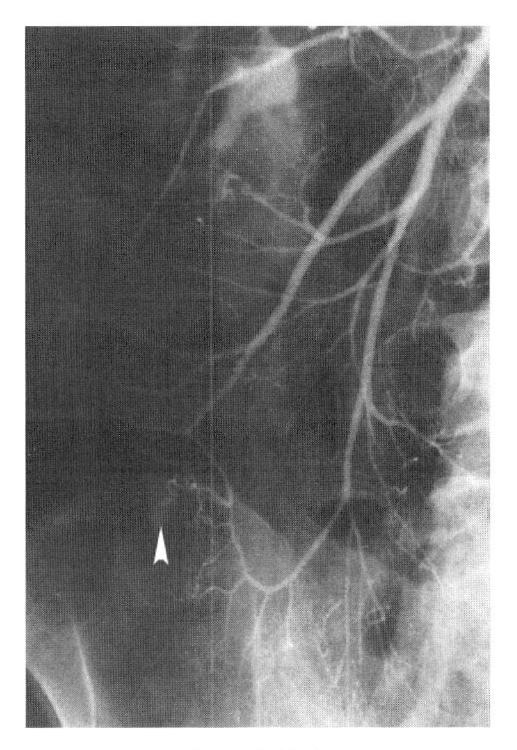

Figure 3.10.1.

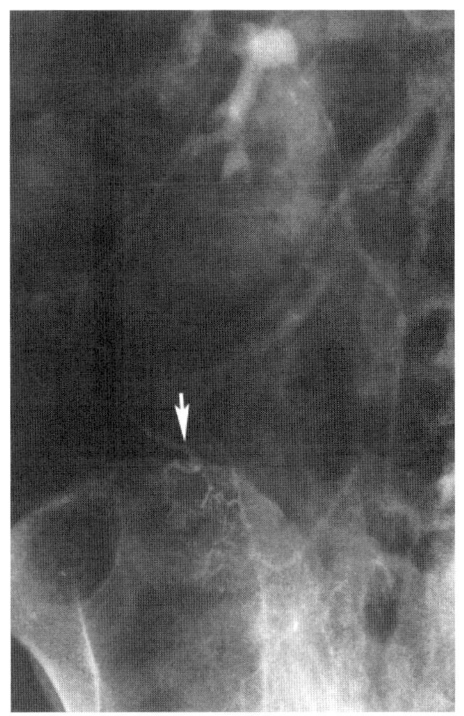

Figure 3.10.2.

Findings. Serial arterial phase (Fig. 3.10.1) and venous phase (Fig. 3.10.2) films from a selective superior mesenteric arteriogram show a small cluster of abnormal arterial vessels (Fig. 3.10.1, *arrowhead*) in the region of the cecum with early, dense, and persistent opacification of a draining vein (3.10.2, *arrow*).

Diagnosis. Angiodysplasia of the colon

Discussion. Angiodysplasia, also called vascular ectasia, is a common etiology of lower intestinal bleeding in patients older than 60 years. Gastrointestinal bleeding caused by angiodysplasia is usually mild and intermittent. Lesions may be single or multiple and most often involve the cecum or ascending colon. They are thought to be acquired, possibly as a result of intermittent partial obstruction of submucosal veins during periods of increased intracolonic pressure. Characteristic angiographic findings include abnormal clusters of small arteries with early, dense, and persistent opacification of the draining veins (17, 18). In elderly patients evaluated for lower gastrointestinal bleeding, angiographic detection of angiodysplasia can be an incidental finding. In the absence of contrast extravasation, indicating active bleeding, other possible causes for the bleeding should be carefully sought. This disorder is seen with increased frequency in patients with a history of aortic stenosis.

Aunt Minnie's Pearls

- *Angiodysplasia is a common cause of bleeding in the lower gastrointestinal tract.*
- *Abnormal clusters of small arteries with early, dense, and persistent opacification of draining veins are characteristic.*
- *Angiodysplasia is associated with aortic stenosis.*

CASE 11

History. 42-year-old alcoholic man with hematemesis after an episode of vomiting and retching

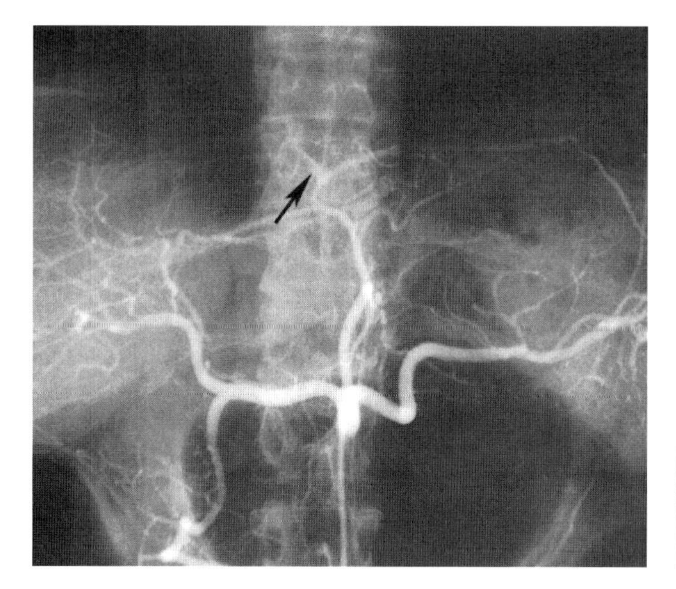

Figure 3.11.1.

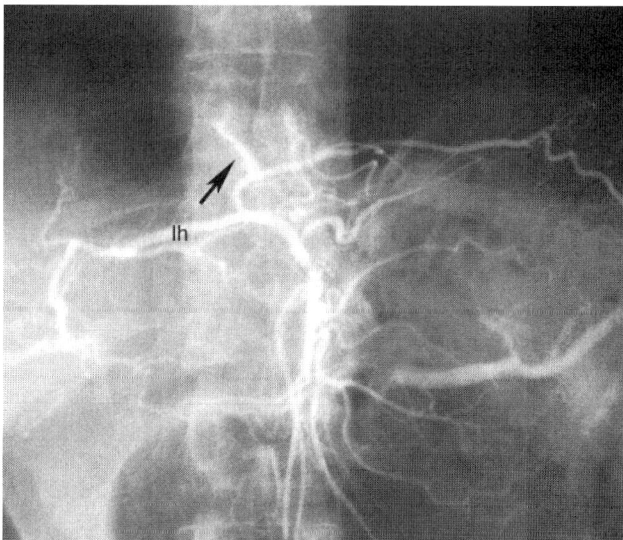

Figure 3.11.2.

Findings. Celiac arteriogram (Fig. 3.11.1) shows a linear collection of extravasated contrast medium at the gastroesophageal junction (*arrow*). Contrast extravasation is seen more prominently on selective injection of the left gastric artery (Fig. 3.11.2, *arrow*). Anomalous origin of the left hepatic artery (lh) from the left gastric artery is noted incidentally.

Diagnosis. Mallory-Weiss laceration

Discussion. The clinical presentation in this case is classic for the Mallory-Weiss syndrome. Bleeding stops spontaneously in most patients, and rebleeding is uncommon. Lesions are usually diagnosed endoscopically. Angiography is indicated for detection and treatment of persistent bleeding. Extravasated contrast material originating near the gastroesophageal junction may be seen to run into the esophagus or gastric fundus. If the lesion is posteriorly located, a linear collection of contrast material will be seen pooling in the laceration as in the index case. Successful treatment includes selective vasopressin infusion or transcatheter embolization (19). Surgery is rarely required.

Aunt Minnie's Pearls

- *Bleeding in the upper gastrointestinal tract after violent vomiting may be due to a Mallory-Weiss laceration of the esophagus.*
- *Linear contrast material extravasation in the tear is a diagnostic angiographic finding.*

CASE 12

History. Elderly hemodialysis patient with unexplained hypotension who complains of persistent severe abdominal pain

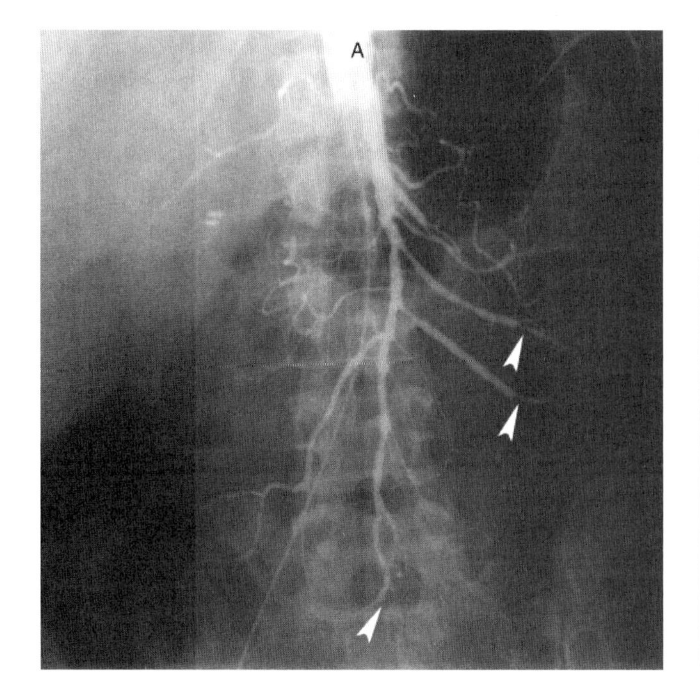

Figure 3.12.1.

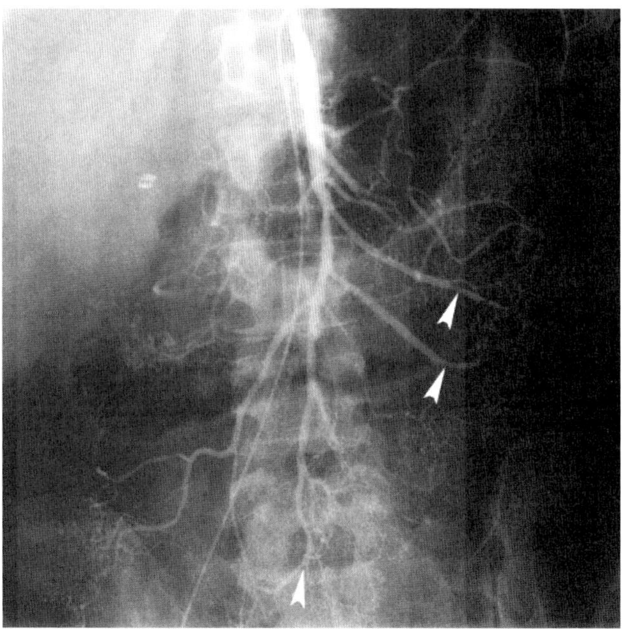

Figure 3.12.2.

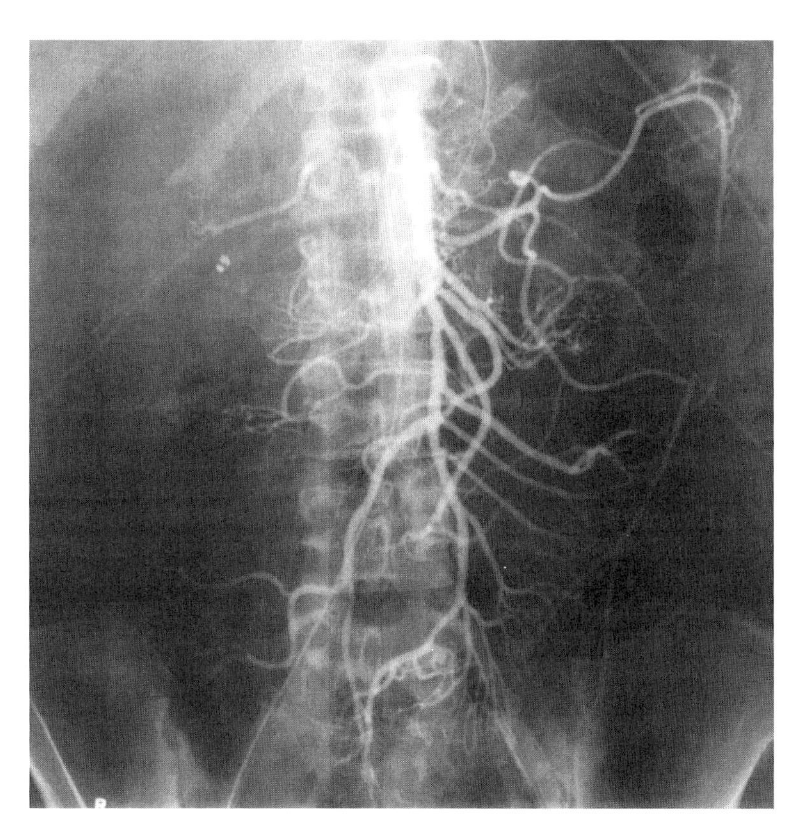

Figure 3.12.3.

Findings. A late-arterial-phase film from a selective superior mesenteric arteriogram (SMA) (Fig. 3.12.1) shows diffusive irregularity of mesenteric arterial branches (*arrowheads*) with severe peripheral arterial constriction and poor opacification of intramural bowel branches. The substantial reflux of contrast medium into the aorta (A) indicates diminished mesenteric arterial flow. A film obtained immediately after selective injection of a vasodilator (Fig. 3.12.2) shows substantial reversal of peripheral arterial spasm (*arrowheads*). After infusion of papaverine into the SMA for 24 hours, the patient's abdominal symptoms resolved, and a final arteriogram (Fig. 3.12.3) shows resolution of the mesenteric vasospasm.

Diagnosis. Nonocclusive mesenteric ischemia

Discussion. The reduction in cardiac output associated with various cardiogenic and noncardiogenic shock states can initiate severe splanchnic vasoconstriction and result in intestinal infarction. When initially examined, patients typically have abdominal pain, often out of proportion to the severity of their physical findings, and a high index of suspicion is required for diagnosis (20). Emergency mesenteric angiography is indicated to exclude SMA thrombosis or embolus (occlusive mesenteric ischemia). In the absence of mesenteric occlusive disease, diffuse constriction of SMA branches with diminished bowel blush and poor visualization of the superior mesenteric vein supports a diagnosis of nonocclusive mesenteric ischemia. Findings of focal segmental areas of spasm, particularly at branch vessel origins, are more specific but less frequently seen (21). If SMA angiography after vasodilator injection shows reversibility of the vasospasm, then selective infusion of papaverine is indicated (22). Patients with clinical signs suggesting intestinal infarction (e.g., rebound abdominal tenderness) require emergency laparotomy and resection of nonviable bowel. Even with optimal therapy, mortality approaches 50%.

Aunt Minnie's Pearls

- *Diffuse mesenteric arterial spasm, especially at branch points, indicates nonocclusive mesenteric ischemia.*
- *If the spasm improves after a test injection of vasodilators, selective papaverine infusion is indicated.*

CASE 13

History. 69-year-old woman with severe abdominal pain and distention 3 days after coronary artery bypass surgery

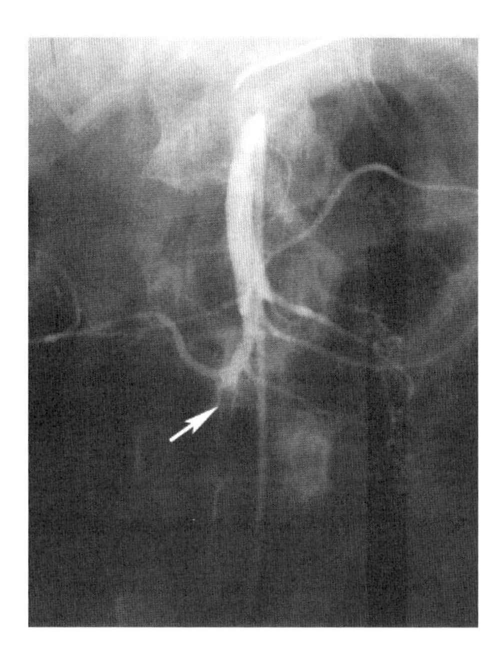

Figure 3.13.1.

Findings. A view from a selective superior mesenteric artery arteriogram (Fig. 3.13.1) shows a radiolucent filling defect (*arrow*) occluding the main lumen just distal to the origin of the right colic artery. Diffuse constriction of visualized jejunal branches is also apparent.

Diagnosis. Acute intestinal ischemia secondary to superior mesenteric artery embolus (occlusive mesenteric ischemia)

Discussion. Superior mesenteric arterial embolism accounts for 40–50% of cases of acute intestinal ischemia (20). Emboli generally originate from the heart and lodge just distal to a major superior mesenteric artery branch. Patients often have a history of peripheral embolism. Emergency angiographic evaluation includes biplane aortography to ascertain patency of the proximal superior mesenteric artery. Selective mesenteric angiography will then reveal an abrupt, rounded vessel cutoff or partial occlusion with an intraluminal filling defect. Mesenteric vasoconstriction is common (21). Survival of the patient generally depends on successful surgical revascularization and resection of nonviable bowel.

Aunt Minnie's Pearls

- *Occlusive mesenteric ischemia is usually due to a superior mesenteric artery embolus.*

CASE 14

History. 24-year-old woman with rapidly worsening ascites

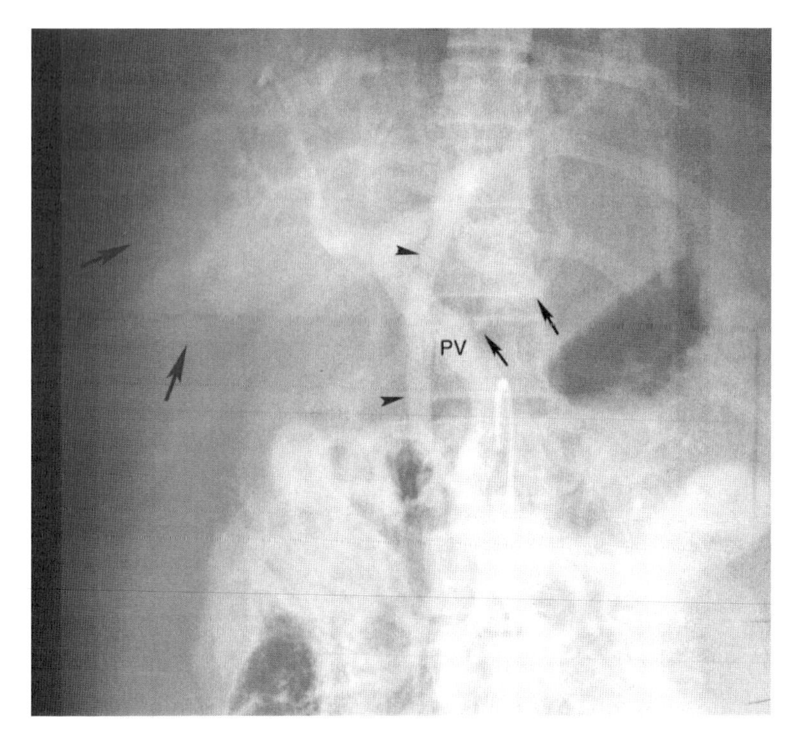

Figure 3.14.1.

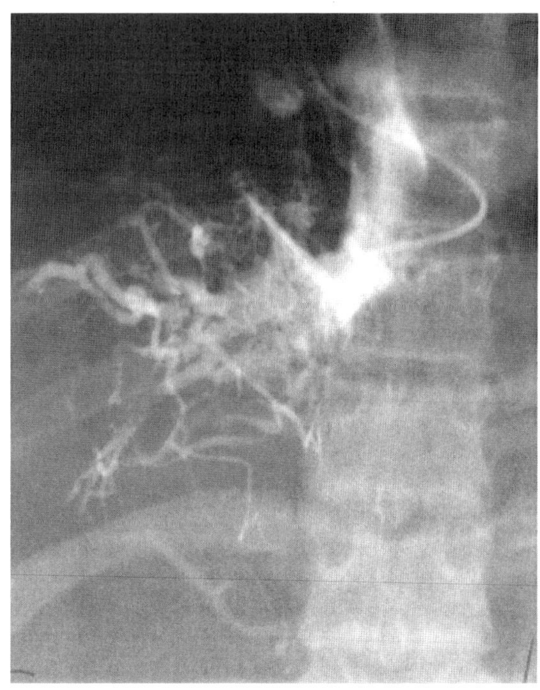

Figure 3.14.2.

Findings. Venous-phase film from superior mesenteric artery arteriogram (Fig. 3.14.1) shows a patent portal vein (PV) with abnormal portosystemic collateral flow via the coronary vein (*small arrows*) and a recanalized umbilical vein (*arrowheads*). Displacement of the liver edge (*large arrows*) from the lateral abdominal wall and centrally located small-bowel loops are indicative of ascites. A wedged hepatic venogram (Fig. 3.14.2) demonstrates a "spider web" pattern of intrahepatic venous collaterals and fails to show a normal hepatic vein.

Diagnosis. Budd-Chiari syndrome

Discussion. Hepatic venous obstruction (Budd-Chiari syndrome) is an uncommon cause of portal hypertension. Patients usually present with hepatosplenomegaly and rapid onset of ascites. Hepatic vein occlusion in adults can be the result of various hypercoagulable states (e.g., polycythemia vera or oral contraceptive use) or tumor invasion, as is seen with hepatocellular or renal cell carcinoma. Often a specific etiology is not determined. Hemodynamic evaluation shows evidence of postsinusoidal venous obstruction, with elevated free and wedged hepatic vein pressures. The spider web appearance of the wedged hepatic venogram is characteristic (23).

Aunt Minnie's Pearls

- *A spider web appearance of intrahepatic venous collaterals is characteristic of Budd-Chiari syndrome.*
- *Hypercoagulable states and tumor invasion of the cava are common causes in adults.*

CASE 15

History. 33-year-old right-handed carpenter with ischemic necrosis of the distal right second, fourth, and fifth fingers

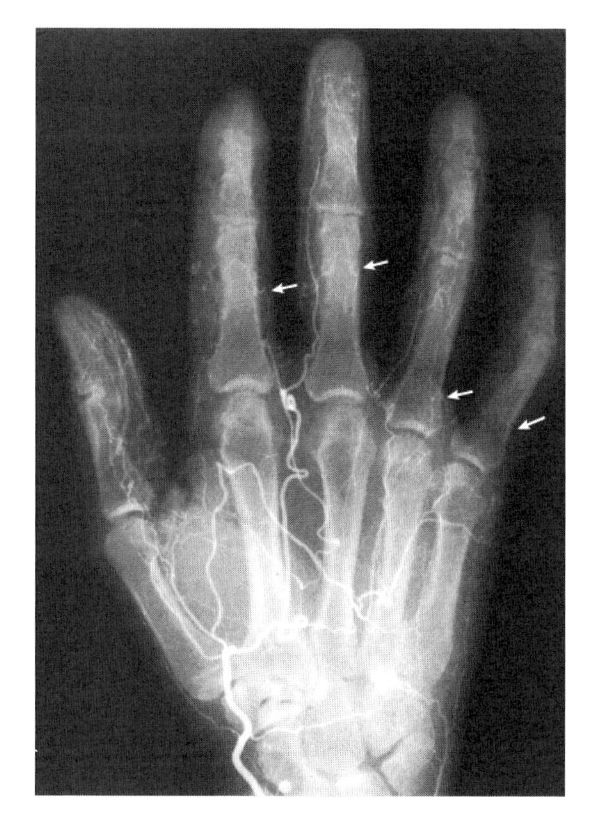

Figure 3.15.1.

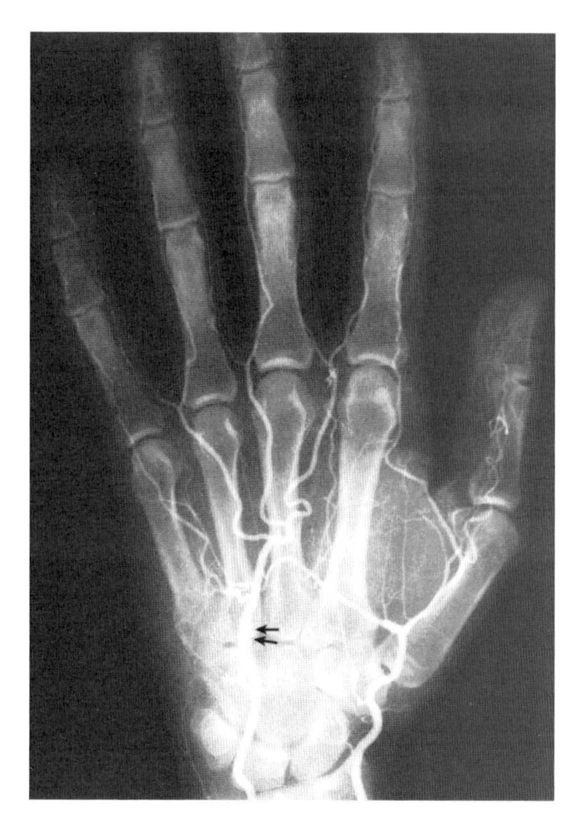

Figure 3.15.2.

Findings. A right-hand arteriogram (Fig. 3.15.1) reveals an occluded distal ulnar artery and superficial palmar arch with proper digital artery occlusions (*arrows*) involving the second through fifth fingers. A left-hand arteriogram (Fig. 3.15.2) shows small ulnar artery aneurysms (*arrows*) located just beyond the hook of the hamate.

Diagnosis. Hypothenar hammer syndrome

Discussion. Repetitive blunt trauma to the palm of the hand resulting in injury to the distal ulnar artery has been termed the hypothenar hammer syndrome (24). Occupational history of repetitive trauma is usually elicited. This patient was a carpenter who repeatedly used a pneumatic nail driver and also used the palms to repeatedly hammer and push against wallboard. Patients may present with digital ischemia, unilateral Raynaud's phenomenon, or a palpable hypothenar mass. Angiography may reveal spasm, occlusion, or an aneurysm of the distal ulnar artery, most commonly located at the level of the carpal hamate bone. These ulnar lesions may serve as the site of origin for distal digital emboli. Surgical therapy has included cervical sympathectomy, ulnar artery aneurysm excision with arterial ligation, and aneurysmectomy with arterial reanastomosis or venous bypass grafting (25).

Aunt Minnie's Pearls

- *Ulnar artery spasm, occlusion, or aneurysms that occur near the hamate bone are diagnostic of hypothenar hammer syndrome.*
- *Patients with hypothenar hammer syndrome usually have a related occupational history.*

CASE 16

History. 12-year-old girl with edema in the left lower extremity; cross-sectional imaging failed to reveal a cause, e.g., retroperitoneal mass

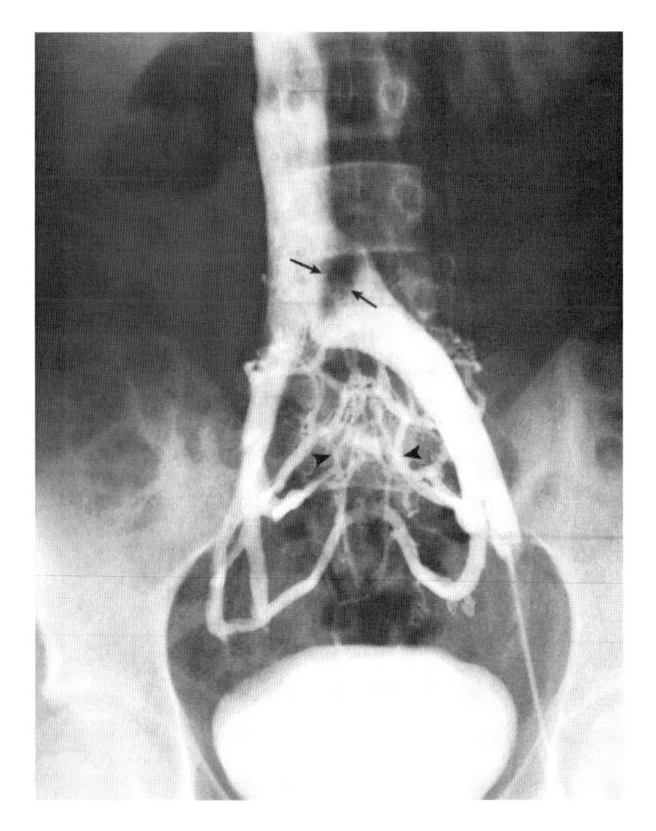

Figure 3.16.1.

Findings. A left iliac venogram (Fig. 3.16.1) demonstrates partial occlusion of the left common iliac vein near its junction with the inferior vena cava (*arrows*). The smoothness of the partial occlusion and the apparent widening of the vein at this site suggest extrinsic compression. A network of pelvic venous collaterals (*arrowheads*) indicates hemodynamically significant venous obstruction.

Diagnosis. Iliac vein compression syndrome (May-Thurner syndrome)

Discussion. Obstruction of flow within the *left* common iliac vein may result from chronic compression by the overlying *right* common iliac artery. Over time, intimal hyperplasia may result in the development of fixed, web-like lesions within the iliac vein lumen. This constellation of clinical and pathologic findings was first described by May and Thurner in 1956. Left iliac venography typically shows a radiolucent defect involving the left common iliac vein near its junction with the inferior vena cava. Radiographic documentation of the presence of transpelvic venous collaterals can be taken as a marker for hemodynamically significant venous obstruction. In the absence of venous collaterals, a measurement of translesional venous pressure gradients both at rest and with exercise may aid in diagnosis (26). Surgical therapy has included transposition of the iliac artery to a position posterior to the vein, along with surgical disruption of intraluminal venous adhesions. If recompression occurs or venous thrombosis is present, a cross-femoral bypass procedure may be necessary. The appropriate role of endoluminal stents in the management of this entity has not yet been defined.

Aunt Minnie's Pearls

- *Symptomatic external compression of the left common iliac vein by the right common iliac artery is known as the May-Thurner syndrome.*

CASE 17

History. 43-year-old man with 2-week history of vertigo, mild left-sided weakness, and absent left upper extremity pulses on physical examination

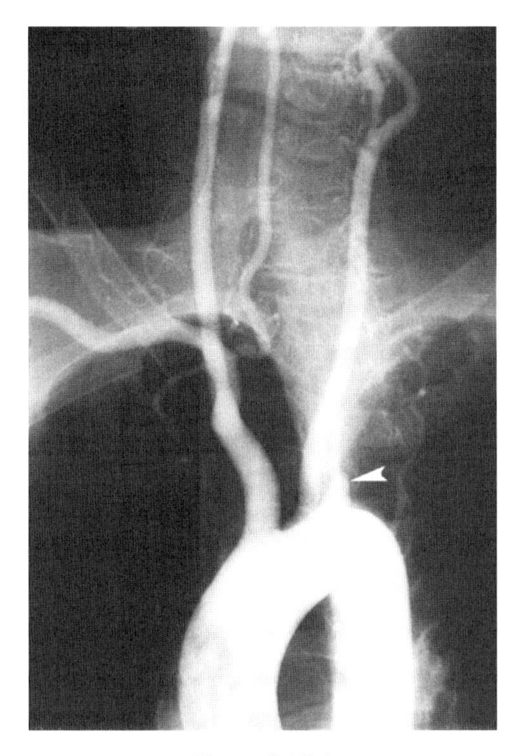

Figure 3.17.1.

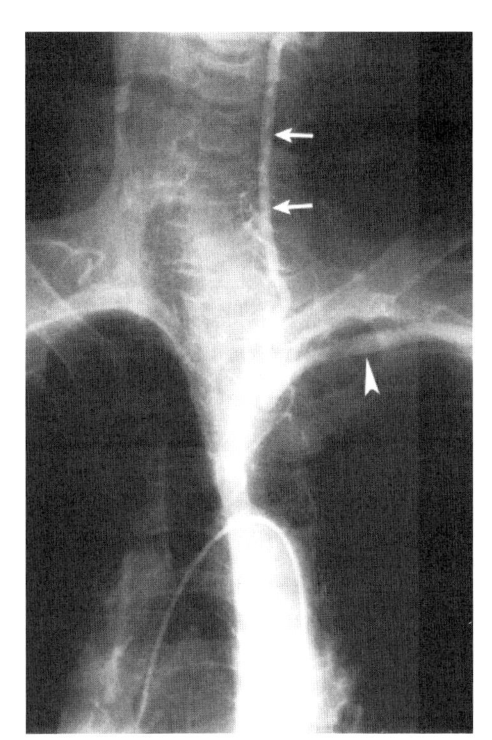

Figure 3.17.2.

Findings. Early film from a thoracic aortogram (Fig. 3.17.1) shows proximal occlusion of the left subclavian artery (*arrowhead*). A proximal right vertebral artery stenosis is also noted. A film obtained late in the aortographic run (Fig. 3.17.2) shows retrograde opacification of the left vertebral artery (*arrows*), which provides collateral flow to the left subclavian artery (*arrowhead*).

Diagnosis. Subclavian steal

Discussion. Occlusion or hemodynamically significant stenosis of the subclavian or innominate artery proximal to the vertebral artery may result in flow reversal in the vertebral artery as a pathway of collateral flow to the ipsilateral upper extremity. This siphoning of blood away from the vertebrobasilar system may result in various neurologic symptoms, including dizziness, vertigo, visual disturbances, or headache. Alternatively, patients may present with upper extremity effort fatigue or signs of microemboli to the hand. Classically the subclavian steal syndrome has been applied to the minority of patients with the characteristic angiographic abnormality who experience symptoms of vertebrobasilar ischemia during upper extremity exercise (27, 28). In patients with significant neurologic or upper extremity ischemic symptoms attributable to the hemodynamic abnormality, conventional treatment has been surgical. Carotid-subclavian bypass, axilloaxillary bypass, or direct repair or bypass from the ascending aorta to a point distal to the lesion have all been applied. A growing body of literature supports the use of balloon angioplasty for treatment of selected patients with subclavian artery stenosis.

Aunt Minnie's Pearls

- *Subclavian steal implies reversal of flow in the vertebral artery caused by a proximal stenosis of the subclavian artery.*
- *Patients have various vertebrobasilar neurologic symptoms with upper extremity exercise.*

CASE 18

History. 40-year-old man with hypertension and intermittent gross hematuria

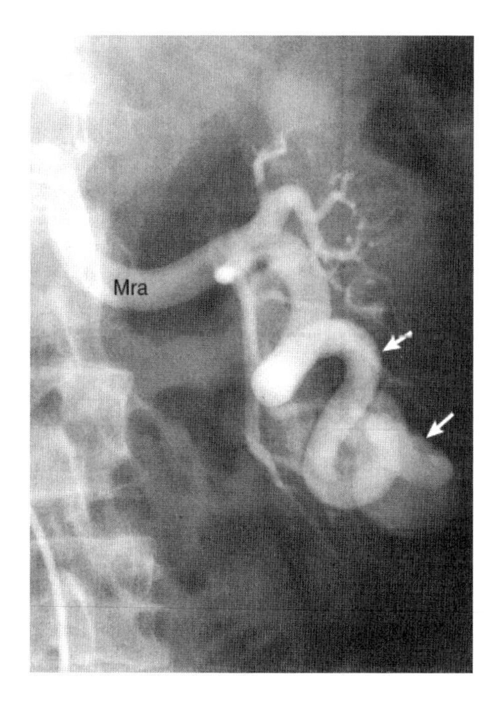

Figure 3.18.1.

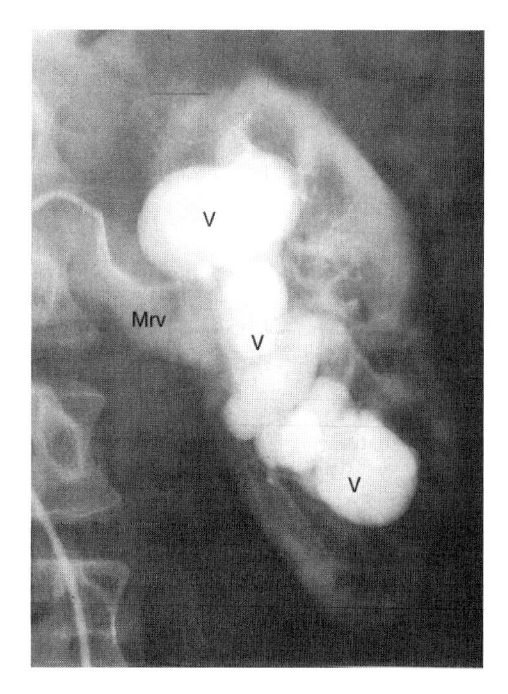

Figure 3.18.2.

Findings. Early (Fig. 3.18.1) and late (Fig. 3.18.2) arterial-phase films from a renal arteriogram reveal marked enlargement of the main renal artery (Mra) with tortuous dilated lower-pole artery (*arrows*). Markedly enlarged venous channels (V) and early opacification of the main renal vein (Mrv) are noted.

Diagnosis. Renal arteriovenous malformation

Discussion. Abnormal arteriovenous communications within the kidney are most commonly iatrogenic and result from percutaneous biopsy or nephrostomy. Such lesions are usually a single abnormal communication between an intrarenal artery and vein and are properly referred to as arteriovenous fistulae. Other acquired causes of arteriovenous fistulae include surgery, trauma, renal cell carcinoma, renal infection, arteritis, and fibromuscular dysplasia. True congenital renal arteriovenous malformations, as in the index case, are rare. A single or multiple arteriovenous communications may be present. Recurrent hematuria is the most common initial symptom. Hypertension, abdominal pain, or a flank bruit may be noted clinically, and large shunts can result in high-output heart failure (29). Larger lesions may be detected with intravenous urography as multinodular impressions on the pelvicaliceal system. Noninvasive modalities, including color Duplex ultrasonography (30) and dynamic contrast-enhanced CT (31), may also show characteristic findings. The definitive diagnosis is made with angiography by detection of tortuous enlarged feeding arteries and early venous opacification, with or without a venous aneurysm. Renal vein and inferior vena cava enlargement are common. Lesions may be amenable to transcatheter embolotherapy, which allows maximal preservation of normal renal parenchyma.

Aunt Minnie's Pearls

- *An enlarged renal artery with early opacification of enlarged renal veins is diagnostic of a renal arteriovenous malformation.*
- *Patients may present with hematuria, hypertension, abdominal pain, or flank bruit.*

CASE 19

History. 40-year-old man without significant risk factors for atherosclerosis presents with claudication of the right calf

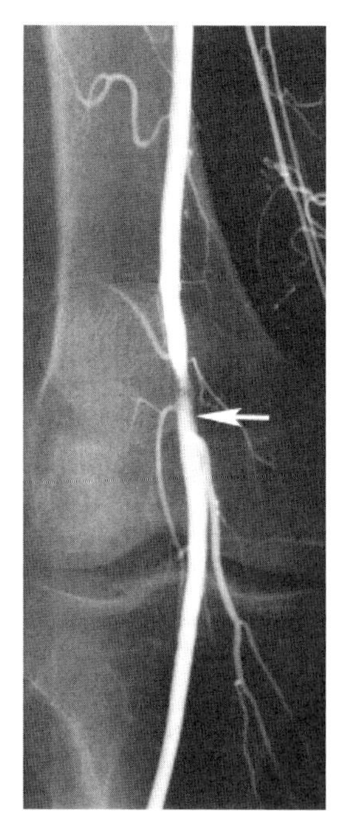

Figure 3.19.1.

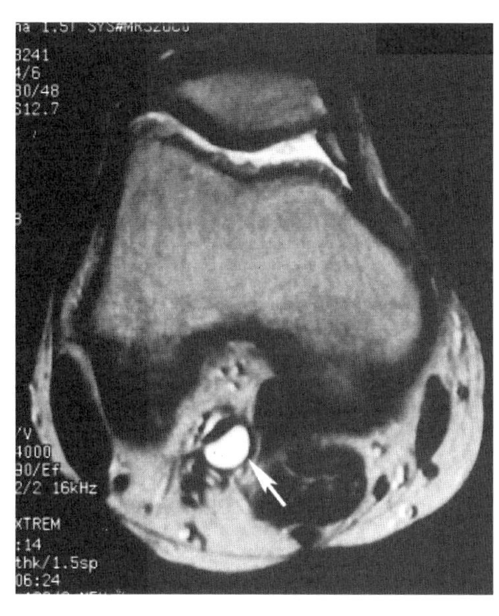

Figure 3.19.2. Fast spin echo 4000/90, ET = 8.

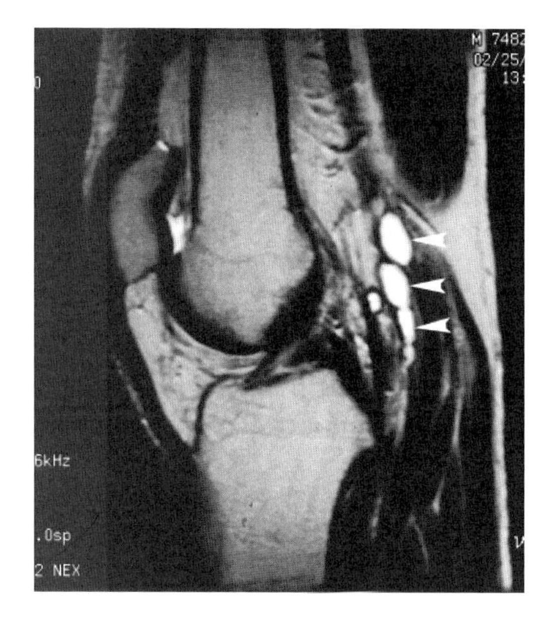

Figure 3.19.3. Fast spin echo 4000/90, ET = 8.

Findings. A popliteal arteriogram s (Fig. 3.19.1) hows focal concentric stenosis (*arrow*) at the level of the patella. The artery above and below the lesion appears normal. An axial T2-weighted MR image reveals hyperintense cystic abnormality (Fig. 3.19.2, *arrow*) within the vessel wall with narrowing of the arterial lumen. A sagittal T2-weighted MR image demonstrates the multilocular nature of the lesion (Fig. 3.19.3, *arrowheads*).

Diagnosis. Cystic adventitial disease of the popliteal artery

Discussion. Cystic adventitial disease of the popliteal artery is a rare entity characterized by subadventitial mucin-containing cysts. The pathologic process causes stenosis or occlusion of the popliteal artery. Patients are most typically young adult men who present with a brief history of severe calf claudication. The etiology of the cystic degeneration is unknown (32). Cross-sectional imaging of the cystic disease and its relationship to the vascular lumen has included ultrasonography, CT (33), and MR imaging (34). Angiography early in the course typically reveals a smoothly tapered concentric stenosis of the midpopliteal artery, classically having an "hourglass" appearance. Alternatively, with an eccentrically placed lesion the artery may be displaced medially or laterally. The vessel proximal and distal to the lesion is characteristically free of luminal irregularity, and signs of more generalized atherosclerosis are typically absent. Patients with advanced disease may present with popliteal artery occlusion. Treatment is surgical—either cystotomy or bypass grafting. Clinical results of image-guided cyst aspiration have been disappointing (32).

Aunt Minnie's Pearls

- *If a smooth popliteal artery stenosis is seen in a young man who has no other evidence of atherosclerosis, think of cystic adventitial disease.*
- *MR images may show diagnostic evidence of this rare disease.*

CASE 20

History. 65-year-old man with unresectable pancreatic carcinoma and an internal/external biliary drainage catheter. The patient presented with gastrointestinal bleeding, fever, and bloody drainage from the biliary catheter.

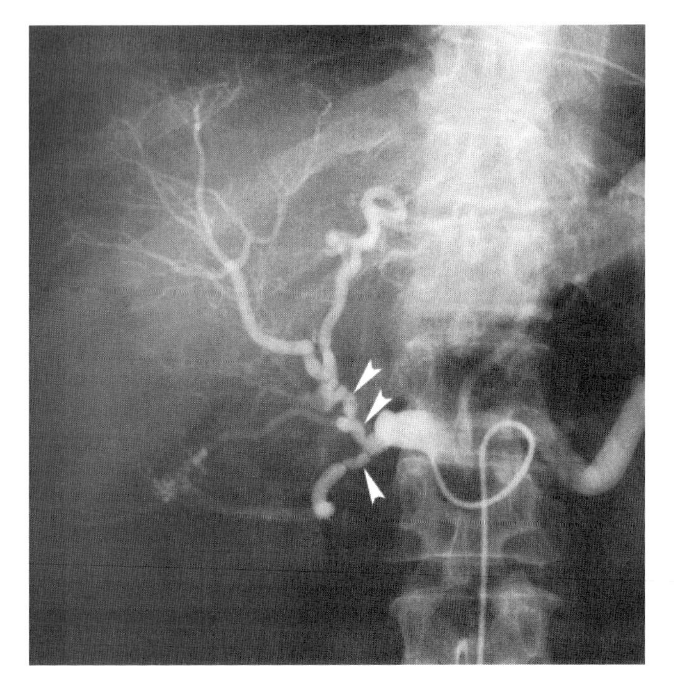

Figure 3.20.1.

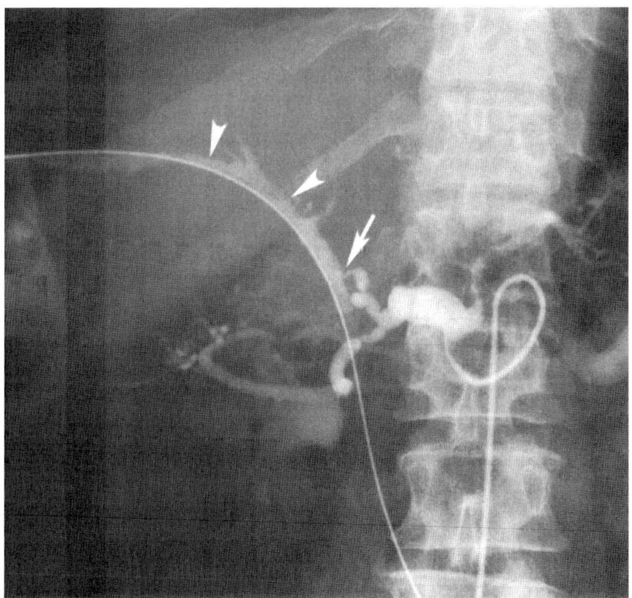

Figure 3.20.2.

Findings. The initial common hepatic artery arteriogram obtained with the faintly radiopaque biliary catheter in place (Fig. 3.20.1) reveals irregular tumor encasement of the proper hepatic and gastroduodenal arteries (*arrowheads*) but no evidence of active bleeding. A repeat hepatic arteriogram acquired after removal of the biliary drainage catheter over a guidewire (Fig. 3.20.2) shows contrast extravasation from the proper hepatic artery into the common bile duct (*arrow*) and drainage of contrast medium along the catheter track (*arrowheads*).

Diagnosis. Arteriobiliary fistula

Discussion. Communication between a branch of the hepatic artery and an adjacent bile duct (an arteriobiliary fistula) results in hemobilia. Arteriobiliary fistulae are most often iatrogenic and may be due to surgery, liver biopsy, or percutaneous transhepatic biliary drainage procedures. They may also result from blunt trauma or may occur spontaneously in patients with hepatic neoplasms (35). In the presence of active bleeding, extravasation of contrast material from a hepatic artery branch into the biliary tree will be seen during hepatic arteriography. Arterial pseudoaneurysms or arterioportal fistulae may be noted in other cases (35). When a percutaneous biliary catheter is present, the tube may temporarily tamponade bleeding, causing a falsely negative study. In this situation, the angiographer may induce bleeding by removing the biliary catheter while maintaining biliary access with a guidewire. Lesions are optimally treated by transcatheter embolotherapy, which allows control of bleeding and preservation of hepatic parenchyma. In the index case, however, the portal vein was found to be occluded, and safe occlusion of the proper hepatic artery was precluded because of the risk of severe hepatic ischemia.

Aunt Minnie's Pearls

- *Hepatic arteriobiliary fistulae occur in the setting of invasive neoplasms or as a result of iatrogenic injuries.*
- *Before embolizing the hepatic artery, always make sure the portal vein is patent so that the liver will have a source of blood flow.*

CASE 21

History. 82-year-old woman with a spontaneous right hemothorax

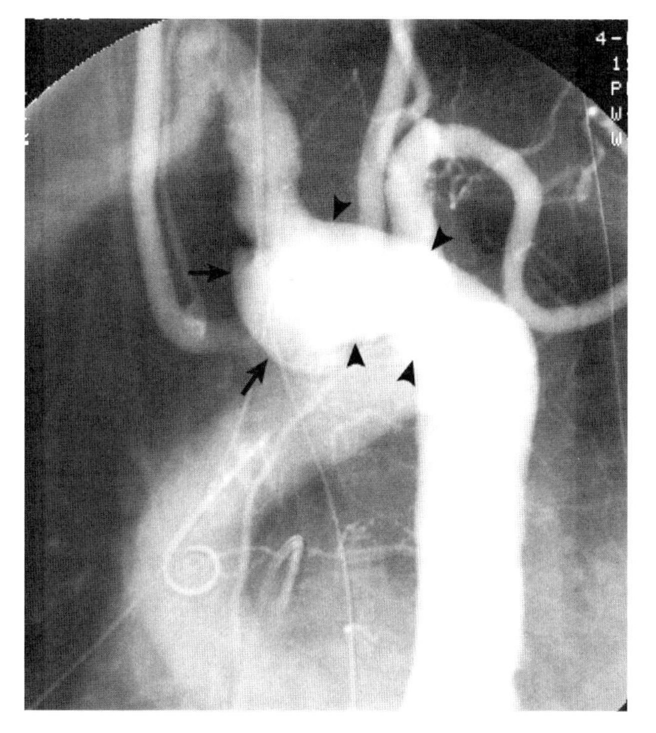

Figure 3.21.1.

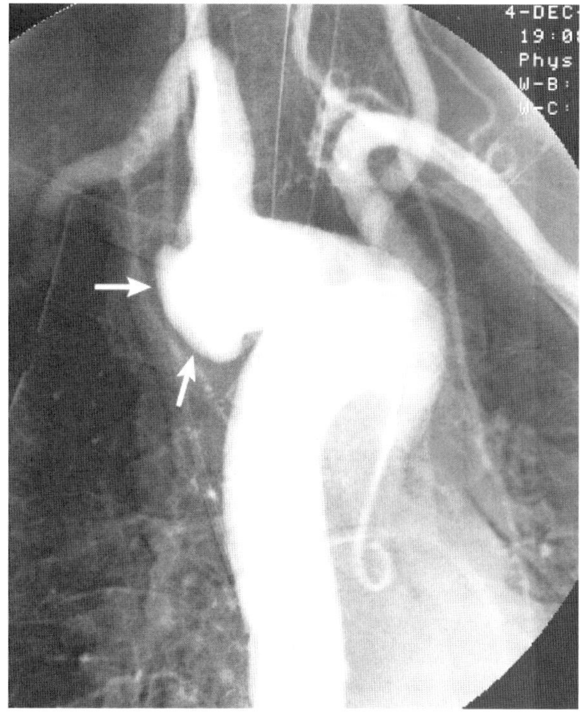

Figure 3.21.2.

Findings. Two views from a thoracic aortogram [Figs. 3.21.1 (RPO) and 3.21.2 (LPO)] reveal a fusiform aneurysm (*arrowheads*) of an aberrant right subclavian artery with a more focal eccentric saccular component (*arrows*).

Diagnosis. Aneurysm of an aberrant right subclavian artery

Discussion. An aberrant right subclavian artery is the most common congenital anomaly of the aortic arch; its incidence is approximately 1% (36). The anomalous vessel, which is always the last great vessel to branch off the aorta, is readily recognized on aortograms as it extends obliquely across the superior mediastinum. The aberrant artery, which is most commonly asymptomatic, rarely compresses the esophagus against the trachea and gives rise to swallowing difficulty, which has been termed "dysphagia lusoria." Even more rarely, atherosclerotic degeneration of the aberrant vessel may result in aneurysmal degeneration. Patients may present with dysphagia, symptoms of airway compression, or chest pain. Death from rupture has been reported, and the patient in the index case presented with intrathoracic hemorrhage. Chest radiography typically reveals a superior mediastinal mass, and this entity can be readily diagnosed with CT or MR imaging. Contrast aortography may be necessary for presurgical planning. Operative treatment involves aneurysm resection and vascular reconstruction (25).

Aunt Minnie's Pearls

- *The aberrant right subclavian artery is the most common anomaly of the great vessels.*
- *Aneurysms of the aberrant vessel occur rarely.*

Case 22

History. 35-year-old man with recent onset of claudication of the right calf and foot

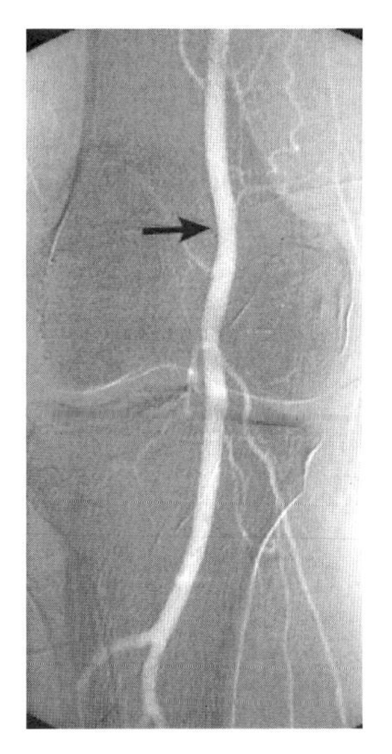

Figure 3.22.1.

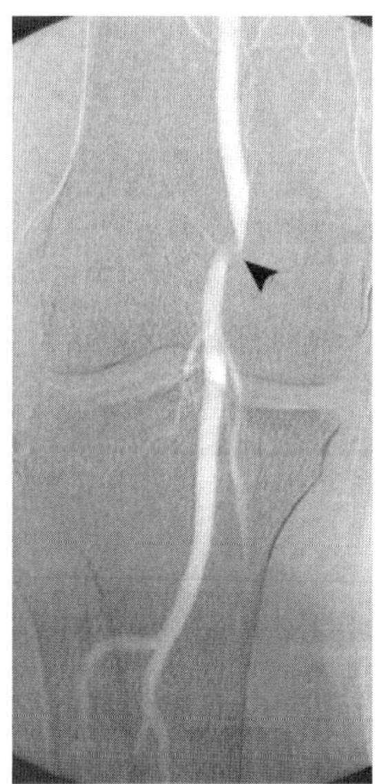

Figure 3.22.2.

Findings. An initial right popliteal arteriogram (Fig. 3.22.1) shows a patent artery without stenosis. However, mild medial deviation of the vessel at the level of the patella is identified (*arrow*). A repeat popliteal arteriogram (Fig. 3.22.2) acquired during active plantar flexion of the right foot against resistance shows further medial deviation and marked luminal compromise (*arrowhead*).

Diagnosis. Popliteal artery entrapment

Discussion. Popliteal artery entrapment is a developmental condition in which the popliteal artery is located medially and deep to the medial head of the gastrocnemius muscle or an abnormal slip of this muscle. Muscular contraction results in arterial luminal compromise. Less commonly, a fibrous band or the popliteus muscle results in compression of the artery. Infrequently, the popliteal vein is also involved. Patients, who are usually men younger than 50 years, generally have no other signs of vascular disease and present with calf and foot claudication that occurs after an episode of vigorous exercise. Although symptoms are usually unilateral, bilateral involvement exists in 25% of cases. Acute onset of symptoms may be due to popliteal artery thrombosis.

The key diagnostic procedure is bilateral lower-extremity angiography. Findings include medial deviation of the proximal popliteal artery, proximal popliteal stenosis with or without poststenotic dilation, or segmental occlusion of the mid-popliteal artery. When initial angiography is not diagnostic, additional stress views during passive dorsiflexion or active plantar flexion of the foot may result in medial deviation and compression of the artery (37). Cystic adventitial disease of the popliteal artery can give a similar appearance in patients with popliteal occlusion (33), and therefore CT (38) or MR imaging (34) may be of value in excluding an adventitial cyst and defining the relationship of the popliteal vessels to adjacent muscles. Treatment involves surgical myotomy, thromboendarterectomy, patch angioplasty, or bypass grafting (37).

Aunt Minnie's Pearls

- *Popliteal artery entrapment is a result of compression of the vessel by the medial head of the gastrocnemius muscle.*
- *In patent vessels, the diagnosis is made by inducing the abnormality with active plantar flexion or passive dorsiflexion during angiography.*

Case 23

History. Young adult man (Figs. 3.23.1 and 3.23.2) involved in a high-speed motor vehicle accident who sustained blunt trauma to the anterior portion of the chest; chest radiograph acquired at admission showed a widened mediastinum

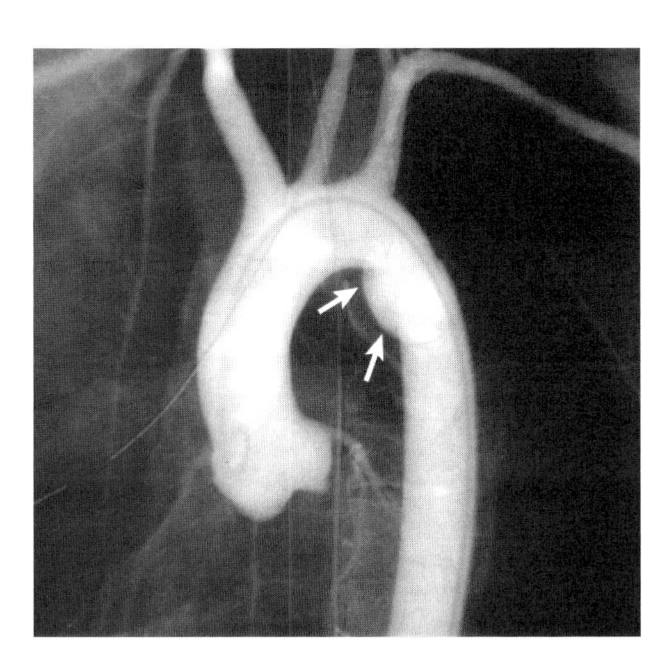

Figure 3.23.1.

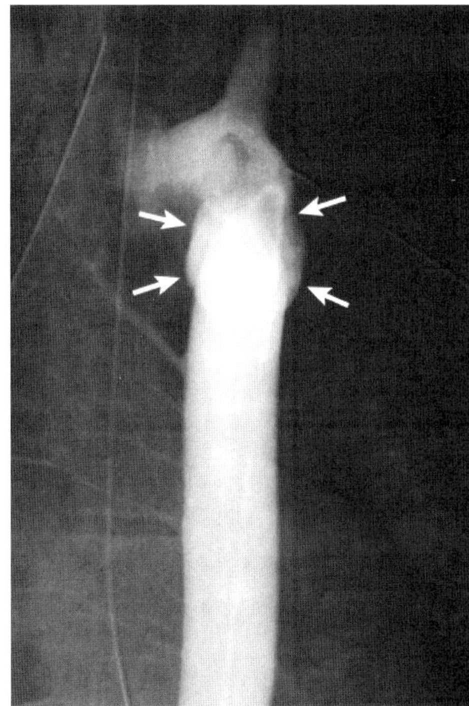

Figure 3.23.2.

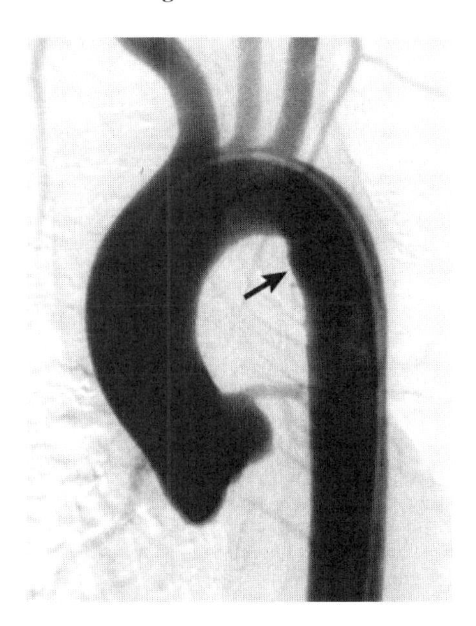

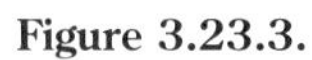

Figure 3.23.3.

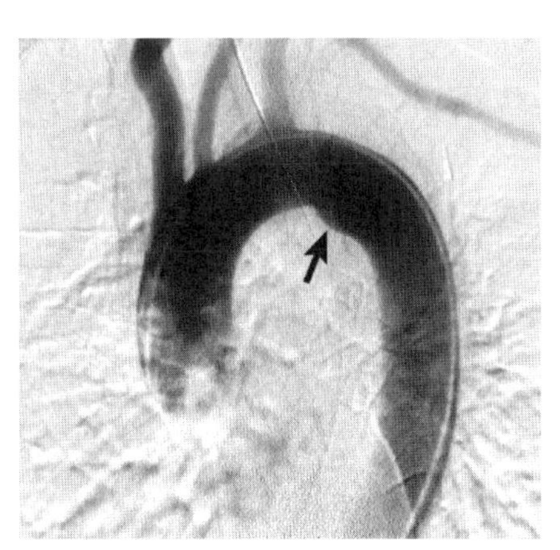

Figure 3.23.4.

Findings. Thoracic aortogram [Figs. 3.23.1 (RPO) and 3.23.2 (AP)] shows a pseudoaneurysm at the aortic isthmus (*arrows*). Thoracic aortograms from two other patients with similar clinical histories (Figs. 3.23.3 and 3.23.4) demonstrate a smoothly contoured luminal convexity along the anteromedial aspect of the aorta at the level of the isthmus (*arrow*), which indicates a ductus diverticulum, a normal variant that can be confused with aortic injury.

Diagnosis. Traumatic rupture of the thoracic aorta

Discussion. Prompt and accurate diagnosis of traumatic rupture of the thoracic aorta is essential. Approximately 90% of the lesions are located at the aortic isthmus, just distal to the origin of the left subclavian artery. Much less commonly, the ascending or distal descending aorta is involved. In autopsy series the percentage of ascending aortic injuries is higher. This disparity may be explained by the fact that ascending aortic injuries are more commonly fatal as a result of aortic valve rupture, coronary artery laceration, severe cardiac contusion, or hemopericardium with cardiac tamponade (39).

Clinical evaluation is an unreliable indicator of aortic injury. Definitive diagnostic tests are necessary. The initial screening test in most cases is a chest radiograph. Various radiographic signs, including mediastinal widening, irregularity of the aortic arch margin, rightward deviation of the trachea or of a nasogastric tube, left apical cap, depression of the left mainstem bronchus, loss of contour of the aorticopulmonary window, widening of the left paraspinal line, loss of contour of the descending thoracic aorta, and thickening of the right paratracheal stripe have all been described as potential signs of aortic injury (40, 41). Chest CT, with or without contrast enhancement, has been used to screen for mediastinal hematoma in patients with equivocal findings on chest radiography (42, 43). Contrast aortography continues to be required for diagnosis of traumatic aortic rupture and should be performed on an emergent basis in patients with clinical or chest radiographic findings suggestive of this injury. Findings may include aortic pseudoaneurysm, intimal tear, complete transection with extravasation, branch vessel injury, posttraumatic dissection, or posttraumatic coarctation (44). False-positive diagnoses have been made in the presence of severe atherosclerosis or as a result of a ductus diverticulum, examples of which are included above. The features of this frequent developmental variant are its smoothly contoured outline, its obtuse margins with the adjoining aortic lumen, and the absence of any luminal irregularity or intraluminal radiolucency (45).

Aunt Minnie's Pearls

- *In patients undergoing angiography, aortic tears occur most commonly just distally to the left subclavian artery.*
- *A ductus diverticulum should have smooth, obtuse margins with the aorta and should never be associated with any intraluminal radiolucencies.*
- *Always be on the lookout for associated great vessel injuries.*

Case 24

History. 63-year-old man with fever and abdominal pain several months after aortobifemoral bypass grafting for aortic aneurysm

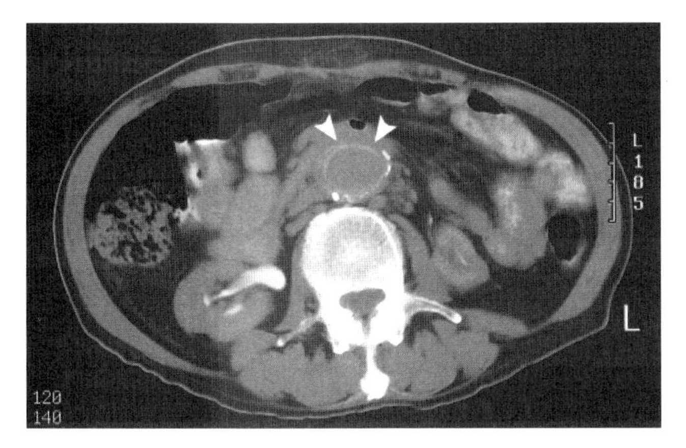

Figure 3.24.1.

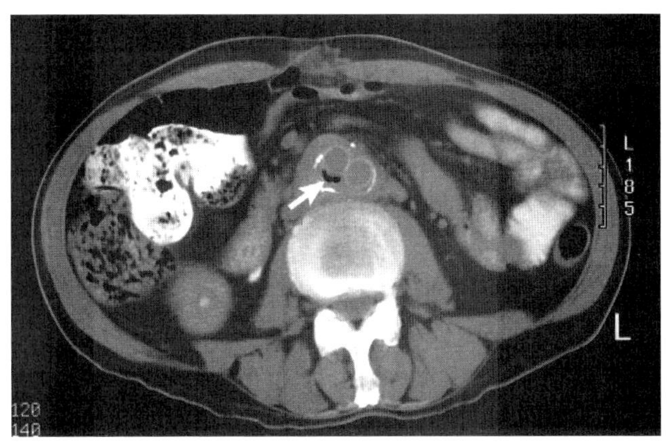

Figure 3.24.2.

Findings. Images from a contrast-enhanced CT scan reveal abnormal perigraft fluid (Fig. 3.24.1, *arrowheads*) outside the aortic wrap and focal gas collections (Fig. 3.24.2, *arrow*) within the perigraft space adjacent to the right limb of the aortofemoral graft.

Diagnosis. Periaortic graft infection

Discussion. Infection of a prosthetic aortic graft is a very serious complication that may lead to limb loss or death. The incidence of such infection ranges from 1 to 2%. The most common cause of graft infection is thought to be contamination of the prosthesis during implantation, although the graft may become infected during a transient bacteremia. When infection extends to involve a graft anastomosis, anastomotic breakdown may lead to formation of an infected pseudoaneurysm. This can result in graft thrombosis, formation of an arterial-enteric fistula, or intraabdominal hemorrhage (46).

CT of infected grafts reveals perigraft fluid collections that are often irregular and septate and are sometimes associated with small pockets of gas. Gas collections, which may normally be seen in the first 10 days after graft placement, are usually single in number and anterior in location. Gas collections that are multiple and posterior in location and that occur more than 10 days after surgery usually indicate perigraft infection (47). They can also indicate an aortoenteric fistula, which presents clinically with gastrointestinal hemorrhage. Management generally involves removal of the infected graft, revascularization by extraanatomic bypass, debridement and drainage of infected tissue, and long-term antibiotic coverage (19).

Aunt Minnie's Pearls

- *Perigraft fluid and gas in a patient more than 10 days after surgery are virtually diagnostic of periaortic graft infection.*
- *Aortoenteric fistulae can have similar imaging findings, but the patient's clinical presentation should exclude this possibility.*

REFERENCES

1. Higgins CB. Essentials of cardiac radiology and imaging. Philadelphia: Lippincott, 1992:184.
2. Williams JE, Honick AB. The great vessels. In: Brant WE, Helms CA, eds. Fundamentals of diagnostic radiology. Baltimore: Williams & Wilkins, 1994:614–617.
3. DeBakey ME, Henley WS, Cooley DA, et al. Surgical management of dissecting aneurysms of the aorta. J Thorac Cardiovasc Surg 1965;49:130–149.
4. Petasnick JP. Radiologic evaluation of aortic dissection. Radiology 1991;180:297–305.
5. Van Praagh R, Van Praagh S, Nebesar RA, Muster AJ, Sinha SN, Paul MH. Tetralogy of Fallot: underdevelopment of the pulmonary infundibulum and its sequelae. Am J Cardiol 1970;26:25–33.
6. Sadler TW. Langman's medical embryology, 5th ed. Baltimore: Williams & Wilkins, 1985:188.
7. Higgins CB. Essentials of cardiac radiology and imaging. Philadelphia: Lippincott, 1992:80.
8. Collett RW, Edward JE. Persistent truncus arteriosus: a classification according to anatomic types. Surg Clin North Am 1949;29: 1245–1270.
9. Van Praagh R. Diagnosis of complex congenital heart disease: morphologic-anatomic method and terminology. Cardiovasc Intervent Radiol 1984;7:115–120.
10. Sadler TW. Langman's medical embryology, 5th ed. Baltimore: Williams & Wilkins, 1985:185.
11. Higgins CB. Essentials of cardiac radiology and imaging. Philadelphia: Lippincott, 1992:84.
12. Higgins CB. Essentials of cardiac radiology and imaging. Philadelphia: Lippincott, 1992:77.
13. Behrman RE, Vaughan VC III. The cardiovascular system. In: Nelson textbook of pediatrics, 13th ed. Philadelphia: Saunders, 1987:976.
14. Goldberg HL, DiMascio A. Psychotropic drugs in pregnancy. In: Lipton MA, DiMascio A, Killam KF, eds. Psychopharmacology: a generation of progress. New York: Raven, 1978:1047–1055.
15. Miller SW. Aortic arch stenoses: coarctation, aortitis, and variants. Appl Radiol 1995;24:15–19.
16. Higgins CB. Essentials of cardiac radiology and imaging. Philadelphia: Lippincott, 1992:174–175.
17. Boley SJ, Sammartano R, Adams A, DiBiase A, Kleinhaus S, Sprayregen S. On the nature and etiology of vascular ectasias of the colon: degenerative lesions of aging. Gastroenterology 1977;72:650–660.
18. Baum S, Athanasoulis CA, Waltman AC, et al. Angiodysplasia of the right colon: a cause of gastrointestinal bleeding. AJR 1977;129:789–794.
19. Reuter SR, Redman HC, Cho KJ. Gastrointestinal angiography, 3rd ed. Philadelphia: Saunders, 1986;1:286–292.
20. Williams LF Jr. Mesenteric ischemia. Surg Clin North Am 1988;68:331–353.
21. Reuter SR, Redman HC, Cho KJ. Gastrointestinal angiography, 3rd ed. Philadelphia: Saunders, 1986;1:109–111.
22. Boley SJ, Sprayregen S, Siegelman SS, Veith FJ. Initial results from an aggressive roentgenological and surgical approach to acute mesenteric ischemia. Surgery 1977;82:848–855.
23. Reuter SR, Redman HC, Cho KJ. Gastrointestinal angiography, 3rd ed. Philadelphia: Saunders, 1986;1:422–425.
24. Conn J Jr, Bergan JJ, Bell JL. Hypothenar hammer syndrome: posttraumatic digital ischemia. Surgery 1970;68:1122–1128.
25. Clagett GP. Upper extremity aneurysms. In: Rutherford RB, ed. Vascular surgery, 3rd ed. Philadelphia: Saunders, 1989;2:957–969.
26. Ferris EJ, Lim WN, Smith PL, Casali R. May-Thurner syndrome. Radiology 1983;147:29–31.
27. Fields WS, Lemak NA. Joint study of extracranial arterial occlusion. VII. Subclavian steal—a review of 168 cases. JAMA 1972;222:1139–1143.
28. Hafner CD. Subclavian steal syndrome: a 12-year experience. Arch Surg 1976; 111:1074–1180.
29. Kadir S. Diagnostic angiography. Philadelphia: Saunders, 1986:445–495.
30. Takebayashi S, Aida N, Matsui K. Arteriovenous malformations of the kidneys: diagnosis and follow-up with color Doppler sonography in six patients. AJR 1991;157:991–995.
31. Honda H, Onitsuka H, Naitou S, et al. Renal arteriovenous malformations: CT features. J Comput Assist Tomogr 1991;15:261–264.
32. Bergan JJ. Adventitial cystic disease of the popliteal artery. In: Rutherford RB. Vascular surgery, 3rd ed. Philadelphia: Saunders, 1989;1:773–779.
33. Fitzjohn TP, White FE, Loose HW, Proud G. Computed tomography and sonography of cystic adventitial disease. Br J Radiol 1986;59:933–935.
34. Berger MF, Weber EE. MR imaging of recurrent cystic adventitial disease of the popliteal artery. J Vasc Interv Radiol 1993;4:695–697.
35. Routh WD, Tatum CM, Lawdahl RB, Rosch J, Keller FS. Tube tamponade: potential pitfall in angiography of arterial hemorrhage associated with percutaneous drainage catheters. Radiology 1990;174:945–949.
36. Kadir S. Regional anatomy of the thoracic aorta. In: Kadir S, ed. Atlas of normal and variant angiographic anatomy. Philadelphia: Saunders, 1991:19–54.
37. Whelon TJ Jr. Popliteal artery entrapment. In: Rutherford RB, ed. Vascular surgery. Philadelphia: Saunders, 1989:779–783.
38. Williams LR, Flinn WR, McCarthy WJ, Yao JS, Bergan JJ. Popliteal artery entrapment: diagnosis by computed tomography. J Vasc Surg 1986;3:360–363.
39. Parmley LF, Mattingly TW, Marion WC, et al. Nonpenetrating traumatic injury of the heart. Circulation 1958;18:371–396.
40. Marnocha KE, Meglinte DDT. Plain film criteria for excluding aortic rupture in blunt chest trauma. AJR 1985;144:19–21.
41. Mirvis SE, Bidwell JK, Buddemeyer EU, et al. Value of chest radiography in excluding traumatic aortic rupture. Radiology 1987;163:487–493.

42. Madayag MA, Kirshenbaum KJ, Nadimpalli SR, Fantus RJ, Cavallino RP, Crystal GJ. Thoracic aortic trauma: role of dynamic CT. Radiology 1991;179:853–855.
43. Richardson P, Mirvis SE, Scorpio R, Dunham CM. Value of CT in determining the need for angiography when findings of mediastinal hemorrhage on chest radiographs are equivocal. AJR 1991;156:273–279.
44. Kadir S. Arteriography of the thoracic aorta. In: Kadir S, ed. Diagnostic angiography. Philadelphia: Saunders, 1986:124–171.
45. Morse SS, Glickman MG, Greenwood LH, et al. Traumatic aortic rupture: false-positive aortographic diagnosis due to atypical ductus diverticulum. AJR 1988;150:793–796.
46. Freischlag JA, Moore WS. Infection in prosthetic vascular grafts. In: Rutherford RB, ed. Vascular surgery. Philadelphia: Saunders, 1989:510–521.
47. Lee JKT. Retroperitoneum: postoperative complications. In: Lee JKT, Sagel SS, Stanley RJ, eds. Computed body tomography with MRI correlation. New York: Raven, 1989:707–753.

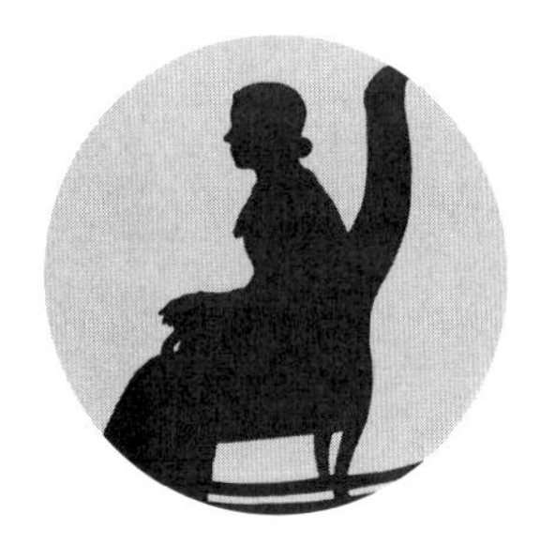

chapter 4

ULTRASOUND

KENNETH L. FORD III, SAM T. AURINGER, TOM C. WINTER III,
SHARLENE A. TEEFEY, AND WILLIAM D. MIDDLETON

CASE 1

History. 34-year-old gravid woman (estimated gestational age = 22.5 weeks) with maternal serum alpha-fetoprotein level of 5.3 multiples of the median

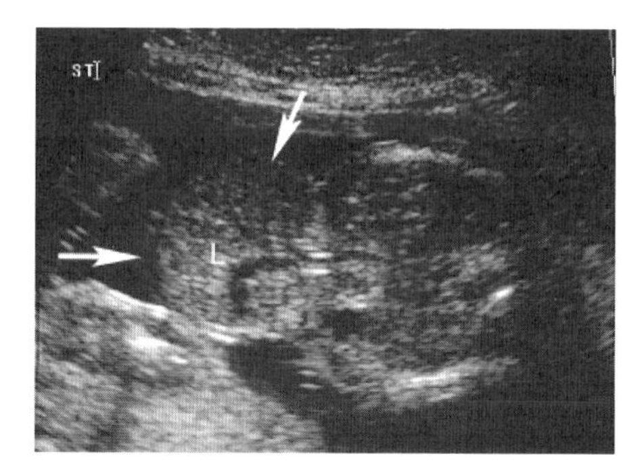

Figure 4.1.1.

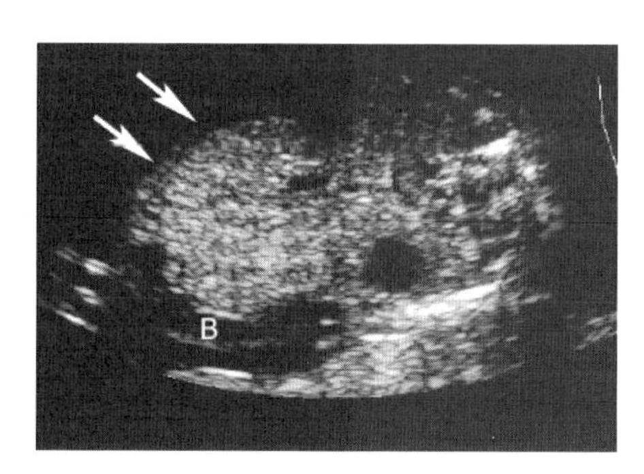

Figure 4.1.2.

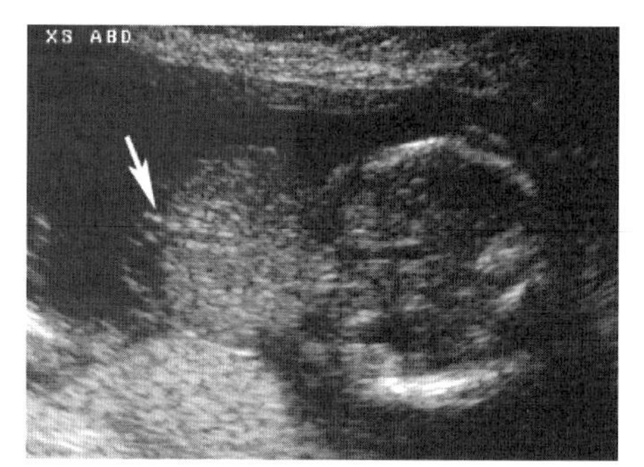

Figure 4.1.3.

Findings. A 3.5-cm defect of the ventral aspect of the fetal anterior abdominal wall is present on these transverse views of the fetal abdomen. Through this defect protrudes a solid mass approximately 4 cm in diameter (Fig 4.1.1, *arrows*). This mass contains both liver (L) and bowel (B) and is covered by a thin membrane (Fig. 4.1.2, *arrows*). Figure 4.1.3 reveals that the umbilical cord inserts into the mass (*arrow*).

Diagnosis. Omphalocele

Discussion. Omphaloceles (exomphalos) occur in one of 4000 live births and are usually detected during routine sonographic examination of the fetal abdomen or in the work-up for elevated alpha-fetoprotein levels. The defect consists of herniation of abdominal contents into the base of the umbilical cord. The cord inserts into the apical-caudal aspect of the mass, unlike gastroschisis, in which the cord inserts normally into the abdominal wall. Although the delineating peritoneal-amniotic membrane is not always easily visible, its presence can be inferred from the smooth surface of the herniated mass. This should be contrasted to gastroschisis, in which there is no delineating membrane and the loops of bowel float freely within the amniotic cavity. The presence of liver within an omphalocele can be inferred by the homogenous appearance of the herniated mass, the presence of intrahepatic vessels, and the large size of the defect (1–3).

Associated anomalies have been reported in 67–88% of fetuses with omphalocele identified prenatally. These anomalies include both karyotype abnormalities and nonchromosomal structural anomalies. Interestingly, chromosome abnormalities have been more strongly associated with small omphalocele sacs that do not contain liver.

Aunt Minnie's Pearls

- *Herniation of abdominal contents into the base of the umbilical cord = omphalocele.*
- *Small omphaloceles that do not contain liver have a stronger association with chromosomal abnormalities than do larger omphaloceles.*

CASE 2

History. 32-year-old gravid woman with maternal serum alpha-fetoprotein of 2.6 multiples of the median

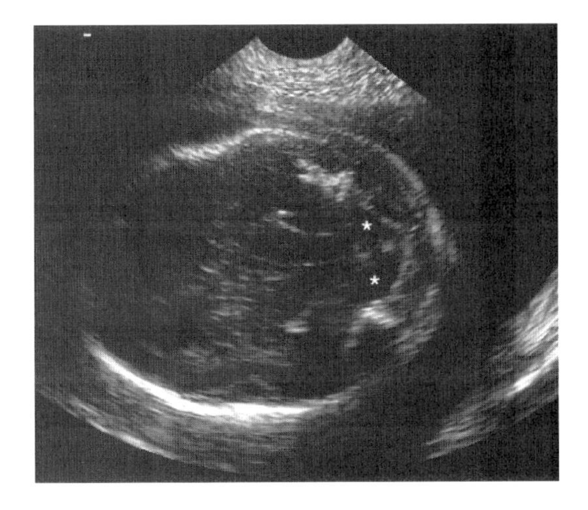

Figure 4.2.1.

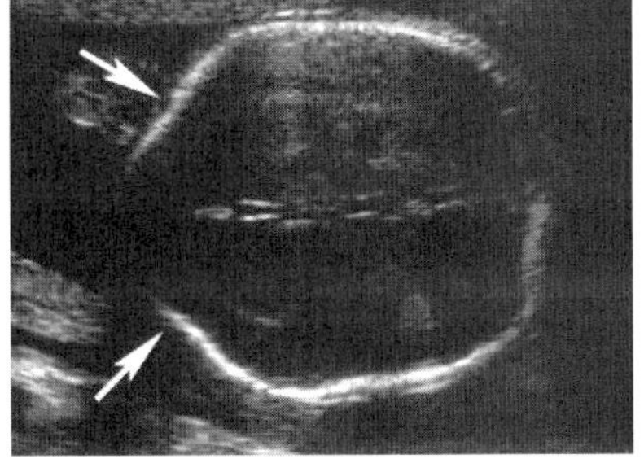

Figure 4.2.2.

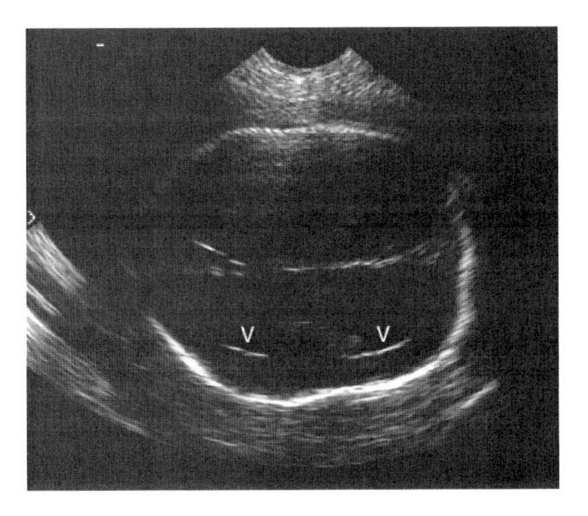

Figure 4.2.3.

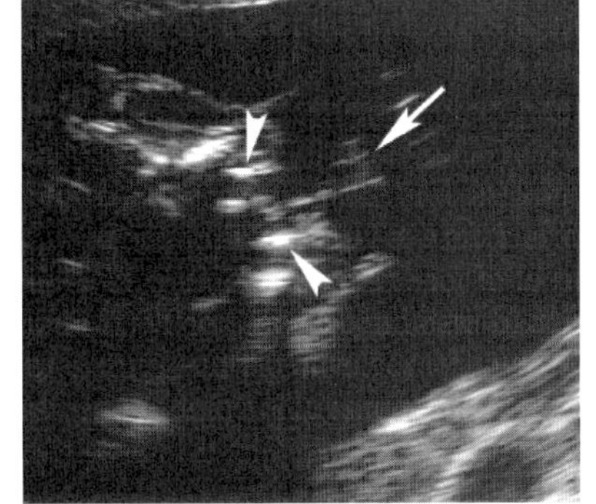

Figure 4.2.4.

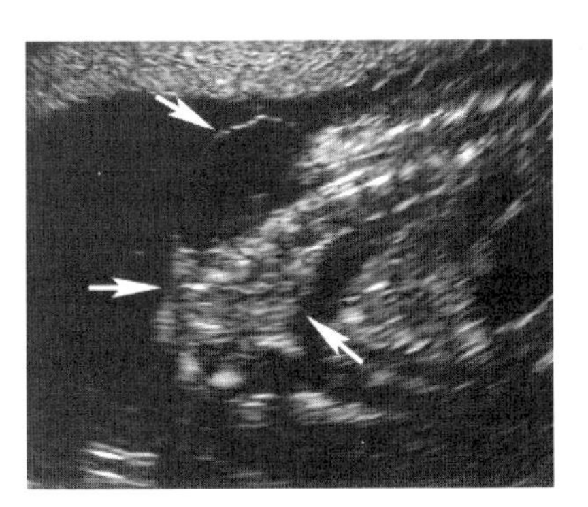

Figure 4.2.5.

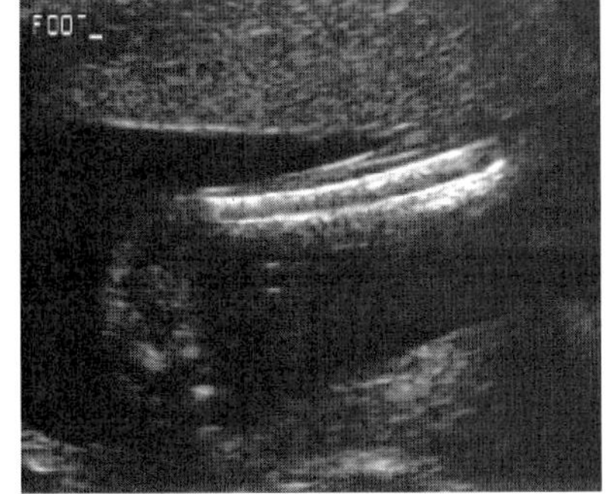

Figure 4.2.6.

Findings. Classic banana sign [obliteration of posterior fossa and curved appearance of the herniated cerebellum (Fig. 4.2.1, *asterisks*)] and lemon sign [abnormal bifrontal concavity (Fig. 4.2.2, *arrows*)] are noted in the cranium of this 20-week-gestation fetus. Mild ventriculomegaly (V) is present (Fig. 4.2.3), and the lateral ventricles measure 13 mm (up to 10 mm is normal). Axial (Fig. 4.2.4) and sagittal (Fig. 4.2.5) views of the spine demonstrate the flared laminae (Fig. 4.2.4, *arrowheads*), which are diagnostic of spina bifida and the associated meningomyelocele (Figs. 4.2.4 and 4.2.5, *arrows*) extending from approximately L3 through S3. Bilateral club feet were also present [only the right foot is shown (Fig. 4.2.6)].

Diagnosis. Chiari II (Arnold-Chiari) malformation and associated meningomyelocele

Discussion. Open neural tube defects are the most common central nervous system malformation (4, 5). Direct visualization of a meningomyelocele may be difficult, however, and even the most skilled examiner may worry about false-negative results. Fortunately for the sonologist, meningomyeloceles are almost always accompanied by the Arnold-Chiari malformation, which has more easily recognizable cranial findings. These include obliteration of the cisterna magna, the lemon sign, ventricular dilatation, and a disproportionately small biparietal diameter. Posterior fossa abnormalities, including obliteration of the cisterna magna and banana-shaped cerebellum, are almost diagnostic of associated open meningomyelocele. Conversely, a normal cisterna magna virtually eliminates the possibility of spina bifida. The lemon sign, although quite useful, is not specific for meningomyelocele (6, 7). In addition, resolution of the lemon sign in fetuses with meningomyelocele invariably occurs by the 34th week of gestation.

The presence of these characteristic cranial findings should serve as a marker for a meningomyelocele. The bony spinal defect should be imaged as should the associated soft-tissue findings (myelomeningocele sac, disruption of the overlying skin, or both). The level and extent of the defect should be reported.

As with all detected prenatal abnormalities, the remainder of the fetus should be carefully examined for associated abnormalities. In particular, neuromuscular anomalies caused by the spinal defect lead to the development of club foot. Meningomyelocele also may be associated with an increased risk of karyotype abnormality (8).

Neural tube defects are usually accompanied by abnormally high levels of maternal serum alpha-fetoprotein. The rate of neural tube defects and the risk of recurrence can be decreased by maternal folate supplementation around the time of conception (9).

Aunt Minnie's Pearls

- *Lemon and banana signs imply meningomyelocele.*

CASE 3

History. 30-year-old woman at 21 weeks gestation; prior sonography was performed in Australia at 8 weeks of gestation (a routine study was requested as part of initial patient evaluation in the United States)

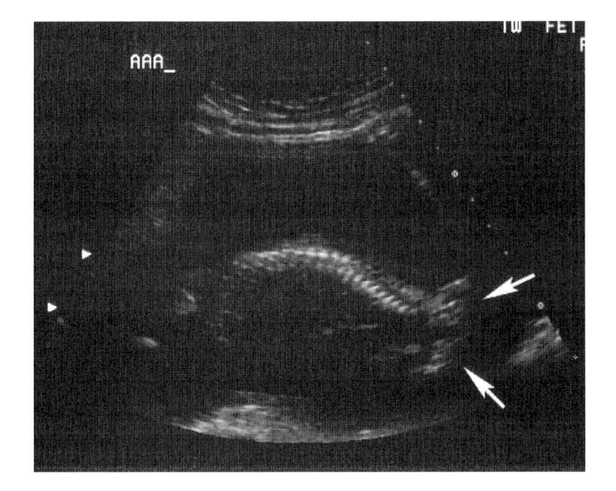

Figure 4.3.1.

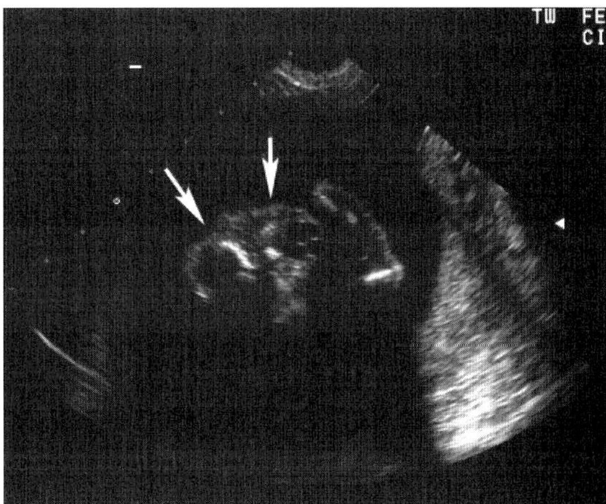

Figure 4.3.2.

Findings. Transabdominal sagittal view of the fetal spine does not demonstrate a normal head (Fig. 4.3.1, *arrows*). Transvaginal coronal view of the face confirms absence of the calvarium and brain cephalad to the orbits (Fig. 4.3.2, *arrows*).

Diagnosis. Anencephaly

Discussion. Anencephaly, which results from failure of the rostral neuropore to close by the 24th day of fetal life, is the single most common type of neural tube defect; it is reported in one in 1000 births (4, 5). A distinct female predominance is seen in anencephaly; the female-to-male ratio is 4:1. Elevated alpha-fetoprotein levels can be detected early in pregnancy, and polyhydramnios is seen in up to half of cases after 26 weeks of gestation. Symmetric loss of both ***brain tissue*** and ***calvarium*** cephalad to the bony orbits is the most reliable feature of this anomaly and is best demonstrated on a coronal image of the fetal face. Angiomatous stroma may be seen above the fetal orbits (area cerebrovasculosa); in such cases, it may be difficult to distinguish this disorder from congenital absence of the calvarium (exencephaly), in which some brain tissue is present above the orbits. Because the bony calvarium cannot be identified with transvaginal sonography before 11.5 weeks of gestation, anencephaly should not be diagnosed before this time.

Up to one-third of cases of anencephaly may have additional anomalies, most commonly spina bifida. If identified, the spinal dysraphism can help to distinguish anencephaly from exencephaly in difficult cases (10). This distinction is important, because the risk of neural tube defects in future pregnancies is greater in mothers of anencephalic children. Again, periconceptional folate acid supplementation decreases the risk of anencephaly.

Aunt Minnie's Pearls

- *Anencephaly = loss of brain tissue and calvarium in a fetus older than 11.5 weeks of gestation.*

CASE 4

History. 32-year-old gravid woman, 33 weeks pregnant, who had two previous cesarean deliveries

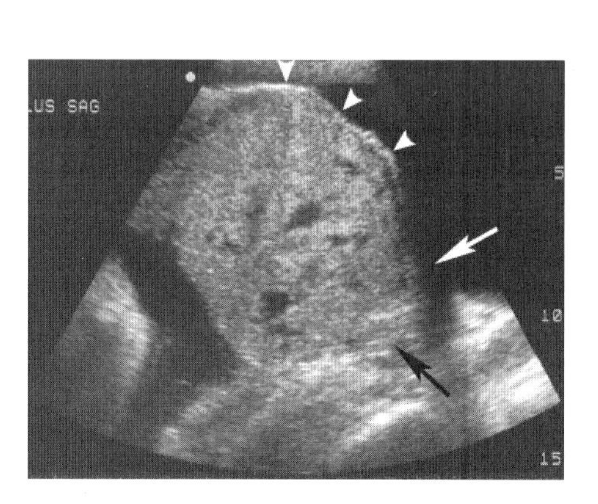

Figure 4.4.1.

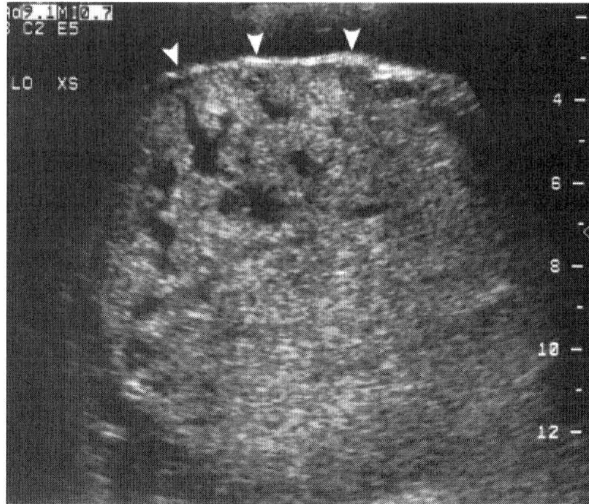

Figure 4.4.2.

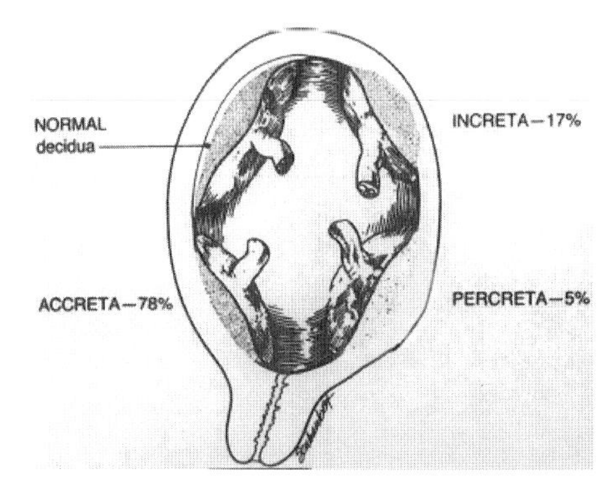

Figure 4.4.3. Differences between normal decidualization and placenta accreta, increta, and percreta along with the relative frequencies of the three subtypes of placenta accreta.

Findings. Sagittal (Fig. 4.4.1) and transverse (Fig. 4.4.2) images of the lower uterine segment demonstrate complete placenta previa (Fig. 4.4.1, *arrows*) and associated absence of the normal hypoechoic myometrium between the placenta and the uterine serosa-bladder wall complex (*arrowheads*).

Diagnosis. Placenta accreta

Discussion. Placenta accreta is defined clinically as an abnormal adherence of the placenta to the uterine wall so that separation does not occur after delivery of the newborn. The pathologic correlate is a partial or complete absence of the decidua and resulting abnormal form of implantation, in which the placental villi adhere directly to (*placenta accreta*), invade into (*placenta increta*), or penetrate through (*placenta percreta*) the myometrium (Fig. 4.4.3). For practical purposes, the term placenta accreta often encompasses all three entities (11).

Although placenta accreta is uncommon (12), predisposing factors include multiparous pregnancies and a history of cesarean section or placenta previa involving the lower anterior uterine wall. In high-risk patients, accurate prospective sonographic diagnosis of placenta accreta may be possible by using (*a*) loss of the normal hypoechoic retroplacental myometrial zone between the placenta and the uterine serosa-bladder wall; (*b*) thinning, irregularity, or disruption of the linear hyperechoic uterine serosa-bladder wall complex interface; or (*c*) presence of focal exophytic masses (extension of placental tissue beyond the uterine serosa) (13).

The morbidity of placenta accreta is related to difficulty in completely extracting the placenta after delivery, which may result in severe hemorrhage, requiring hysterectomy. Therefore, prospective sonographic diagnosis is important, particularly in high-risk patients.

Aunt Minnie's Pearls

- *Abnormal attachment of the placenta to the uterine wall = placenta accreta.*
- *Failure to prospectively diagnose this anomaly may result in severe maternal hemorrhage.*

CASE 5

History. 27-year-old gravid woman with a history of a second trimester spontaneous abortion

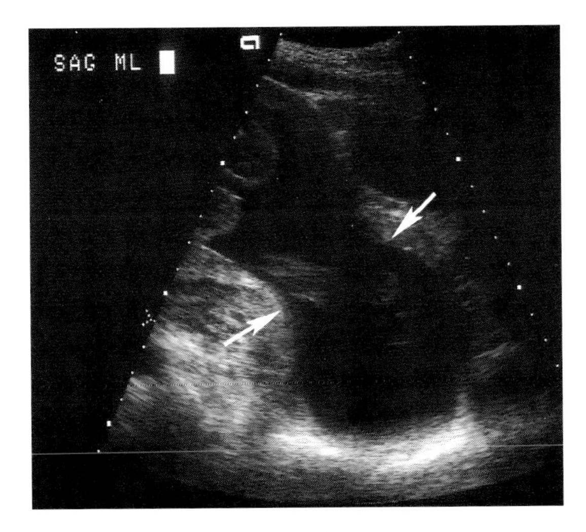

Figure 4.5.1.

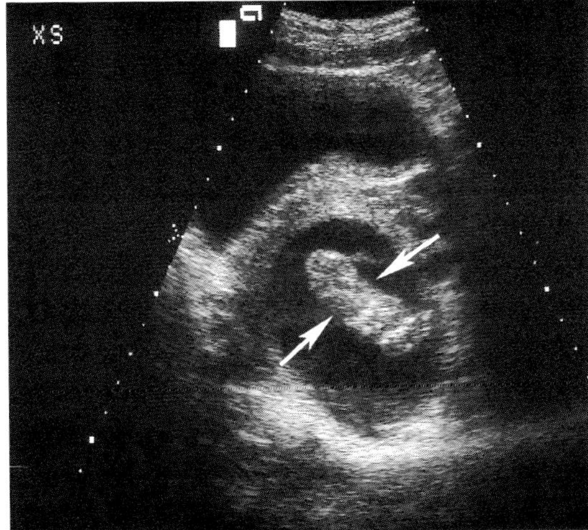

Figure 4.5.2.

Findings. A sagittal image reveals that the cervix is dilated to 3 cm, and classic hourglass bulging membranes protrude into the vagina (Fig. 4.5.1, *arrows*). In addition, the fetal foot is seen on a transverse image of the cervix (Fig. 4.5.2, *arrows*).

Diagnosis. Cervical incompetence

Discussion. Cervical incompetence is a functional condition in patients who often present with a history of recurrent, usually painless second-trimester spontaneous abortions. Sonographic findings of a cervix less than 3 cm long, a gaping internal os, and funneling or tunneling of the patient's membranes into the endocervical canal can be associated with preterm delivery (15). The shorter the cervix, the more likely the patient will deliver prematurely. Cervical cerclage is the treatment of choice.

The cervix can change, often dramatically, during the sonographic examination. The cervix may appear completely normal at one point in the examination and grossly abnormal at another. Therefore, in high-risk patients, the cervix should be imaged more than once and observed continuously for several minutes (16).

Aunt Minnie's Pearls

- *Hourglass membranes gaping through cervical os = severe cervical incompetence.*

CASE 6

History. Uncertain dates

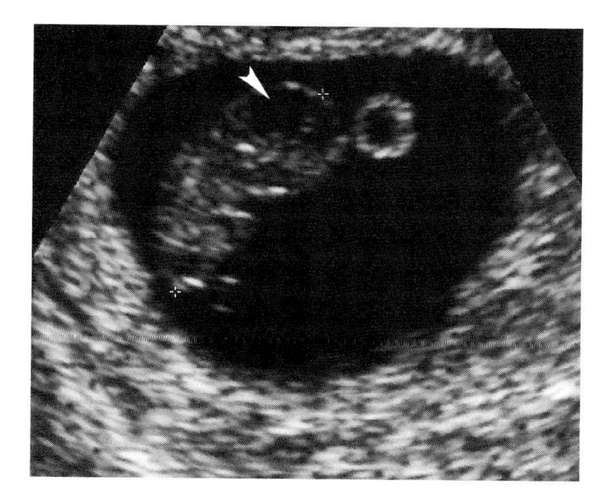

Figure 4.6.1.

Findings. Transvaginal image in the sagittal plane (Fig. 4.6.1) shows a 4-mm smoothly marginated anechoic cystic mass in the posterior aspect of the fetal head (*arrowheads*) in this 8-week-gestation fetus

Diagnosis. Normal rhombencephalon

Discussion. The introduction of transvaginal probes and accompanying equipment improvements allows for exquisite visualization of first-trimester fetal anatomy. The cystic structure demonstrated here in the posterior aspect of the first-trimester embryonic cranium represents the rhomboid fossa (part of the rhombencephalon complex). This is a normal structure that can be routinely seen on ultrasonographic images between the 8th and 12th menstrual weeks and typically measures 3–4 mm in diameter (17). It should not be confused with an abnormal cystic posterior fossa structure, such as a Dandy-Walker cyst or other neural anomalies.

Aunt Minnie's Pearls

- *The rhombencephalon is a normal cystic structure in the fetal cranium between 8 and 12 menstrual weeks.*

CASE 7

History. Repeated bouts of urinary colic

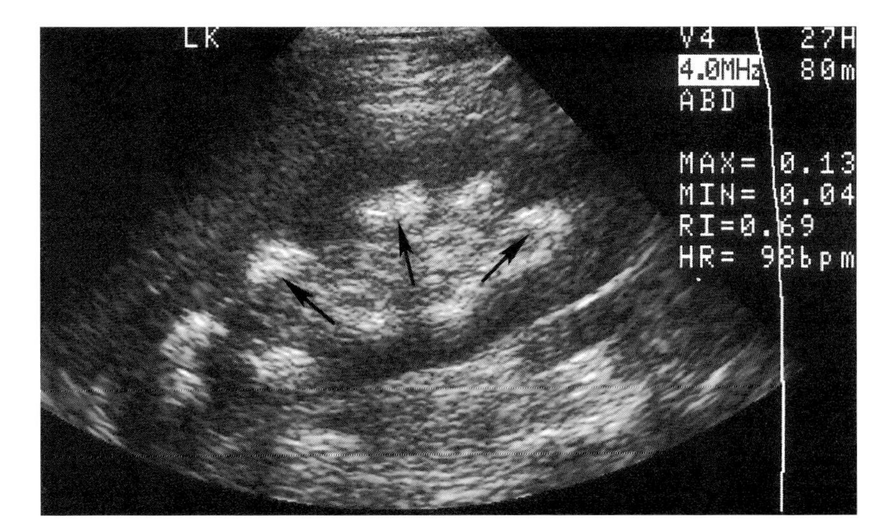

Figure 4.7.1.

Findings. A longitudinal view of the kidney (Fig. 4.7.1) demonstrates markedly increased echogenicity in the renal pyramids (*arrows*). The renal cortex is normal in echogenicity, and no hydronephrosis is identified. The kidneys are normal in shape and are otherwise unremarkable.

Diagnosis. Medullary nephrocalcinosis

Discussion. Nephrocalcinosis is defined as abnormal deposition of calcium salts in the renal cortex (cortical nephrocalcinosis) or pyramids (medullary nephrocalcinosis). This should be distinguished from urinary stone formation, which is termed urolithiasis. Medullary nephrocalcinosis can be recognized on ultrasonography as markedly hyperechoic renal pyramids, which may produce distal acoustic shadowing. Early medullary nephrocalcinosis may appear as hyperechoic rings around the pyramids. Sonography is more sensitive than plain films for the diagnosis of nephrocalcinosis; therefore, correlation with a KUB is not always helpful (18).

The three leading causes of medullary nephrocalcinosis include hyperparathyroidism (40%), medullary sponge kidney (20%), and distal type I renal tubular acidosis (20%) (19). Other causes of hypercalcemia that can produce medullary nephrocalcinosis include drugs (steroids and furosemide), sarcoidosis, immobilization, milk alkali syndrome, paraneoplastic syndromes, hypervitaminosis D, and hyperthyroidism. If the calcification is noticeably segmental, medullary sponge kidney is the primary consideration because other leading causes of medullary nephrocalcinosis typically produce diffuse and bilateral renal involvement. The combination of cortical and medullary nephrocalcinosis strongly suggests primary oxaluria.

Aunt Minnie's Pearls

- *Hyperechoic renal pyramids with or without distal acoustic shadowing = medullary nephrocalcinosis.*
- *Hyperparathyroidism, medullary sponge kidney, and distal renal tubular acidosis are the leading causes.*

CASE 8

History. Patient with a renal transplant that was recently evaluated because of elevating creatinine

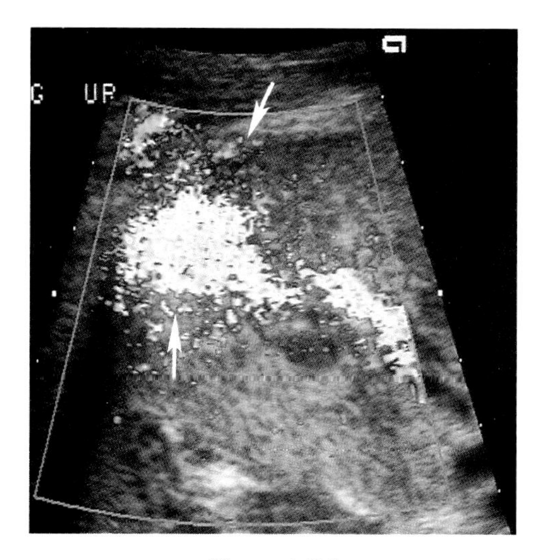

Figure 4.8.1.

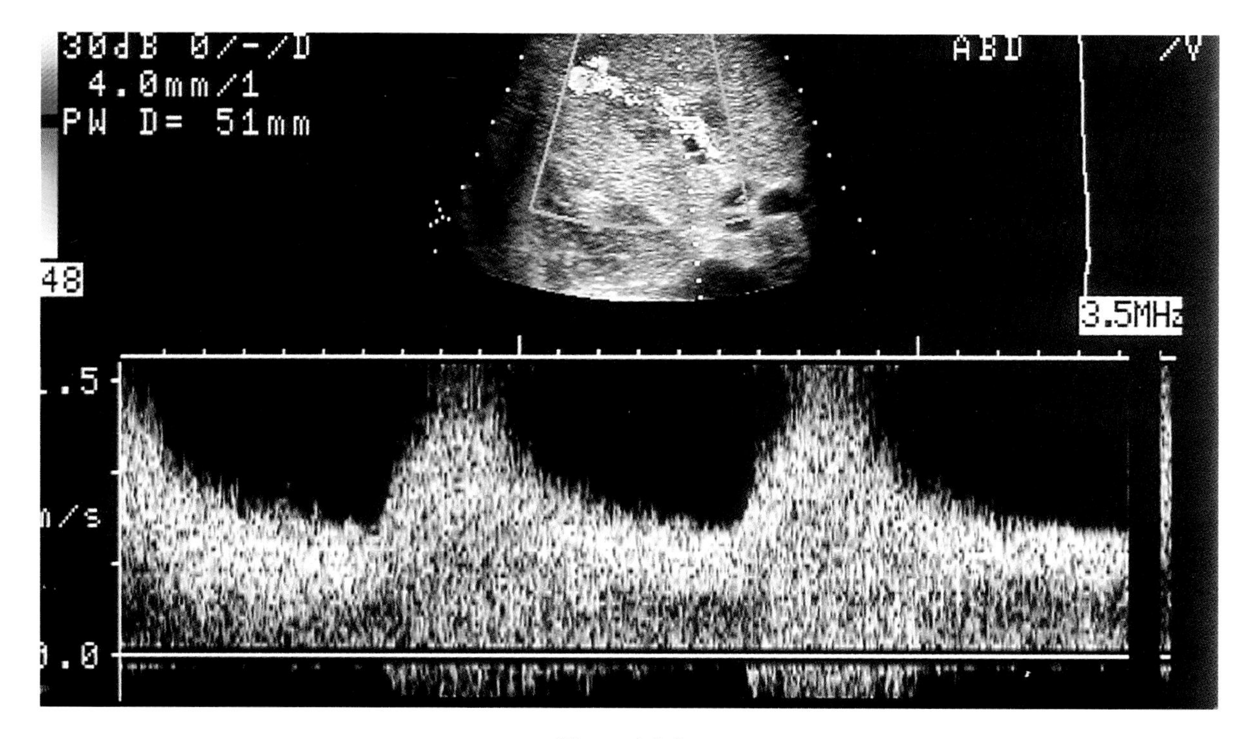

Figure 4.8.2.

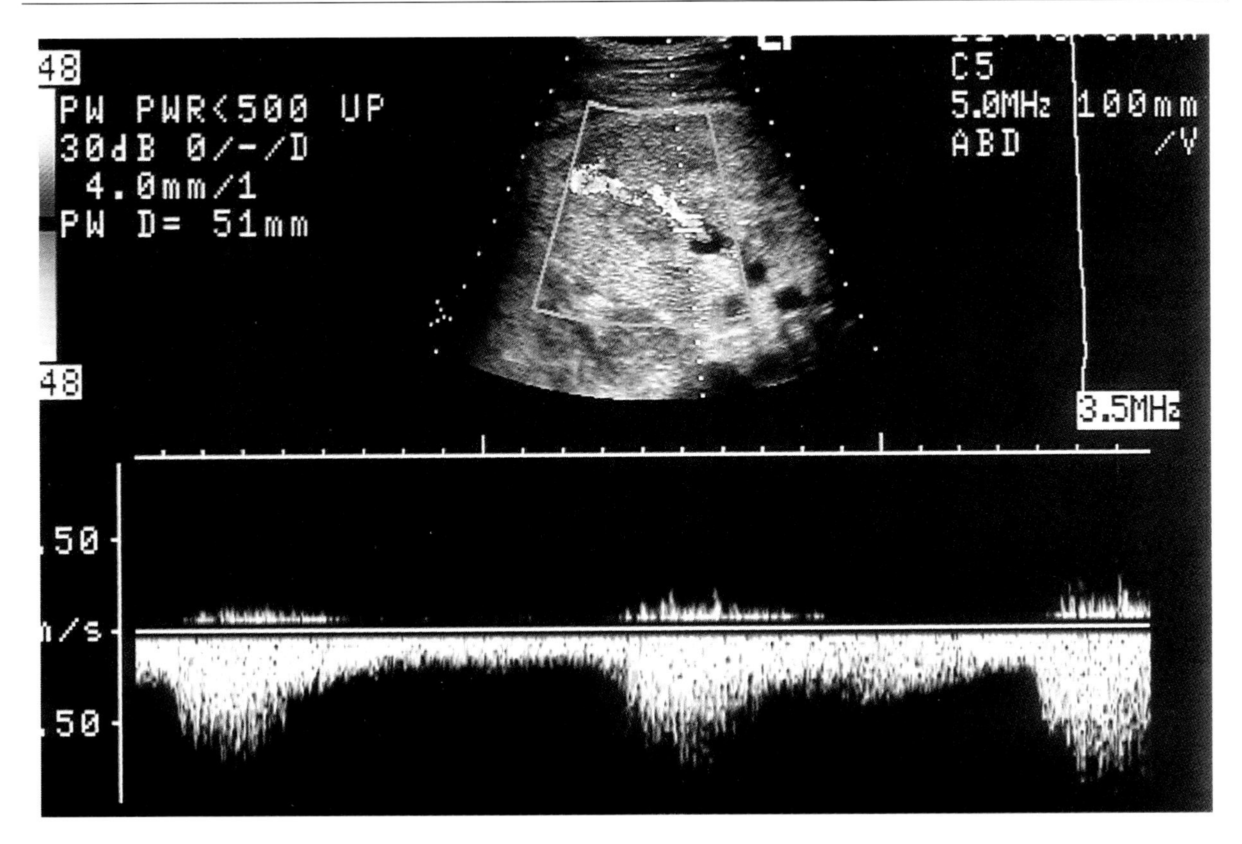

Figure 4.8.3.

Findings. Color Doppler examination of the transplant kidney demonstrates marked perivascular tissue vibration in the upper pole parenchyma (Fig. 4.8.1, *arrows*). Doppler waveform of a renal artery in the same region (Fig. 4.8.2) reveals abnormally high peak systolic and end-diastolic velocities (peak systolic flow in this case is >150 cm/s; the normal range is ≈20–50 cm/s) (20). The renal vein in this region has an arterialized waveform (Fig. 4.8.3).

Diagnosis. Traumatic (postbiopsy) arteriovenous fistula (AVF) in a renal transplant

Discussion. An AVF is an abnormal direct communication between an artery and a vein. The most common etiology for a renal transplant AVF is percutaneous biopsy. Characteristic color and pulse-wave Doppler findings allow specific diagnosis of this entity in many instances. Because of the rapid and turbulent blood flow in the AVF, the surrounding soft tissues vibrate with an amplitude that varies with the cardiac cycle (20). The vibrating tissue interfaces produce a Doppler frequency shift that is the Doppler equivalent of a bruit. The result is random red and blue color assignment in the soft tissues surrounding the AVF (21). Abundant and fast flow in both systole and diastole in the feeding artery leads to abnormally high peak systolic and end diastolic velocities, as in the case demonstrated. Because arterial blood is in direct communication with a draining vein, the venous Doppler waveform may be pulsatile or "arterialized." This latter finding is conclusive evidence of an AVF (22).

Aunt Minnie's Pearls

- *Perivascular tissue vibration, high peak-systolic and end-diastolic velocities, and arterialized venous waveform are diagnostic of an AVF.*
- *AVF in a renal transplant is usually due to percutaneous biopsy.*

CASE 9

History. Mentally challenged patient who gives a history of a left nephrectomy

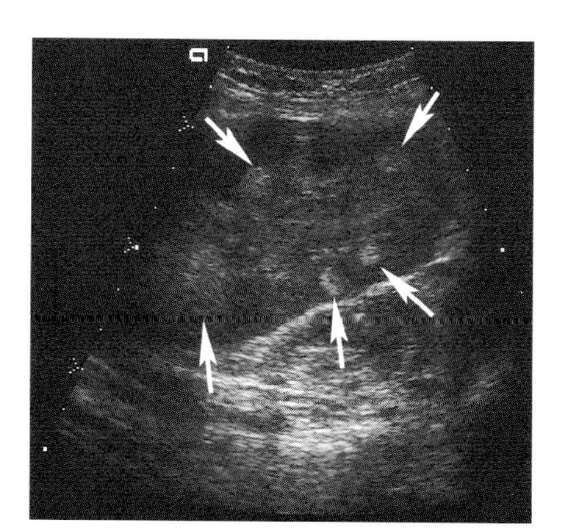

Figure 4.9.1.

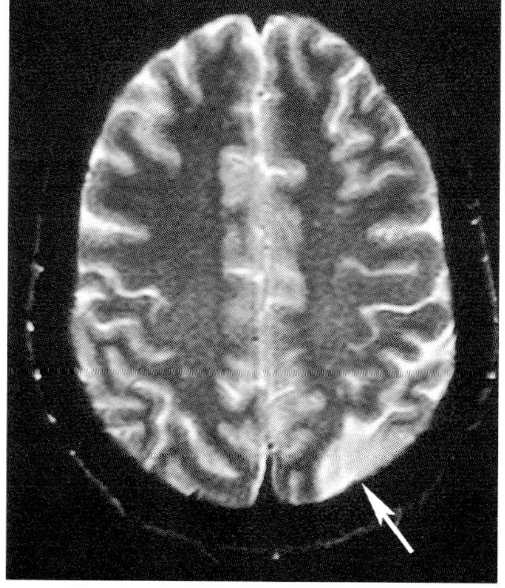

Figure 4.9.2. Axial SE 3000/90.

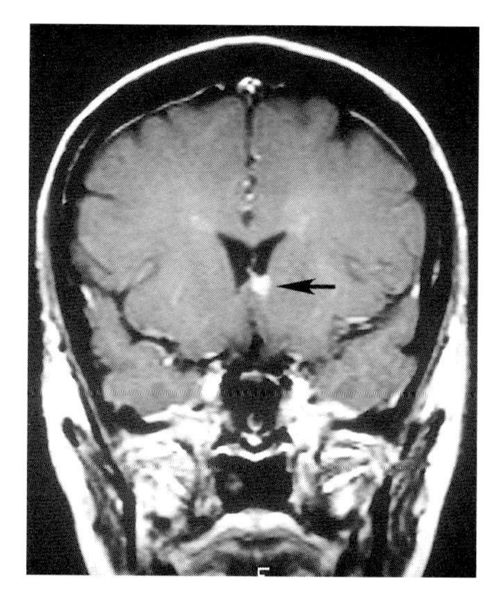

Figure 4.9.3. Coronal MRI with gadolinium, SE 817/30.

Findings. A longitudinal ultrasound image of the right kidney (Fig. 4.9.1) demonstrates numerous homogenously hyperechoic masses originating in the renal cortex (*arrows*). A previously acquired MR image of the brain reveals findings of cortical tubers (Fig. 4.9.2, *arrow*) and a giant cell astrocytoma near the foramen of Monro (Fig. 4.9.3, *arrow*).

Diagnosis. Renal angiomyolipomas in a patient with tuberous sclerosis

Discussion. A solitary hyperechoic mass in the kidney can be caused by several benign and malignant processes. When innumerable well-defined hyperechoic masses are seen, however, the differential diagnosis is more limited; most of these cases represent angiomyolipomas in patients with tuberous sclerosis. However, approximately 5% of patients with innumerable renal angiomyolipomas do not have stigmata of tuberous sclerosis (23). To make a confident imaging-specific diagnosis, correlation with other imaging modalities is necessary, such as CT of the fatty renal lesions or MR imaging for the characteristic brain findings in tuberous sclerosis. Rarely, multiple fatty renal lesions are due to lipomas or teratomas, but in such cases the characteristic imaging features of tuberous sclerosis would be absent elsewhere in the body.

Tuberous sclerosis, or Bourneville disease (24), is an autosomal dominant neurocutaneous disorder that leads to renal anomalies in most patients. Angiomyolipomas are seen in approximately 80% and renal cysts in 20–40%. Larger angiomyolipomas (≥4 cm) have a tendency to bleed and therefore may require urgent nephrectomy, as in this patient, or embolization (25). Renal masses are the most common cause of spontaneous perinephric hemorrhage, and renal cell carcinoma and angiomyolipoma lead the list. Angiography of angiomyolipomas reveals characteristic microaneurysms in the mass.

Aunt Minnie's Pearls

- *Multiple, bilateral hyperechoic renal masses in a patient with tuberous sclerosis are almost certainly angiomyolipomas.*

CASE 10

History. Patient with longstanding history of portal vein thrombosis

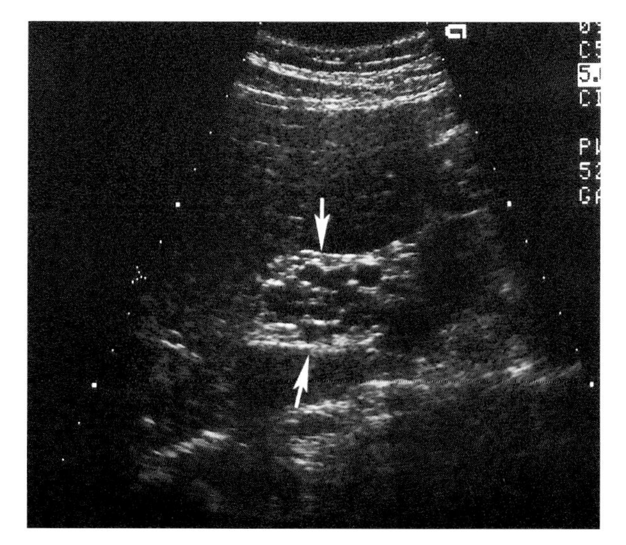

Figure 4.10.1.

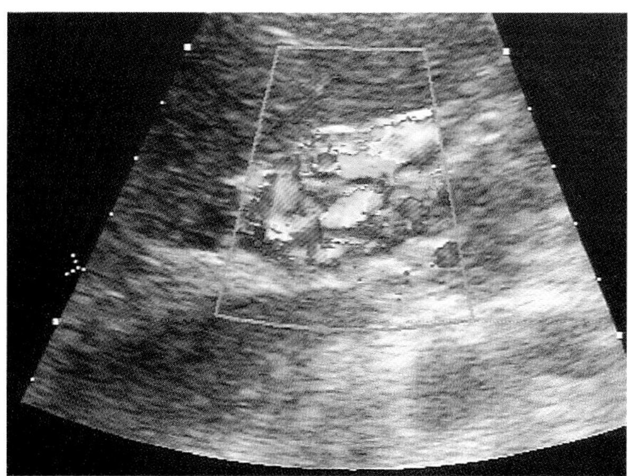

Figure 4.10.2.

Findings. Gray scale (Fig 4.10.1) and color Doppler (Fig. 4.10.2) images at the level of the porta hepatis demonstrate small, tortuous vessels (*arrows*) in the expected location of the main portal vein. The main portal vein was not visualized during the exam.

Diagnosis. Cavernous transformation of the portal vein

Discussion. Cavernous transformation of the portal vein represents dilatation of periportal veins in response to portal vein thrombosis. The main causes of portal vein thrombosis in adults include hepatocellular carcinoma, cirrhosis, pancreatitis, hypercoagulable states, and splenectomy. Although typically identified in patients with chronic portal vein thrombosis, periportal collaterals may form within days or weeks of the initial thrombotic event (26). The collateral vessels run in the free edge of the lesser omentum (hepatoduodenal ligament). Blood flow in these vessels is hepatopetal or bidirectional, with Doppler waveforms characteristic of portal venous flow (low velocity with minimal phasicity with respiration or cardiac activity) (27). When one dominant collateral vessel forms, it is sometimes confused with a patent main portal vein. Recognition that the collateral vessel is anterior to a nonreplaced hepatic artery helps to correctly identify the vessel as a collateral.

Aunt Minnie's Pearls

- *Tortuous collateral vessels in the expected location of the main portal vein are diagnostic of cavernous transformation of the portal vein.*

CASE 11

History. Patient with history of gallstones and recent weight loss

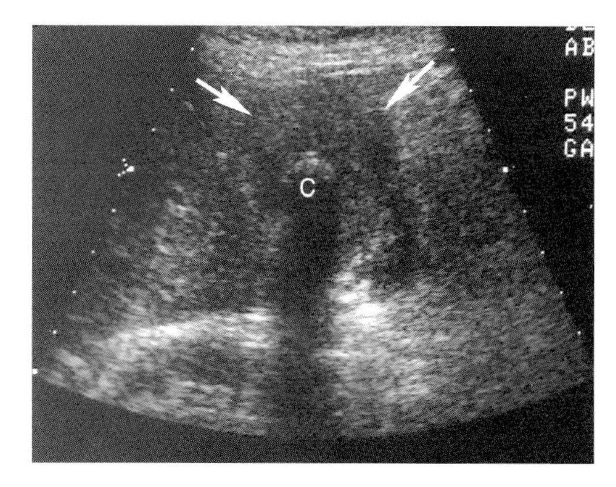

Figure 4.11.1.

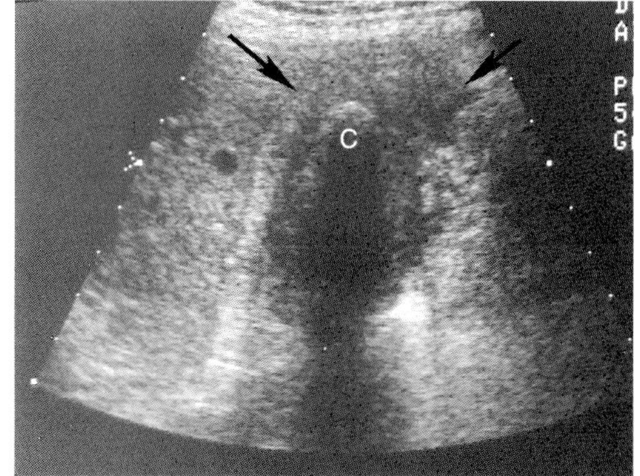

Figure 4.11.2.

Findings. Transverse (Fig. 4.11.1) and longitudinal (Fig. 4.11.2) images through the gallbladder show a soft tissue mass in the expected location of the gallbladder (*arrows*). A dense round structure in the center of the soft tissue mass casts a clean acoustic shadow and therefore is most likely a gallbladder calculus (C). The patient had no tenderness over the gallbladder (negative Murphy's sign) and no history suggestive of cholecystitis.

Diagnosis. Cholelithiasis and gallbladder carcinoma

Discussion. Approximately 75% of patients with gallbladder carcinoma have gallstones. Although poorly understood, the chronic inflammation associated with gallstones is believed to result in epithelial dysplasia and the development of adenocarcinoma. One of the most common imaging presentations of gallbladder carcinoma is that of a soft tissue mass in the gallbladder surrounding a gallstone. Other presentations include a polypoid intraluminal mass or focal wall thickening. Calcification of the gallbladder wall (porcelain gallbladder) also predisposes to carcinoma (28). Although the quoted risk for developing carcinoma ranges from 16 to 60%, most agree that a porcelain gallbladder is an indication for cholecystectomy.

Because of early spread of tumor to the liver or regional lymph nodes, gallbladder carcinoma carries a dismal 20% 5-year survival rate. Hematogenous dissemination to distal organs is unusual. Invasion of the tumor into the hepatoduodenal ligament may result in obstruction of the common bile duct, and the hepatic flexure of the colon is sometimes involved.

Aunt Minnie's Pearls

- *A soft tissue mass that replaces the gallbladder lumen and is associated with a gallstone = gallbladder carcinoma in almost all cases.*
- *Look for liver invasion or metastases and regional lymph node enlargement.*

CASE 12

History. Two patients with postprandial colic

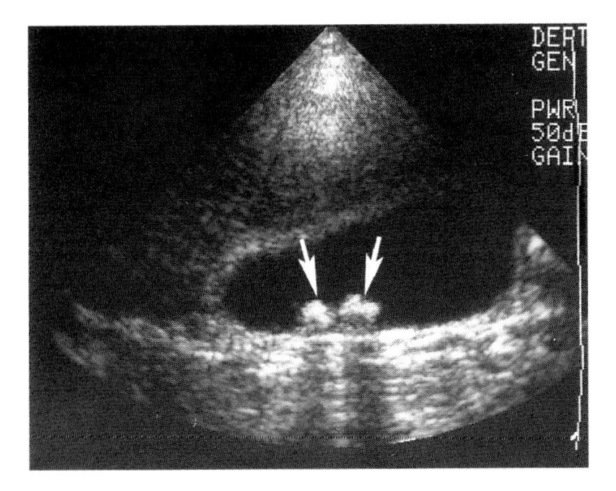

Figure 4.12.1.

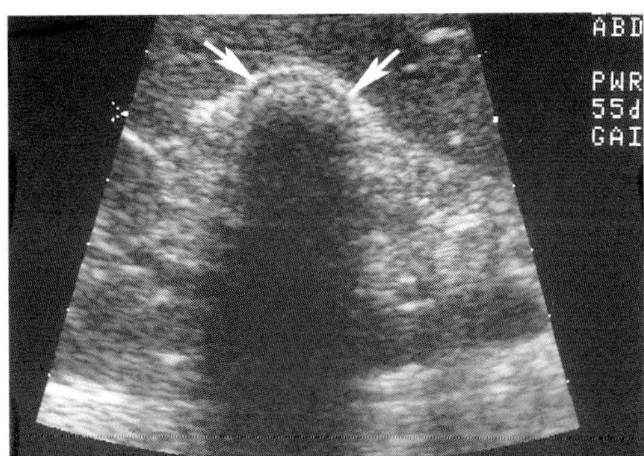

Figure 4.12.2.

Findings. The gallbladder in patient A contains several foci of dense calcification (Fig. 4.12.1, *arrows*) that produce an intense acoustic shadow. The foci are also mobile and surrounded by anechoic bile. In patient B (Fig. 4.12.2), a transverse view of the gallbladder fossa demonstrates a region of intense acoustic shadowing suggestive of stones, but the patient's gallbladder is contracted and not well seen. Closer analysis of this area reveals a hypoechoic band (*arrows*) anterior to the echogenic material that is producing the acoustic shadow.

Diagnosis. Cholelithiasis in distended (patient A) and contracted (patient B) gallbladder

Discussion. The ultrasonographic diagnosis of gallstones requires demonstrating an intensely echogenic focus that produces a "clean" posterior acoustic shadow. Maximizing the production of an acoustic shadow requires utilization of a high-frequency transducer with a single focal zone set at the same depth as the stone. Occasionally, stones that are less than 3 mm in diameter may not shadow, and in these cases differentiating a stone from sludge or a polyp can be problematic, especially if the stone is adherent to the gallbladder wall.

Demonstrating gallstones in a contracted gallbladder is difficult, but a useful sign has been described to aid in the diagnosis of cholelithiasis in these patients. The WES triad refers to demonstration of the hypoechoic band of the gallbladder wall juxtaposed with the echogenic line of the gallstones and their shadow (29). Care must be exercised in using this sign, because a gas-filled duodenum can closely mimic the WES triad. Careful temporal observation of the area, or giving the patient water to drink, usually prevents confusing the duodenum for a true WES triad.

Aunt Minnie's Pearls

- *Gallstones are mobile echogenic foci that produce acoustic shadows.*
- *If the gallbladder is contracted, use the WES triad to diagnose cholelithiasis.*

CASE 13

History. Patient with intermittent pelvic pain

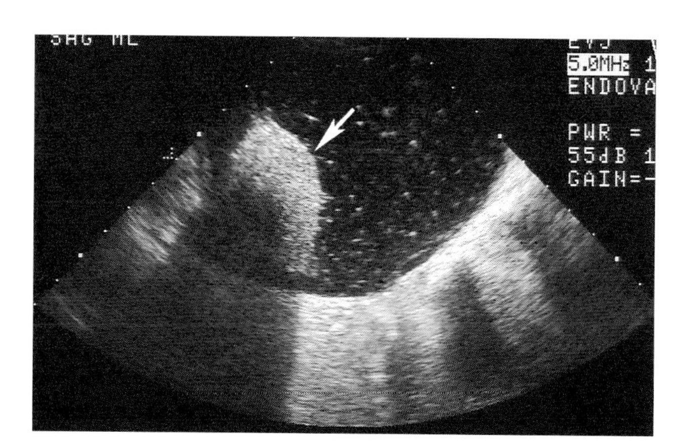

Figure 4.13.1.

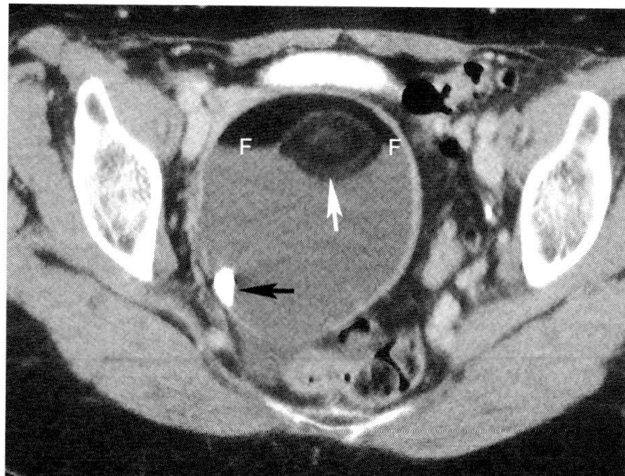

Figure 4.13.2.

Findings. A transverse ultrasound image in the region of the right adnexa (Fig. 4.13.1) reveals a cystic mass that contains diffuse low-level internal echogenicity. In addition, a hyperechoic nodule inside the mass (*arrow*) produces marked posterior acoustic shadowing. A contrast-enhanced CT scan at the same level (Fig. 4.13.2) shows the soft tissue nodule floating inside the lesion (*white arrow*) as well as an internal calcification (*black arrow*) and fat-fluid level (F).

Diagnosis. Ovarian dermoid

Discussion. This benign germ-cell tumor of the ovary is named dermoid because the internal lining of the cystic mass contains skin and dermal appendages. Ovarian teratoma may be a more appropriate name because these masses contain elements from all three primitive germ-cell lines. Although ovarian dermoids are histologically benign, their clinical behavior is not always benign. These neoplasms can cause ovarian torsion, and malignant degeneration (usually into squamous cell carcinoma) occurs rarely in older individuals. Therefore these masses are usually removed at the time of diagnosis.

Dermoids may be diagnosed with various imaging modalities by identifying the characteristic ectodermal elements of hair, teeth, and bone. A specific sonographic diagnosis can be made by identifying plugs of hair, fat, and calcium floating within the cystic mass. These Rokitansky plugs are hyperechoic on sonograms and often produce prominent posterior acoustic shadowing. The identification of a sebum-fluid level and calcification is also diagnostic of this tumor (30).

Aunt Minnie's Pearls

- *A cystic adnexal mass with fat-fluid level and Rokitansky plug = ovarian dermoid.*
- *These masses are removed because they predispose to ovarian torsion and may undergo malignant degeneration.*

CASE 14

History. Two patients with vague scrotal discomfort

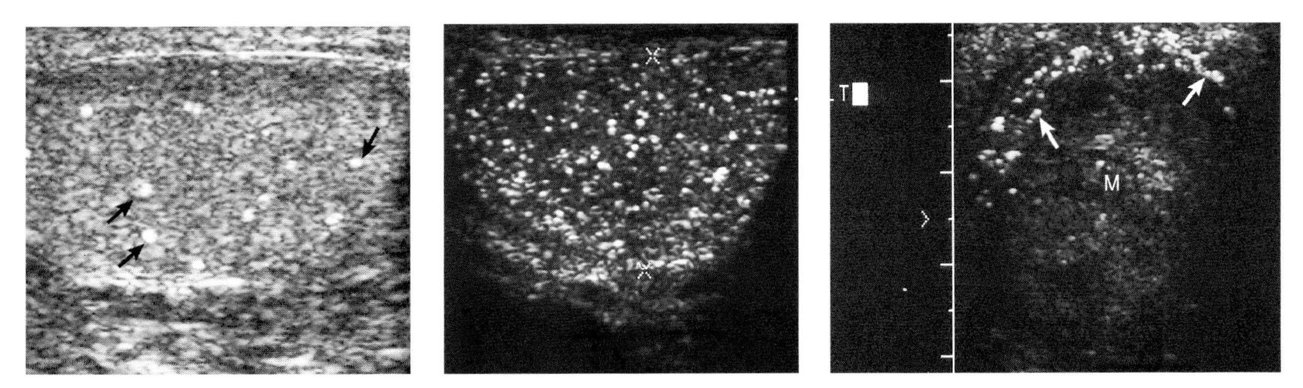

Figure 4.14.1. **Figure 4.14.2.** **Figure 4.14.3.**

Findings. A single longitudinal view of the left testicle in patient A (Fig. 4.14.1) reveals numerous tiny hyperechoic, non-shadowing foci (*arrows*). This appearance was present in the other testicle as well. The testicles are otherwise normal in echogenicity and size. A longitudinal view of the right testicle in patient B (Fig. 4.14.2) again demonstrates tiny hyperechoic foci. However, in this patient a transverse view of the left testicle (Fig. 4.14.3) reveals numerous tiny hyperechoic foci displaced to the periphery of the testicle (*arrows*) by a large heterogeneous mass (M).

Diagnosis. Testicular microlithiasis (patient A) and testicular microlithiasis with seminoma (patient B)

Discussion. Testicular microlithiasis occurs when degenerated tubular epithelium sloughs into the lumen of the seminiferous tubule and calcifies. These tiny (<2 mm) hyperechoic foci produce no acoustic shadowing and are almost always bilateral. Testicular microlithiasis can be differentiated from other causes of testicular calcification by its characteristic appearance and distribution. Associated conditions include cryptorchidism, Klinefelter's and Down's syndromes, male pseudohermaphroditism, and pulmonary alveolar microlithiasis (31).

Testicular microlithiasis may coexist with an overt testicular neoplasm, as in patient B, or with the premalignant condition of intratubular germ cell neoplasia. Although various malignant germ cell tumors have been found in patients with testicular microlithiasis, the degree of increased risk for the development of neoplasm is unknown (31, 32). Therefore, when testicular microlithiasis is discovered with ultrasonography, the testicles should be carefully surveyed for neoplasm in all patients, and ultrasonographic follow-up in 6 months to 1 year should be performed until the degree of increased risk for neoplasm is better defined.

Aunt Minnie's Pearls

- *Numerous tiny foci of calcium in both testicles = testicular microlithiasis.*
- *Be aware of the association of testicular microlithiasis with testicular neoplasms.*
- *Whenever a testicular mass is discovered, always survey the retroperitoneum for metastatic adenopathy.*

CASE 15

History. Patient with scrotal mass

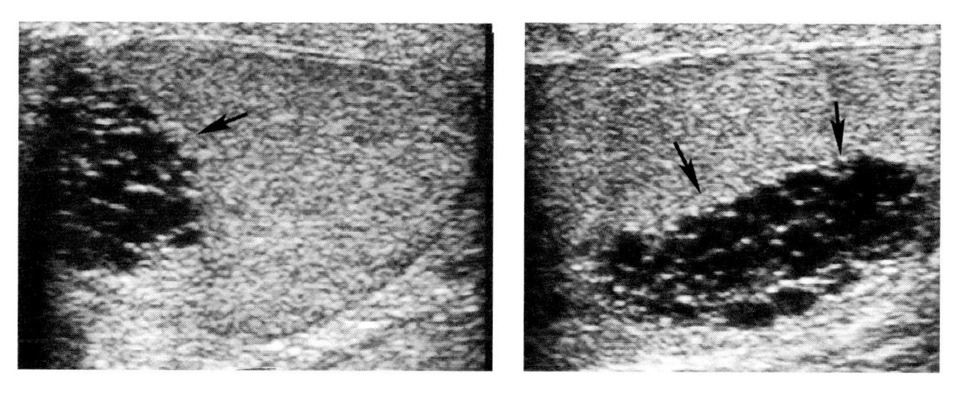

Figure 4.15.1. Figure 4.15.2.

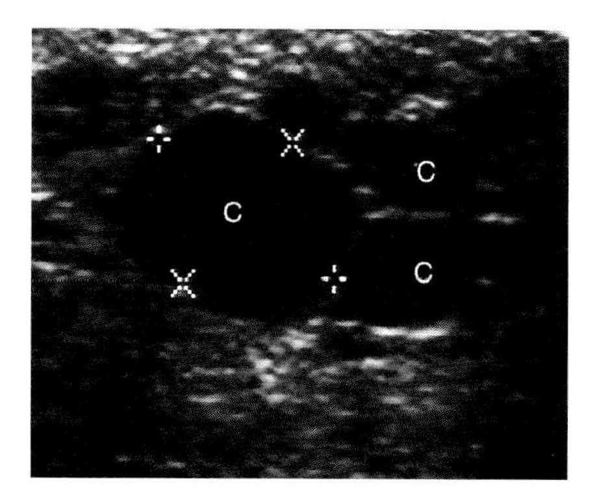

Figure 4.15.3.

Findings. A transverse (Fig. 4.15.1) and longitudinal (Fig. 4.15.2) view of the left testicle reveals numerous small cystic structures adjacent to the mediastinum testis (*arrows*). Also demonstrated (Fig. 4.15.3) are bilateral cysts originating in the epididymis (C), which likely accounted for the patient's palpable mass. The testes are otherwise normal.

Diagnosis. Tubular ectasia of the rete testis and spermatoceles

Discussion. The rete testis is a latticework of tubules that are located in the mediastinum testes and connect the seminiferous tubules to the efferent ductules. If the rete testis becomes abnormally dilated, a unique appearance of dilated, serpiginous tubules near the mediastinum is seen on sonograms. In most cases this tubular ectasia of the rete testis is associated with spermatoceles, intratesticular cysts, or both. The process is usually bilateral but may be asymmetric (33). Although the etiology is obscure, the association of testicular cysts with previous trauma or infection has led to the assumption that tubular ectasia has a similar etiology (34).

The sonographic appearance of tubular ectasia parallels a spectrum of severity from mild serpiginous dilatation of the tubules to cysts in the region of the mediastinum. The condition is usually identified in middle-aged men, and the lesion itself is nonpalpable and usually asymptomatic. No serious sequelae of the abnormality are known.

Aunt Minnie's Pearls

- *Small cystic spaces in the mediastinum testis = tubular ectasia of the rete testis.*
- *Almost all cases are associated with spermatoceles or testicular cysts.*

CASE 16

History. Woman with swelling sensation around vagina and dyspareunia

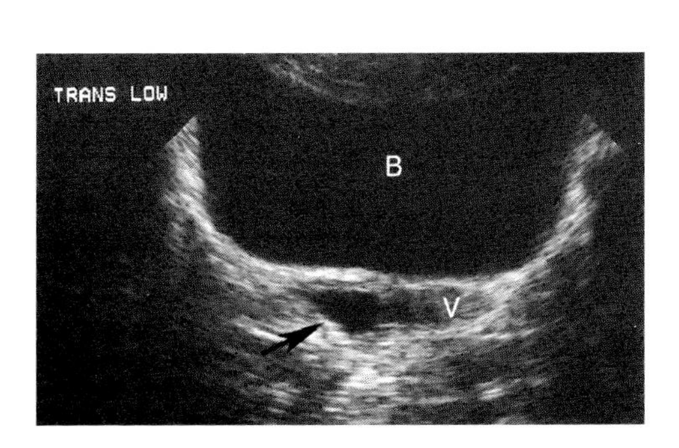

Figure 4.16.1.

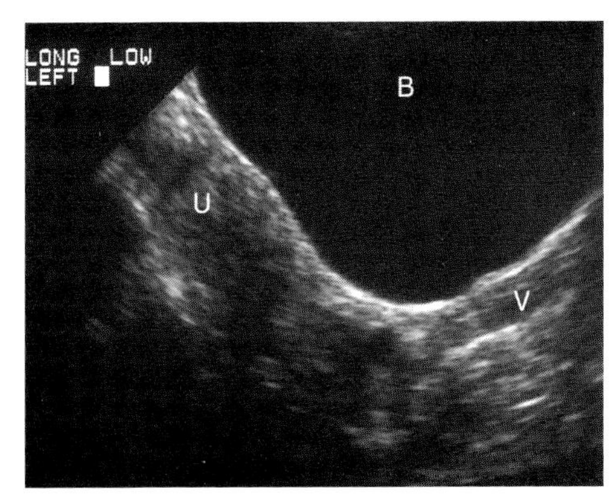

Figure 4.16.2.

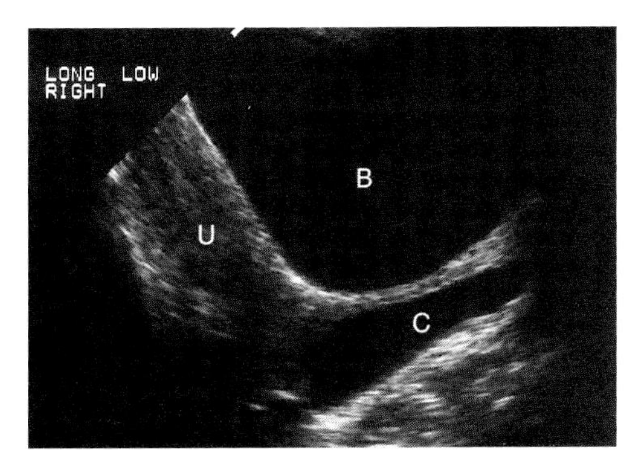

Figure 4.16.3.

Findings. Transvesical ultrasonography at the level of the vagina (Fig. 4.16.1) reveals a simple cystic mass (*arrow*) situated behind the bladder (B) and adjacent to the vagina (V). A longitudinal view obtained in the midline (Fig. 4.16.2) demonstrates the uterus (U), bladder (B), and vagina (V). Another longitudinal view (Fig. 4.16.3) angled slightly to the right of Figure 4.16.2 reveals an elongated cyst (C) that parallels the vagina.

Diagnosis. Gartner's duct cyst

Discussion. Although the mesonephric (wolffian) duct in the male population is responsible for formation of the internal genital tract, this structure normally involutes in women. A Gartner's duct cyst represents cystic dilatation of a remnant of the mesonephric duct. The abnormality is characteristically located in the lateral or anterolateral wall of the vagina. They tend to parallel the course of the vagina and therefore are elongated. The cyst may be asymptomatic or it may be associated with swelling, pain, or dyspareunia. Other cysts that occur in this region (e.g., epidermal inclusion cysts) are much less common and are differentiated from a Gartner's duct cyst by their point of origin. Gartner's duct cysts are associated with ipsilateral renal agenesis in some cases (35).

Another common cystic lesion incidentally discovered during pelvic ultrasonography includes the nabothian cyst, which is a common simple cyst located in the cervix. It is usually asymptomatic, often multiple, and of no clinical significance.

Aunt Minnie's Pearls

- *A simple cyst arising in the anterolateral vaginal wall = Gartner's duct cyst.*
- *Gartner's duct cyst is a cystic wolffian duct remnant.*
- *A simple cyst in the cervix is known as a nabothian cyst.*

CASE 17

History. Patient who underwent a cardiac catheterization 1 day ago

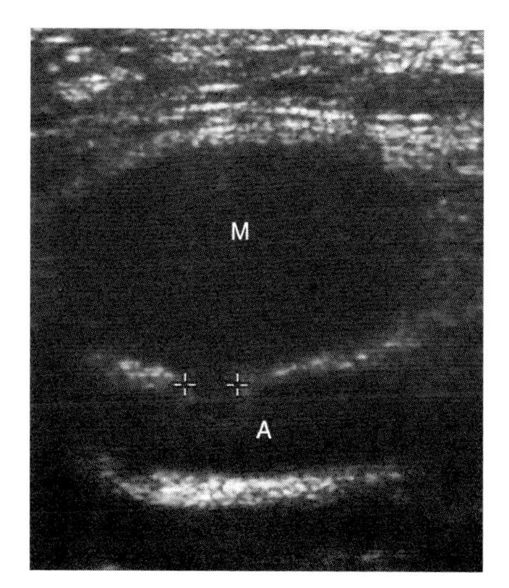

Figure 4.17.1.

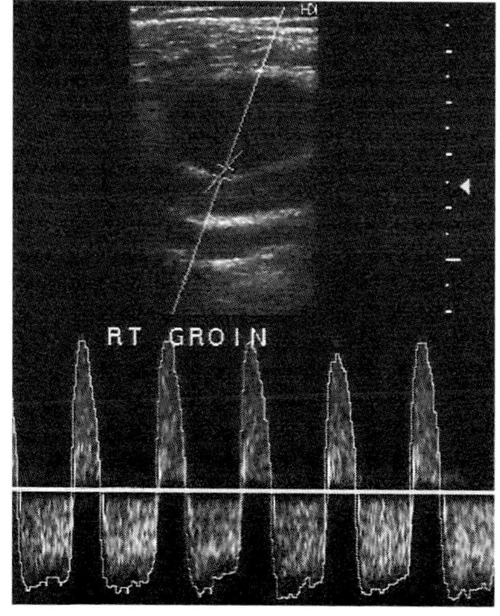

Figure 4.17.2.

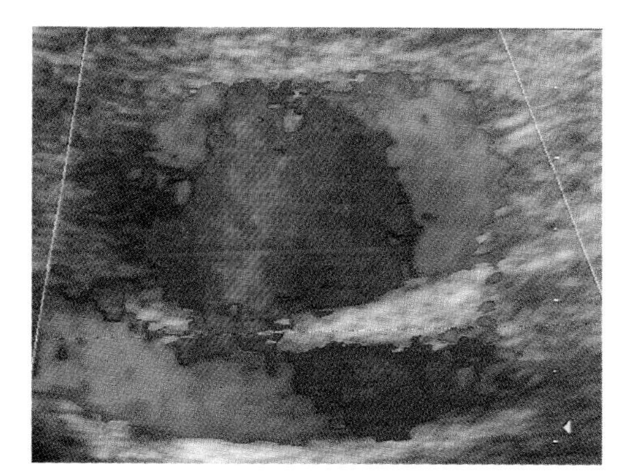

Figure 4.17.3.

Findings. On this single longitudinal gray scale image of the right common femoral artery (Fig. 4.17.1), a round anechoic mass (M) is present anterior to the artery (A). A Doppler waveform (Fig. 4.17.2) obtained in an area of communication between the artery and the anechoic mass demonstrates flow both toward (above baseline) and then away from (below baseline) the transducer or a "to-and-fro" appearance. A corresponding color Doppler image (Fig. 4.17.3) reveals a swirling color flow pattern in the cystic mass.

Diagnosis. Postcatheterization femoral artery pseudoaneurysm

Discussion. A pseudoaneurysm is a localized rupture of an artery contained by the surrounding soft tissues. The wall of the aneurysm does not contain intima, media, and adventitia and is therefore termed a pseudoaneurysm. Femoral artery pseudoaneurysm is a well-known complication of percutaneous angiography that occurs when arterial blood communicates with an extravascular collection of blood via the puncture site. Ultrasonography is used to differentiate between a pseudoaneurysm and a periarterial hematoma. The pseudoaneurysm can sometimes be treated with ultrasound by compressing the area until complete thrombosis of the pseudoaneurysm occurs.

A characteristic Doppler finding is the to-and-fro waveform obtained at the neck of the pseudoaneurysm. Blood entering the pseudoaneurysm during systole produces flow above the baseline, and blood exiting during diastole produces flow below the baseline (36). The normal transient diastolic flow reversal seen from small arterial branches of the femoral artery should not be confused with the pandiastolic flow reversal seen at pseudoaneurysm necks. Color Doppler examination of the area reveals the swirling color pattern similar to the yin-yang symbol in Chinese dualistic philosophy.

Aunt Minnie's Pearls

- *A pseudoaneurysm has a characteristic to-and-fro waveform at its neck.*
- *A characteristic yin-yang swirling color Doppler flow pattern is seen within the pseudoaneurysm.*

CASE 18

History. Young woman with a positive pregnancy test, pelvic pain, vaginal bleeding, and history of a right ectopic pregnancy requiring salpingectomy

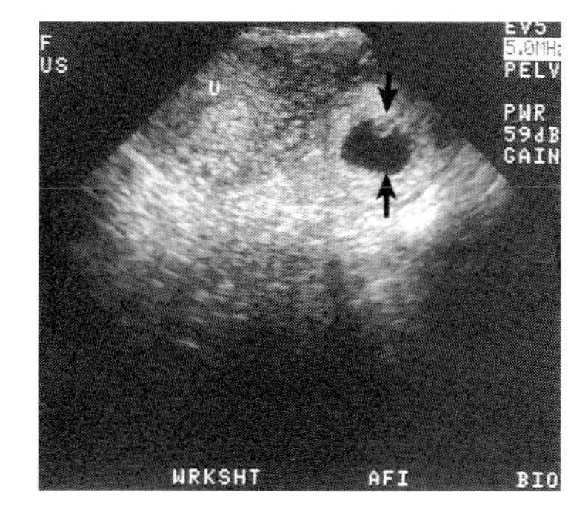

Figure 4.18.1.

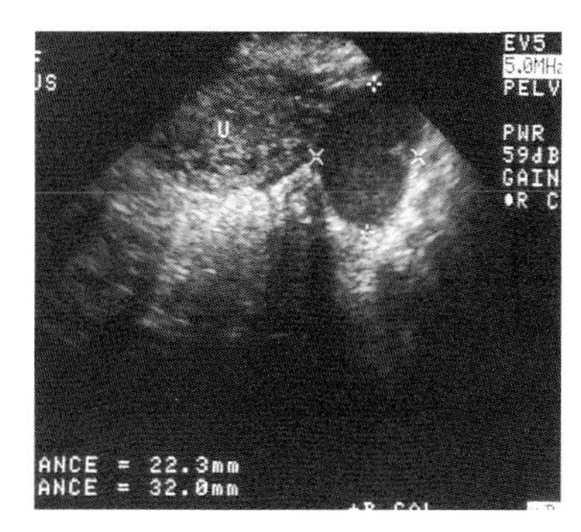

Figure 4.18.2.

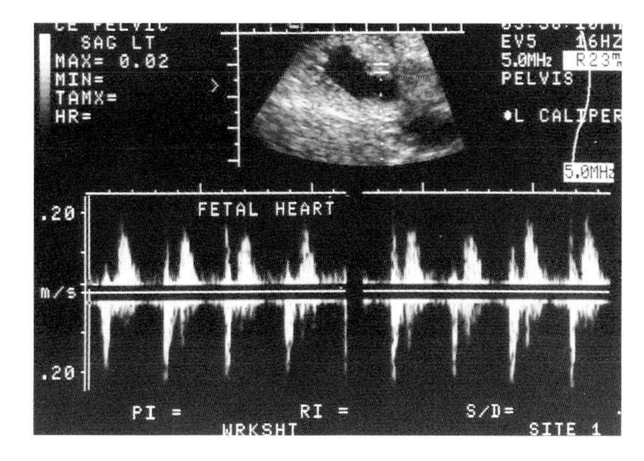

Figure 4.18.3.

Findings. A transverse, transabdominal view through the left adnexa (Fig. 4.18.1) shows a gestational sac and yolk sac (*arrows*) adjacent to the uterus (U). A heterogeneous cystic mass is seen just superior to the gestational sac (Fig. 4.18.2, calipers). Transvaginal sonography of the gestational sac (Fig. 4.18.3) reveals a fetal heartbeat within an embryonic pole.

Diagnosis. Live ectopic pregnancy associated with an adnexal hematoma

Discussion. When embryonic implantation occurs in any location other than the uterus, an ectopic pregnancy exists. Patients who are at risk for this abnormality include those with a history of previous ectopic pregnancy, in vitro fertilization, pelvic inflammatory disease, previous tubal ligation or reconstruction, and women with intrauterine devices in place. Patients with ectopic pregnancies may be asymptomatic but more commonly present with pain and vaginal bleeding. Also remember that patients who are undergoing ovulation induction therapy may present with concomitant intrauterine and ectopic pregnancies (1 in 4000 patients).

The diagnosis of ectopic pregnancy relies on correlation of transvaginal ultrasonographic findings with serum B-hCG levels. When the serum B-hCG level reaches 1000 mIU/mL (second IS), pregnancies should be identifiable as intrauterine with modern transvaginal equipment. Findings that suggest an ectopic pregnancy include absence of an intrauterine gestation, pseudogestational intrauterine sac, adnexal masses or rings, and free cul-de-sac fluid. Visualization of an embryonic pole outside the uterus, as in the example case, allows diagnosis with 100% accuracy (37).

Aunt Minnie's Pearls

- *In the first trimester, adnexal pain and vaginal bleeding suggest the diagnosis of ectopic pregnancy.*
- *If the serum B-hCG level is $\geq$1000 mIU/mL, an intrauterine pregnancy should be identified with transvaginal sonography.*

CASE 19

History. Newborn infant girl with a right renal cyst noted on a prenatal sonogram

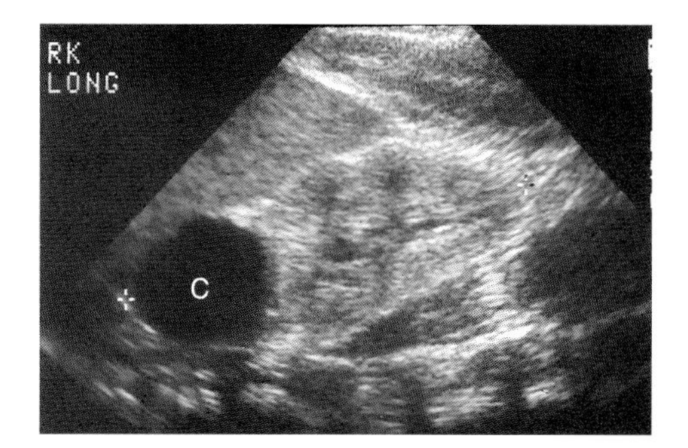

Figure 4.19.1.

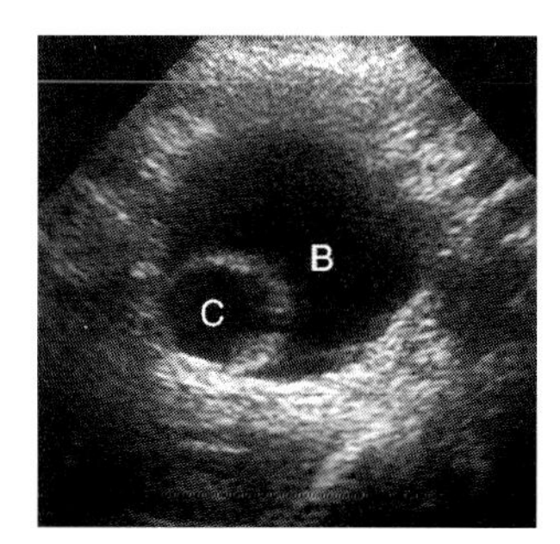

Figure 4.19.2.

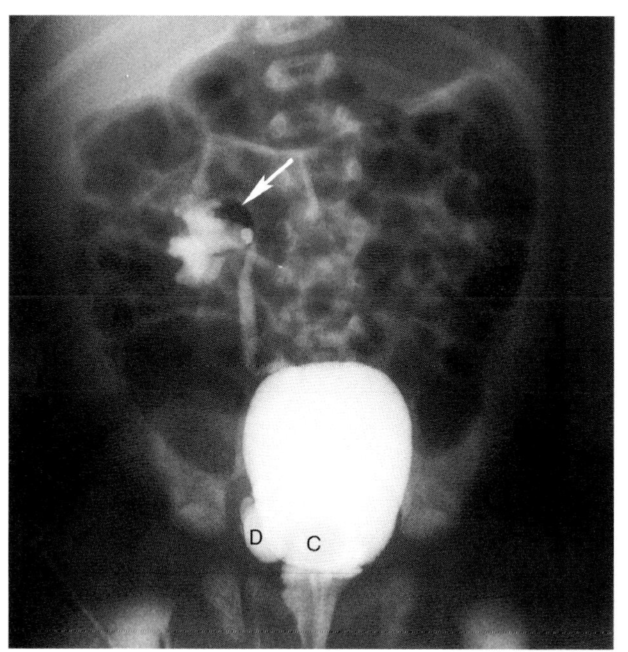

Figure 4.19.3.

Findings. A sagittal ultrasound image of the right kidney (Fig. 4.19.1) demonstrates a right upper pole cyst (C). A transverse view (Fig. 4.19.2) of the bladder (B) shows a cystic structure (C) in the inferolateral right bladder producing a classic cyst-within-a-cyst appearance. The voiding cystoureterogram (Fig. 4.19.3) shows a filling defect (C) in the bladder, right paraureteral diverticulum (D), and right vesicoureteral reflux into the lower moiety of a duplicated right intrarenal collecting system, also known as the famous drooping-lilly sign (*arrow*).

Diagnosis. Ureteropelvic duplication with an ectopic ureterocele

Discussion. Ureteropelvic duplication complicated by an ectopic ureterocele is an important surgical cause of urinary tract infections in infants and young children. The Weigert-Meyer rule dictates that the upper pole ureter inserts into the bladder inferomedially to the lower pole ureter, which inserts in the normal anatomic location. The ectopic ureter may also insert into the urethra, vagina, or vestibule in female patients, leading to continuous urinary incontinence. In the male population, the ectopic ureter may insert into the posterior urethra, seminal vesicles, or prostate, and because these structures are proximal to the urethral sphincter, incontinence does not occur. In general, the upper pole ureter is obstructed by an ectopic ureterocele, and the lower pole ureter refluxes. Further, the ectopic ureterocele may obstruct either the ipsilateral lower pole ureter, the contralateral ureter, or even the bladder outlet. Therefore one should remember that an ectopic ureterocele is a common cause of bilateral hydronephrosis, especially in the infant girl (38).

Aunt Minnie's Pearls

- *Ureteropelvic duplication may be complicated by an ectopic ureterocele.*
- *The ureterocele obstructs the upper pole collecting system and may obstruct the lower pole ureter, the opposite ureter, or the bladder outlet.*

CASE 20

History. 6-week-old boy with nonbilious vomiting

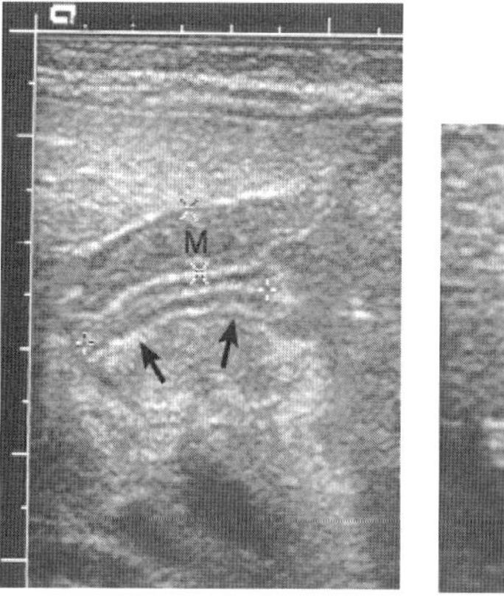

Figure 4.20.1.

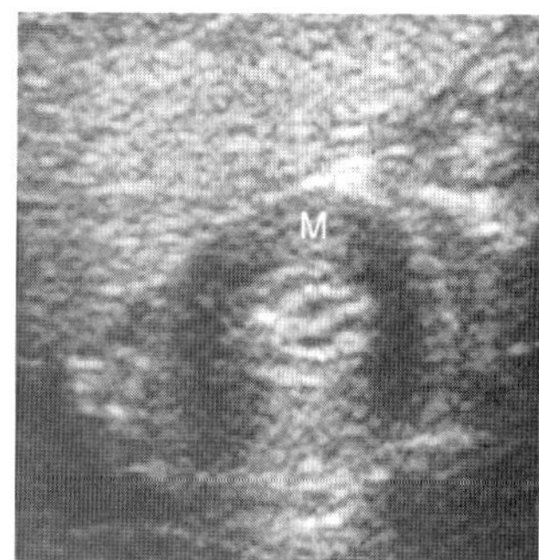

Figure 4.20.2.

Findings. Sagittal (Fig. 4.20.1) and transverse (Fig. 4.20.2) views through the epigastrium show that the circular muscle (M) of the pylorus is thickened and measures 6.1 mm. The pyloric canal appears elongated *(arrows)*, measuring 19.3 mm.

Diagnosis. Hypertrophic pyloric stenosis

Discussion. Ultrasonography allows direct visualization of the pathologic hypertrophic circular muscle rather than infer its presence by the upper gastrointestinal series. Hypertrophic pyloric stenosis is more common in males and has a familial predisposition. The most common presentation is nonbilious vomiting in an infant 2–6 weeks old. In general, a pyloric channel length of ≥17 mm is considered abnormal. Although a pyloric muscle thickness of ≥3.0 mm is reported as diagnostic evidence of hypertrophic pyloric stenosis, slightly greater measurements of 3.5 or even 4.0 mm are preferred at some institutions. If the pylorus is difficult to localize, the infant may be given a small amount of water to distend the gastric antrum. Hypertrophic pyloric stenosis is differentiated from pylorospasm by the constancy of the thickened pylorus during the entire examination and the lack of normal peristalsis in the thickened pyloric channel. Surgical treatment is a Ramstedt pyloromyotomy in which the hypertrophic circular muscle is split longitudinally. Muscle thickness usually returns to normal by 3 months (39).

Aunt Minnie's Pearls

- *Nonbilious vomiting in an infant 2–6 weeks old suggests hypertrophic pyloric stenosis.*
- *Sonographic findings include a pyloric muscle thickness of ≥3–4 mm and canal length of >17 mm.*
- *Make sure the pylorus is abnormal during the entire examination to eliminate the possibility of pylorospasm.*

CASE 21

History. Infant girl delivered in breech presentation with an abnormal physical examination

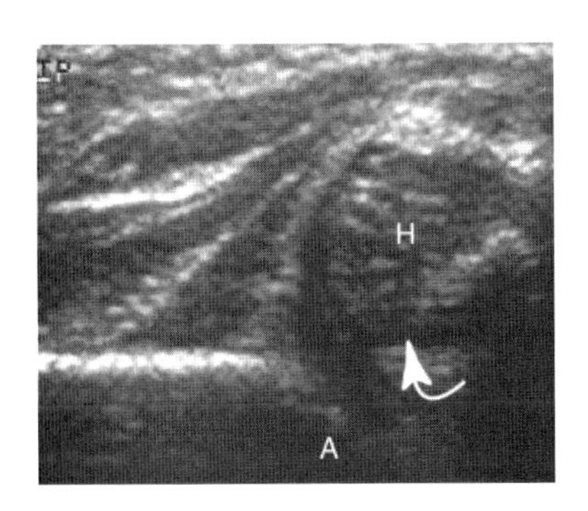

Figure 4.21.1. Left hip.

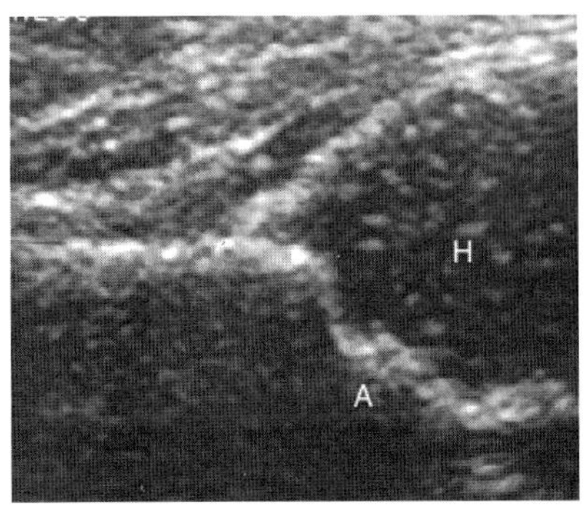

Figure 4.21.2. Right hip.

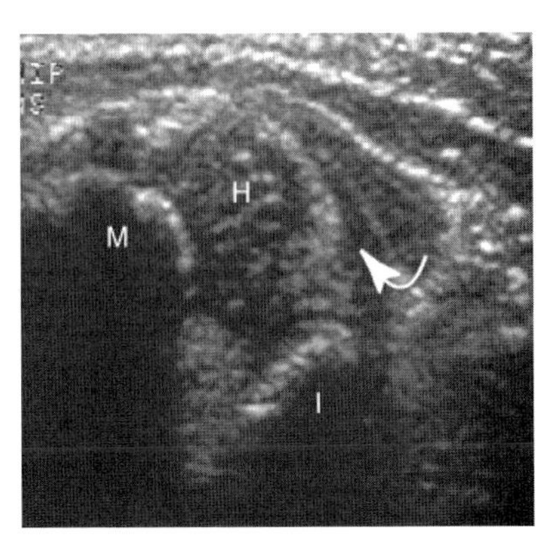

Figure 4.21.3. Left hip.

Findings. A coronal flexion view (Fig. 4.21.1) demonstrates superolateral subluxation (*arrow*) of the left hip (H) relative to the acetabulum (A). The right hip (Fig. 4.21.2) appears normal. The transverse flexion view demonstrates posterior subluxation of the left hip (Fig. 4.21.3), which is recognized on this view by the posterior displacement (*arrow*) of the epiphysis (H) relative to the ischium (I), producing an abnormal gap between the hip and ileum. The femoral metaphysis (M) obscures the pubis on this view.

Diagnosis. Developmental dysplasia of the left hip (DDH)

Discussion. Early diagnosis of DDH is critical for a successful outcome. Sonographic imaging is indicated for the infant with an abnormal physical examination or risk factors for DDH. Risk factors for DDH include a positive family history, breech presentation, congenital torticollis, foot and knee deformities suggesting intrauterine crowding, and neuromuscular diseases associated with teratogenic dislocation of the hips, e.g., myelodysplasia and arthrogryposis. As in the case presented, DDH more commonly affects girls than boys, and the left hip is involved more frequently than the right.

To decrease false-positive studies, screening examinations are preferably performed at 4–6 weeks of age when maternal estrogenic effect is waning. The routine examination consists of axial and coronal views of both hips and determination of the angle formed by the superior acetabulum and a vertical line that parallels the lateral margin of the iliac bone (alpha-angle). Stress maneuvers mimicking the Barlow clinical test are sometimes used to dynamically demonstrate the abnormal posterior and superior subluxation of the hip (40).

Aunt Minnie's Pearls

- *DDH is diagnosed when the femoral head subluxes posteriorly and superiorly with respect to the acetabulum.*
- *Risk factors include female gender, breech delivery, intrauterine crowding, and some neuromuscular diseases.*

CASE 22

History. 5-year-old girl with fever, leukocytosis, and abdominal pain

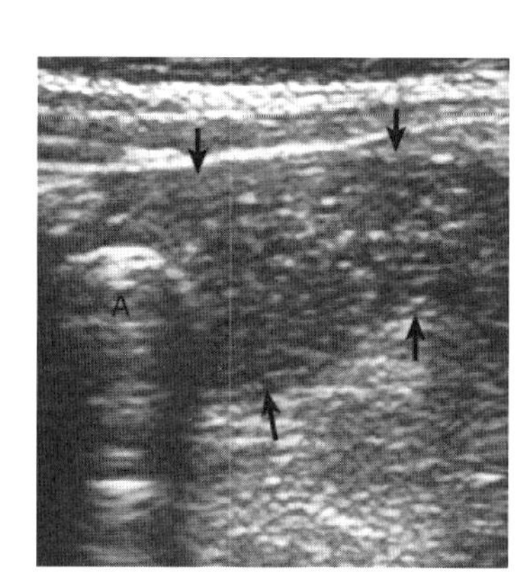

Figure 4.22.1.

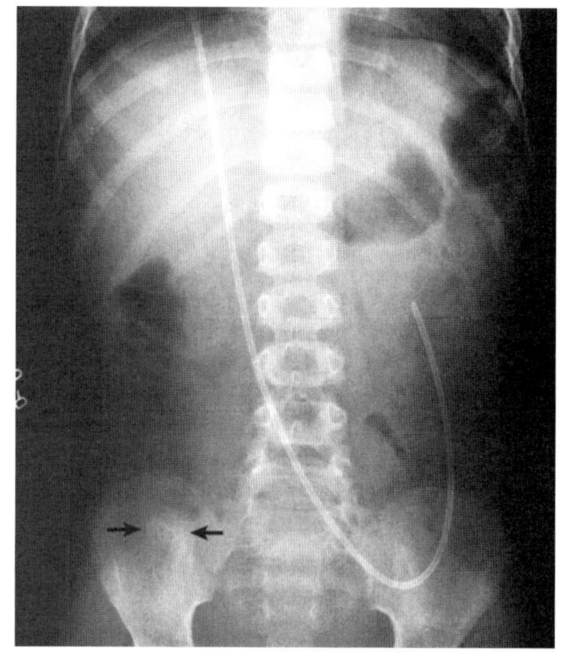

Figure 4.22.2.

Findings. A longitudinal (Fig. 4.22.1) image of the right lower quadrant demonstrates a tubular structure measuring 15 mm in diameter (*arrows*) that contains an 11-mm echogenic focus (A) that produces distal acoustical shadowing. An anteroposterior plain film of the abdomen reveals a laminated calcification in the right lower quadrant (Fig. 4.22.2, *arrows*).

Diagnosis. Appendicitis with an appendicolith

Discussion. Sonography for the diagnosis of appendicitis is best reserved for the clinically indeterminate case or patient with an intermediate probability of disease. Criteria for the sonographic diagnosis of nonperforated appendicitis include a hyperemic noncompressible blind-ending tubular structure with an outer diameter of >6 mm. Perforated appendicitis occurs in 20–30% of children and decreases the overall sensitivity and accuracy of the sonographic study. The most reliable sonographic features of perforation are loss of the echogenic submucosal layer, increased periappendiceal echogenicity, and periappendiceal fluid collections. An appendiceal abscess may present as a hypoechoic or complex mass elsewhere in the abdomen or in the pelvic cul-de-sac. Scanning the patient's point of maximal tenderness often facilitates finding the appendix. Also, using graded compression allows the examiner to gradually displace overlying bowel gas from the region of the appendix (41).

Aunt Minnie's Pearls

- *Ultrasound criteria for appendicitis include a noncompressible appendix with an outer diameter of >6 mm; an appendicolith may also be seen in few cases.*
- *Always check for fluid collections that suggest perforation or abscess formation.*

Case 23

History. 4-year-old child with abdominal pain and thick, bloody stools

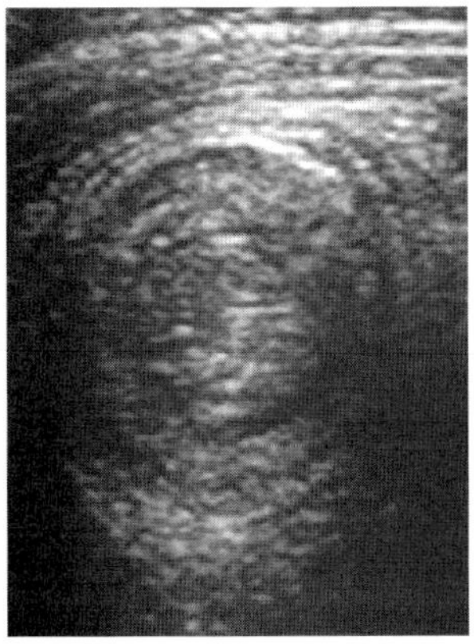

Figure 4.23.1.

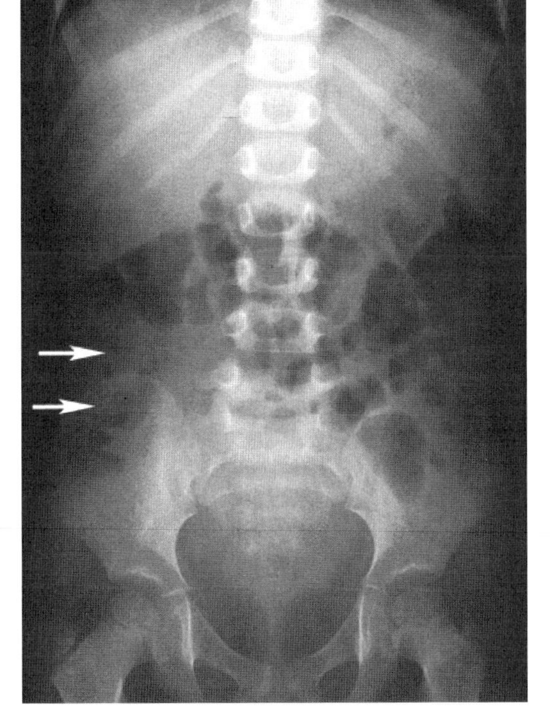

Figure 4.23.2.

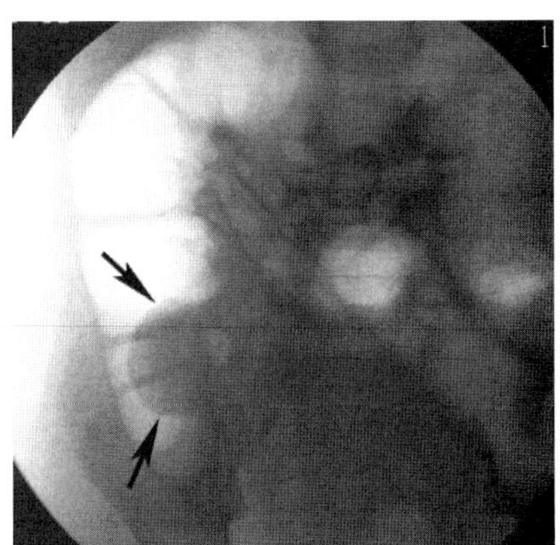

Figure 4.23.3.

Findings. A transverse sonogram of the right lower quadrant reveals a target sign with multiple concentric rings surrounding an echogenic center (Fig. 4.23.1). The plain film reveals a relative paucity of gas in the right abdomen (Fig. 4.23.2, *arrows*). The air enema not only revealed a soft tissue mass inside the colon, diagnostic of an intussusception (Fig. 4.23.3, *arrows*), but also was successful in treating the patient.

Diagnosis. Intussusception

Discussion. Typically, idiopathic ileocolic intussusception occurs in children 3 months to 3 years old with crampy abdominal pain, bloody "currant jelly" stools, or a palpable abdominal mass. The possibility of a pathologic lead point should be considered in children outside the usual age range. Common pathologic lead points include Meckel's diverticula, duplication cysts, and lymphoma. Classic sonographic findings include the target, doughnut, and multiple concentric ring signs in the transverse plane and the pseudokidney and "sandwich" signs on longitudinal images. An air or contrast enema can confirm the diagnosis and possibly treat the patient. Free intraperitoneal fluid may be observed, but because it is not necessarily associated with peritonitis or perforation, it should not alone be considered a contraindication to radiologic reduction (42).

Aunt Minnie's Pearls

- *Idiopathic ileocolic intussusception occurs in children 3 months to 3 years old, and occurrence outside this age range suggests a lead point.*
- *Ultrasonography is very sensitive in the diagnosis of this disorder, and air or contrast enemas are diagnostic and often therapeutic.*

Case 24

History. 13-year-old girl with cyclic lower abdominal pain

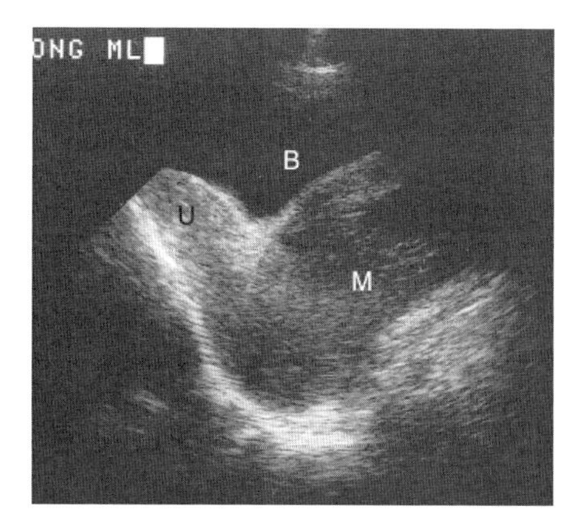

Figure 4.24.1.

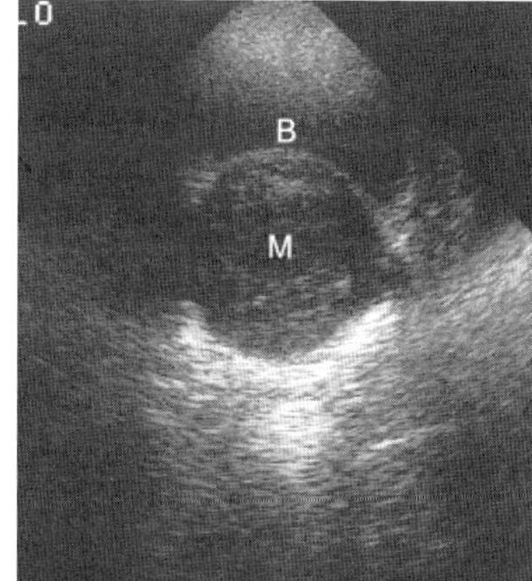

Figure 4.24.2.

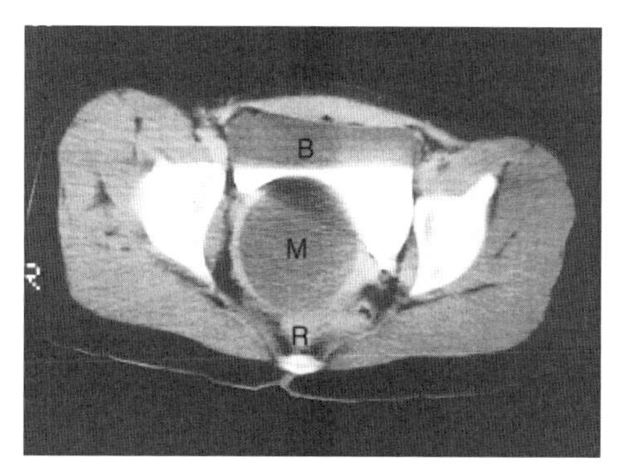

Figure 4.24.3. Axial CT with contrast.

Findings. A longitudinal sonographic image through the pelvis (Fig. 4.24.1) reveals a tubular mass (M) that is contiguous with the uterus (U). Transverse ultrasonography (Fig. 4.24.2) and CT (Fig. 4.24.3) images of the pelvis reveal a fluid- and debris-filled midline mass (M) between the bladder (B) and rectum (R). The mass is therefore in the expected location of the vagina.

Diagnosis. Hematocolpos

Discussion. Vaginal obstruction may be encountered in the neonate or adolescent female. Neonatal vaginal obstruction is associated with major structural anomalies, such as vaginal atresia or persistent urogenital sinus. In these patients, associated congenital anomalies (e.g., anorectal malformations, congenital heart disease, renal and spinal anomalies) must be excluded. Adolescent vaginal obstruction is most often due to a simple imperforate hymen without associated anomalies. Cyclic lower abdominal pain with primary amenorrhea is the classic clinical presentation. In general, the vagina is thin-walled and more distensible than the uterus, which has thick muscular walls, although in some cases the uterus may distend as well (hematometrocolpos). There may be associated hematosalpinx or hydrosalpinx and hydroureteronephrosis. Simple hymenectomy is curative in the uncomplicated adolescent form (43).

Aunt Minnie's Pearls

- *Buildup of secretions and blood in the vagina = hematocolpos.*
- *If this abnormality occurs in neonates, always exclude other congenital anomalies.*

CASE 25

History. Neonate with jaundice, decreased hematocrit, and a right flank mass

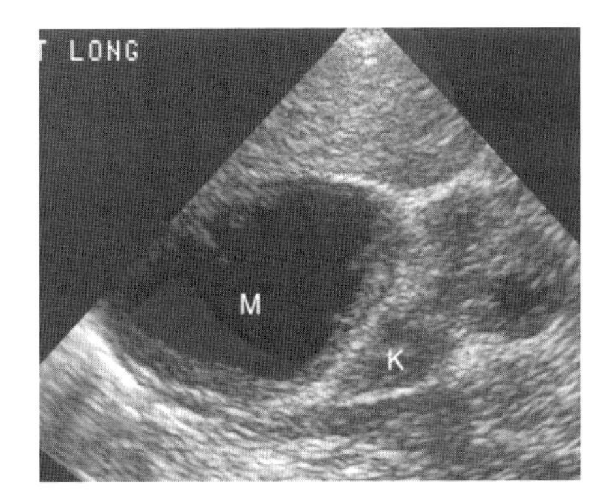

Figure 4.25.1.

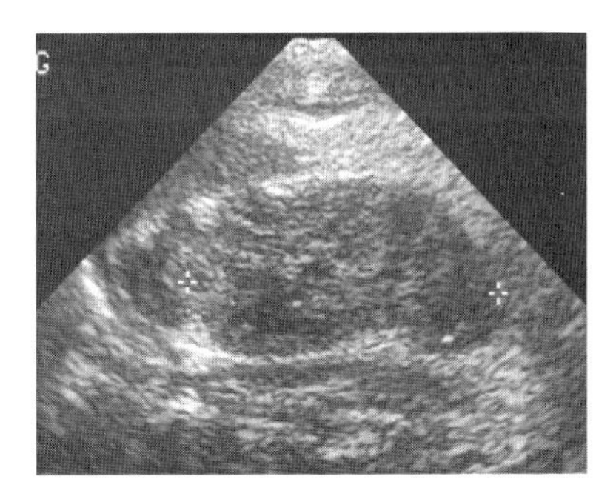

Figure 4.25.2.

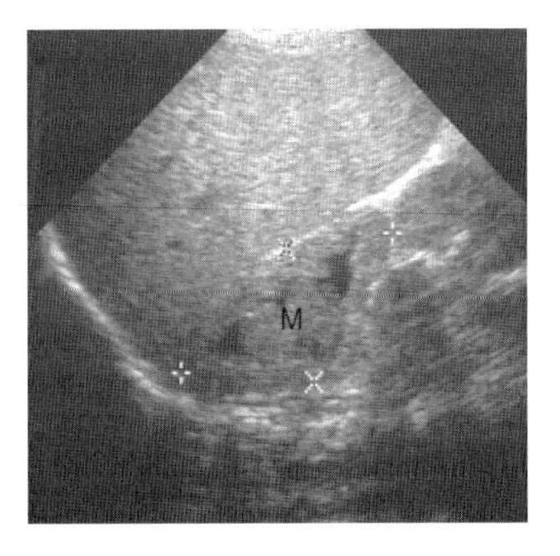

Figure 4.25.3.

Findings. An initial longitudinal image of the right flank (Fig. 4.25.1) reveals a right adrenal mass (M) with peripheral solid and central cystic components located superior to the kidney (K). Left kidney and adrenal are normal (Fig. 4.25.2); 1 month later, the right adrenal mass (M) is smaller (Fig. 4.25.3).

Diagnosis. Adrenal hemorrhage

Discussion. Adrenal hemorrhage is the most common neonatal adrenal mass. Patients at increased risk include infants of diabetic mothers and babies experiencing perinatal stress from conditions such as sepsis, hypoxia, birth trauma, shock, renal-vein thrombosis, and extracorporeal membrane oxygenation. Adrenal hemorrhage is more frequently right-sided than left-sided and may be bilateral. Adrenal insufficiency is rarely observed. Significant complications include extracapsular hemorrhage with shock and renal vein thrombosis with diminished renal function. The major differential diagnostic consideration is congenital adrenal neuroblastoma. There are no pathognomonic sonographic features that allow differentiation between the two lesions on the initial examination. Adrenal hemorrhage, however, will decrease in size and become more homogeneous on follow-up examinations, whereas neuroblastoma will show interval growth (44).

Aunt Minnie's Pearls

- *Think adrenal hemorrhage in a newborn with jaundice, anemia, and an abdominal mass.*
- *Follow-up examinations are critical to distinguish adrenal hemorrhage from congenital adrenal neuroblastoma.*

Case 26

History. Neonate with abnormal prenatal sonography

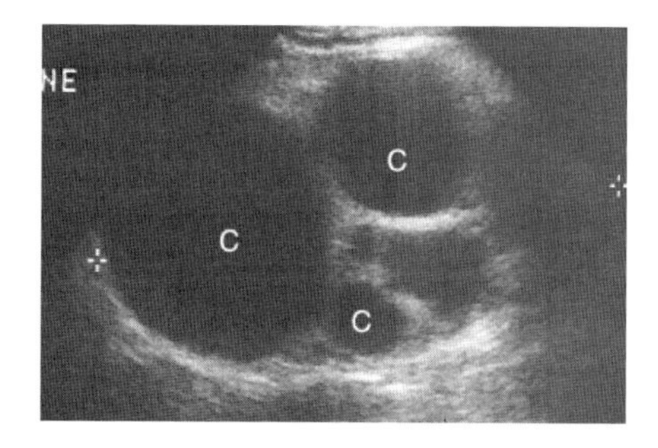

Figure 4.26.1.

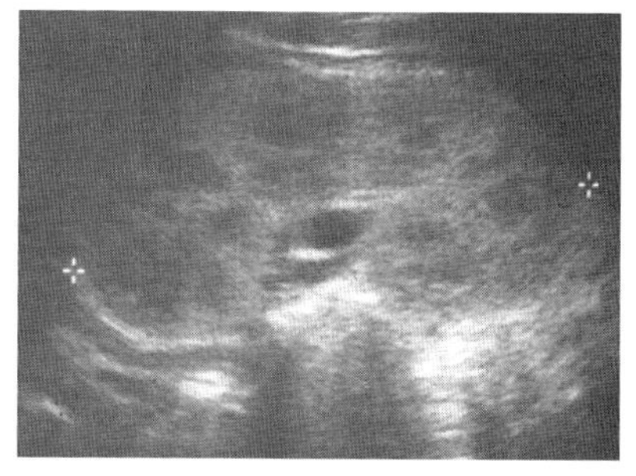

Figure 4.26.2.

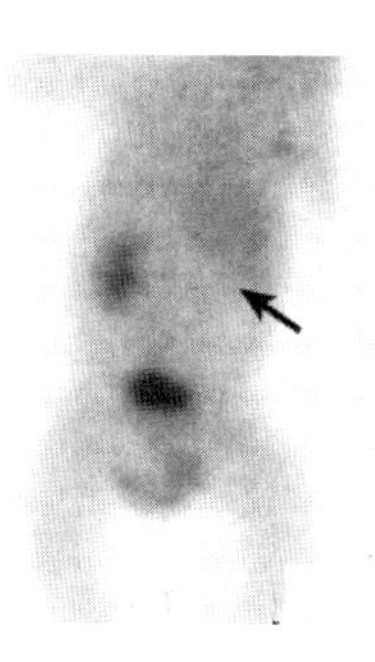

Figure 4.26.3.

Findings. The right kidney (Fig. 4.26.1) is replaced by multiple cysts (C) of varying sizes that do not intercommunicate and are separated by echogenic parenchyma. The left kidney (Fig. 4.26.2) is sonographically normal. A posterior image from a renogram shows a normally functioning left kidney and absent renal function on the right (Fig. 4.26.3, *arrow*).

Diagnosis. Right multicystic dysplastic kidney (MCDK)

Discussion. Classic MCDK is thought to be due to early in utero atresia of the proximal ureter, renal pelvis, and infundibula. MCDK is the second most common neonatal abdominal mass after congenital ureteropelvic junction obstruction, and most cases now present with an abnormal prenatal sonogram. One easy and reliable ultrasonographic sign of MCDK is that the largest cyst will never be central, as is the case with congenital ureteropelvic junction obstruction in which the largest cyst is central and represents the dilated renal pelvis. Nuclear medicine can also assist in differentiating between these two diagnoses by showing no function in the MCDK, and it is also helpful in examining the contralateral kidney, which is abnormal in up to 20% of patients. The most frequent abnormalities observed in the contralateral kidney are vesicoureteral reflux and ureteropelvic junction obstruction. Obviously, bilateral MCDK is not compatible with life.

Although MCDKs were traditionally resected because of initial studies suggesting that the masses may be responsible for the development of hypertension, MCDK is now managed nonoperatively because it usually decreases in size, calcifies, and does not produce symptoms. Serial imaging studies are indicated for surveillance of regression or enlargement, and nephrectomy is an option for enlarging, complicated, or atypical cystic renal masses (45, 46).

Aunt Minnie's Pearls

- *MCDK causes numerous cysts that are not connected on ultrasound images.*
- *Nuclear medicine studies will confirm the diagnosis by showing no function on the affected side.*
- *Look for anomalies involving the contralateral kidney.*

CASE 27

History. 10-week-old infant with jaundice and acholic stools

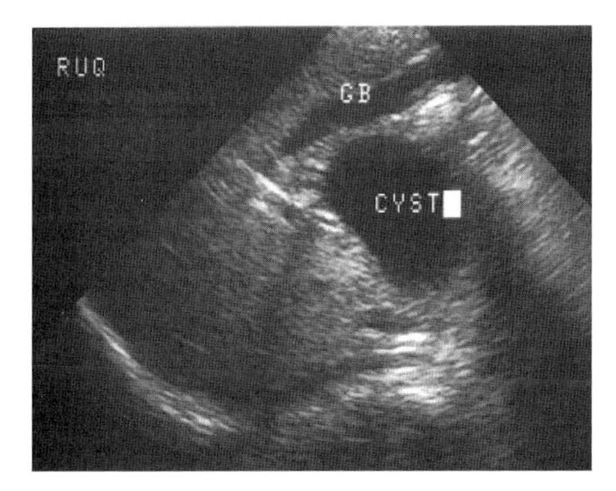

Figure 4.27.1.

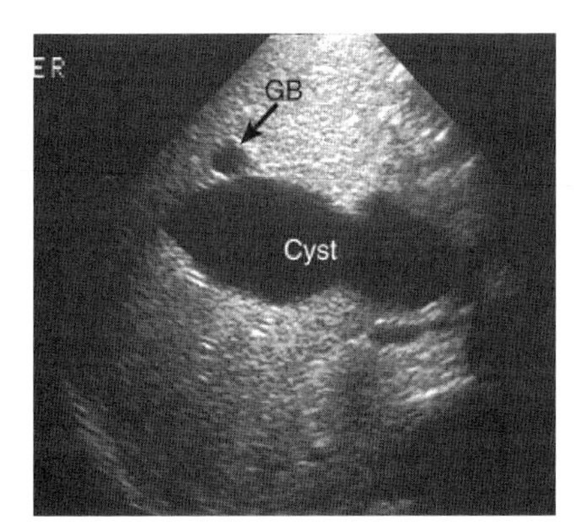

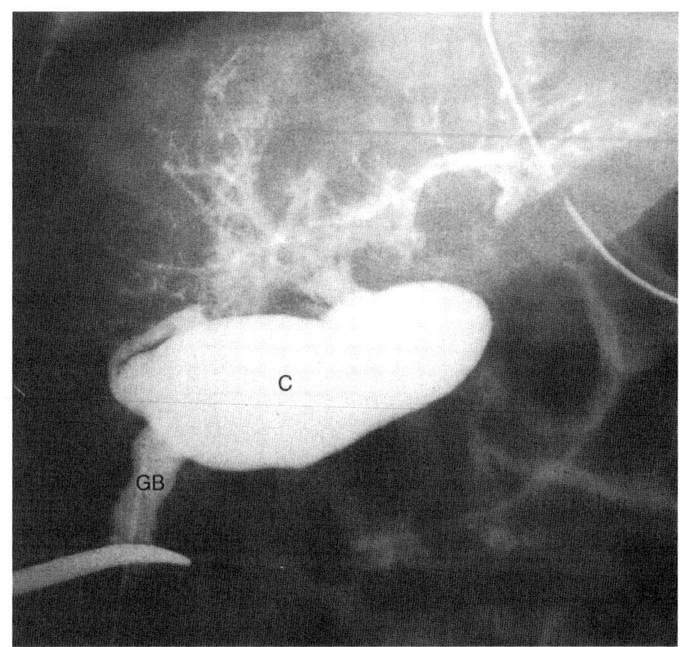

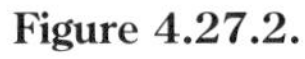

Figure 4.27.2.

Figure 4.27.3.

Findings. Longitudinal (Fig. 4.27.1) and transverse (4.27.2) images through the porta hepatis reveal a bilobed cystic mass (Cyst) located in the porta hepatis and separate from the gallbladder (GB). An operative cholangiogram (Fig. 4.27.3) obtained by injection of the gallbladder shows the large bilobed cyst (C) communicating with the gallbladder and an attenuated intrahepatic biliary tree. Note the absence of contrast distally in the gastrointestinal tract.

Diagnosis. Choledochal cyst associated with distal extrahepatic biliary atresia

Discussion. The neonatal choledochal cyst is congenital in origin and is often associated with extrahepatic biliary atresia. The clinical presentation is indistinguishable from that of neonatal hepatitis and biliary atresia. Children with choledochal cysts not associated with biliary atresia present later in life with an abdominal mass, pain, or jaundice. Sonography, hepatobiliary scintigraphy, and operative cholangiography are required for complete evaluation of the neonate. Nuclear scintigraphy may reveal only the lack of excretion of radionuclide into the gastrointestinal tract, consistent with biliary atresia, but may fail to visualize the choledochal cyst. Early diagnosis of biliary atresia is crucial, because performance of a Kasai procedure (portoenterostomy) before 12 weeks of age improves the prognosis (47).

Aunt Minnie's Pearls

- *Choledochal cysts are seen on sonograms as cystic portal structures that are separate from the gallbladder.*
- *In neonates, this disorder may be associated with extrahepatic biliary atresia.*

CASE 28

History. 12-year-old girl with acute abdominal pain

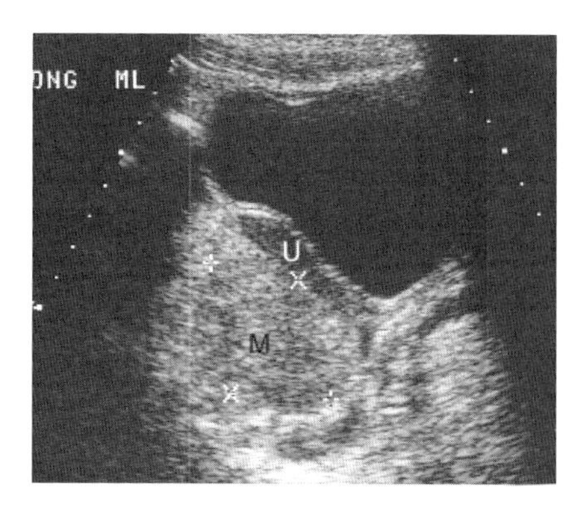

Figure 4.28.1.

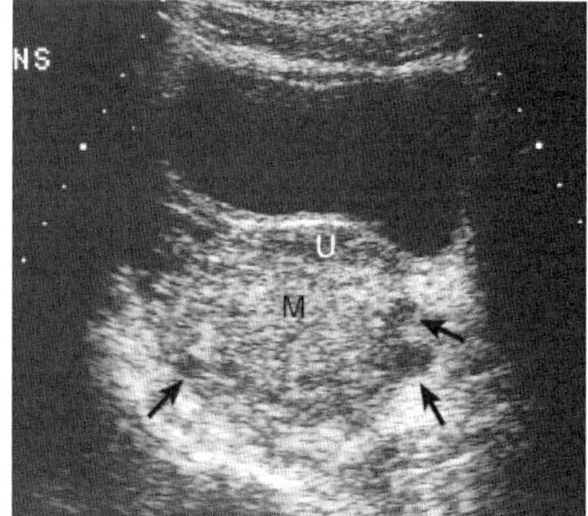

Figure 4.28.2.

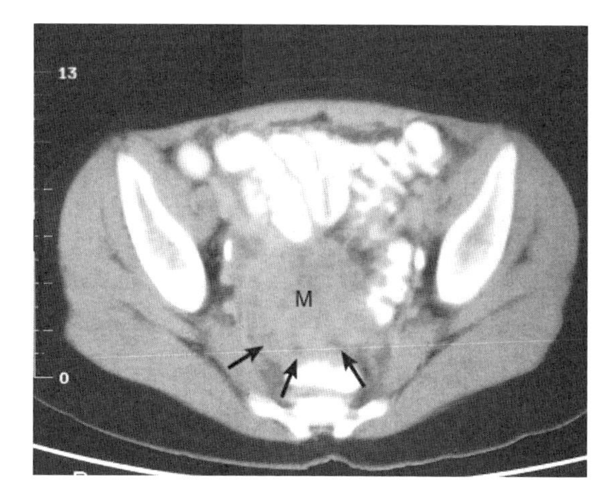

Figure 4.28.3. Axial CT with contrast.

Findings. Longitudinal (Fig. 4.28.1) and transverse (Fig. (4.28.2) ultrasound images demonstrate a mass (M) in the pelvic cul-de-sac with good through transmission of sound and multiple, small, peripheral cysts (*arrows*). The mass is separate from the uterus (U). Color Doppler interrogation of the mass revealed no blood flow within the mass. An axial CT image (4.28.3) confirms the presence of peripheral low attenuation areas in the mass (*arrows*).

Diagnosis. Ovarian torsion

Discussion. Ovarian torsion typically occurs in the premenarchal girl who presents with the acute onset of abdominal pain, nausea, vomiting, and leukocytosis. Half of patients have a palpable mass and give a previous history of similar episodes. Torsion may be due to a lesion in the ovary (e.g., tumor or cyst), or it may occur spontaneously in an anatomically normal ovary. The sonographic appearance of ovarian torsion may vary from that of an enlarged edematous ovary to a complex adnexal mass. When pelvic cul-de-sac fluid is encountered in a premenarchal girl with a tender adnexal mass, this diagnosis should be strongly considered. The finding considered specific for ovarian torsion in this age group is the presence of multiple peripheral cysts that represent edematous fluid-filled follicles. The peripheral cysts are often subtle and hypoechoic rather than truly anechoic. Prompt surgical treatment is required to salvage the ovary before necrosis occurs (48). Another cause of peripheral ovarian cysts is the Stein-Leventhal syndrome, but that diagnosis would present in an older woman with the characteristic history of obesity and hirsutism.

Aunt Minnie's Pearls

- *Always think ovarian torsion in a young girl with pelvic pain.*
- *Although various findings may be seen, multiple small peripheral cysts are specific for ovarian torsion in the pediatric age group.*

CASE 29

History. Infant born prematurely

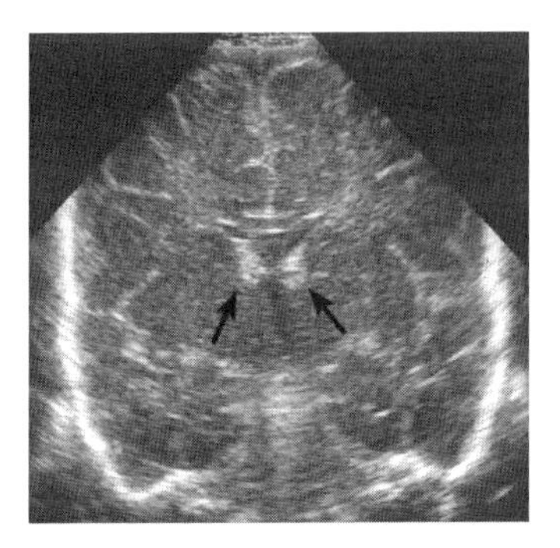

Figure 4.29.1.

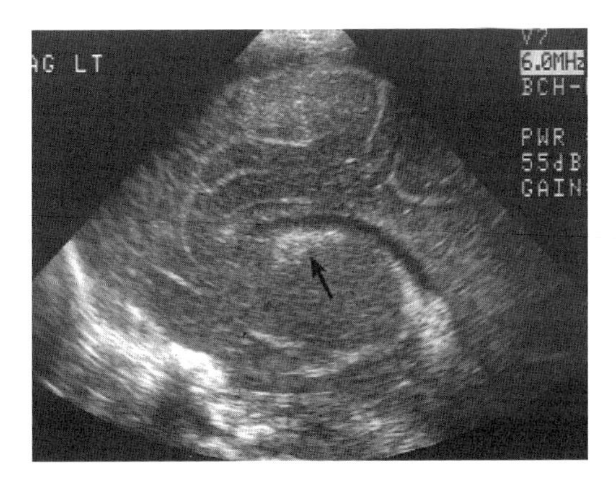

Figure 4.29.2. Left side.

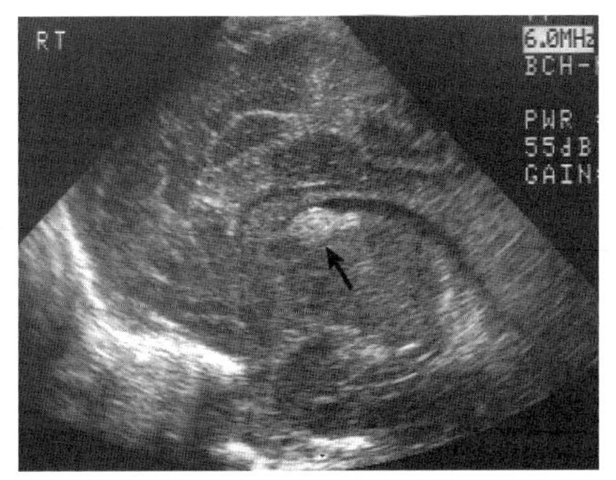

Figure 4.29.3. Right side.

Findings. A coronal image of the neonatal brain (Fig. 4.29.1) shows bilateral hyperechoic masses (*arrows*) that are inferolateral to the floors of the frontal horns and medial to the caudate. On the sagittal images (Figs. 4.29.2 and 4.29.3), the hyperechoic masses appear as a bulge anterior to the caudothalamic groove (*arrows*).

Diagnosis. Bilateral germinal matrix/subependymal hemorrhages

Discussion. The germinal matrix is a bed of highly vascular subependymal tissue that is located adjacent to the lateral ventricles in the caudothalamic groove. In premature infants, the stresses of delivery and extrauterine life can lead to thrombosis, bleeding, and infarction in the delicate tissues of the germinal matrix. In fact, intracranial hemorrhage occurs in 25–40% of premature infants born at <32 weeks of gestation and weighing <1500 grams. Hyperechoic masses that are centered on the caudothalamic groove are characteristic of germinal matrix hemorrhages. Look for ventricular and parenchymal extension of the hemorrhage and hydrocephalus because prognosis is affected by the presence of these complicating features. As the hemorrhagic areas evolve, they become less echogenic and may even result in cystic encephalomalacia.

Screening sonography of the head is usually performed in this population at days 7 and 14 of life, because approximately 90% of intracranial hemorrhages occur by day 6 of life, and most cases of posthemorrhagic hydrocephalus present by day 14. A discharge study is also performed for prognostic assessment, and neurodevelopmental outcome is generally proportional to the severity of the intracranial hemorrhage and degree of ventricular dilatation (49).

Aunt Minnie's Pearls

- *Hyperechoic masses in the caudothalamic groove in a premature infant (<32 weeks or <1500 grams) are germinal matrix hemorrhages.*
- *Check for ventricular and parenchymal extension and for the development of hydrocephalus.*

Case 30

History. Full-term infant with low Apgar scores, hypotonia, seizures, and metabolic acidosis

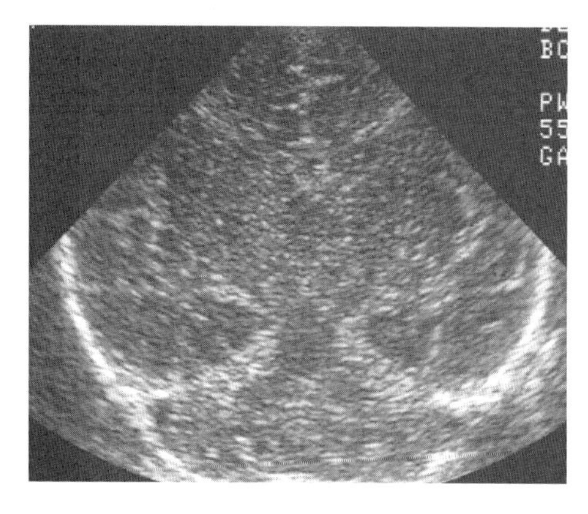

Figure 4.30.1. Coronal view.

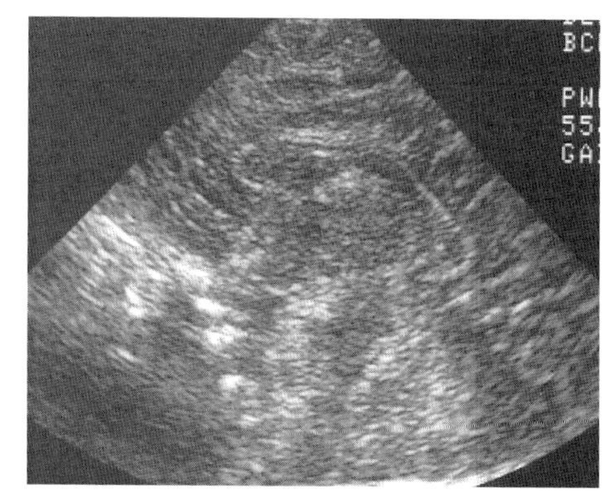

Figure 4.30.2. Sagittal view.

Findings. Coronal (Fig. 4.30.1) and sagittal (Fig. 4.30.2) images of the neonatal brain demonstrate diffusely increased brain echogenicity, poor sulcal-gyral differentiation, and small ventricles.

Diagnosis. Perinatal asphyxia/diffuse hypoxic-ischemic injury

Discussion. Perinatal asphyxia is a common cause of diffuse hypoxic-ischemic injury in the full-term infant. Neurologic outcome correlates with the sonographic appearance, because 90% of patients with abnormal brain echogenicity progress to death or neurologic sequelae. The sonographic findings of diffuse echogenicity and sulcal effacement reflect neuronal necrosis and mass effect from cerebral edema. In addition, focal areas of infarction may be seen as increased echogenicity in the basal ganglia, middle cerebral artery territories, and watershed areas. Late findings of diffuse injury include cystic encephalomalacia, parenchymal calcifications, and atrophy with ventriculomegaly (50).

Aunt Minnie's Pearls

- *Diffuse increased echogenicity and sulcal effacement are diagnostic of hypoxic-ischemic injury.*
- *Focal areas of infarction may be seen in the basal ganglia, middle cerebral artery territory, or watershed areas.*

REFERENCES

1. Goncalves LF, Jeanty P. Ultrasound evaluation of fetal abdominal wall defects. In: Callen PW, ed. Ultrasonography in obstetrics and gynecology, 3rd ed. Philadelphia: Saunders, 1994:370–388.
2. Nyberg DA, Mack LA. Abdominal wall defects. In: Nyberg DA, Mahony BS, Pretorius DH, eds. Diagnostic ultrasound of fetal anomalies: text and atlas. Chicago: Year Book, 1990:395–432.
3. Emanuel PG, Garcia GI, Angtuaco TL. Prenatal detection of anterior abdominal wall defects with US. RadioGraphics 1995;15:517–530.
4. Filly RA. Ultrasound evaluation of the fetal neural axis. In: Callen PW, ed. Ultrasonography in obstetrics and gynecology, 3rd ed. Philadelphia: Saunders, 1994:189–234.
5. Nyberg DA, Mack LA. The spine and neural tube defects. In: Nyberg DA, Mahony BS, Pretorius DH, eds. Diagnostic ultrasound of fetal anomalies: text and atlas. Chicago: Year Book, 1990:146–202.
6. Nyberg DA, Mack LA, Hirsch J, Mahony BS. Abnormalities of fetal cranial contour in sonographic detection of spina bifida: evaluation of the "lemon" sign. Radiology 1988;167:387–392.
7. Ball RH, Filly RA, Goldstein RB, Callen PW. The lemon sign: not a specific indicator of meningomyelocele. Ultrasound Med 1993;12:131–134.
8. Harmon JP, Hiett AK, Palmer CG, Golichowski AM. Prenatal ultrasound detection of isolated neural tube defects: is cytogenetic evaluation warranted? Obstet Gynecol 1995;86:595–599.
9. Czeizel AE. Prevention of congenital abnormalities by periconceptional multivitamin supplementation. Br Med J 1993;306:1645–1648.
10. Hendricks SK, Cyr DR, Nyberg DA, Raabe R, Mack LA. Exencephaly: clinical and ultrasonic correlation to anencephaly. Obstet Gynecol 1988;72:898–901.
11. Gersell DJ, Kraus FT, Riffle MB. Diseases of the placenta. In: Kurman RJ, ed. Blaustein's pathology of the female genital tract, 3rd ed. New York: Springer-Verlag, 1987:769–834.
12. Townsend RR. Ultrasound evaluation of the placenta and umbilical cord. In: Callen PW, ed. Ultrasonography in obstetrics and gynecology, 3rd ed. Philadelphia: Saunders, 1994:440–465.
13. Finberg HJ, Williams JW. Placenta accreta: prospective sonographic diagnosis in patients with placenta previa and prior cesarean section. Ultrasound Med 1992;11:333–343.
14. Benedetti TJ. Obstetric hemorrhage. In: Gabbe SG, Niebyl JR, Simpson JL, eds. Obstetrics: normal and problem pregnancies, 2nd ed. New York: Churchill Livingstone, 1991:588.
15. Hall DA, Yoder IC. Ultrasound evaluation of the uterus. In: Callen PW, ed. Ultrasonography in obstetrics and gynecology, 3rd ed. Philadelphia: Saunders, 1994:586–614.
16. Hertzberg BS, Kliewer MA, Farrell TA, DeLong DM. Spontaneously changing gravid cervix: clinical implications and prognostic features. Radiology 1995;196:721–724.
17. Cyr DR, Mack LA, Nyberg DA, Shepard TH, Shuman WP. Fetal rhombencephalon: normal US findings. Radiology 1988;166:691–692.
18. Glazer GM, Callen PW, Filly RA. Medullary nephrocalcinosis: sonographic evaluation. AJR 1982;138:55–57.
19. Amis ES Jr, Newhouse JH. Essentials of uroradiology. Boston: Little, Brown, 1991:216.
20. Middleton WD, Kellman GM, Melson GL, Madrazo BL. Postbiopsy renal transplant arteriovenous fistulas: color Doppler US characteristics. Radiology 1989;171:253–257.
21. Perrella RR. Renal transplantation: use of sonography. Urol Radiol 1992;14:43–48.
22. Kurtz AB, Middleton WD. Ultrasound: the requisites. St. Louis: Mosby, 1995:115.
23. Amis ES Jr, Newhouse JH. Essentials of uroradiology. Boston: Little, Brown, 1991:124.
24. Bourneville DM. Sclerose tubereuse des circonvolutions cerebrales: idiotie et epilepsie hemiplegique. Arch Int Neurol 1880;1:81–91.
25. Oesterling JE, Fishman EK, Goldman SE, Marshall FF. The management of renal angiomyolipoma. J Urol 1986;135:1121–1124.
26. De Gaetano AM, Lafortune M, Patriquin H, De Franco A, Aubin B, Paradis K. Cavernous transformation of the portal vein: patterns of intrahepatic and splanchnic collateral circulation detected with Doppler sonography. AJR 1995;165:1151–1155.
27. Parvey HR, Raval B, Sandler CM. Portal vein thrombosis: imaging findings. AJR 1994;162:77–81.
28. Berk RN, Armbuster TG, Saltzstein SL. Carcinoma in the porcelain gallbladder. Radiology 1973;106:29–31.
29. MacDonald FR, Cooperberg PL, Cohen MM. The WES triad: a specific sonographic sign of gallstones in the contracted gallbladder. Gastrointest Radiol 1981;6:39–41.
30. Dodd GD III, Budzik RF Jr. Lipomatous tumors of the pelvis in women: spectrum of imaging findings. AJR 1990;155:317–322.
31. Backus ML, Mack LA, Middleton WD, King BF, Winter TC III, True LD. Testicular microlithiasis: imaging appearances and pathologic correlation. Radiology 1994;192:781–785.
32. Patel MD, Olcott EW, Kerschmann RL, Callen PW, Gooding GAW. Sonographically detected testicular microlithiasis and testicular carcinoma. J Clin Ultrasound 1993;21:447–452.
33. Weingarten BJ, Kellman GM, Middleton WD, Gross ML. Tubular ectasia within the mediastinum testis. J Ultrasound Med 1992;11:349–353.
34. Hamm B, Fobbe F, Loy V. Testicular cysts: differentiation with US and clinical findings. Radiology 1988;168:19–23.
35. Li YW, Sheih CP, Chen WJ. MR imaging and sonography of Gartner's duct cyst and single ectopic ureter with ipsilateral renal dysplasia. Pediatr Radiol 1992;22:472–473.
36. Polak JF. The peripheral vessels. In: Rumack CM, Wilson SR, Charboneau JW, eds. Diagnostic ultrasound. St. Louis: Mosby/Year Book, 1991;1:678–681.

37. Filley RA. Ectopic pregnancy. In: Callen PW, ed. Ultrasonography in obstetrics and gynecology. Philadelphia: Saunders, 1994:641–659.
38. Nussbaum AR, Dorst JP, Jeffs RD, Gearhart JP, Sanders RC. Ectopic ureter and ureterocele: their varied sonographic manifestations. Radiology 1986;159:227–235.
39. O'Keeffe FN, Stansberry SD, Swischuk LE, Hayden CK Jr. Antropyloric muscle thickness at US in infants: what is normal? Radiology 1991;178:827–830.
40. Harcke HT, Grissom LE. Performing dynamic sonography of the infant hip. AJR 1990;155:837–844.
41. Siegel MJ. Gastrointestinal tract. In: Siegel MJ, ed. Pediatric sonography, 2nd ed. New York: Raven, 1995:288–294.
42. Verschelden P, Filiatrault D, Garel L, et al. Intussusception in children: reliability of US in diagnosis—a prospective study. Radiology 1992;184:741–744.
43. Blask ARN, Sanders RC, Rock JA. Obstructed uterovaginal anomalies: demonstration with sonography. Part II: teenagers. Radiology 1991;179:84–88.
44. Shackelford GD. Adrenal glands, pancreas, and other retroperitoneal structures. In: Siegel MJ, ed. Pediatric sonography, 2nd ed. New York: Raven, 1995:306–310.
45. Strife JL, Souza AS, Kirks DR, Strife CF, Gelfand MJ, Wacksman J. Multicystic dysplastic kidney in children: US follow-up. Radiology 1993;186:785–788.
46. Atiyeh B, Husmann D, Baum M. Contralateral renal abnormalities in multicystic dysplastic kidney disease. J Pediatr 1992;121:65–67.
47. Torrisi JM, Haller JO, Velcek FT. Choledochal cyst and biliary atresia in the neonate: imaging findings in five cases. AJR 1990;155:1273–1276.
48. Siegel MJ. Pediatric gynecologic sonography. Radiology 1991;179:593–600.
49. Siegel MJ. Brain. In: Siegel MJ, ed. Pediatric sonography, 2nd ed. New York: Raven, 1995:40–49.
50. Siegel MJ, Shackelford GD, Perlman JM, Fulling KH. Hypoxic-ischemic encephalopathy in term infants: diagnosis and prognosis evaluated by ultrasound. Radiology 1984;152:395–399.

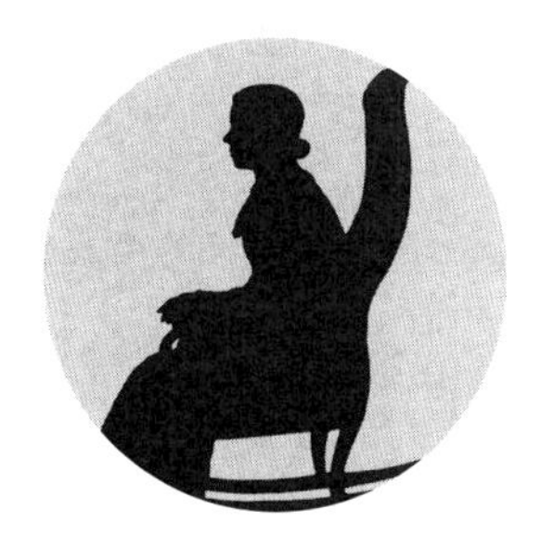

chapter 5

NUCLEAR MEDICINE

EDWARD K. GRISHAW AND JAMES D. BALL

CASE 1

History. 68-year-old man with dementia, ataxia, and incontinence

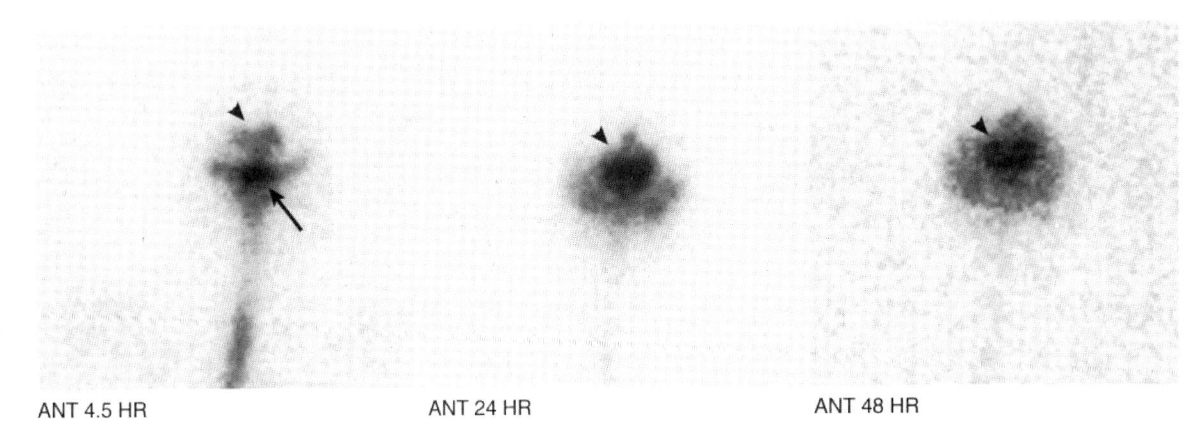

Figure 5.1.1. Anterior views at 4.5, 24, and 48 hours.

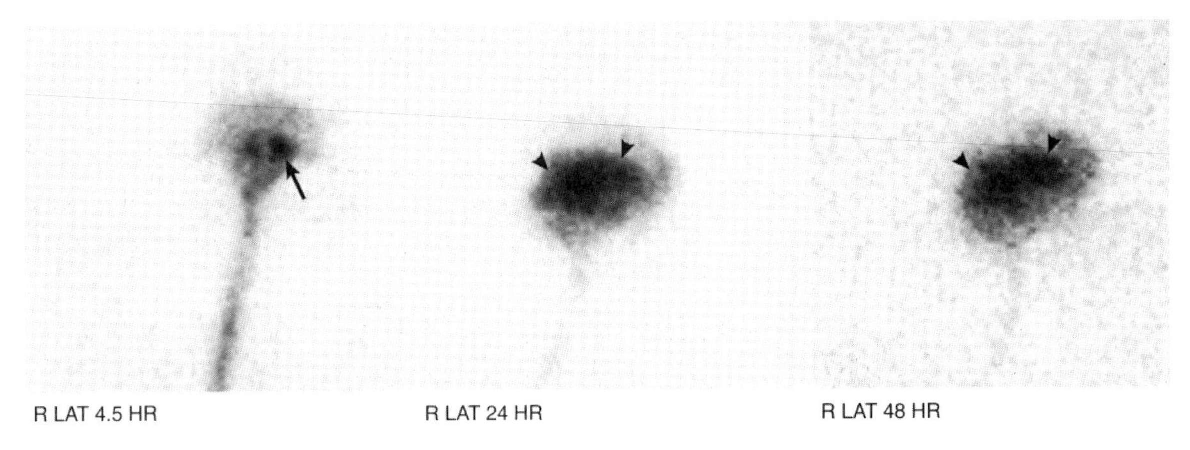

Figure 5.1.2. Right lateral views at 4.5, 24, and 48 hours.

Findings. Multiple frontal (Fig. 5.1.1) and lateral (Fig. 5.1.2) images from an ^{111}In DTPA cisternography study are presented. Activity is present in the basal cisterns at 4.5 hours (*arrows*). Mild lateral ventricular activity is also seen at this time and is more prominent at 24 and 48 hours (*arrowheads*). Flow over the convexities is delayed.

Diagnosis. Normal-pressure hydrocephalus

Discussion. Clinically, normal-pressure hydrocephalus is characterized by the triad of ataxia, dementia, and incontinence. Cerebrospinal fluid flow reversal is useful in distinguishing this entity from other causes of dementia associated with ventriculomegaly (i.e., hydrocephalus ex vacuo). Surgical shunting can alleviate a patient's symptoms; however, not all patients respond to this treatment (1). The amount of response is dependent on the amount of activity in the ventricles compared with that over the convexities and on the duration of neurologic symptoms and signs (2).

Normally, the radiotracer reaches the basal cisterns within 1 hour after administration via lumbar puncture. Between 2 and 6 hours the activity ascends into the interhemispheric and sylvian fissures. Radiotracer flows over the cerebral convexities by 24 hours. Normally, no lateral ventricular activity is seen. In classic normal-pressure hydrocephalus, radiotracer reflux into the lateral ventricles occurs and persists for 24, 48, or even 72 hours after injection.

Aunt Minnie's Pearls

- *In normal-pressure hydrocephalus, radiotracer refluxes into the lateral ventricles and persists for 24, 48, or even 72 hours.*
- *Clinical triad of dementia, ataxia, and incontinence.*

CASE 2

History. 42-year-old man with a seizure disorder

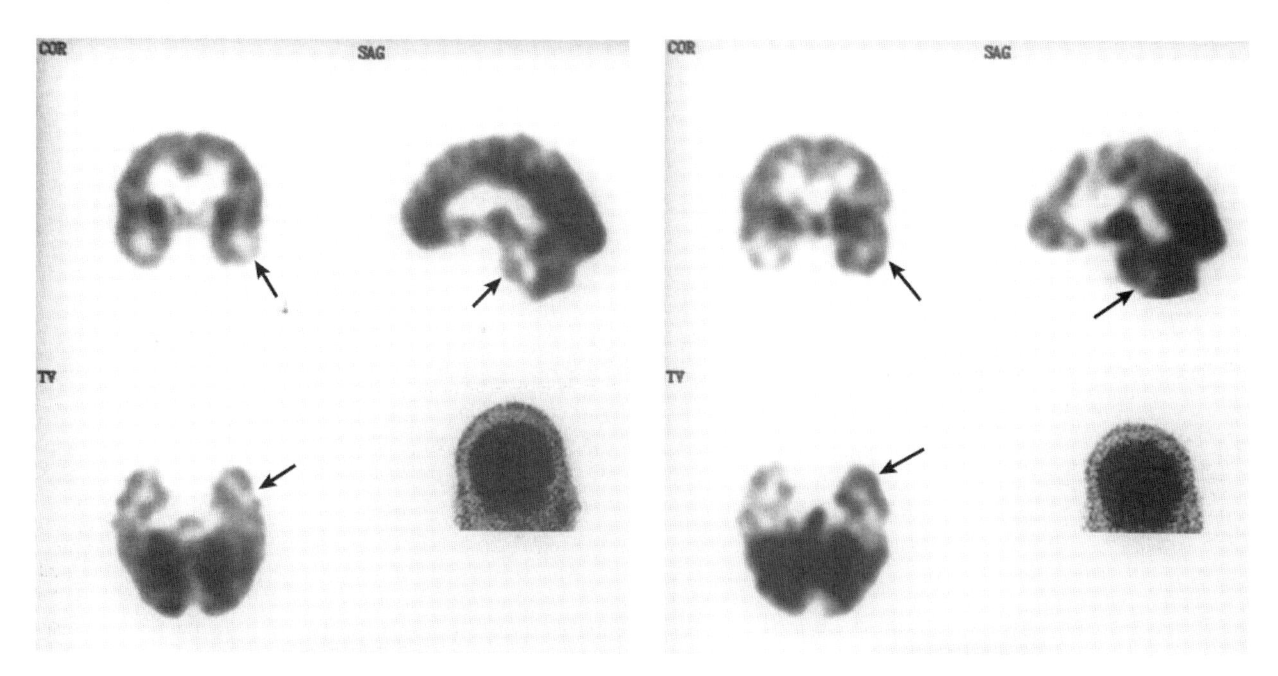

Figure 5.2.1. Interictal single photon emission CT.

Figure 5.2.2. Ictal single photon emission CT.

Findings. An interictal ^{99m}Tc hexamethylpropyleneamine oxime brain single photon emission CT study (Fig. 5.2.1) shows subtle decreased activity of left temporal lobe laterally (*arrows*). A repeat study obtained during a seizure (Fig. 5.2.2) reveals increased activity of left temporal lobe (*arrows*).

Diagnosis. Left temporal lobe seizure focus

Discussion. Thirty to sixty percent of patients with complex partial seizures do not respond to medical therapy (3). Because most complex partial seizures arise in the temporal lobes, these patients may benefit from temporal lobectomy; however, relatively few undergo the procedure because of difficulty in seizure focus localization. Scalp, cortical, and depth electroencephalography (EEG) had been the mainstay of seizure focus localization. Scalp EEG, however, has poor spatial resolution. Surface EEG has limited sampling and is insensitive to deep seizure foci. Depth EEG, although sensitive to deep seizure foci, requires invasive placement and is limited to a small area of sampling (3). CT and MR imaging have only 17 and 34% sensitivity, respectively (4).

Conversely, single photon emission CT imaging has been used to identify 70–80% of complex partial seizure patients with a resectable seizure focus (5). Classically, the seizure focus is seen as an area of increased perfusion ictally and decreased perfusion interictally. Although clinical images may be obtained after the patient's seizure, the radiopharmaceutical for the ictal study must be injected while the patient is actively seizing, because the area of increased activity may quickly "switch" to decreased activity shortly after ictus.

Aunt Minnie's Pearls

- *Seizure foci show increased perfusion ictally and decreased perfusion interictally.*

CASE 3

History. 62-year-old man who suffered a major cerebrovascular accident

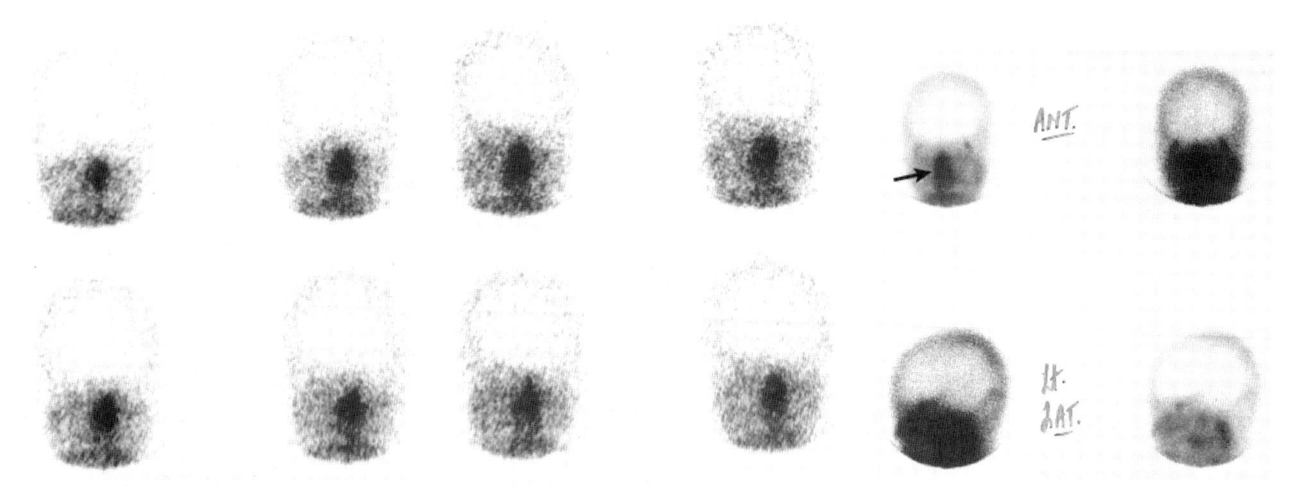

Figure 5.3.1.

Figure 5.3.2. ANT, anterior; lT LAT, left lateral.

Findings. The initial flow images from this ^{99m}Tc hexamethylpropyleneamine oxime (HMPAO) cerebral perfusion study (Fig. 5.3.1) show that no arterial flow is present in either cerebral hemisphere. The delayed static images (Fig. 5.3.2) confirm that no cerebral activity is seen. Prominent activity is identified in the patient's face and scalp (*arrow*).

Diagnosis. Absent cerebral perfusion

Discussion. Although the diagnosis of brain death is made on clinical criteria, the radionuclide cerebral perfusion study is often used for confirmation. Unlike electroencephalography, radionuclide evaluation does not produce false-positive studies in patients with hypothermia or a metabolic disturbance, i.e., anoxia, uremia, hepatic encephalopathy, severe sepsis, or high doses of fentanyl, diazepam, or barbiturates (6). The scintigraphic appearance of brain death involves absence of both intracranial arterial and major dural sinus flow. Controversy exists regarding whether faint visualization of the sagittal or transverse sinuses precludes this diagnosis (6). The "hot nose" sign described with absent cerebral perfusion represents the shunting of blood from the internal to the external carotid arteries.

Unlike DTPA, pertechnetate, and glucoheptonate, HMPAO is less dependent on bolus injection (6, 7). In addition, cerebral perfusion can be evaluated on static as well as flow images, because HMPAO normally crosses the blood-brain barrier.

Aunt Minnie's Pearls

- *Absent cerebral perfusion is accompanied by the "hot nose" sign.*
- *Nuclear studies are not limited by hypothermia or metabolic disturbance.*

CASE 4

History. 70-year-old woman with low back pain

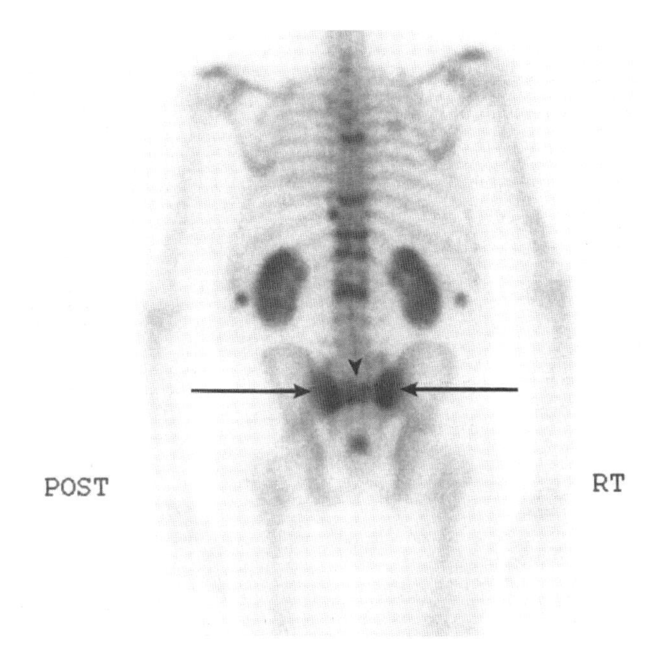

Figure 5.4.1. POST, posterior; RT, right.

Findings. A posterior view from a whole body bone scan (Fig. 5.4.1) shows vertical areas of increased activity involving both sacral alae (*arrows*). A horizontal region of increased activity also extends across the body of the sacrum (*arrowhead*). Also identified are numerous areas of abnormal activity in the spine that likely represent vertebral body fractures.

Diagnosis. Sacral and vertebral body insufficiency fractures

Discussion. Insufficiency fractures are stress fractures that occur when normal stress is applied to bone with abnormal elastic resistance or deficient mineralization. Conversely, fatigue fractures are stress fractures that occur from abnormal stresses on normal bone. Common causes of insufficiency fractures include osteoporosis (as in the index case), osteomalacia/rickets, steroid use, radiation therapy, Paget's disease, rheumatoid arthritis, hyperparathyroidism, and fibrous dysplasia. The "H" or "Honda" sign, which includes both the vertical and horizontal fractures in the sacrum, is characteristic of a sacral insufficiency fracture (8). The vertical lines of increased activity represent fractures through the sacral alae, and the transverse area of uptake is secondary to a fracture through the sacral body (9). The bone scan is more sensitive than plain films for the detection of sacral insufficiency fractures.

Aunt Minnie's Pearls

- *The H or Honda sign is a specific sign for sacral insufficiency fractures.*
- *Insufficiency fractures occur from normal stress on abnormal bone.*

CASE 5

History. 27-year-old woman with pain in the right hand who recently underwent open reduction and internal fixation of a distal right radial fracture

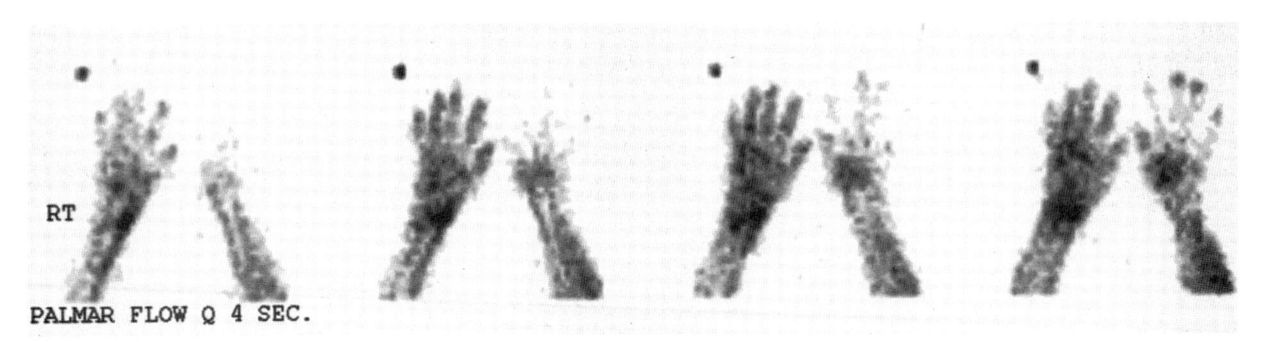

Figure 5.5.1.

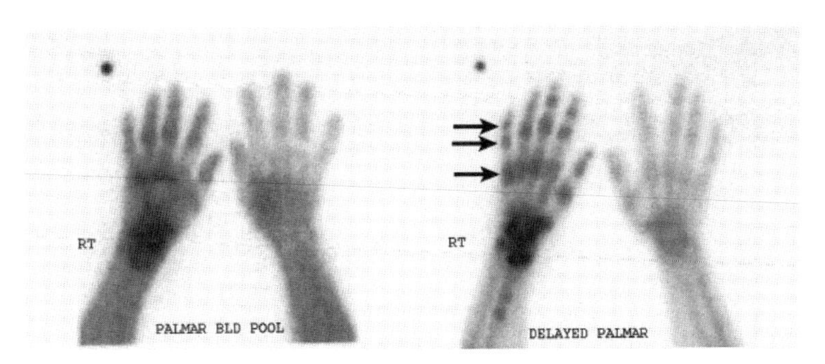

Figure 5.5.2. BLD POOL, blood pool.

Findings. Images from a three phase bone scan demonstrate increased blood flow (Fig. 5.5.1) to the right wrist and hand. Immediate and delayed static images (Fig. 5.5.2) show diffuse increased bony uptake in a periarticular distribution (*arrows*). The two focal areas of abnormal increased activity in the distal right radius represent the region of fracture and operative fixation.

Diagnosis. Reflex sympathetic dystrophy

Discussion. Reflex sympathetic dystrophy, or Sudeck's atrophy, presents clinically as local pain, soft-tissue swelling, and vasomotor instability of the involved extremity. The most common etiologies include trauma (often minor), immobilization, infection, myocardial infarction, and neurologic disease (10). Symptoms are thought to occur because of an abnormal sympathetic nervous system response to the traumatic insult (11). The disorder is less frequent in children than in adults (12). Radiographically there is periarticular soft-tissue swelling and regional osteoporosis. Classically, bone scintigraphy demonstrates increased flow and periarticular uptake in the involved extremity, with delayed images being the most sensitive for the diagnosis of reflex sympathetic dystrophy. Radionuclide imaging is not as sensitive in diagnosing this entity if symptoms have been present for more than 1 year because delayed images may have normal or reduced activity (13).

Aunt Minnie's Pearls

- *Increased flow + periarticular uptake + patient with history of trauma and vasomotor instability = reflex sympathetic dystrophy.*

CASE 6

History. Infant with hypothyroidism

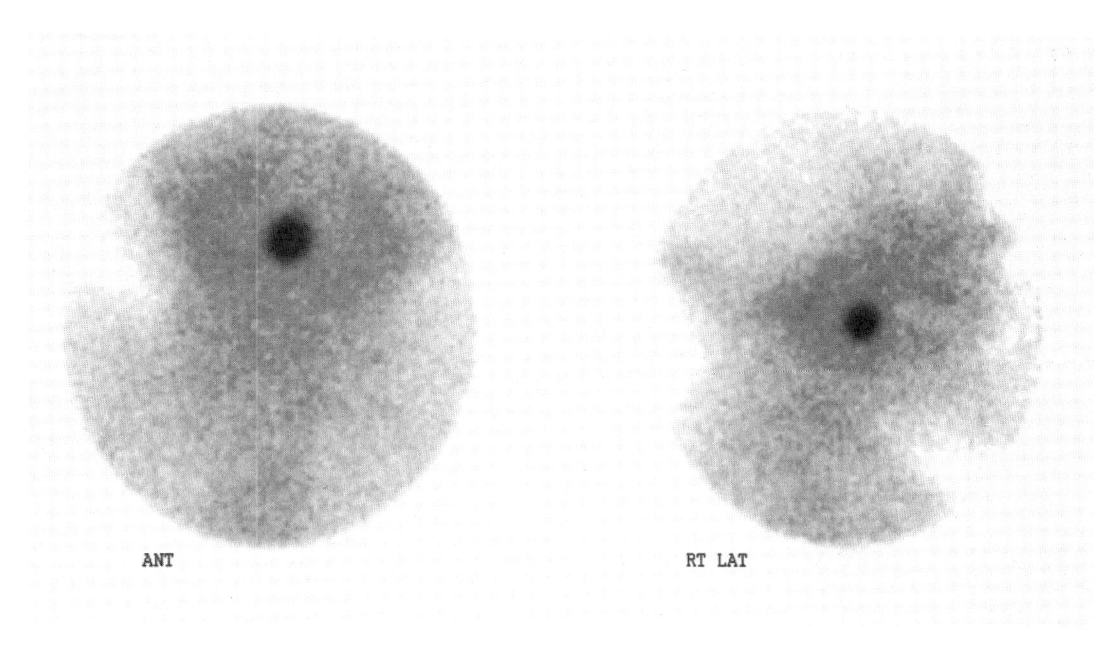

Figure 5.6.1.

Findings. A focal area of increased activity is present in the midline in the region of the tongue base on anteroposterior (ANT) and right lateral (RT LAT) views from a ^{99m}Tc pertechnetate thyroid scan (Fig. 5.6.1). No activity is seen in the thyroid bed.

Diagnosis. Lingual thyroid

Discussion. Lingual thyroid results from failure of the thyroid gland to descend during embryogenesis. The ectopic gland is typically hypofunctional. Hypothyroidism associated with ectopic thyroid tissue occurs sporadically, whereas hypothyroidism secondary to biosynthetic defects is inherited (14). In addition to hypothyroidism, the lingual thyroid may present as a mass in the tongue or upper neck. This abnormality must be diagnosed shortly after birth because failure to begin replacement therapy promptly will adversely affect intellectual development.

Aunt Minnie's Pearls

- *An ectopic or lingual thyroid is typically hypofunctional.*
- *Screening for hypothyroidism is routine in newborns because failure to diagnose hypothyroidism may result in severe intellectual impairment.*

CASE 7

History. 40-year-old woman with hypertension refractory to medical therapy

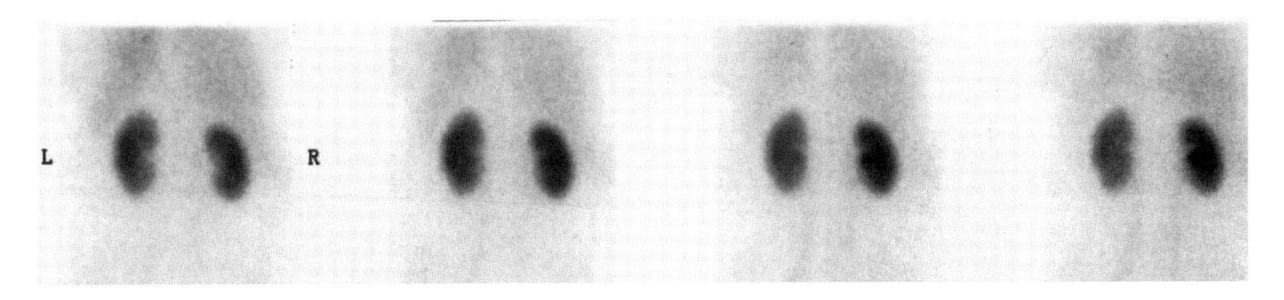

Figure 5.7.1.

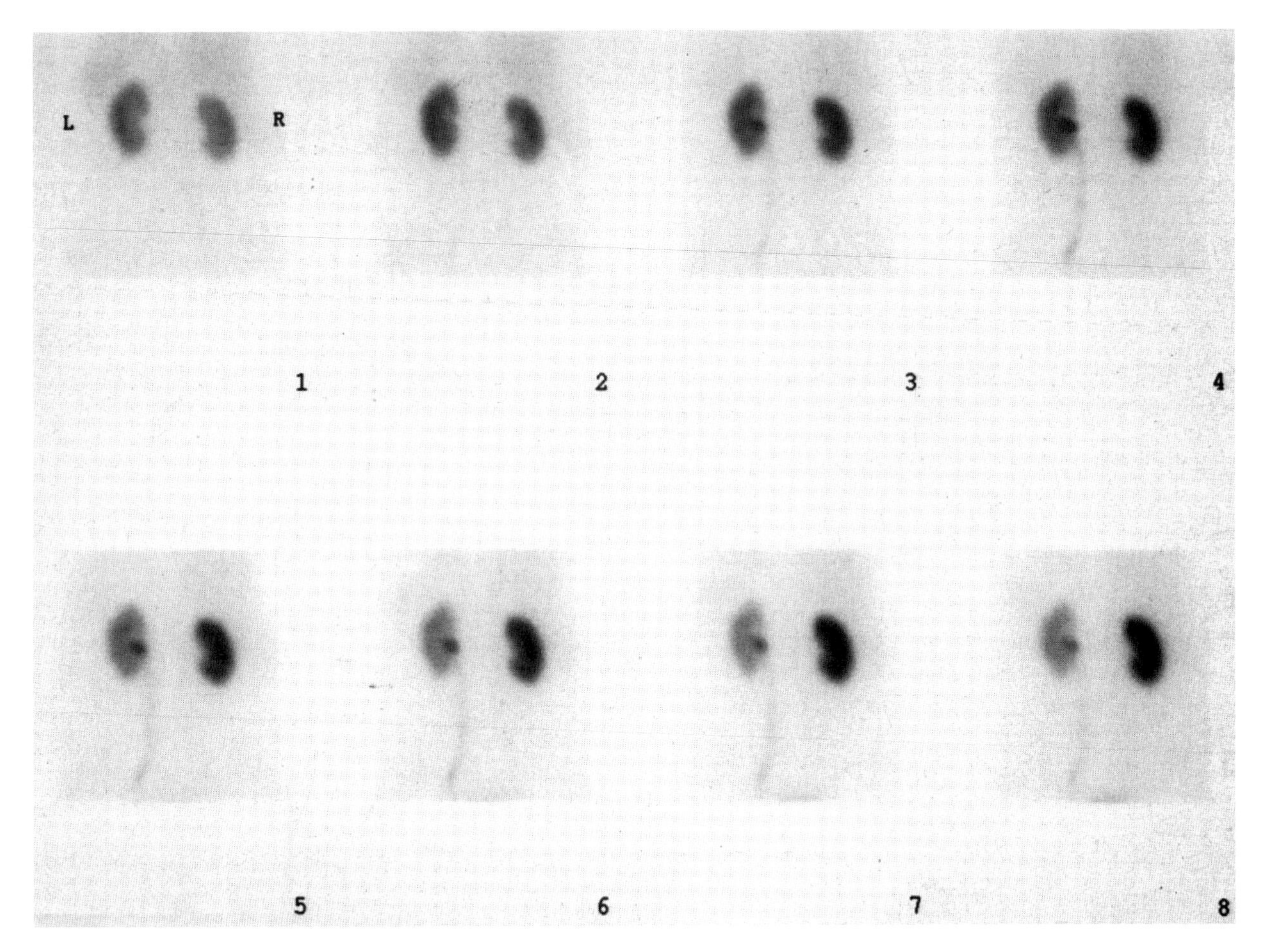

Figure 5.7.2.

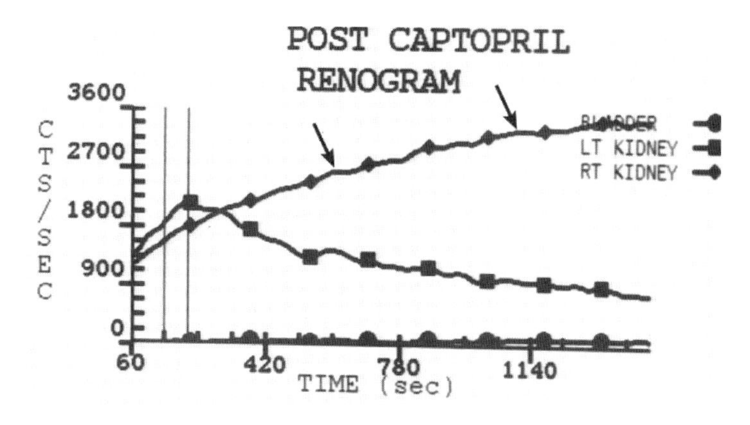

Figure 5.7.3.

Findings. Images acquired during a precaptopril ^{99m}Tc MAG3 renogram (Fig. 5.7.1) demonstrate slightly increased cortical activity retention in the right kidney. After captopril administration (Fig. 5.7.2), this asymmetry becomes pronounced. Right renal cortical activity retention is significant, and excretion of radiopharmaceutical into the collecting system is minimal. The abnormal response of the right kidney to captopril administration is also demonstrated on a time-activity curve of the renogram (Fig. 5.7.3, *arrows*).

Diagnosis. Right renovascular hypertension

Discussion. Renovascular hypertension is caused by hypoperfusion-induced stimulation of the renin-angiotensin system. It accounts for approximately 1–2% of all hypertensive patients (15). The most common causes of renal hypoperfusion are atherosclerosis and fibromuscular dysplasia.

The involved kidney maintains glomerular filtration rate by compensatory vasoconstriction of the efferent arteriole by angiotensin II, the end product of the renin-angiotensin system. Captopril, an inhibitor of angiotensin-converting enzyme, prevents efferent arteriole constriction. If a hemodynamically significant lesion of the renal artery is present, glomerular filtration rate will drop on administration of captopril when compared with the precaptopril examination. Scintigraphically, this difference is seen as delayed radiotracer uptake and cortical retention (16).

Aunt Minnie's Pearls

- *Renovascular hypertension mediated by the renin-angiotensin system.*
- *After captopril administration, delayed radiotracer uptake and cortical retention will be seen in the affected kidney.*

CASE 8

History. 2-year-old female with multiple urinary tract infections

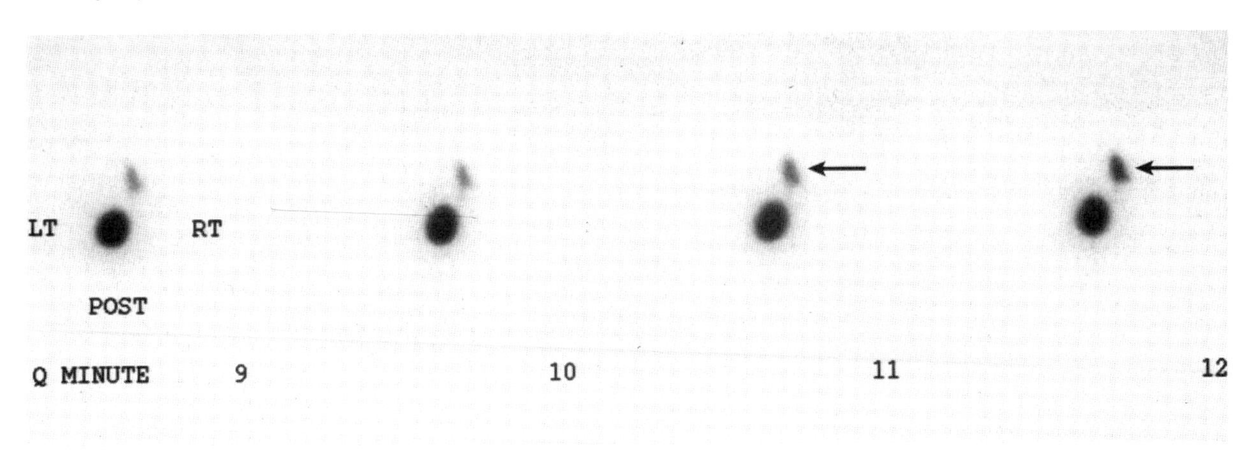

Figure 5.8.1.

Findings. Posterior (POST) images from a ^{99m}Tc pertechnetate cystogram (Fig. 5.8.1) reveal activity extending from the bladder to the right renal collecting system (*arrows*).

Diagnosis. Vesicoureteral reflux

Discussion. Radionuclide cystography is becoming increasingly popular for the detection and follow-up of vesicoureteral reflux. The radiation absorbed dose is significantly lower than that associated with conventional voiding cystourethrography (17–19). As little as 1 ml of refluxed urine can be detected with this technique. Reflux is considered mild when it is confined to the ureter, moderate when it involves the pelvicaliceal system, and severe when a distended pelvicaliceal system and/or tortuous ureter is identified (17). Reflux may be seen during either filling or voiding.

Sterile, low-pressure reflux does not cause renal injury. However, untreated reflux of infected urine can lead to chronic renal failure and hypertension (18). As the child ages, the distal ureteral submucosal tunnel lengthens, and in 80% of patients the reflux resolves spontaneously.

Aunt Minnie's Pearls

- *Nuclear cystography is more sensitive and exposes the patient to less radiation than contrast voiding cystourethrography.*

CASE 9

History. 39-year-old man with an acute onset of chest pain and dyspnea

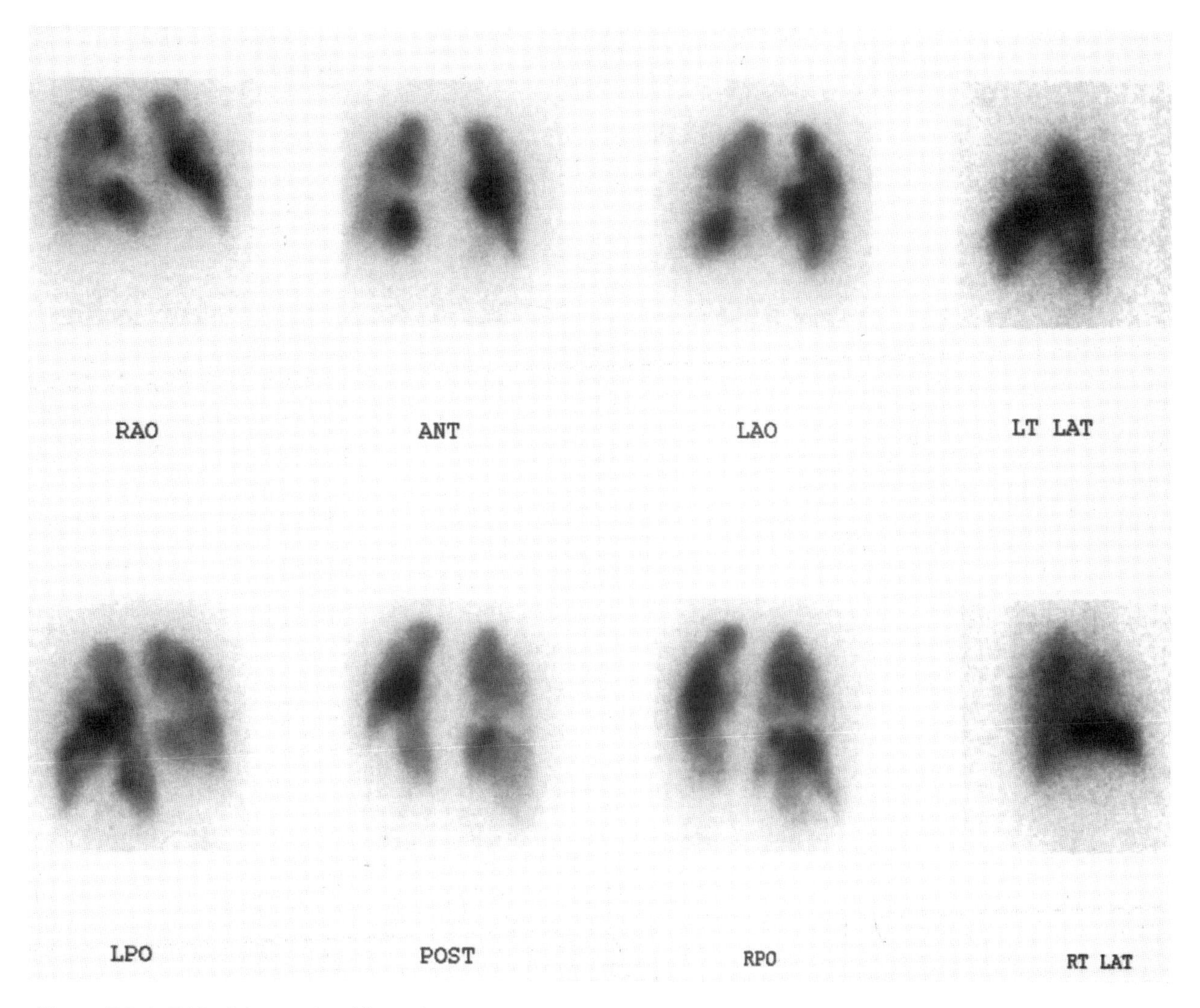

Figure 5.9.1. RAO, right anterior oblique; ANT, anterior; LAO, left anterior oblique; LT LAT, left lateral; LPO,left posterior oblique; POST, posterior; RPO, right posterior oblique; RT LAT, right lateral.

Findings. Pulmonary perfusion images obtained after injection of ^{99m}Tc MAA (Fig. 5.9.1) reveal multiple segmental perfusion defects. Posterior ventilation images utilizing ^{133}Xe (Fig. 5.9.2) demonstrate normal ventilation during first breath, equilibrium, and washout images.

Diagnosis. Multiple pulmonary emboli

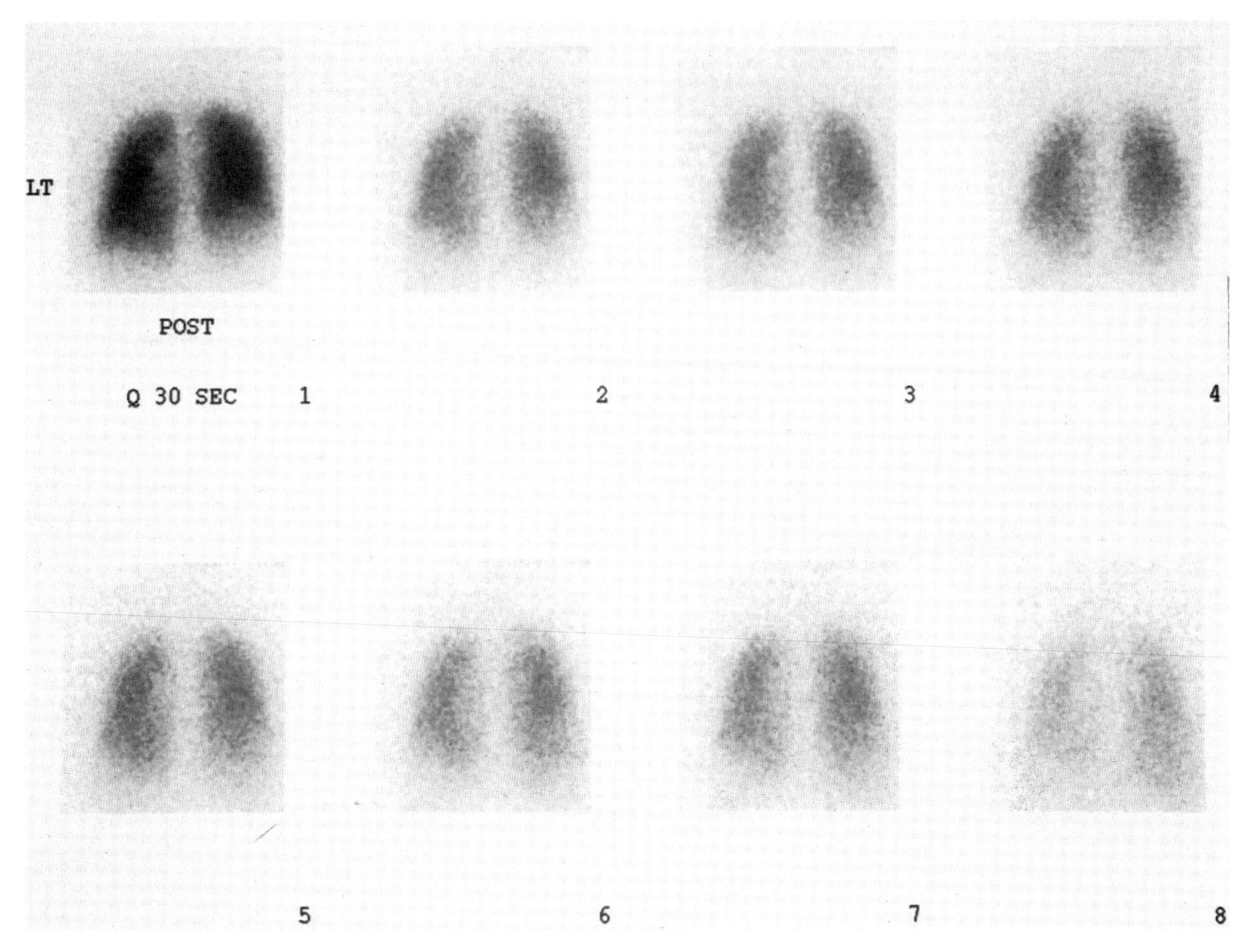

Figure 5.9.2. LT, left.

Discussion. Pulmonary embolic disease is typically a sequelae of deep venous thrombosis. Patients can present with a multitude of nonspecific findings, including pleuritic chest pain, hemoptysis, dyspnea, hypoxia, and tachypnea. Radiographic analysis is often nonspecific, with findings including a normal chest, atelectasis, and small pleural effusion. Less commonly, focal oligemia (Westermark sign), pulmonary artery enlargement, or a pleural-based wedge-shaped density indicative of pulmonary infarction (Hampton's hump) can be seen.

If multiple (≥2) segmental ventilation-perfusion mismatches are identified in areas where there is no corresponding chest radiographic abnormality, pulmonary embolism is diagnosed with high probability in all classification schemes. Rarely, vasculitides can produce a similar pattern with segmental mismatches in several lobes of the lung, but the patient's clinical presentation and medical history should allow accurate diagnosis of these patients. Recently, PIOPED investigators have updated diagnostic criteria for probability of pulmonary embolus (20). The reader is referred to this source for further discussion.

Aunt Minnie's Pearls

- *If multiple (≥2) segmental ventilation-perfusion mismatches are identified in areas where there is no corresponding chest radiographic abnormality, pulmonary embolism is diagnosed with high probability in all classification schemes.*

CASE 10

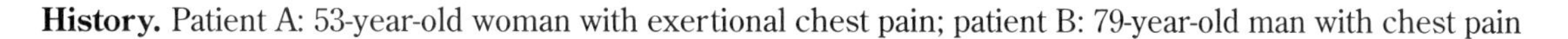

History. Patient A: 53-year-old woman with exertional chest pain; patient B: 79-year-old man with chest pain

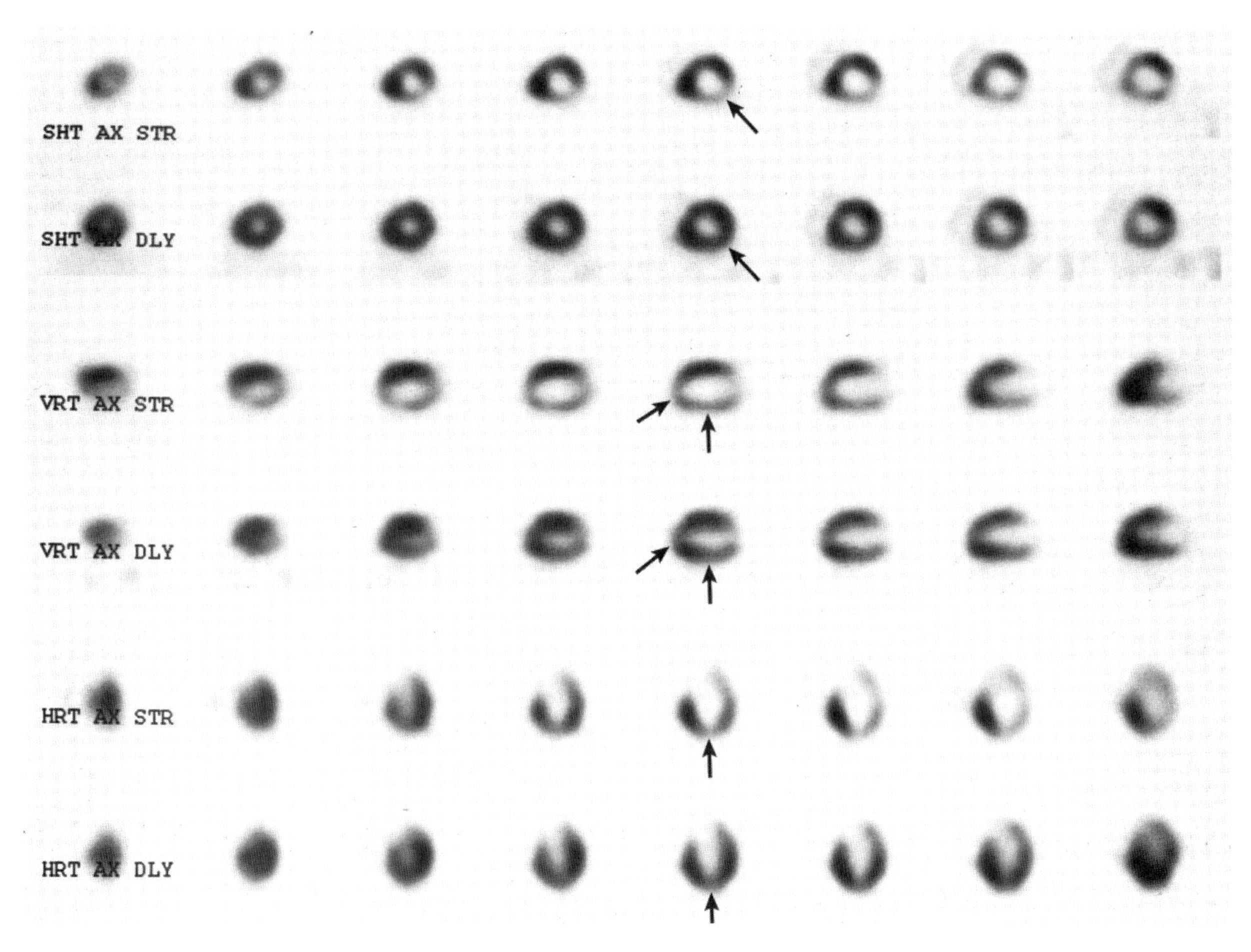

Figure 5.10.1. Patient A.

Findings. Two patients are presented who underwent ^{201}Tl-chloride myocardial perfusion imaging with single photon emission CT. In patient A (Fig. 5.10.1), a reversible perfusion defect involves the inferolateral wall and apex (*arrows*). In contrast, patient B (Fig. 5.10.2) shows a fixed perfusion defect inferolaterally (*arrows*).

Diagnosis. Myocardial ischemia (patient A) and infarct (patient B)

Discussion. The three most commonly used radiopharmaceuticals for myocardial perfusion imaging are ^{201}Tl chloride, ^{99m}Tc sestamibi, and ^{99m}Tc teboroxime. ^{201}Tl chloride is a potassium analog that localizes by active transport across the cell membrane. Its distribution results from initial myocardial uptake and subsequent equilibration with the blood pool. Approximately 5% of the administered dose localizes within the myocardium, with approximately 88% of the agent being extracted on the first pass (21). ^{99m}Tc sestamibi is a lipophilic cation that localizes passively within the mitochondria because of a large negative transmembrane potential. Its extraction fraction is lower than that of the other agents; however, myocardial uptake is similar. Compared with ^{201}Tl chloride, no significant redistribution occurs. ^{99m}Tc teboroxime is a neutral lipophilic boronic acid adduct of technetium dioxime. It has the highest extraction fraction (>90%) of the three compounds; however, the agent rapidly washes out. No significant redistribution occurs (22).

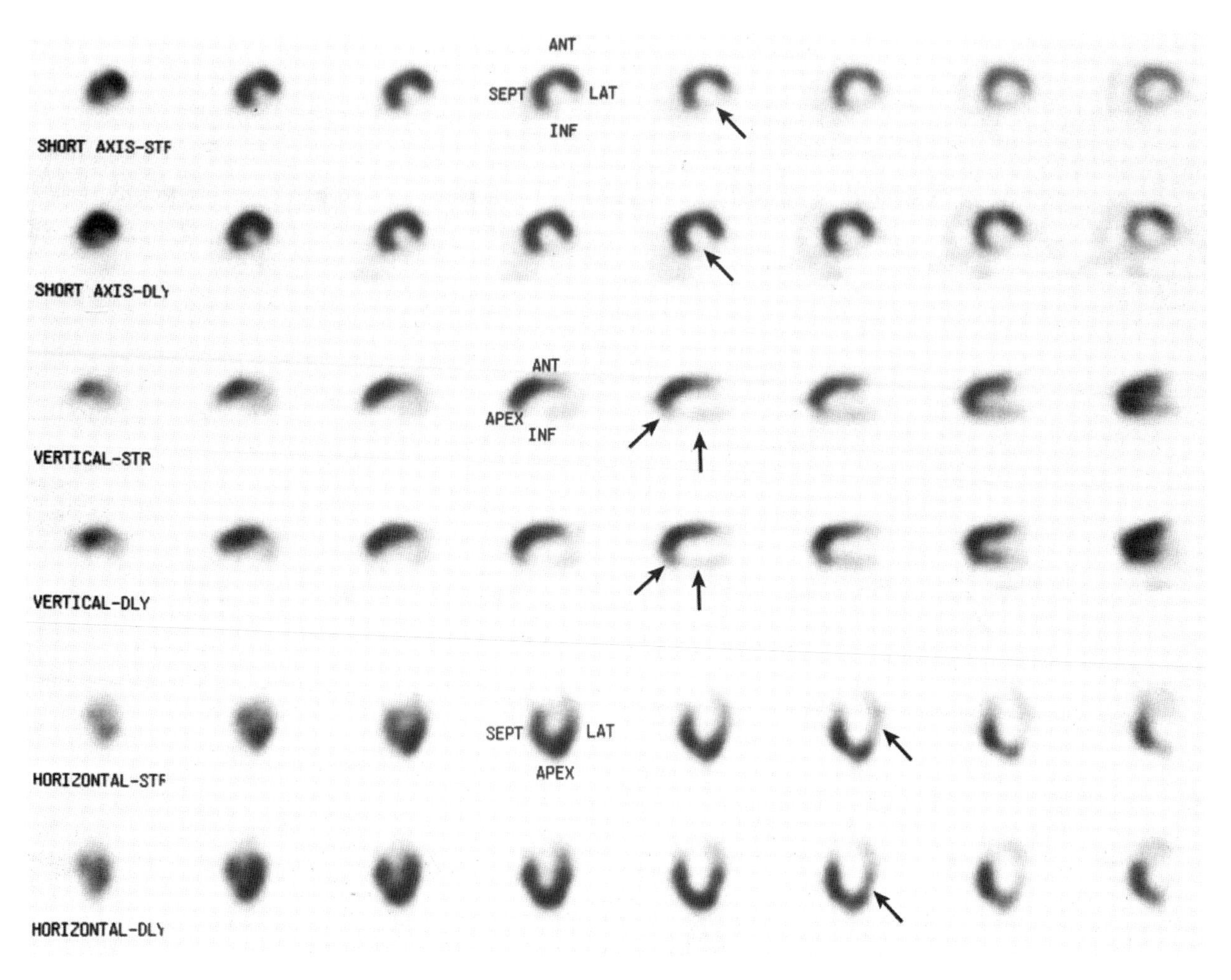

Figure 5.10.2. Patient B. STR, stress; DLY, delay; ANT, anterior; SEPT, septum; LAT, lateral; INF, inferior.

Myocardial perfusion imaging assesses the viability of myocardial tissue. The study is performed under resting and stress conditions. Stress may be produced mechanically, i.e., through exercise or by pharmacological means such as with dipyridamole or adenosine, both of which are potent vasodilators. Areas of ischemia demonstrate a region of relatively decreased activity on poststress images, which improves on rest/redistribution images. Nonreversible abnormalities represent areas of acute or remote myocardial infarction. A third pattern of abnormal activity, known as reverse redistribution, appears as relatively diminished activity on rest/redistribution images and normal on stress images. The cause of reverse redistribution is unknown, but this finding may correlate with myocardial ischemia in some patients.

Many lesions can produce positive thallium stress tests in the absence of coronary artery disease. These lesions include mitral valve prolapse, valvular aortic stenosis, aortic regurgitation, left bundle branch block, idiopathic hypertrophic subaortic stenosis, cardiomyopathy, and hypertensive myocardial hypertrophy. Specific areas of artifact include the apex with aortic regurgitation and the septum with left bundle branch block. In idiopathic hypertrophic subaortic stenosis and hypertensive myocardial hypertrophy, increased count density in the region of the septum produces a relative decrease in the lateral wall, which can be mistaken for infarction (23).

Aunt Minnie's Pearls

- *Ischemia: reversible perfusion defect.*
- *Infarct: fixed perfusion defect.*

CASE 11

History. 78-year-old man with bright red blood per rectum

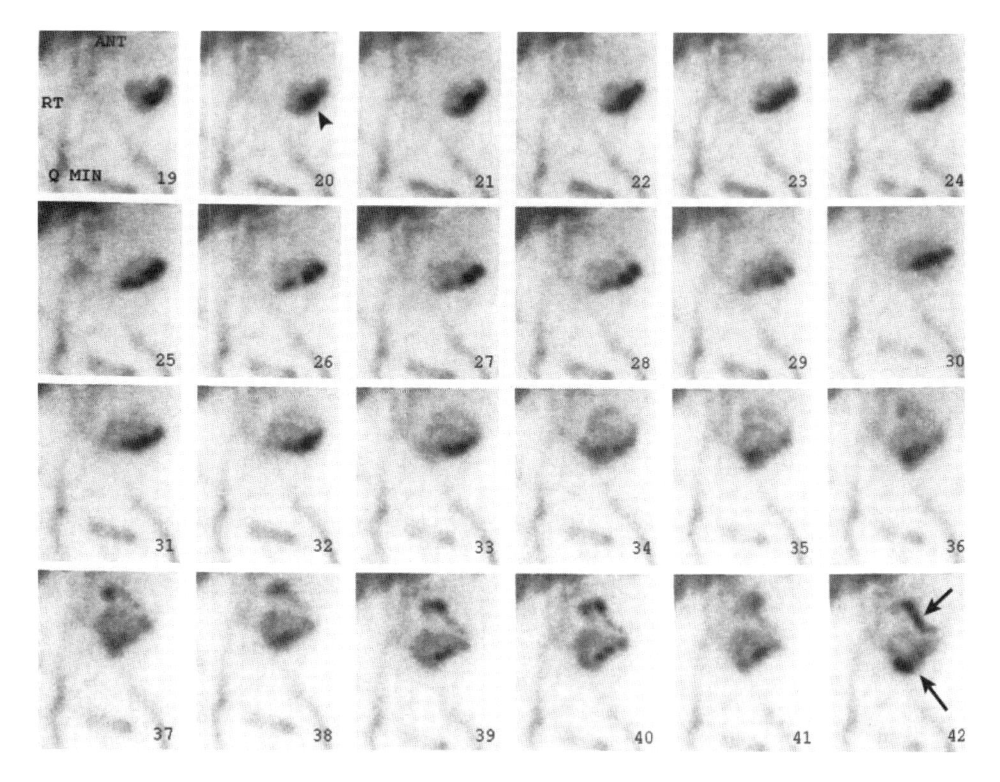

Figure 5.11.1. ANT, anterior; RT, right.

Findings. Dynamic images obtained during a ^{99m}Tc red blood cell scan (Fig. 5.11.1) reveal an abnormal focus of activity in the left-lower-quadrant (*arrowhead*). Activity migrated through small bowel loops during the examination (*arrows*).

Diagnosis. Gastrointestinal bleeding

Discussion. The principal use of the ^{99m}Tc red blood cell scan has been in the evaluation of patients with active but not life-threatening lower gastrointestinal bleeding. This study is helpful in the detection and localization of the bleeding site. The use of this test is limited in the evaluation of upper gastrointestinal bleeding, for which fiberoptic endoscopy is more appropriate. Bleeding rates as low as 0.1–0.2 mL/min can be detected with ^{99m}Tc-labeled red blood cell scintigraphy compared with 0.5–1.0 mL/min with angiography (24). An additional benefit is its ability to detect intermittent bleeding for up to 24 hours.

Gastrointestinal bleeding is seen as a focal area of progressively increasing activity that migrates with time as a result of bowel peristalsis. Vascular lesions that are not actively bleeding can also be detected on the flow phase. The most common causes of lower gastrointestinal bleeding include diverticulosis, neoplasia, angiodysplasia, and enterocolitis. Many diagnostic pitfalls have been identified. The more common causes are gastrointestinal activity attributable to free pertechnetate as well as genitourinary activity, including ectopic kidney, activity in the renal pelvis, ureter, or bladder, and genital blush (25). None of these possibilities would produce migration of activity in the bowel as seen in the index case.

Aunt Minnie's Pearls

- Focal ^{99m}Tc red blood cell activity that migrates along the expected course of the bowel represents active gastrointestinal bleeding.

CASE 12

History. Two patients with peritoneovenous shunts

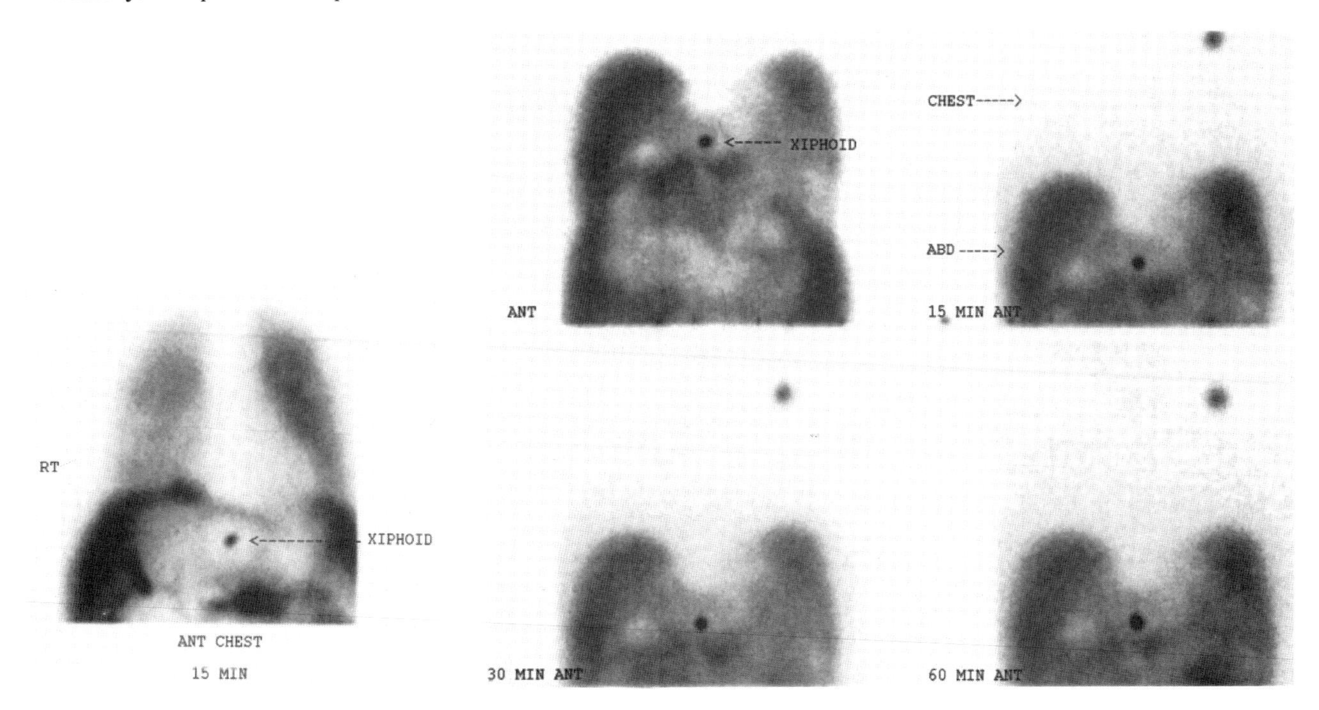

Figure 5.12.1. RT, right; ANT, anterior.

Figure 5.12.2. ABD, abdomen; ANT, anterior.

Findings. In patient A (Fig. 5.12.1), activity is seen within the lungs 15 minutes after administration of ^{99m}Tc MAA into the peritoneal cavity. In patient B (Fig. 5.12.2), no activity is identified within the lungs 15, 30, or 60 minutes after administration of ^{99m}Tc MAA into the peritoneal cavity.

Diagnosis. Patient A: normally functioning peritoneovenous shunt; patient B: obstructed peritoneovenous shunt

Discussion. In patients with ascites that is refractory to medical therapy, peritoneovenous shunts are used to drain the ascitic fluid from the peritoneal cavity into the central venous system. Occlusion or malfunction of the shunt occurs in 5–15% of patients (26). Shunt patency is evaluated by sequential imaging after administration of particulate material into the peritoneal cavity. Two agents, ^{99m}Tc MAA and ^{99m}Tc sulfur colloid, are commonly used. ^{99m}Tc MAA deposits within the lung, and ^{99m}Tc sulfur colloid is taken up by the liver and spleen. ^{99m}Tc MAA is preferred because lung deposition is a better end point than liver-spleen activity. Lung activity is normally seen within 10 minutes after injection and indicates shunt patency. Visualization of efferent shunt tubing, however, is not necessarily indicative of shunt patency. When visualization of lung activity is used as the sole criterion of patency, a sensitivity of 100%, specificity of 92.2%, and accuracy of 98.5% have been demonstrated (27).

Aunt Minnie's Pearls

- *With ^{99m}Tc MAA, lung activity is seen in a normally functioning shunt.*
- *Visualization of efferent shunt tubing is not conclusive evidence of a patent shunt.*

CASE 13

History. 33-year-old woman status-post right hemithyroidectomy for thyroid carcinoma and radioiodine ablation of residual thyroid tissue. Patient presents 6 months after therapy with an enlarging neck mass.

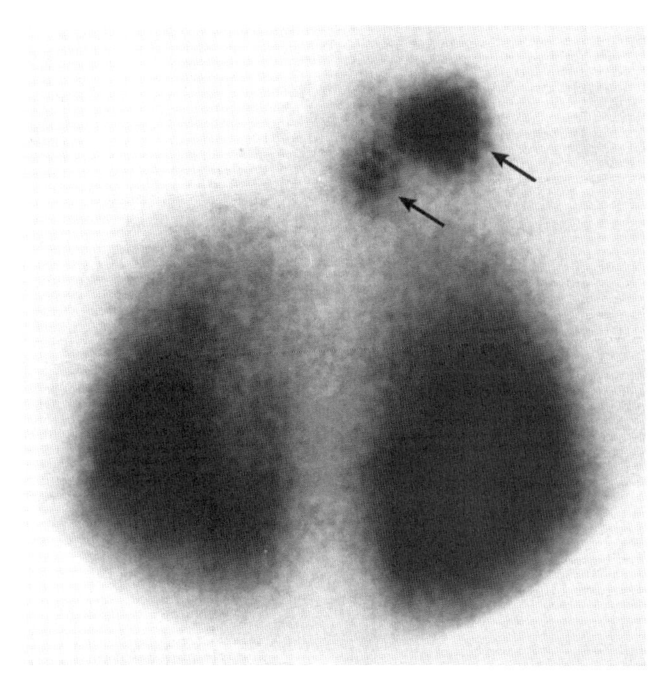

Figure 5.13.1.

Findings. A ^{131}I whole-body scan (Fig. 5.13.1) demonstrates diffuse abnormal activity in both lungs. Additional foci of abnormal activity are seen in the left side of the neck (*arrows*).

Diagnosis. Thyroid carcinoma with pulmonary metastases and cervical adenopathy

Discussion. Thyroid cancer is categorized into four major histologic types: papillary, follicular, medullary, and anaplastic. After a total thyroidectomy, radioiodine concentrates in follicular carcinoma and, to a variable degree, in papillary carcinoma. Medullary and anaplastic carcinomas do not concentrate radioiodine. Papillary carcinoma is the most common type; 30–55% of patients with papillary carcinoma have local nodal metastases at the time of initial surgery. Follicular carcinoma constitutes 20–25% of thyroid cancers and spreads hematogenously. Medullary carcinoma, which causes elevated serum calcitonin levels, may be found in the setting of multiple endocrine neoplasia syndromes Type IIA and IIB. Approximately 50% of patients with medullary carcinoma have metastatic disease at the time of diagnosis. Anaplastic carcinomas constitute approximately 10% of thyroid cancers, and prognosis with this type of tumor is dismal (28, 29).

Preparation for whole-body imaging requires withdrawal of thyroid hormone therapy for 2–4 weeks to allow maximal stimulation by endogenous thyroid-stimulating hormone. Placing the patient on a low-iodide diet for the final 2 weeks is helpful in decreasing the body's iodide pool and thereby enhancing uptake of radioactive iodide. Recent thyroid-stimulating hormone and thyroglobulin levels should be reviewed immediately before the patient is dosed for the total body ^{131}I study.

Aunt Minnie's Pearls

- *Radioiodine concentration occurs in follicular and variably in papillary carcinoma; medullary and anaplastic carcinomas do not take up radioiodine.*
- *Inadequate endogenous thyroid-stimulating hormone stimulation may result in poor tracer uptake and false-negative studies.*

CASE 14

History. 27-year-old woman with acute shortness of breath and chest pain

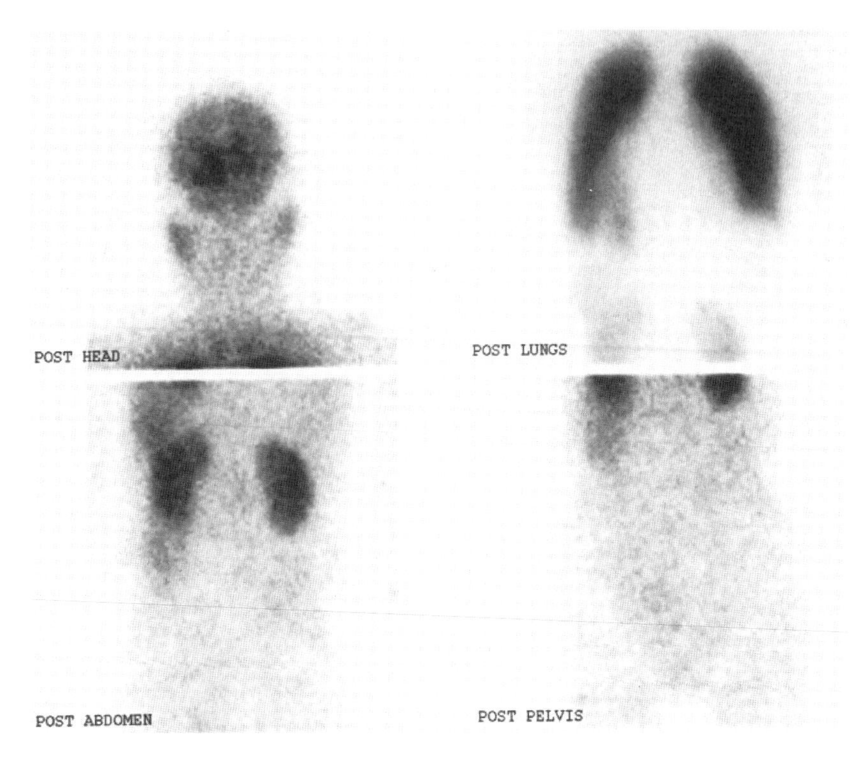

Figure 5.14.1. POST, posterior.

Findings. After administration of ^{99m}Tc MAA to the patient, abnormal uptake is identified within the brain and kidneys (Fig. 5.14.1). Normal uptake is seen in the lungs, and the heart is markedly enlarged.

Diagnosis. Right-to-left shunt

Discussion. Right-to-left shunting is demonstrated by systemic embolization of ^{99m}Tc MAA particles as part of a pulmonary perfusion study or shunt evaluation. Normally, first-pass pulmonary uptake of ^{99m}Tc MAA is nearly complete, because only 4% of the administered dose undergoes physiologic shunting. Normally, this small amount of physiologic shunting is not visually detectable (30).

Particle embolization secondary to cardiac or pulmonary shunts is most often seen in the kidneys, brain, extremities, and thyroid. Brain and extremity uptake is definitive evidence of right to left shunting. Care must be taken in attributing thyroid and renal uptake to a shunt, because thyroid and kidney activity may be seen if free pertechnetate is present. Also, normal renal excretion of the radiotracer occurs as ^{99m}Tc MAA is metabolized (30).

Aunt Minnie's Pearls

- *Brain and extremity uptake is definitive evidence of a right-to-left shunt.*

CASE 15

History. Young African-American woman with a history of a hemolytic anemia

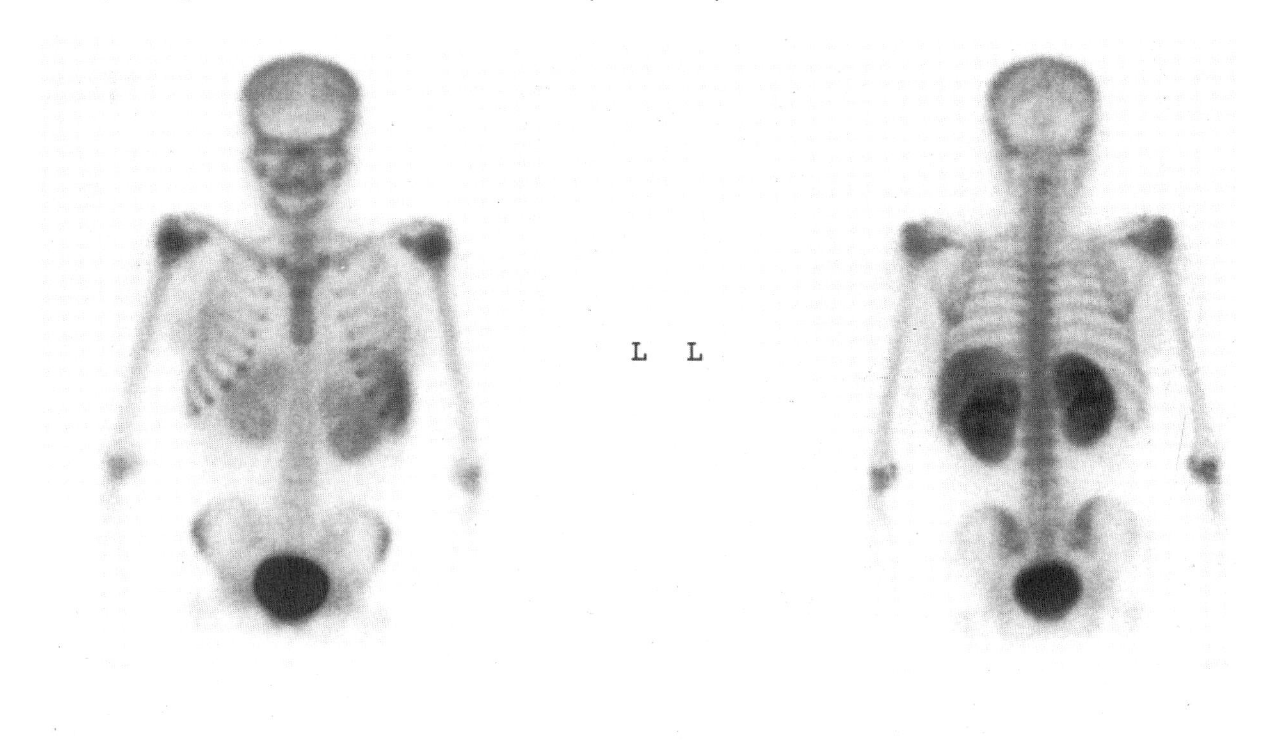

Figure 5.15.1. L, left.

Findings. Anterior and posterior images from a whole body bone scan (Fig. 5.15.1) reveal marked radionuclide uptake in the spleen and kidneys. The spleen appears small, whereas the kidneys are enlarged. Increased activity in the humeral heads is also identified.

Diagnosis. Sickle cell disease

Discussion. Sickle cell disease is a homozygous hereditary anemia that occurs because of chromosomal defect in the beta hemoglobin chain. Red blood cells form into an abnormal sickle shape in response to low oxygen tension. Owing to their abnormal shape, the sickled cells cause small vessel occlusions that result in tissue infarction and pain crises. The spleen is usually severely affected in older patients with sickle cell disease, and the repeated infarcts lead to dystrophic calcium deposition in the organ. A characteristic appearance of a small densely calcified spleen can be discovered on bone scans, as well as plain films or CT. Other findings on bone scan include increased or decreased activity in areas of bony infarction and increased activity in the diaphyses of the long bones caused by bone marrow expansion. The kidneys may be slightly enlarged and demonstrate increased activity, as in the index case. The cause for the abnormality in the kidneys is not completely understood, but it does not appear to correlate with altered clinical renal function. (31)

Aunt Minnie's Pearls

- *Markedly increased activity in a small spleen on bone scintigraphy = sickle cell disease.*
- *Look for bone infarcts or for increased activity in the long bone diaphyses from bone marrow expansion.*

CASE 16

History. Noncontributory

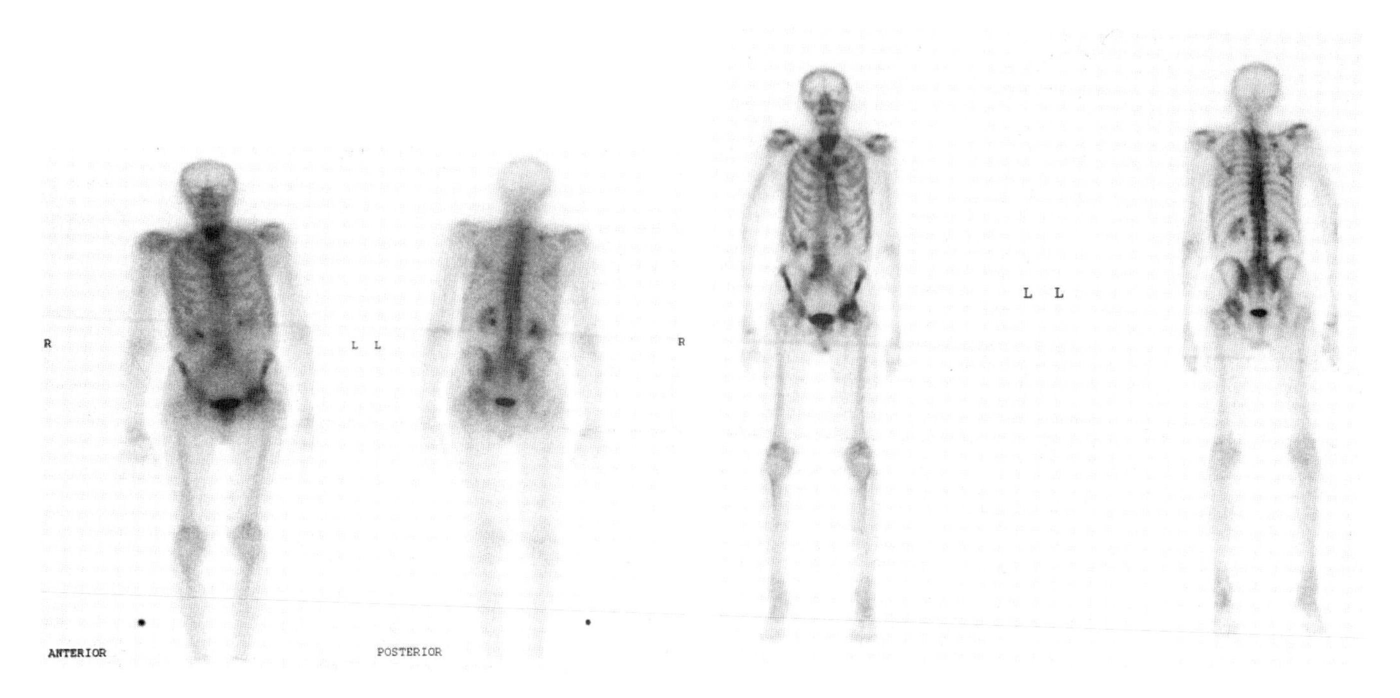

Figure 5.16.1.

Figure 5.16.2.

Findings. The initial whole body bone scan image (Fig. 5.16.1) demonstrates poor detail and contrast (note sharpness of the cobalt side marker). After technical adjustments, the repeat whole body bone scan image (Fig. 5.16.2) shows improved detail and contrast and less soft tissue activity.

Diagnosis. Off-peak imaging with window set at the energy of the cobalt 57 (122 kev) side marker

Discussion. Peaking the gamma camera is a process that involves appropriately centering the camera's single channel analyzer windows to the radionuclide in use. Although the camera may have an automatic peaking feature, the technologist should always view the spectral display of the radionuclide being imaged to be sure that the correct energy window is selected and that it is centered on the radionuclide of interest. Off-peak imaging results from incorrect energy window selection. If the window is centered too high, available photons will be excluded. If centered too low, the images will contain increased amounts of scatter, which may be evident in increased visualization of soft tissue activity. Nonuniformity also affects the response of the photomultiplier tubes, which may result in geometric hot and cold regions in the image, which correspond to the location of photomultiplier tubes (32). The camera should be peaked daily and upon any switch to a different radionuclide (33). In the index case, the radiologist correctly identified the problem by noticing the poor resolution of the image, increased soft tissue activity, and unusually sharp image of the cobalt marker.

Aunt Minnie's Pearls

- *Off-peak imaging = incorrect energy window selection.*
- *Peak the gamma camera daily and whenever a different radionuclide is used.*

CASE 17

History. Quality control

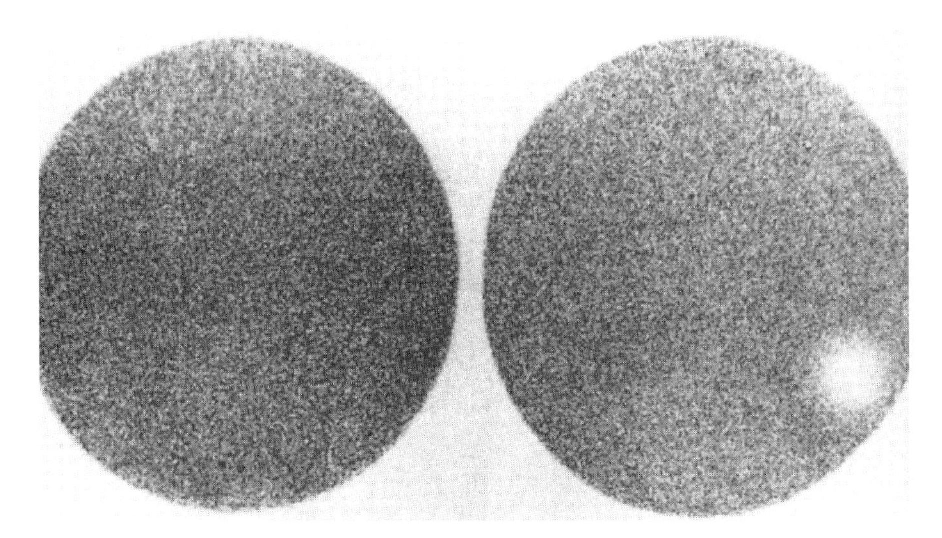

Figure 5.17.1. From Bushberg JT, Seibert JA, Leidholdt EM Jr, Boone JM. The essential physics of medical imaging. Baltimore: Williams & Wilkins, 1994:550.

Findings. Two ^{99m}Tc pertechnetate flood-field images are submitted (Fig. 5.17.1). Image on the left demonstrates normal uniformity. Image on the right is from the same camera with a nonfunctioning photomultiplier tube.

Diagnosis. Nonfunctioning photomultiplier tube

Discussion. Field uniformity represents the ability of an imaging system to provide a uniform image across the entire crystal face. A properly functioning camera produces a homogeneous flood-field image or, at most, mild heterogeneity with areas of slightly increased activity corresponding to photomultiplier tubes. Drift or nonfunction of a photomultiplier tube shows as an area of decreased activity on clinical or flood-field images (34). Field uniformity is assessed daily by utilizing test images obtained with either a point source or flood-field source of radioactivity (technetium or cobalt sources are commonly used). Intrinsic flood tests are performed without the collimator in place, and extrinsic flood images are obtained with the collimator attached. When the collimator is in place, only sheet sources can be used. It is also important to have a general idea of how many counts are necessary to achieve a good flood image with the camera. The values needed range from a few million counts for standard cameras to more than 100 million counts for single photon emission CT cameras.

Aunt Minnie's Pearls
- *Field uniformity must be assessed daily.*

CASE 18

History. 56-year-old woman with dyspnea

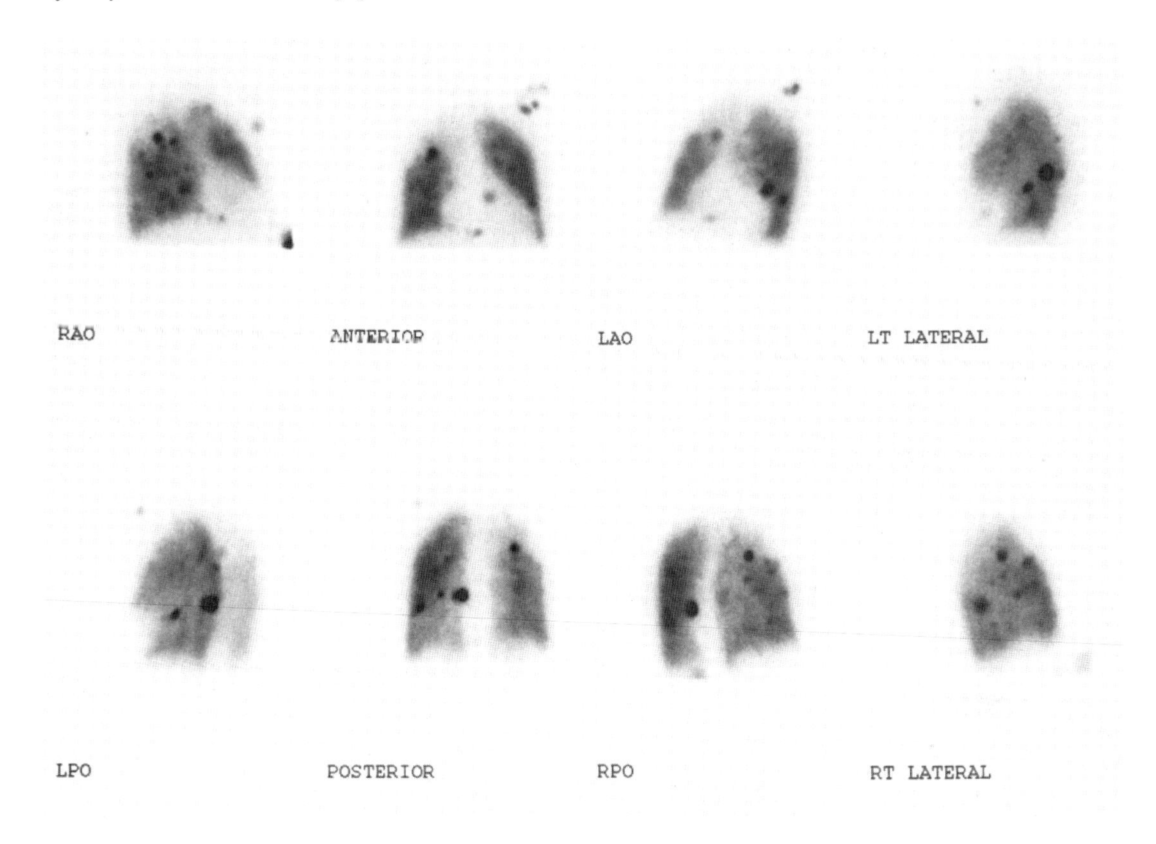

Figure 5.18.1. RAO, right anterior oblique; LAO, left anterior oblique; LT, left; LPO, left posterior oblique; RPO, right posterior oblique; RT, right.

Findings. A ^{99m}Tc pulmonary perfusion study (Fig. 5.18.1) shows multiple abnormal foci of increased activity in both lungs.

Diagnosis. Aggregated ^{99m}Tc MAA

Discussion. Pulmonary perfusion imaging depends on capillary blockade. If blood is withdrawn into the syringe containing ^{99m}Tc MAA and is allowed to coagulate, the radiolabeled compound will aggregate within blood clots. Aggregation can also occur if the syringe is not agitated before injection. The injected radiolabeled clots will obstruct vessels corresponding to the size of the clot and will appear as hot spots on images. The large concentrations of activity incorporated into the clots may result in a statistically significant reduction in counts to the other areas of the lung, possibly resulting in missed abnormalities (35).

Aunt Minnie's Pearls

- *Aggregated ^{99m}Tc MAA shows up as hot spots on pulmonary perfusion imaging.*

CASE 19

History. Noncontributory

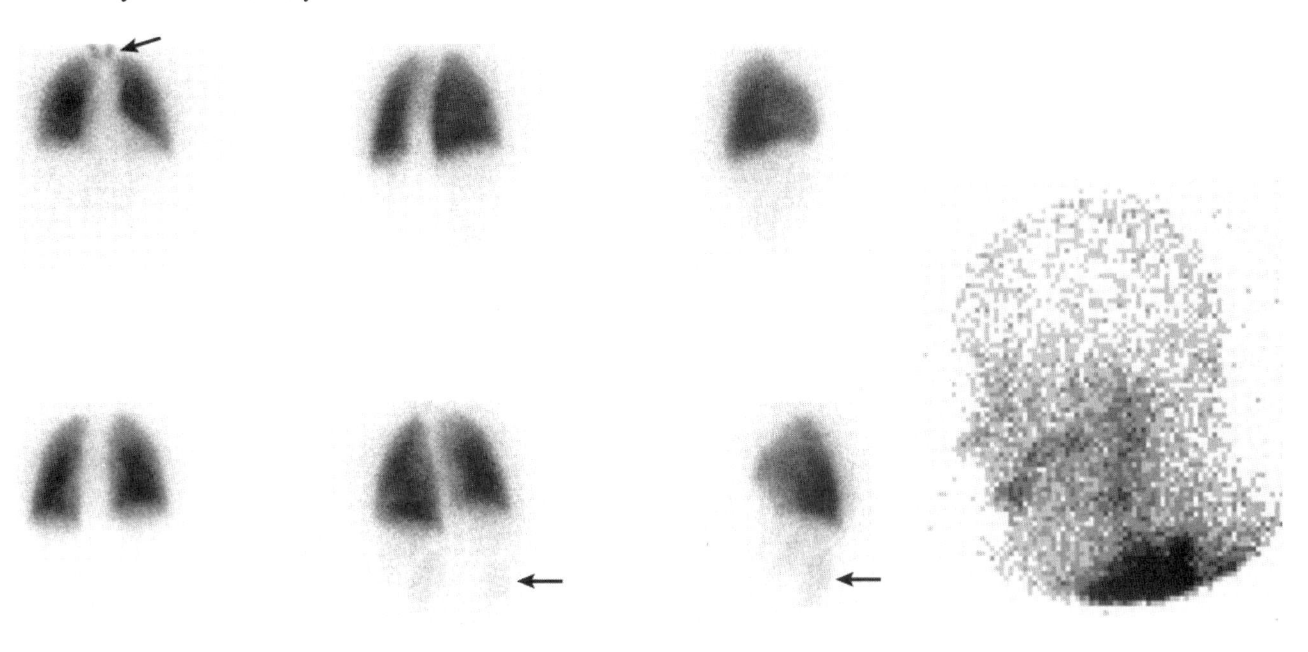

Figure 5.19.1. Figure 5.19.2.

Findings. Multiple images[13] from a pulmonary perfusion study (Fig. 5.19.1) reveal normal pulmonary perfusion. However, unexpected activity is seen in the thyroid gland and faintly in the kidneys (*arrows*). A lateral static view of the head shows scalp and facial soft tissue activity but no brain activity. This differentiates this diagnosis from the one shown in case 14.

Diagnosis. Radiochemical impurity (image reveals the presence of free pertechnetate)

Discussion. Radiochemical impurity exists when a portion of the radionuclide being imaged is in an undesired chemical form. The most common radiochemical impurity encountered in clinical practice is free pertechnetate. This impurity forms when oxygen or water is inadvertently allowed to mix with the contents of the radiopharmaceutical kit. Stannous chloride ions, which are needed to reduce technetium to its reactive state (from +7 to +4 valence), become oxidized by the contaminate. Oxidized technetium ions will not combine with the desired carrier molecules (MAA, albumin, DTPA, diphosphonate, or glucoheptonate) (36).

Free pertechnetate can be confirmed by thin layer chromatography. When an organic solvent is placed on a chromatography strip with a small amount of the radiopharmaceutical, the free ^{99m}Tc will migrate with the solvent. The amount of activity that migrates divided by the total amount of activity placed on the test strip represents the fraction of free pertechnetate. The acceptable amount of radiochemical impurity is usually less than 5%. Another radiochemical impurity not discussed here is hydrolyzed technetium or technetium dioxide. This impurity can be discovered by performing thin layer chromatography with a saline solvent.

Aunt Minnie's Pearls

- *Suspect free pertechnetate when gastric mucosa, renal, and thyroid activity is unexpectedly seen on the nuclear medicine study.*
- *The presence of free pertechnetate can be confirmed with thin layer chromatography.*

CASE 20

History. Patient undergoing a whole body ^{131}I scan

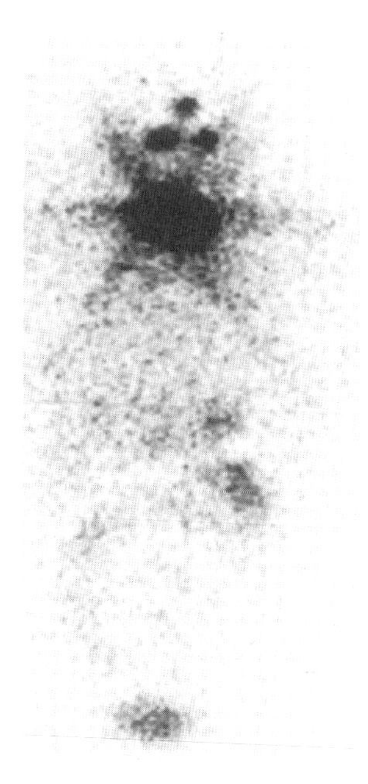

Figure 5.20.1.

Findings. A frontal view from the whole body ^{131}I scan (Fig. 5.20.1) shows a radiating "star" pattern of activity over the expected region of the thyroid gland.

Diagnosis. Septal penetration

Discussion. Just as in conventional radiography, collimators are used in nuclear medicine to absorb unwanted scattered photons before they reach the image. Scattered photons impact the scintillation camera in an area that does not correspond to their anatomic point of origin on the patient, resulting in images that are poor in resolution and contrast (37). Most modern nuclear collimators use a system of hexagonal holes bordered by septa. Normally the photons will penetrate the holes if their incident angle on the collimator is appropriate. Scattered photons will encounter the collimator from an angle of incidence that makes them hit and absorb into the septa. When the scattered photons have high energy or occur in very large numbers (high photon flux), they may penetrate the thinnest portions of the septa. The characteristic six-point star pattern results because septal penetration occurs most easily through the six walls that directly face the opening of the hexagonal holes in the collimator.

Positron emission tomography and high dose ^{131}I are common sources of septal penetration in clinical imaging because of the high energy and photon flux associated with them. If a low dose of ^{131}I is used and this artifact is observed, the physician should suspect that an inappropriate collimator (low or medium energy) has been mistakenly used.

Aunt Minnie's Pearls

- *Six-point star = septal penetration.*
- *This artifact is seen with inappropriate collimator selection or whenever very high photon flux occurs.*

REFERENCES

1. Larsson A, Moonen M, Bergh AC, Lindberg S, Wikkelso C. Predictive value of quantitative cisternography in normal pressure hydrocephalus. Acta Neurol Scand 1990;81:327–332.
2. Palmer EL, Scott JA, Strauss HW. Practical nuclear medicine. Philadelphia: Saunders, 1992:382.
3. Devous MD Sr, Leroy RF, Homan RW. Single photon emission computed tomography in epilepsy. Semin Nucl Med 1990;20:325–341.
4. Thrall JH, Ziessman HA. Nuclear medicine: the requisites. St. Louis: Mosby, 1995:272.
5. Palmer EL, Scott JA, Strauss HW. Practical nuclear medicine. Philadelphia: Saunders, 1992:378.
6. Laurin NR, Driedger AA, Hurwitz GA, et al. Cerebral perfusion imaging with technetium-99m HM-PAO in brain death and severe central nervous system injury. J Nucl Med 1989;30:1627–1635.
7. Wilson K, Gordon L, Selby JB Sr. The diagnosis of brain death with Tc-99m HMPAO. Clin Nucl Med 1993;18:428–434.
8. Ries T. Detection of osteoporotic sacral fractures with radionuclides. Radiology 1983;146:783–785.
9. Balseiro J, Brower AC, Ziessman HA. Scintigraphic diagnosis of sacral fractures. AJR 1987;148:111–113.
10. Resnick D. Bone and joint imaging. Philadelphia: Saunders, 1989:575–577.
11. Palmer EL, Scott JA, Strauss HW. Practical nuclear medicine. Philadelphia: Saunders, 1992:164.
12. Goldsmith DP, Vivino FB, Eichenfield AH, Athreya BH, Heyman S. Nuclear imaging and clinical features of childhood reflex neurovascular dystrophy: comparison with adults. Arthritis Rheum 1989;32:480–485.
13. O'Mara RE. Benign bone disease. In: Sandler MP, Coleman RE, Whackers FJT, Patton JA, Gottschalk A, Hoffer PB, eds. Diagnostic nuclear medicine, 3rd ed. Baltimore: Williams & Wilkins, 1996:693.
14. Datz FL, Patch GG, Arias JM, Morton KA. Nuclear medicine: a teaching file. St. Louis: Mosby, 1992:3.
15. Barron BJ, Lamk ML, Kim EE. Genitourinary nuclear medicine II. In: Sandler MP, Coleman RE, Whackers FJT, Patton JA, Gottschalk A, Hoffer PB, eds. Diagnostic nuclear medicine, 3rd ed. Baltimore: Williams & Wilkins, 1996:1212.
16. Sfakinakis GN, Bourgoignie JJ. Renal scintigraphy following angiotensin-converting enzyme inhibition in the diagnosis of renovascular hypertension (captopril scintigraphy). In: Nuclear medicine annual. New York: Raven, 1988:125–170.
17. Thrall JH, Ziessman HA. Nuclear medicine: the requisites. St. Louis: Mosby, 1995:313–315.
18. Eggli DF, Tulchinsky M. Scintigraphic evaluation of pediatric urinary tract infection. Semin Nucl Med 1993;23:199–218.
19. Rothwell DL, Constable AR. Radionuclide cystography in the management of vesico-ureteric reflux. Br J Urol 1977;49:621–627.
20. Gottschalk A, Sostman HD, Coleman RE, et al. Ventilation-perfusion scintigraphy in the PIOPED study. Part II. Evaluation of the scintigraphic criteria and interpretations. J Nucl Med 1993;34:1119–1126.
21. Gerson MC, ed. Cardiac nuclear medicine. New York: McGraw-Hill, 1987:2–4.
22. Beller GA, Watson DD. Physiological basis of myocardial perfusion imaging with the technetium-99m agents. Semin Nucl Med 1991;21:173–181.
23. Mettler FA Jr, Guiberteau MJ. Essentials of nuclear medicine imaging, 3rd ed. Philadelphia: Saunders, 1991:116–117.
24. Baum S. Angiography and the gastrointestinal bleeder. Radiology 1982;143:569–572.
25. Thrall JH, Ziessman HA. Nuclear medicine: the requisites. St. Louis: Mosby, 1995:246.
26. Madeddu G, D'Ovidio NG, Casu AR, et al. Evaluation of peritoneovenous shunt patency with Tc-99m labeled microspheres. J Nucl Med 1983;24:302–307.
27. Stewart CA, Sakimura IT, Applebaum DM, Siegel ME. Evaluation of peritoneovenous shunt patency by intraperitoneal Tc-99m macroaggregated albumin: clinical experience. AJR 1986;147:177–180.
28. DeLellis RA. The endocrine system. In: Cotran RS, Kumar V, Robbins SL, eds. Robbins pathologic basis of disease, 4th ed. Philadelphia: Saunders, 1989:1233.
29. Freitas JE, Gross MD, Ripley S, Shapiro B. Radionuclide diagnosis and therapy of thyroid cancer: current status report. Semin Nucl Med 1985;15:106–131.
30. Palmer EL, Scott JA, Strauss HW. Practical nuclear medicine. Philadelphia: Saunders, 1992:238–239.
31. Sty JR, Babbitt DP, Sheth K. Abnormal Tc-99m-methylene diphosphonate accumulation in the kidneys of children with sickle cell disease. Clin Nucl Med 1992;17:236.
32. Palmer EL, Scott JA, Strauss HW. Practical nuclear medicine. Philadelphia: Saunders, 1992:51–52.
33. Patton JA. Quality assurance. In: Sandler MP, Coleman RE, Whackers FJT, Patton JA, Gottschalk A, Hoffer PB, eds. Diagnostic nuclear medicine, 3rd ed. Baltimore: Williams & Wilkins, 1996:164.
34. Thrall JH, Ziessman HA. Nuclear medicine: the requisites. St. Louis: Mosby, 1995:26.
35. Mettler FA Jr, Guiberteau MJ. Essentials of nuclear medicine imaging, 3rd ed. Philadelphia: Saunders, 1991:146–147.
36. Mettler FA Jr, Guiberteau MJ. Essentials of nuclear medicine imaging, 3rd ed. Philadelphia: Saunders, 1991:34–35.
37. Sorenson JA, Phelps ME. Physics in nuclear medicine, 2nd ed. Orlando: Grune & Stratton, 1987:372–374.

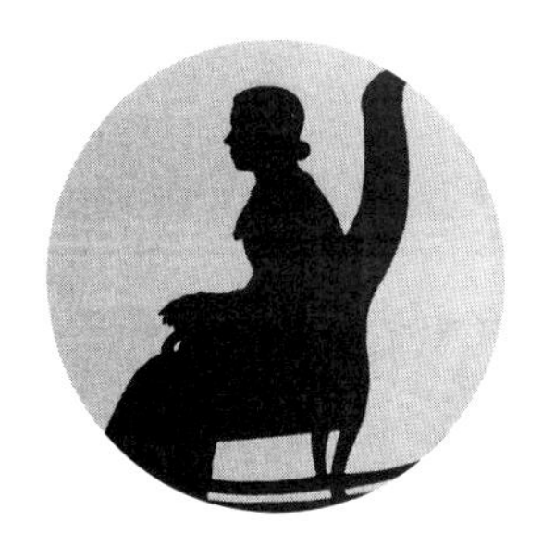

chapter 6

NEURORADIOLOGY

CHRISTOPHER A. SCHLARB AND DANIEL W. WILLIAMS III

CASE 1

History. 33-year-old woman with postural headache

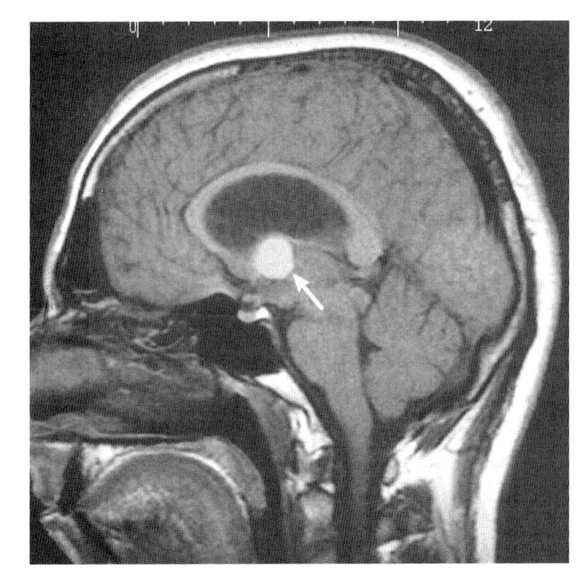

Figure 6.1.1. SE 450/16 without gadolinium.

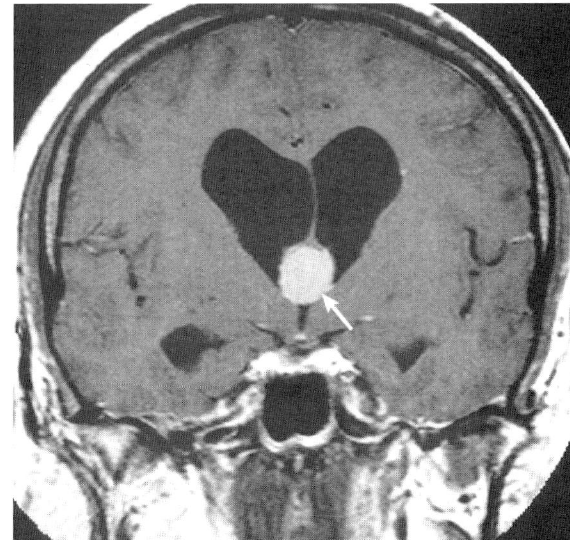

Figure 6.1.2. SE 600/20 with gadolinium.

Findings. A midline sagittal T1-weighted MR image (Fig. 6.1.1) demonstrates a well-defined homogeneously hyperintense mass (*arrow*) located at the foramen of Monro. A coronal T1-weighted MR image after gadolinium administration (Fig. 6.1.2) reveals that the mass is unchanged in signal intensity (*arrow*). Enlargement of the lateral ventricles is also present.

Diagnosis. Colloid cyst

Discussion. Third ventricular colloid cysts are rare masses accounting for less than 1% of all intracranial tumors (1). The origin of this benign lesion remains controversial, although a widely accepted theory suggests an origin from the primitive neuroepithelium of the tela choroidea. Patients typically present with postural headaches (Brun's syndrome) secondary to a ball-valve effect at the foramen of Monro with associated obstructive hydrocephalus. Acute ventricular obstruction resulting in death has been reported. Colloid cysts usually do not enhance and are either isodense or hyperdense to brain on CT. The signal characteristics on MR vary, but the most common appearance is a hyperintense mass on T1-weighted images secondary to a high cholesterol content (2, 3).

Aunt Minnie's Pearls

- *On T1-weighted MR images, a colloid cyst usually presents as a high signal intensity mass at the foramen of Monro.*
- *Postural headaches (Brun's syndrome) or death from ventricular obstruction may occur.*

CASE 2

History. 14-year-old boy with a seizure disorder

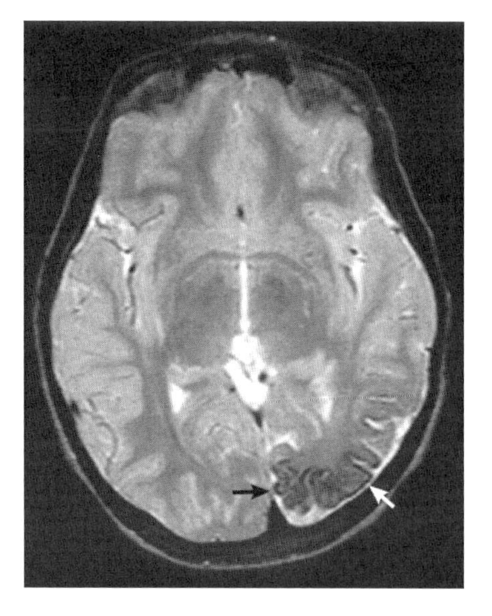

Figure 6.2.1. SE 3000/90 without gadolinium.

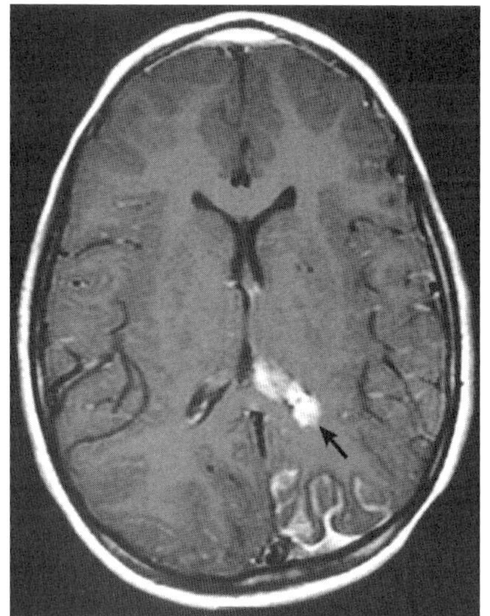

Figure 6.2.2. SE 600/16 with gadolinium.

Findings. Gyriform low signal within the atrophic cortex of the left occipital lobe (*arrows*) is seen on this axial T2-weighted MR image (Fig. 6.2.1). An axial postcontrast T1-weighted MR image (Fig. 6.2.2) demonstrates enhancement of the leptomeninges and an enlarged ipsilateral choroid plexus (*arrow*).

Diagnosis. Sturge-Weber syndrome (encephalotrigeminal angiomatosis)

Discussion. Sturge-Weber syndrome is a sporadically occurring neurocutaneous syndrome first described by W. Allen Sturge (1879) with the first radiographic depiction by Parkes Weber (1929) (4). The hallmark of this disease is the vascular angiomatous lesion involving the face in the distribution of the trigeminal nerve ("port-wine" stain or nevus flammeus) and ipsilateral brain and meninges. Imaging findings include cortical calcifications, lobar atrophy with secondary calvarial changes (Dyke-Davidoff-Masson syndrome), leptomeningeal enhancement, choroid plexus angiomas, and venous abnormalities (5, 6). The evaluation of patients with suspected Sturge-Weber syndrome should include contrast enhanced MR imaging because the full extent of the cortical vascular lesions may not be apparent on unenhanced imaging (7).

Aunt Minnie's Pearls

- *Unilateral cortical atrophy and calcifications associated with enhancing leptomeningeal and choroid plexus angiomas = Sturge-Weber syndrome.*
- *MR with contrast is necessary to evaluate the full extent of the disease.*

CASE 3

History. 5-month-old girl with a sacral skin defect

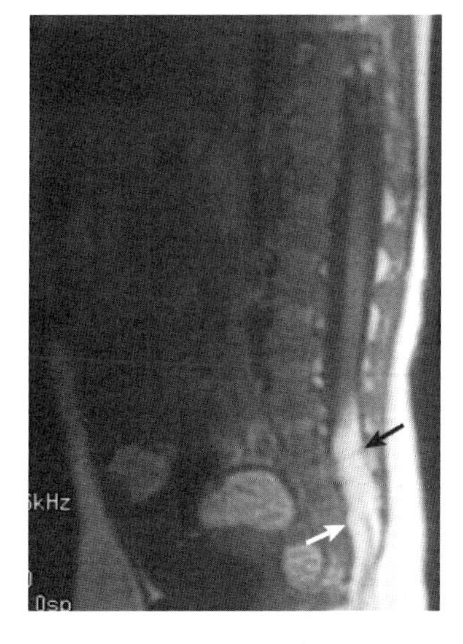

Figure 6.3.1. SE 500/17 without gadolinium.

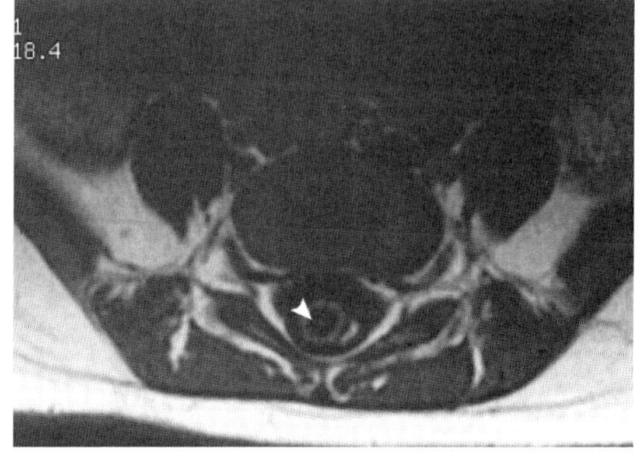

Figure 6.3.2. SE 700/19 without gadolinium.

Findings. A sagittal T1 weighted MR image (Fig. 6.3.1) reveals a low-lying spinal cord that terminates into a high signal lipomatous mass (*arrows*). The lipoma extends posteriorly through the dysraphic spine and is in continuity with the subcutaneous fat. Hydrosyringomyelia is present within the tethered cord as demonstrated on the axial T1-weighted image at the level of the lower lumbar spine (Fig. 6.3.2, *arrowhead*).

Diagnosis. Lipomyelomeningocele

Discussion. A lipomyelomeningocele likely arises from premature disjunction of the neuroectoderm from cutaneous ectoderm. This anomaly accounts for 20% of skin covered lumbosacral masses and up to half of occult spinal dysraphisms (8). Although these lesions are similar to myelomeningoceles, in this disorder, the distal spinal cord is dorsally contiguous with a lipomatous mass that extends to the subcutaneous tissues. The nerve roots do not pass through the fatty mass, which is dorsal to the cord and extradural in location. A tethered cord is almost always present, and up to 25% of patients have associated hydrosyringomyelia (9). Skin tags or dimples, dermal sinuses, and other cutaneous defects are found in up to 50% of patients. Of note, this disorder is not associated with the Chiari II malformation, while meningomyeloceles are synonymous with the Chiari II malformation.

Aunt Minnie's Pearls

- *A lipomyelomeningocele is an occult spinal dysraphism in which the distal spinal cord is contiguous dorsally with a large fatty mass.*
- *A tethered cord, hydrosyringomyelia, and cutaneous abnormalities are common findings associated with lipomyelomeningocele.*
- *This lesion is not associated with the Chiari II malformation.*

CASE 4

History. 15-year-old woman with hearing loss

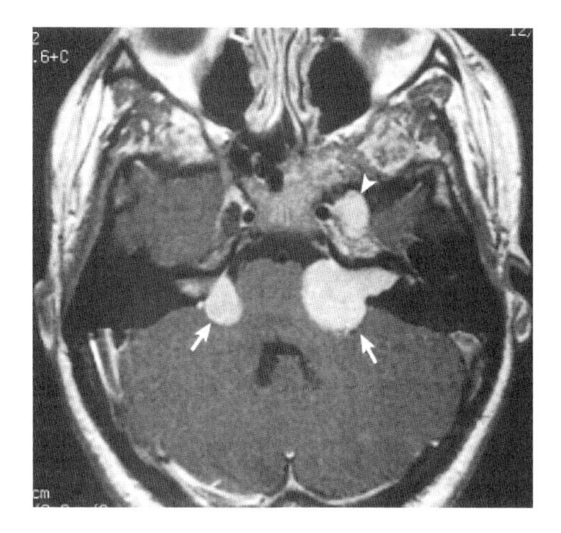

Figure 6.4.1. SE 500/26 with gadolinium.

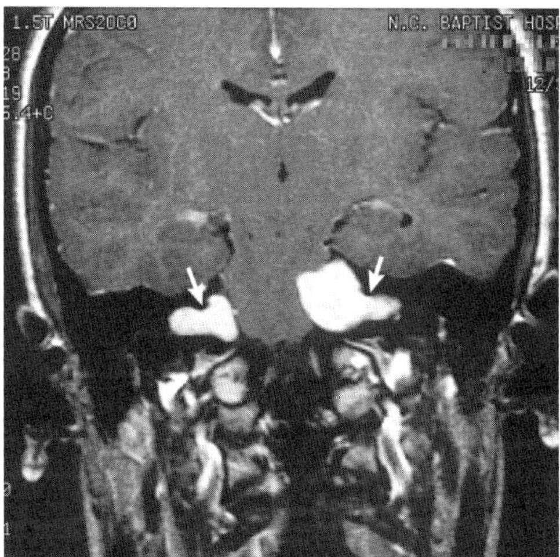

Figure 6.4.2. SE 500/26 with gadolinium.

Findings. Axial (Fig. 6.4.1) and coronal (Fig. 6.4.2) postcontrast T1-weighted MR images demonstrate enhancing masses (*arrows*) within both internal auditory canals that extend into the cerebellopontine angles. The brainstem is displaced to the right. Also note an enhancing mass within Meckel's cave on the left (*arrowhead*).

Diagnosis. Neurofibromatosis type 2

Discussion. Neurofibromatosis type 2 (NF-2) is an autosomal dominant disorder that is recognized as a distinct form of the disease separated genetically, clinically, and radiographically from neurofibromatosis type 1. The incidence of neurofibromatosis type 2 is approximately 1/50,000 live births as opposed to 1/2000 to 3000 live births for neurofibromatosis type 1. Bilateral acoustic schwannomas are the hallmark of this disease, commonly presenting during or soon after puberty (10). Schwannomas of other cranial and spinal nerves, intracranial and spinal meningiomas, and spinal cord ependymomas may also be present (5, 6, 11).

Aunt Minnie's Pearls

- *Bilateral acoustic schwannomas = neurofibromatosis type 2.*

CASE 5

History. 5-year-old girl with short stature, delayed dentition, delayed skeletal maturation, and endocrine abnormalities

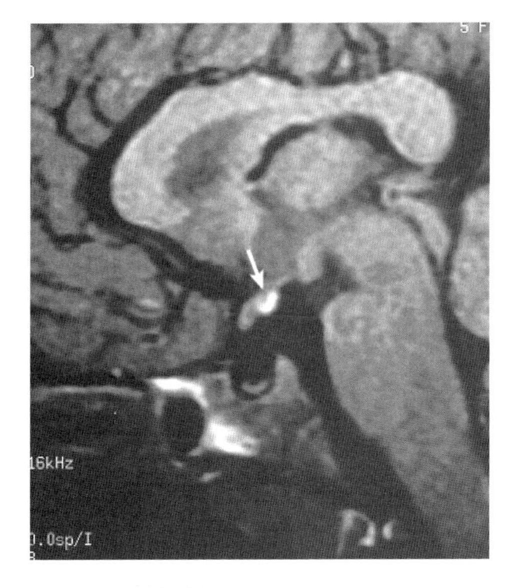

Figure 6.5.1. SE 650/19 without gadolinium.

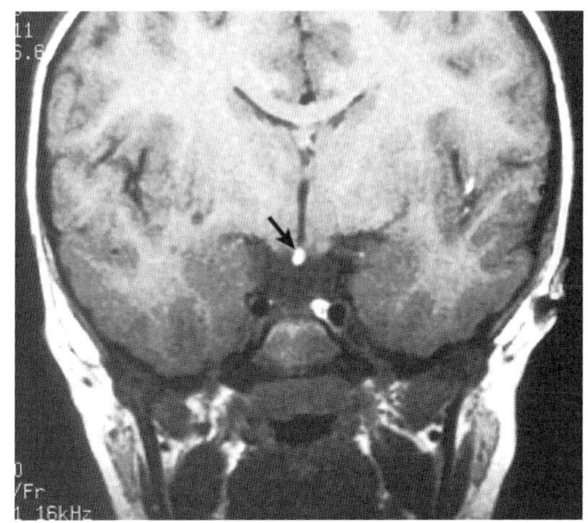

Figure 6.5.2. SE 500/15 without gadolinium.

Findings. Midline bright signal (*arrow*) is present in the region of the tuber cinereum on midline sagittal (Fig. 6.5.1) and coronal (Fig. 6.5.2) T1-weighted MR images. Also demonstrated is a small sella turcica, diminutive pituitary gland, and an atretic pituitary stalk.

Diagnosis. Primary panhypopituitarism with translocation of the pituitary bright spot (ectopic posterior pituitary)

Discussion. Because the posterior pituitary bright spot is felt to be due to the inherent signal intensity of neurosecretory granules in the neurohypophysis, an ectopic bright spot may be found in any process that disrupts the transport of antidiuretic hormone from the hypothalamus to the posterior pituitary lobe (12). Primary panhypopituitarism occurs when the pituitary gland is congenitally hypoplastic or absent. In the clinical setting of panhypopituitarism, a high correlation exists between the hormonal disorder and ectopia of the neurohypophysis. Growth disturbances may predominate the clinical picture, as in the index case. A history of traumatic or breech delivery is present in many patients, with the presumed association being perinatal rupture of the pituitary infundibulum (13). Characteristic MR findings of primary panhypopituitarism include a small sella turcica, diminutive pituitary gland, atretic pituitary stalk, and an ectopic posterior pituitary bright spot (14).

Aunt Minnie's Pearls

- *An ectopic posterior pituitary arises from disruption of the normal transport of neurosecretory granules from the hypothalamus to the posterior pituitary.*
- *Characteristic MR findings of primary panhypopituitarism include a small sella turcica, diminutive pituitary gland, atretic pituitary stalk, and an ectopic posterior pituitary bright spot.*

CASE 6

History. Head, neck, and shoulder pain in a 37-year-old woman

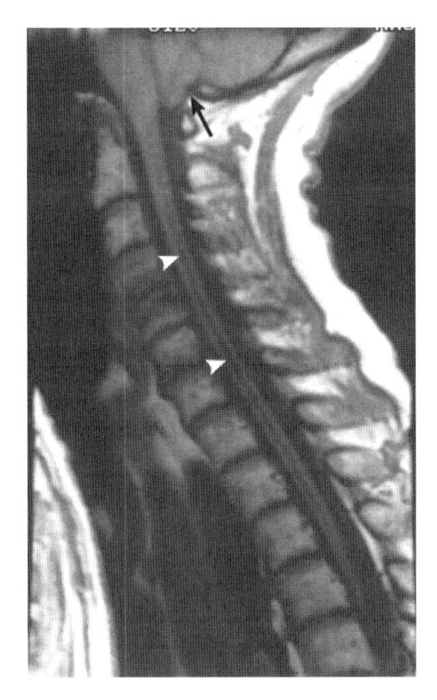

Figure 6.6.1. SE 500/11 without gadolinium.

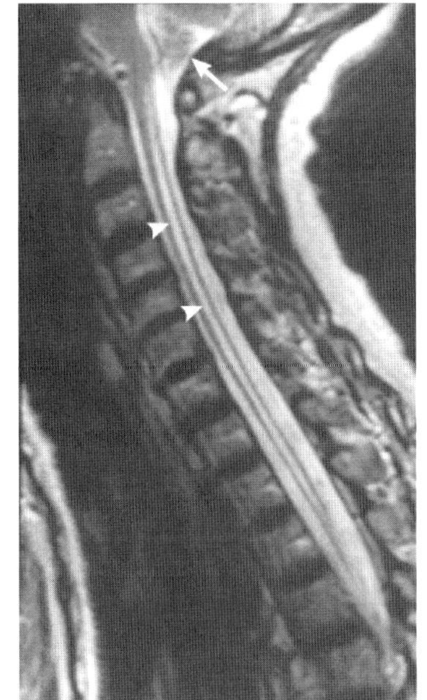

Figure 6.6.2. SE 4000/102 without gadolinium.

Findings. Midline sagittal T1- (Fig. 6.6.1) and T2-weighted (Fig. 6.6.2) MR images demonstrate tonsillar herniation (*arrows*) and a syrinx involving the cervical cord (*arrowheads*).

Diagnosis. Chiari I malformation

Discussion. In 1891, Hans Chiari first described a congenital hindbrain deformity consisting of downward displacement of the cerebellar tonsils through the foramen magnum and into the cervical canal (15). The amount of tonsillar herniation needed to make the diagnosis varies depending on the patient's age. However, more than 5–6 mm of tonsillar herniation, as in the index case, is abnormal in all age groups. Unlike the Chiari II malformation, the medulla, vermis, and fourth ventricle are usually normal or only slightly deformed. Patients may be asymptomatic or may present in adulthood with a wide range of symptoms. Approximately 30% of patients with tonsillar herniation from 5–10 mm below the foramen magnum are asymptomatic, but tonsillar displacement greater than 12 mm is invariably symptomatic (16). A syrinx is present in up to 40% of patients with Chiari I malformation, and associated skeletal anomalies such as Klippel-Feil syndrome and atlantooccipital assimilation are detected in approximately 25% of patients.

Aunt Minnie's Pearls
- *The Chiari I malformation consists of herniation of the cerebellar tonsils through the foramen magnum.*
- *A cervical syrinx and skeletal anomalies are associated findings.*

CASE 7

History. 2-year-old boy with developmental delay, nystagmus, and blindness

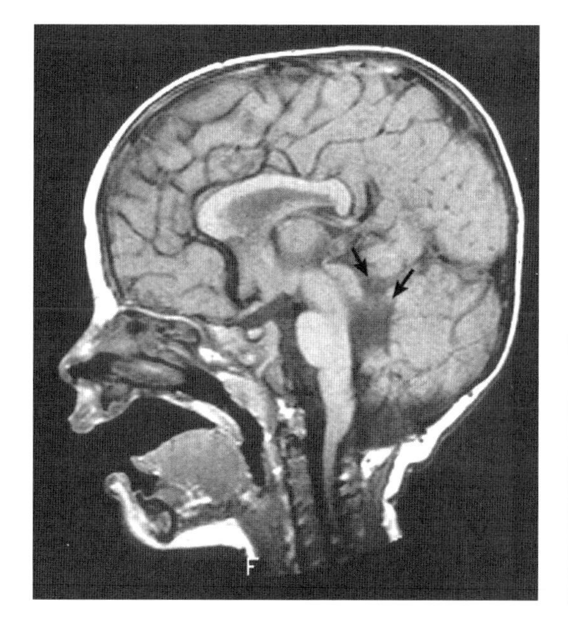

Figure 6.7.1. SE 500/16 without gadolinium.

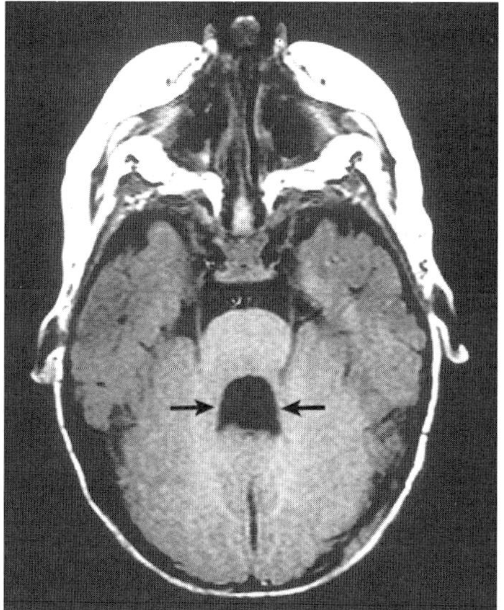

Figure 6.7.2. SE 700/16 without gadolinium.

Findings. Dysplasia of the vermis and slight enlargement of the fourth ventricle are demonstrated on the midline sagittal T1-weighted MR image (Fig. 6.7.1). The roof of the fourth ventricle is convex superiorly (*arrows*). An axial T1-weighted MR image at the level of the pons (Fig. 6.7.2) shows an unusual "batwing" configuration of the fourth ventricle (*arrows*), which is convex anteriorly. Thinning of the superior cerebellar peduncles (not shown) was also present.

Diagnosis. Joubert's syndrome

Discussion. Joubert's syndrome is an autosomal recessive disorder frequently associated with profound global developmental delay, neonatal tachypnea, congenital retinal dystrophy, and supranuclear ocular motor abnormalities (17). Dysgenesis of the vermis with a distinctive "batwing" configuration to the enlarged fourth ventricle at the level of the upper pons is the cardinal morphologic feature of this syndrome (18). The brainstem and superior and inferior cerebellar peduncles are often hypoplastic. Agenesis of the corpus callosum, occipital encephaloceles, polydactyly, cystic renal disease, and optic disc colobomas have less frequently been associated.

Aunt Minnie's Pearls

- *Batwing configuration of the fourth ventricle = Joubert's syndrome.*

CASE 8

History. 29-year-old woman with mild mental retardation

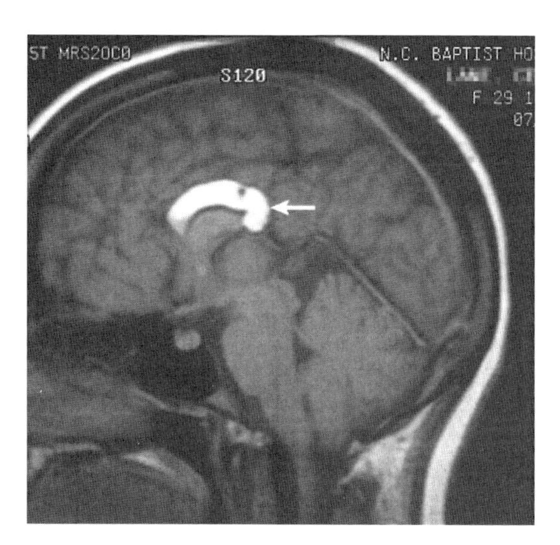

Figure 6.8.1. SE 550/24 without gadolinium.

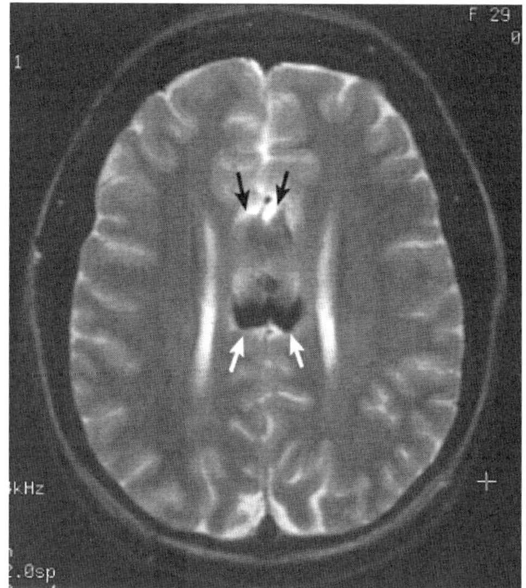

Figure 6.8.2. SE 3000/90 without gadolinium.

Findings. A sagittal T1-weighted MR image (Fig. 6.8.1) demonstrates a large midline hyperintense mass (*arrow*) associated with partial callosal agenesis. An axial T2-weighted image (Fig. 6.8.2) reveals a large lobulated mass following the signal intensity of fat located along the interhemispheric fissure. Note the chemical shift artifact at the margins of the mass (*arrows*).

Diagnosis. Partial corpus callosum agenesis with associated callosal lipoma

Discussion. Intracranial lipomas are relatively rare congenital malformations that are due to abnormal persistence of the meninx primativa, which is a primitive neural crest tissue responsible for formation of the leptomeninges (19). Many patients with intracranial lipomas will be completely asymptomatic. Lipomas that originate in the corpus callosum may occur anteriorly or posteriorly in that structure. Anterior or "tubulonodular" lipomas are large lesions associated with agenesis of the rostral corpus callosum and forebrain abnormalities (20). Posterior lipomas, like that in the index case, are thin and comma-shaped in appearance and are associated with mild agenesis of the genu or body of the corpus callosum.

On MR, these lesions follow the signal intensity of fat, appearing hyperintense on T1-weighted images (21). Characteristic low attenuation fatty density is readily detected on CT, as is the dystrophic calcification that may occur at the margins of the lipoma. On plain films of the skull, a characteristic picture of the tubulonodular variety may be seen as a large lucent mass anterior in the brain with striking calcification located around the periphery of the mass.

Aunt Minnie's Pearls

- *Lipomas are often associated with partial agenesis of the corpus callosum.*

CASE 9

History. 7-year-old boy with mental retardation and seizures

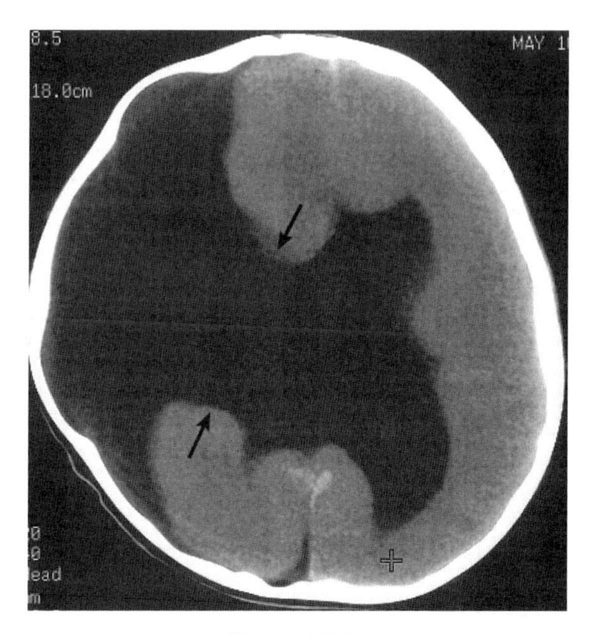

Figure 6.9.1.

Findings. An axial CT image at the level of the lateral ventricles (Fig. 6.9.1) shows a large cerebrospinal fluid-filled cleft (*arrows*) extending from the inner table of the skull to the lateral ventricle. Note the asymmetry of the skull and absence of the septum pellucidum.

Diagnosis. Schizencephaly (open-lip type)

Discussion. Schizencephaly, which is a disorder of sulcation and cellular migration, refers to gray matter-lined cerebrospinal fluid-filled clefts that span from the peripheral surface of the cerebral cortex to the ventricle (22). The pial covering of the peripheral brain surface therefore extends inward to fuse with the ependyma of the lateral ventricle. The "closed-lip" type of schizencephaly refers to a cleft that is narrow with apposition of the edges lined with gray matter. A widely separated cleft is referred to as an "open-lip" schizencephaly. The heterotopic gray matter lining the cleft is usually abnormal, often demonstrating polymicrogyria or pachygyria. Associated anomalies include absence of the septum pellucidum (in up to 90% of cases) and septooptic dysplasia.

Aunt Minnie's Pearls

- *A hemispheric cleft lined with gray mater = schizencephaly.*
- *Associated anomalies include absence of the septum pellucidum and septooptic dysplasia.*

CASE 10

History. 15-month-old girl with seizures

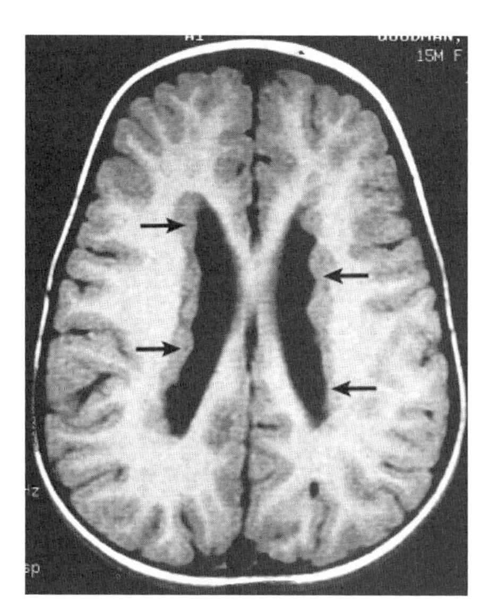

Figure 6.10.1. SE 600/14 without gadolinium.

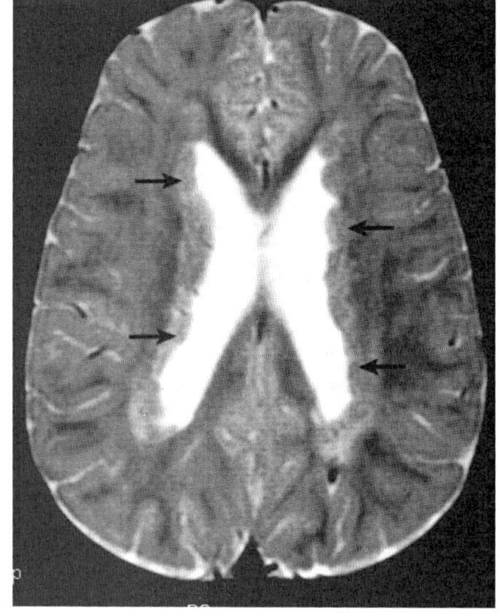

Figure 6.10.2. SE 3000/90 without gadolinium.

Findings. Axial T1- (Fig. 6.10.1) and T2-weighted (Fig. 6.10.2) MR images show diffuse subependymal nodules (*arrows*) lining both lateral ventricles. The nodules maintain isointensity with cortical gray matter on both pulse sequences.

Diagnosis. Gray matter heterotopia

Discussion. Gray matter heterotopia is a relatively common congenital abnormality that results from an in utero arrest of neuronal migration (23). The abnormally located gray matter is usually found in the subependymal region of the lateral ventricles, especially around the trigones. Occasionally, the heterotopias will be more peripherally located near the cerebral cortex. Patients come to clinical attention because of seizures and developmental retardation.

Heterotopias may be classified into three groups: subependymal heterotopia, focal subcortical heterotopia, and diffuse (band) heterotopia (24). The imaging hallmark is the isointensity with cortical gray matter on all imaging sequences and the lack of contrast enhancement. These characteristics allow the radiologist to distinguish this abnormality from the subependymal nodules that occur in tuberous sclerosis. On CT, heterotopias may be difficult to visualize.

Aunt Minnie's Pearls

- *To diagnose gray matter heterotopia, the nodules must follow the signal intensity of gray matter on all pulse sequences and show no enhancement after contrast administration.*

CASE 11

History. 2-month-old girl with a craniofacial abnormality

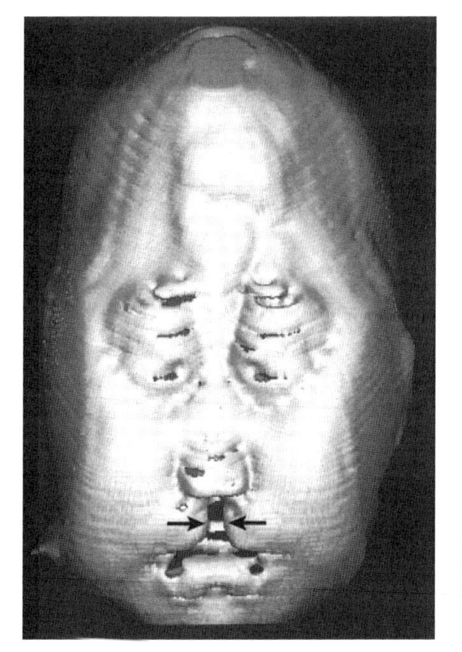

Figure 6.11.1.

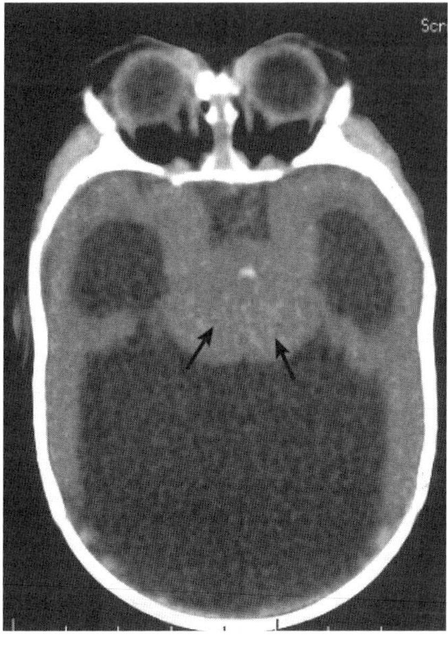

Figure 6.11.2.

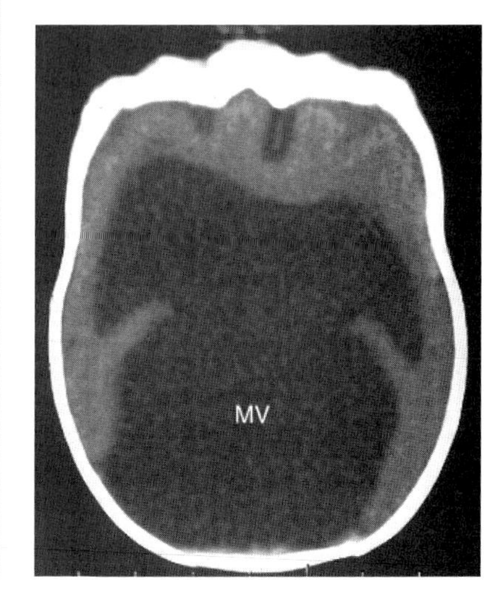

Figure 6.11.3.

Findings. Three-dimensional CT with soft tissue algorithm (Fig. 6.11.1) shows a cleft lip (*arrows*), abnormal nares, and hypotelorism. Axial CT images demonstrate fusion of the thalami (Fig. 6.11.2, *arrows*) and a large monoventricle (MV) (Fig. 6.11.3).

Diagnosis. Alobar holoprosencephaly

Discussion. Holoprosencephaly refers to a continuum of congenital malformations occurring from failure of induction of the prosencephalon and absent or incomplete cleavage of the brain into distinct cerebral hemispheres (25). Three subtypes have been proposed according to the severity of cerebral and facial anomalies. These include alobar, semilobar, and lobar holoprosencephaly (26). In the most severe subtype, alobar holoprosencephaly, there is complete or near complete lack of hemispheric cleavage. A primitive midline monoventricle, fused thalami, and absence of the falx cerebri and interhemispheric fissure are the typical imaging features. Midline facial anomalies ranging from hypotelorism to cyclopia are usually present. A multitude of extracranial and chromosomal abnormalities may occur in association with alobar holoprosencephaly, frequently resulting in a stillborn infant or death in the neonatal period.

Aunt Minnie's Pearls

- *Midline monoventricle with fused thalami = alobar holoprosencephaly.*

CASE 12

History. 26-year-old man with hydrocephalus since birth

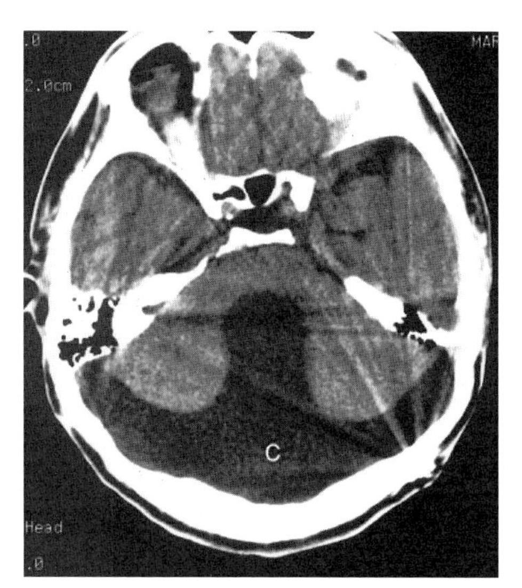

Figure 6.12.1.

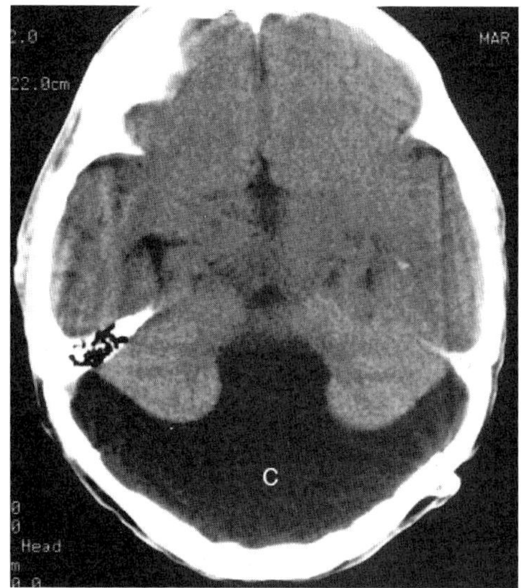

Figure 6.12.2.

Findings. Axial CT scans (Figs. 6.12.1 and 6.12.2) without contrast demonstrate agenesis of the vermis and hypoplasia of the cerebellum. A large posterior fossa cyst (C) is present that is in direct communication with the fourth ventricle.

Diagnosis. Dandy-Walker syndrome

Discussion. The Dandy-Walker syndrome, accounting for approximately 15% of cystic posterior fossa masses, consists of dysgenesis of the vermis, cystic dilatation of the fourth ventricle, absence of the foramina of Magendie and Luschka, absence of communication between the subarachnoid space and the fourth ventricle, and enlargement of the posterior fossa (27). The cerebellar hemispheres are hypoplastic, and dysgenesis of the vermis ranges from hypoplasia to complete agenesis (28). Obstructive hydrocephalus is present in approximately 80% of patients. An enlarged posterior fossa with the torcular herophili lying far above the lambdoid suture (torcular-lambdoid inversion) is a classic finding on plain films. Associated central nervous system anomalies and extracranial abnormalities are present in approximately 70 and 25% of patients, respectively (28). The Dandy-Walker variant, accounting for 30% of cystic posterior fossa masses (27), consists of mild vermian hypoplasia, slight to moderate fourth ventricle enlargement, and a normal or only mildly enlarged posterior fossa.

Aunt Minnie's Pearls

- *Vermian dysgenesis with cystic enlargement of the fourth ventricle = Dandy-Walker syndrome.*

CASE 13

History. 19-year-old woman in motor vehicle accident

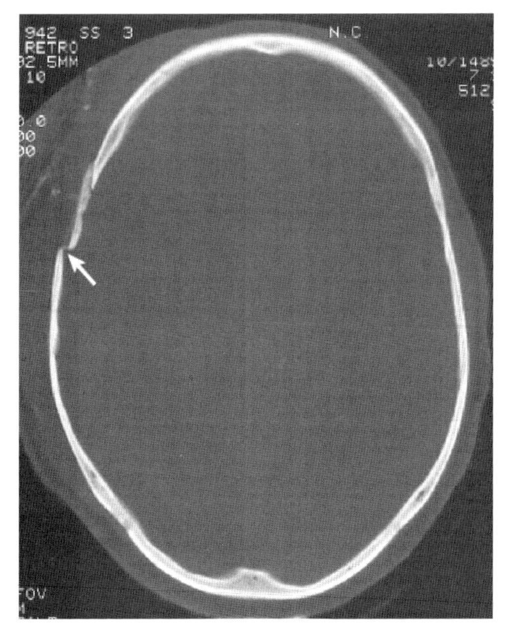

Figure 6.13.1.

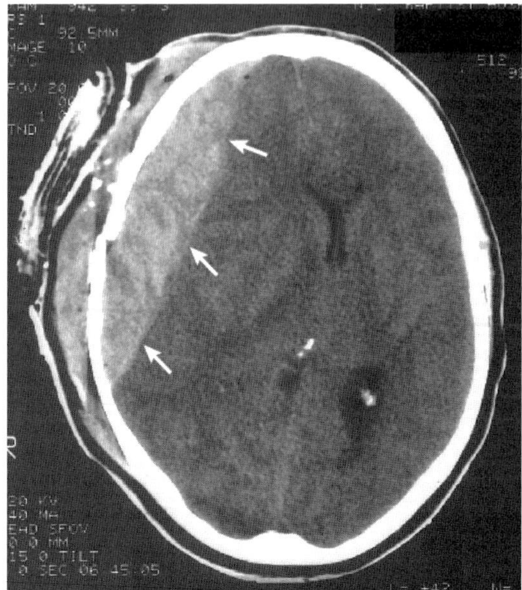

Figure 6.13.2.

Findings. An axial CT scan with bone reconstruction (Fig. 6.13.1) shows a depressed right parietal skull fracture (*arrow*). The same image rewindowed for soft tissue structures (Fig. 6.13.2) reveals a biconvex hyperdense extraaxial mass (*arrows*). There is also subfalcial herniation with leftward displacement of the gray-white matter interface of the right parietal lobe.

Diagnosis. Acute epidural hematoma

Discussion. Epidural hematomas are the result of bleeding into the potential space between the outer or periosteal layer of the dura mater and the inner table of the skull. They are present in less than 5% of patients imaged for cranial trauma. Epidural bleeding most commonly arises from disruption of the meningeal arteries, although laceration of a dural venous sinus and venous "oozing" from meningeal venous injury may have similar results. Skull fractures are present in approximately 90% of patients with epidural hematomas (29). Because epidural hematomas are located external to the outer or periosteal dural layer (which is firmly bound at the suture margin) they rarely cross sutures and typically appear biconvex. CT without contrast is the examination of choice for suspected epidural hematomas. Typical imaging features include a hyperdense biconvex extraaxial mass displacing brain with secondary brain herniation. Active bleeding is indicated by areas of inhomogeneity within an epidural hematoma. Clinically, epidural hematomas are usually managed by emergent surgical evacuation. Interestingly, a patient with an epidural hematoma may initially be neurologically intact, only to develop the rapid onset of severe neurologic compromise (the so-called "lucid interval"). Because of the morbidity and mortality associated with untreated epidural hematomas, all patients with severe head trauma or unconsciousness after head trauma are imaged for this and other brain injuries.

Aunt Minnie's Pearls

- *90% of epidural hematomas are associated with a skull fracture.*
- *These lesions are usually biconvex and do not cross sutures.*

CASE 14

History. 1-month-old girl with seizures

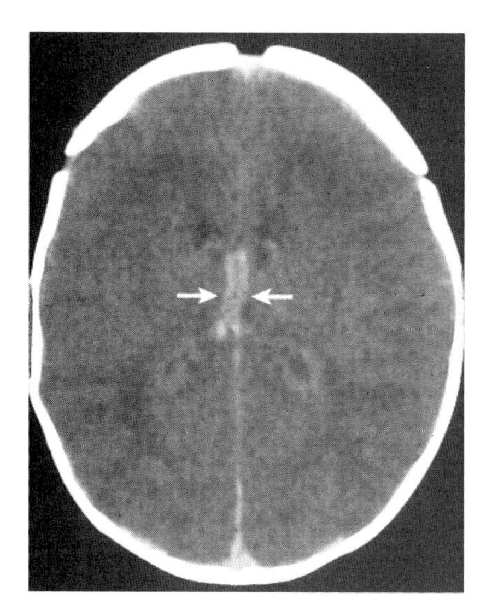

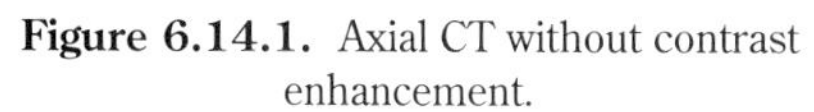

Figure 6.14.1. Axial CT without contrast enhancement.

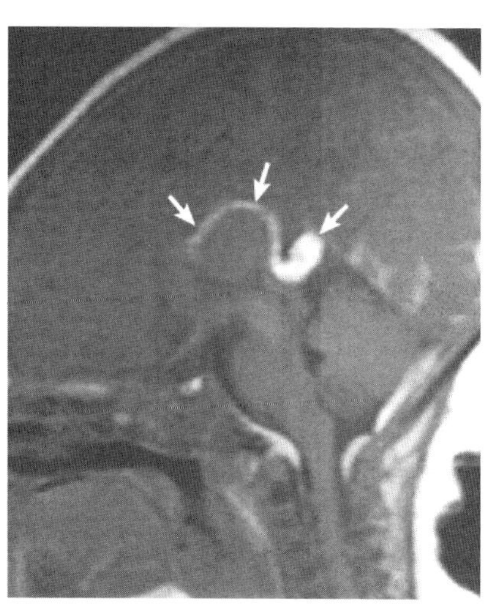

Figure 6.14.2. SE 500/11 without gadolinium.

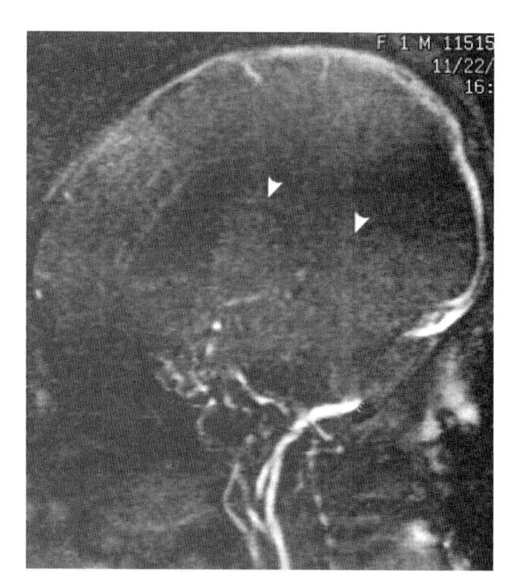

Figure 6.14.3. Phase contrast venogram, FV = 15.0 cm/s, without gadolinium.

Findings. Axial noncontrast CT (Fig. 6.14.1) shows high density in the internal cerebral veins (*arrows*). Sagittal T1-weighted MR image (Fig. 6.14.2) demonstrates abnormal high signal within the internal cerebral veins and vein of Galen (*arrows*). No flow is present within the deep venous system on phase contrast magnetic resonance venography (Fig. 6.14.3, *arrowheads*).

Diagnosis. Deep cerebral venous thrombosis

Discussion. Deep cerebral venous thrombosis is an uncommon disorder frequently resulting in severe neurological disability or death. Diagnosis and appropriate management are often delayed because of the nonspecific clinical manifestations. This condition is most common in infants with dehydration or septicemia. Oral contraceptives, pregnancy, and hematologic disorders are etiologic factors associated with venous thrombosis in adults. Alteration in the level of consciousness with progression to a comatose state is the classic presentation in deep cerebral venous thrombosis. CT findings include hyperdense thrombus within the internal cerebral veins, vein of Galen, or straight sinus on noncontrast studies. Hypodensity in the basal ganglia representing edema or infarction may be also seen (30). Nonfilling of the deep cerebral veins with enlarged collaterals is present at angiography. MRI may be used as the definitive investigation, initially demonstrating absence of flow within the affected venous structures. After several days, the thrombosed vessel becomes hyperintense on T1- and T2-weighted images as the thrombus becomes replete with extracellular methemoglobin. Antithrombotic therapy is now considered to be safe and effective treatment, particularly when hemorrhage has not been demonstrated (31).

Aunt Minnie's Pearls

- *Absence of flow and hyperintensity in the internal cerebral veins, vein of Galen, or straight sinus = deep cerebral venous thrombosis.*

CASE 15

History. 10-month-old girl with midline facial anomalies and a mass in the nasopharynx

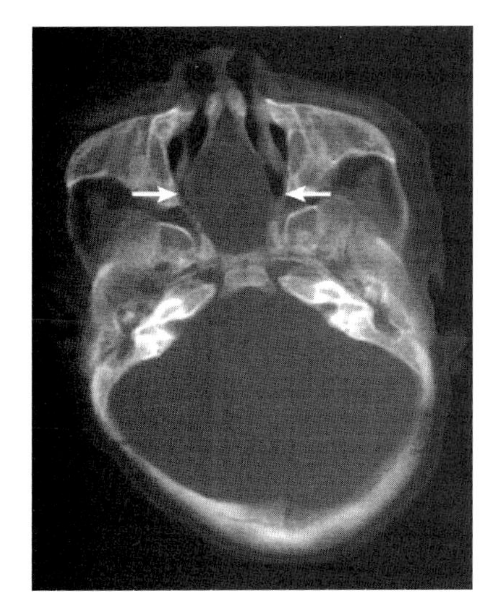

Figure 6.15.1.

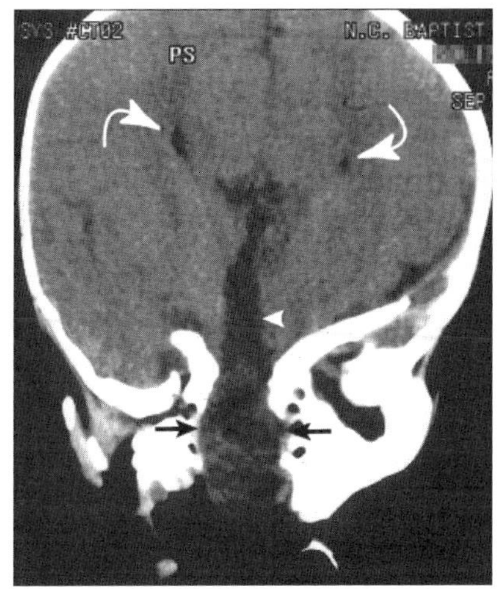

Figure 6.15.2.

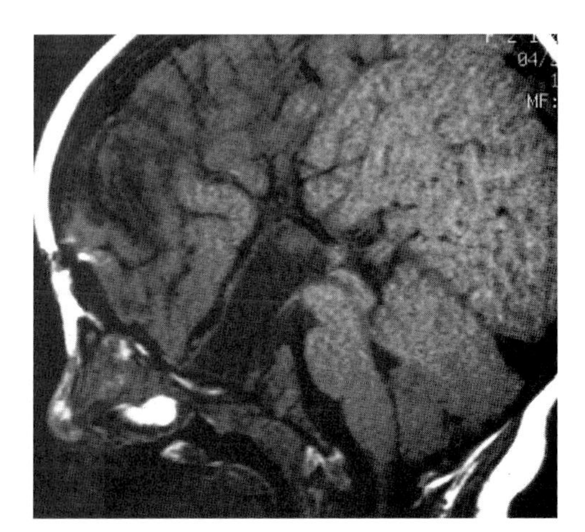

Figure 6.15.3. SE 600/17 without gadolinium.

Findings. Axial (Fig. 6.15.1) and coronal (Fig. 6.15.2) CT images with bone and soft tissue reconstruction, respectively, show a cerebrospinal fluid attenuation mass (*arrows*) extending into the nasopharynx that is directly contiguous with the third ventricle (*arrowhead*). A wide defect is present in the basisphenoid, and there is separation and angulation of the lateral ventricles producing a "Viking horn" appearance (*curved arrows*), indicating agenesis of the corpus callosum. A sagittal MR image (Fig. 6.15.3) also reveals the cerebrospinal fluid-filled mass and shows to better advantage the lack of brain tissue within it.

Diagnosis. Basal (transphenoidal) meningocele

Discussion. Congenital malformations consisting of a defect in the cranium and dura with extracranial extension of intracranial structures are referred to as cephaloceles. A meningocele is present if the herniated sac contains only leptomeninges filled with cerebrospinal fluid. If the herniated sac contains brain elements, the malformation is termed an encephalocele. Bifidum occultum designates the uncommon condition of a simple skull defect without prolapse of the leptomeninges or brain. Cephaloceles occur at multiple locations in the cranium, and significant race, gender, and geographic variations occur with the different types of cephaloceles (32). Basal cephaloceles (transphenoidal, sphenoethmoidal, transethmoidal) are the rarest types and are commonly associated with optic malformations, endocrine dysfunction, and anomalies of the corpus callosum (33). CT is sensitive in the evaluation of the bony defect, but MRI is much more accurate in determining the contents within the herniated sac (34).

Aunt Minnie's Pearls

- *MRI is more accurate than CT in determining the contents of a cephalocele.*

CASE 16

History. 58-year-old man with deafness and ataxia

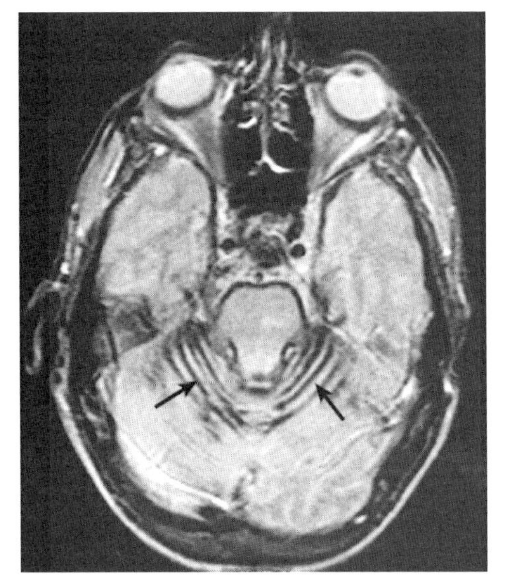

Figure 6.16.1. SE 2300/60 without gadolinium.

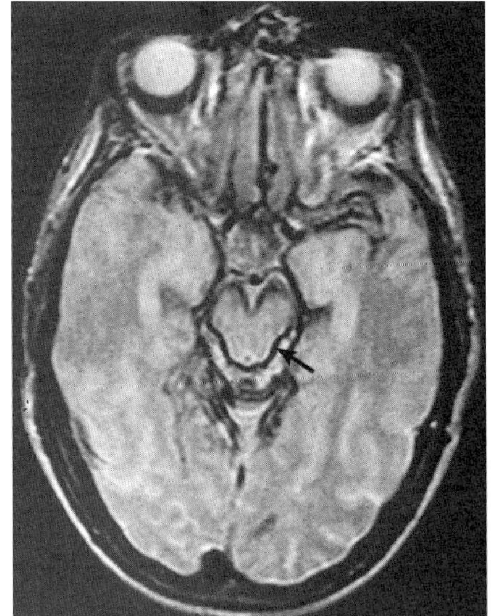

Figure 6.16.2. SE 2300/60 without gadolinium.

Findings. Axial T2-weighted MR images at the level of the brainstem (Figs. 6.16.1 and 6.16.2) demonstrate low signal coating the surface of the brainstem and cerebellum (*arrows*).

Diagnosis. Superficial siderosis

Discussion. Superficial siderosis is a rare disorder characterized by the deposition of hemosiderin in the leptomeninges covering the cerebrum, cerebellum, brainstem, cranial nerves, and spinal cord. Chronic subarachnoid hemorrhage is the etiology of superficial siderosis, and the source of bleeding is found in over 50% of patients (35). The clinical triad of sensorineural hearing loss, cerebellar ataxia, and pyramidal signs along with hemorrhagic or xanthochromic cerebrospinal fluid permits a clinical diagnosis (36). MR imaging readily confirms the hemosiderin deposition and provides a diagnosis at an earlier stage of the disease (37). T2-weighted images demonstrate a rim of marked hypointensity along the surface of affected structures (36). CT occasionally suggests the diagnosis by showing a rim of mild hyperdensity around the brainstem; however, MR demonstrates this abnormality to better advantage (38). Therapeutic management includes surgical ablation of the bleeding source. When interpreting fast spin echo images, an artifactual low signal rim around the brain may be seen and should not be confused with superficial siderosis that will persist on spin echo imaging.

Aunt Minnie's Pearls

- *A marked hypointense rim on T2-weighted MR images coating the brain and spinal cord = superficial siderosis.*
- *The etiology of this disorder is subarachnoid hemorrhage.*

CASE 17

History. 2-month-old boy with cranial asymmetry

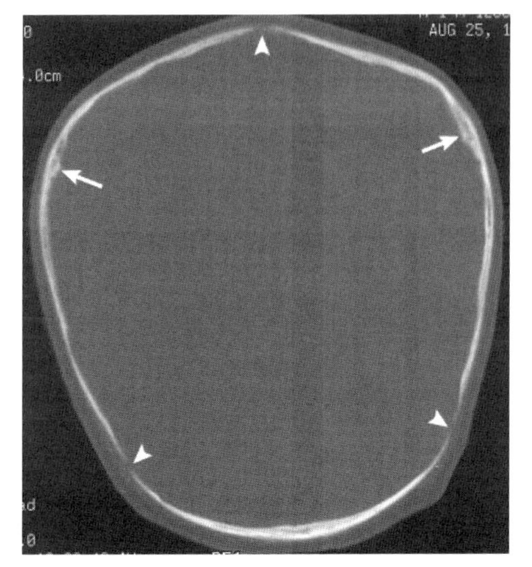

Figure 6.17.1.

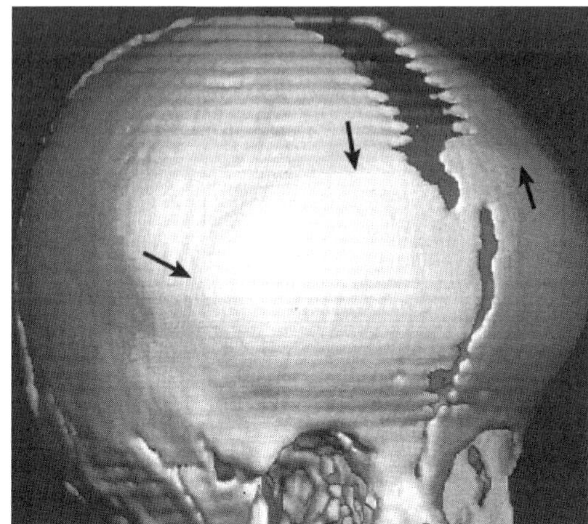

Figure 6.17.2.

Findings. Axial CT with bone algorithm (Fig. 6.17.1) shows fusion of both coronal sutures (*arrows*). Sagittal and lambdoid sutures are open (*arrowheads*). Note the rounded and foreshortened appearance of the head. Three-dimensional CT in the frontal oblique projection (Fig. 6.17.2) demonstrates bony bridging and obliteration of both coronal sutures (*arrows*).

Diagnosis. Bilateral coronal craniosynostosis (brachycephaly)

Discussion. Craniosynostosis is the premature closure of a cranial suture. Cessation of growth at a suture leads to a decrease in the diameter of the skull perpendicular to the plane of the affected suture. Premature closure may be idiopathic (primary craniosynostosis) or secondary to metabolic diseases, bony dysplasias, hematologic disorders, or alterations in intracranial pressure. The sagittal suture is the most common suture involved. The coronal suture is the second most commonly involved suture, and craniosynostosis may be unilateral or bilateral. With bilateral coronal synostosis, the skull is brachycephalic, demonstrating a wide cranium that is short in the anteroposterior dimension. CT is superior in the detection of suture closure as well as demonstrating the shape of the skull (39). Three-dimensional CT is highly accurate in the diagnosis and assessment of craniosynostosis and may facilitate surgical planning by precisely localizing the proper site for craniectomy (40, 41).

Aunt Minnie's Pearls

- *Three-dimensional CT is accurate in the detection and assessment of craniosynostosis.*

CASE 18

History. 32-year-old man with ataxia, nausea, and vomiting

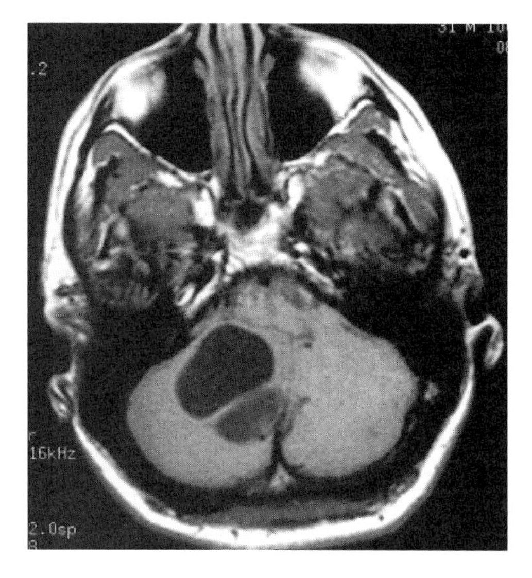

Figure 6.18.1. SE 766/13 without gadolinium.

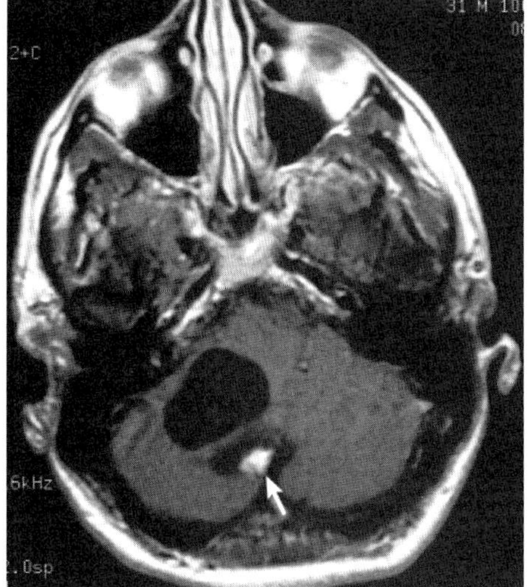

Figure 6.18.2. SE 500/19 with gadolinium

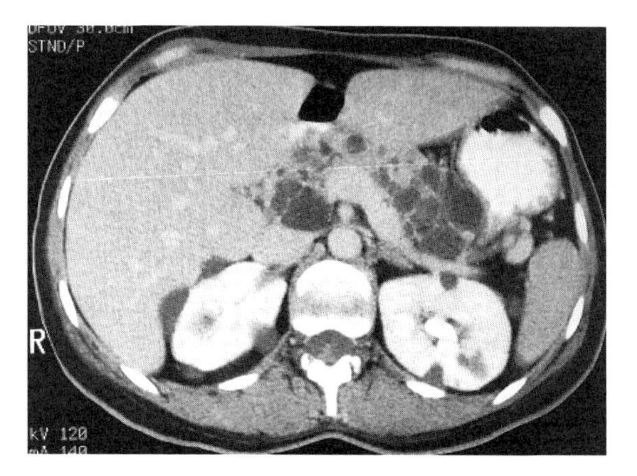

Figure 6.18.3.

Findings. An axial T1-weighted image (Fig. 6.18.1) shows a large cystic mass within the cerebellum that demonstrates intense enhancement of a mural nodule after contrast administration (Fig. 6.18.2, *arrow*). A contrast enhanced CT image of the abdomen (Fig. 6.18.3) reveals numerous cysts within the kidneys and pancreas.

Diagnosis. Cerebellar hemangioblastoma in a patient with von Hippel-Lindau syndrome

Discussion. Hemangioblastomas are rare tumors accounting for <3% of all intracranial neoplasms and typically occur in patients 20–50 years old. Hemangioblastomas occur either sporadically or as a manifestation of von Hippel-Lindau syndrome). Von Hippel-Lindau syndrome is inherited as an autosomal dominant disorder linked to a defect on chromosome 3. In addition to hemangioblastomas of the cerebellum, brainstem, and cord, non–central nervous system manifestations of von Hippel-Lindau syndrome include cysts of the kidneys, pancreas, and liver as well as renal cell carcinoma, microcystic adenoma of the pancreas, and pheochromocytoma. Hemangioblastomas in von Hippel-Lindau syndrome are multiple in up to 40% of cases and typically present at least 10 years earlier than those occurring in patients without the syndrome (42). To diagnose von Hippel-Lindau syndrome, multiple hemangioblastomas or one hemangioblastoma with other visceral manifestations of the disease are required. Greater than 50% of hemangioblastomas are cystic, with a mural nodule that demonstrates intense enhancement. If the cyst wall is thick or enhanced, other neoplasms should be considered (6). A pilocytic astrocytoma or metastasis may also present as a cystic mass of the fourth ventricle, but patients with these tumors would not be expected to have the other manifestations of von Hippel-Lindau syndrome.

Aunt Minnie's Pearls

- Multiple cystic masses with an enhancing mural nodule or one mass with specific visceral manifestations = von Hippel-Lindau syndrome.
- Visceral manifestations of von Hippel-Lindau syndrome = renal, pancreatic, and liver cysts, renal cell carcinoma, pheochromocytoma, and retinal hemangioblastomas.

CASE 19

History. 77-year-old woman with left proptosis

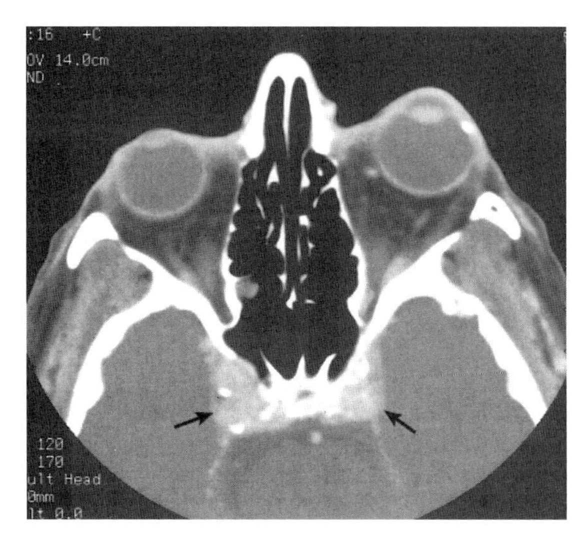

Figure 6.19.1.

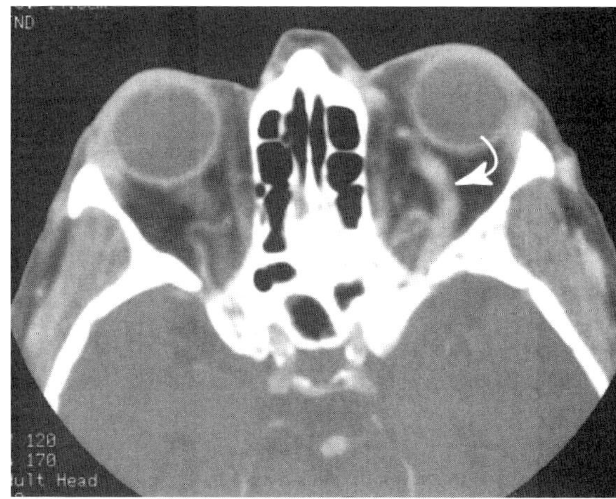

Figure 6.19.2.

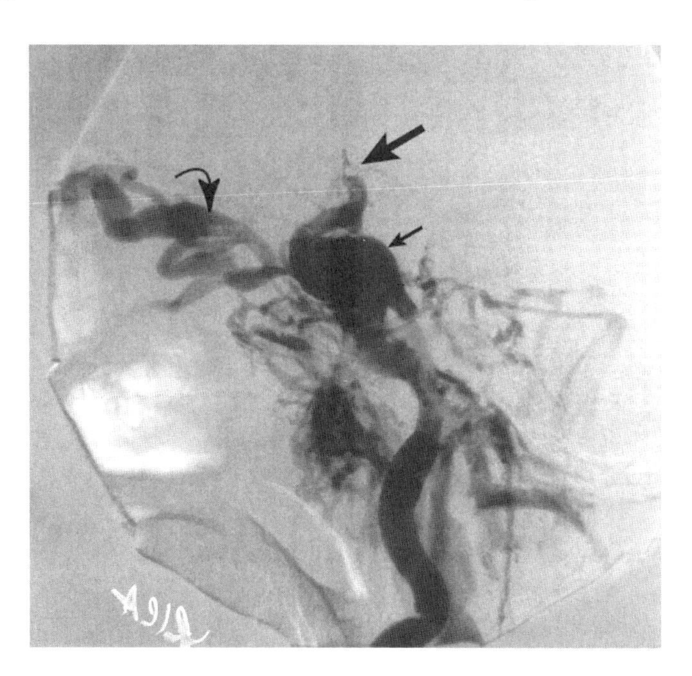

Figure 6.19.3.

Findings. Two images from an axial contrast enhanced CT scan of the orbits (Figs. 6.19.1 and 6.19.2) demonstrate mild bulging of the cavernous sinuses bilaterally (*arrows*) and a markedly enlarged left superior ophthalmic vein (*curved arrow*). A lateral view from a right internal carotid artery angiogram (Fig. 6.19.3) demonstrates lack of filling of the supraclinoid carotid (*large arrow*) with early opacification of both cavernous sinuses (*small arrow*) with multiple draining veins, including the left superior ophthalmic vein (*curved arrow*).

Diagnosis. Carotid cavernous fistula

Discussion. Carotid artery cavernous sinus fistulas can be classified as either direct or indirect (43). Direct carotid cavernous fistulas are usually posttraumatic and involve a tear in the wall of the carotid artery as it passes through the cavernous sinus (44). Indirect carotid cavernous fistulas are dural arteriovenous malformations involving meningeal branches of the external and occasionally the internal carotid arteries and the cavernous sinus. Indirect carotid cavernous fistulas are usually spontaneous and occur in older women. Symptoms include pulsatile exophthalmos, chemosis, and occasionally blurred vision. Direct type fistulas have similar but often more dramatic symptoms. CT and/or MR findings include proptosis with a bulging cavernous sinus and a dilated superior ophthalmic vein (45). MRI may demonstrate abnormal flow voids within or between the cavernous sinuses (46). Cerebral angiography is diagnostic, and treatment is usually transcatheter embolization.

Aunt Minnie's Pearls

- *Abnormal vascular communication between the internal carotid artery and the veins of the cavernous sinus = carotid cavernous fistula.*
- *Typical symptoms include exophthalmos, chemosis, and blurred vision.*

CASE 20

History. 12-year-old girl with lower extremity weakness, bladder dysfunction, and worsening scoliosis

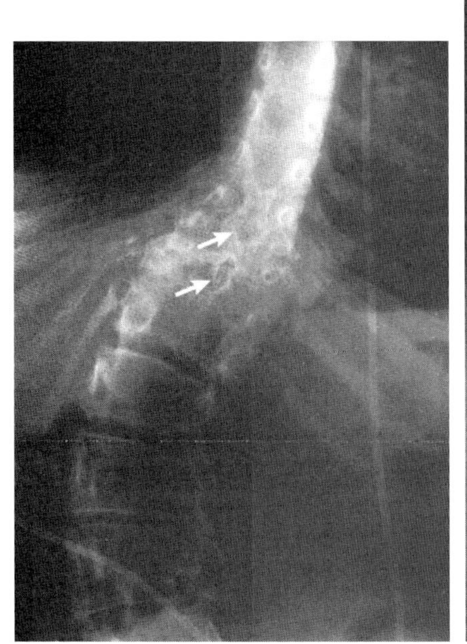

Figure 6.20.1.

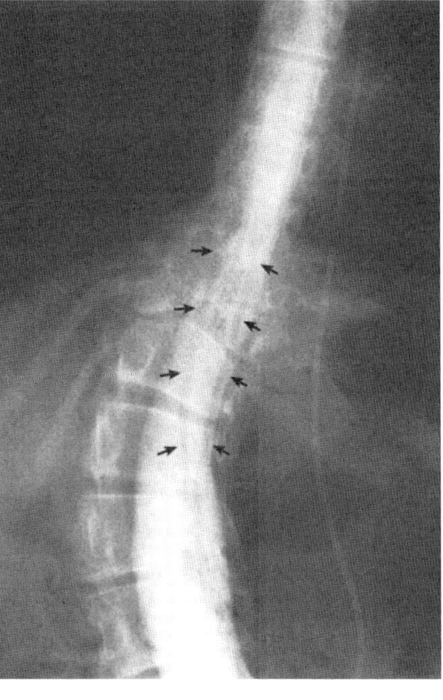

Figure 6.20.2.

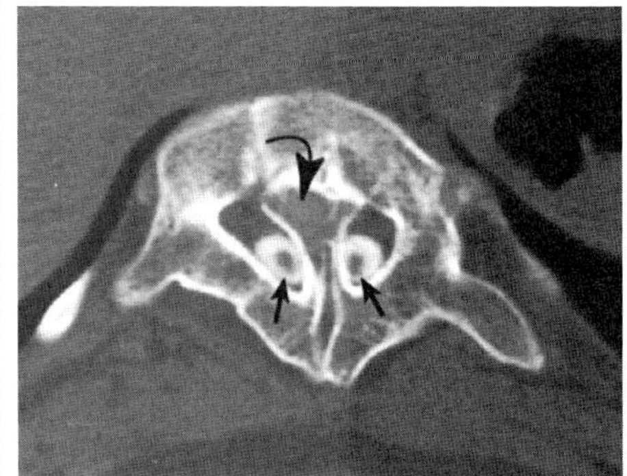

Figure 6.20.3.

Findings. A frontal plain film of the thoracolumbar spine (Fig. 6.20.1) demonstrates marked scoliosis, multiple low thoracic segmentation anomalies, and a central bony spur (*arrows*). A frontal view from a myelogram (Fig. 6.20.2) shows contrast surrounding two hemicords (*arrows*). An axial postmyelogram CT scan through the lower thoracic region (Fig. 6.20.3) reveals the bony septum (*curved arrow*) separating the two hemicords (*arrows*), each within its own dural tube. The two hemicords rejoined below this bony spur and were tethered in the low lumbar region.

Diagnosis. Diastematomyelia

Discussion. Diastematomyelia is an occult dysraphic state in which the spinal cord is divided into two hemicords by a sagittal cleft (47). This congenital anomaly most commonly occurs in females (80–85%) and usually involves the low thoracic or upper lumbar region (48). It is associated with various other abnormalities including scoliosis, vertebral segmentation anomalies, cutaneous stigmata overlying the spine, Chiari II malformation, tethered cord, and hydromyelia (which may be confined to one hemicord). In half of the cases the hemicords share a dural sac; in the other half each hemicord has its own dural sac (49). A fibrous or bony spur separating the two hemicords is present in 50% of cases.

Aunt Minnie's Pearls

- *Diastematomyelia is an occult dysraphic state in which the spinal cord is divided into two hemicords by a sagittal cleft.*

CASE 21

History. 1-month-old girl with a lumbosacral abnormality

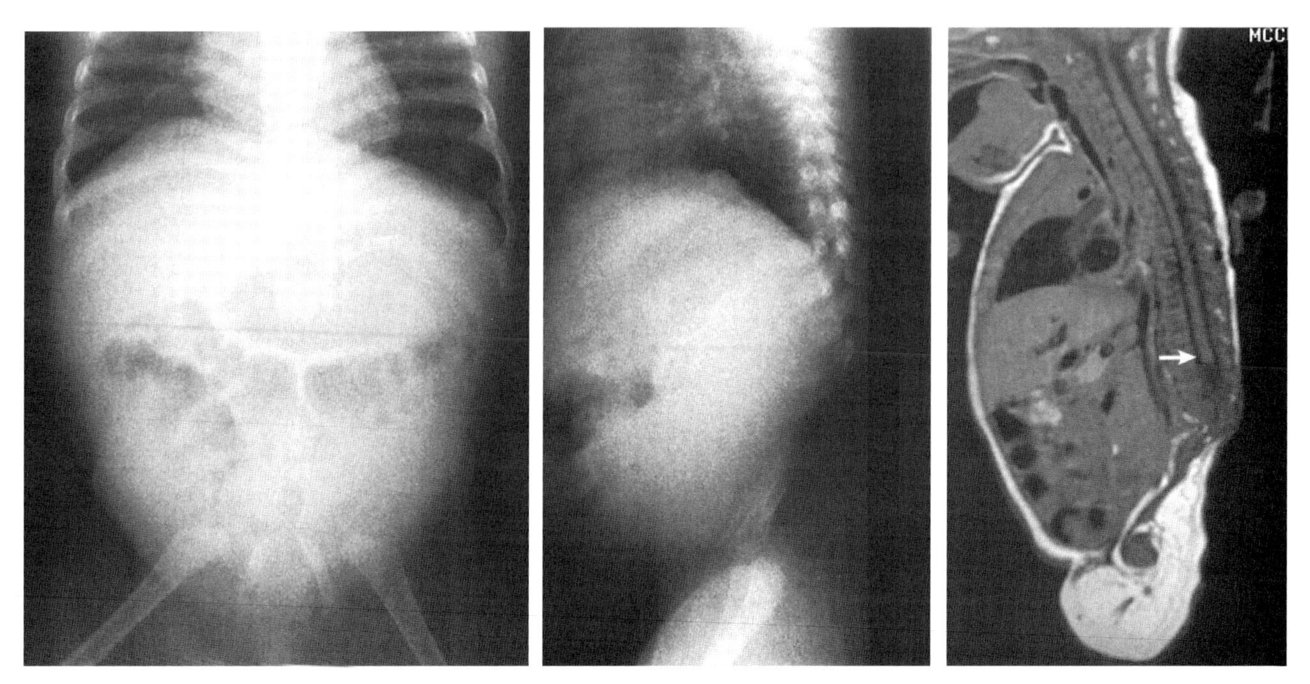

Figure 6.21.1. **Figure 6.21.2.** **Figure 6.21.3.** SE 500/14 without gadolinium.

Findings. AP (Fig. 6.21.1) and lateral (Fig. 6.21.2) plain films of the abdomen demonstrate agenesis of the lumbar spine and severe hypoplasia of the sacrum with fused iliac bones. A sagittal T1 MRI scan (Fig. 6.21.3) shows the lumbosacral abnormality as well as a blunted cord (*arrow*) that ends at the T10–T11 level.

Diagnosis. Caudal regression syndrome with lumbosacral agenesis

Discussion. The caudal regression syndrome is a congenital anomaly in which there is abnormal formation of the lower portion of the spine and spinal cord (50). There is a spectrum of abnormality with varying degrees of lumbosacral hypoplasia or aplasia. This anomaly is frequently associated with abnormalities of the genitourinary system and with lower extremity sensory and motor abnormalities. A high percentage of infants with this condition are born to diabetic mothers. The distal spinal cord typically has a blunted appearance (51). The cause for this condition is unknown but appears to be the result of some disturbance in the caudal mesoderm early in gestation (52).

Aunt Minnie's Pearls

- *Sacral agenesis with fused iliac bones and associated cord anomalies = caudal regression syndrome.*
- *Many infants with this disorder are born to diabetic mothers.*

CASE 22

History. 15-year-old girl with acute onset of numbness and weakness in both lower extremities and a T4 sensory level

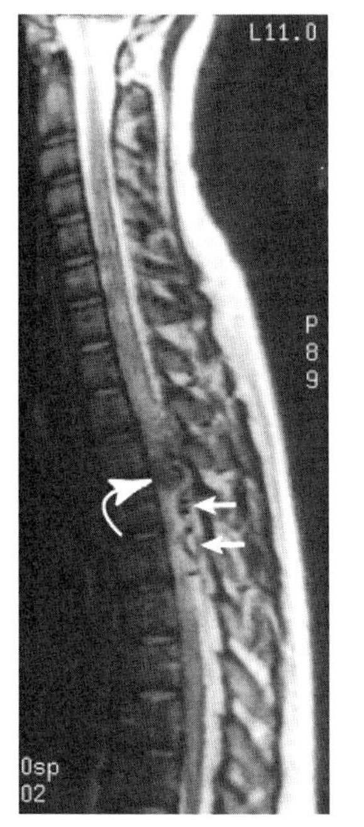

Figure 6.22.1. SE 4000/96 without gadolinium.

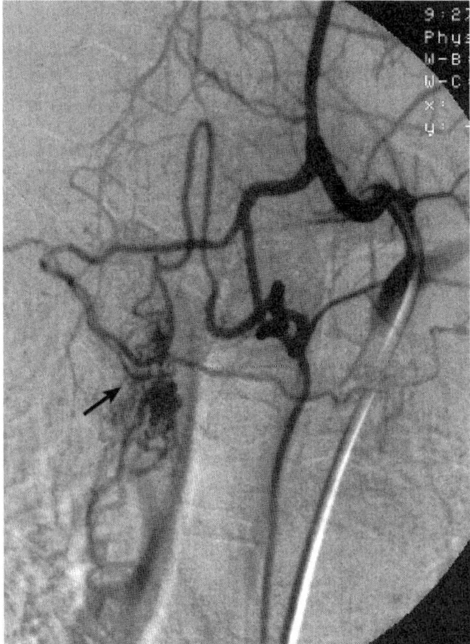

Figure 6.22.2.

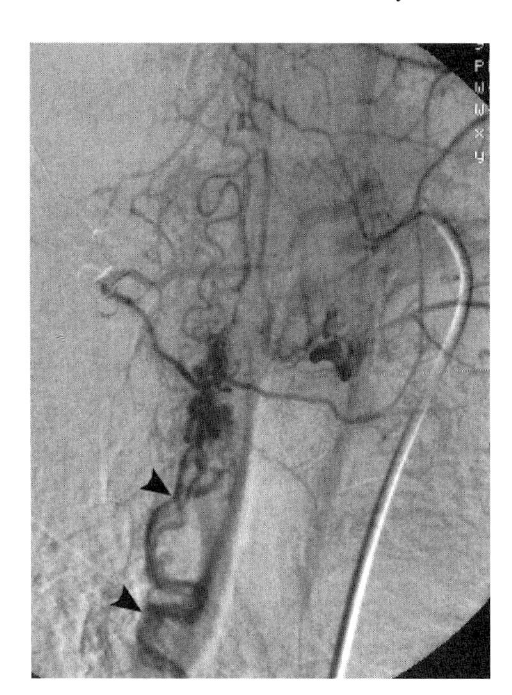

Figure 6.22.3.

Findings. A sagittal T2-weighted MR image of the cervicothoracic region (Fig. 6.22.1) demonstrates a heterogeneous intramedullary lesion at the T3–T4 level (*curved arrow*) and multiple serpentine flow voids on the surface of the cord, predominantly posteriorly (*arrows*). Early (Fig. 6.22.2) and late (Fig. 6.22.3) frontal arterial films from a spinal arteriogram reveal an abnormal tangle of vessels projecting over the spinal canal (*arrow*) with large, early draining veins (*arrowheads*).

Diagnosis. Spinal arteriovenous malformation

Discussion. Vascular malformations of the spinal cord have been classified according to the anatomic location of the malformation nidus or shunt (53). Type 1 malformations are dural arteriovenous fistulas. These typically occur in the low thoracic region in middle-aged and older men who present with progressive neurologic deterioration. Type 2 malformations are intramedullary arteriovenous malformations with a compact nidus supplied by multiple feeders from the spinal arteries. These occur in younger patients who frequently develop symptoms acutely from intramedullary hemorrhage. Type 3 arteriovenous malformations are rare lesions that extensively involve both intramedullary and extramedullary compartments with multiple feeders. Type 4 arteriovenous malformations are intradural, extramedullary arteriovenous fistulas that usually occur near the conus medullaris in middle-aged patients with progressive neurologic deficits.

Myelography usually demonstrates enlarged, tortuous vessels associated with these arteriovenous malformations, which show up as serpentine flow voids on MRI (54). Abnormal cord signal is also present if there has been intramedullary hemorrhage or ischemia/infarction from chronic venous congestion. Spinal arteriography is the gold standard for evaluating spinal arteriovenous malformations. Therapy consists of intravascular embolization occasionally combined with surgery (55).

Aunt Minnie's Pearls

- *Spinal arteriovenous malformations occur in several types that vary by location and age group involved.*

CASE 23

History. 45-year-old man with phantom pain after traumatic right arm amputation

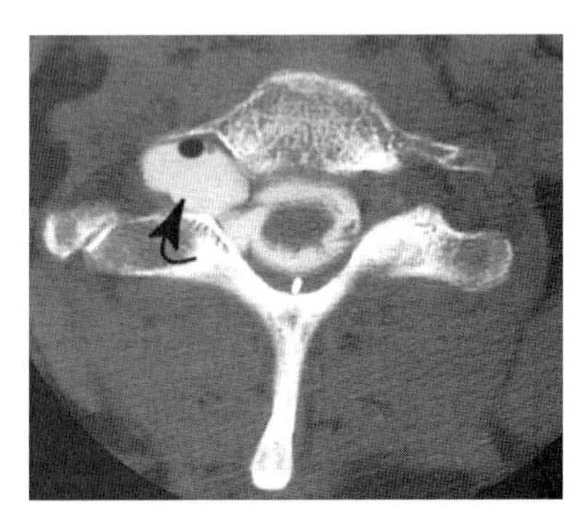

Figure 6.23.2.

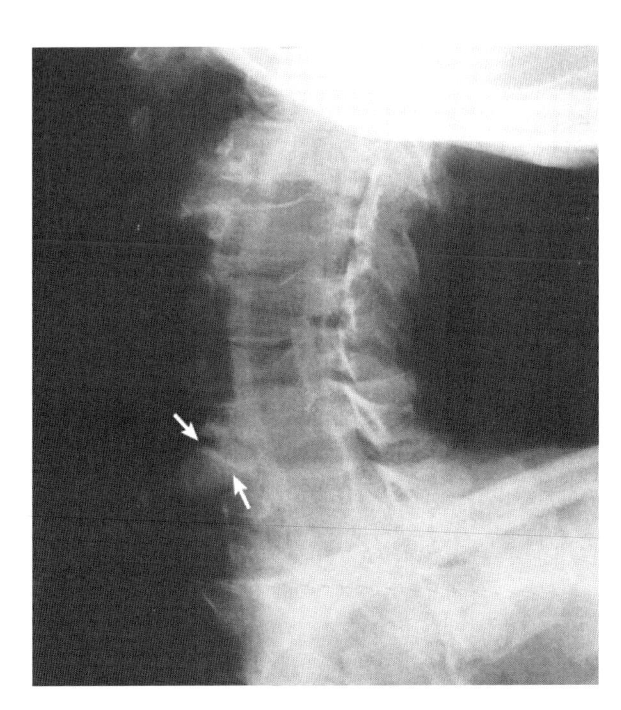

Figure 6.23.1.

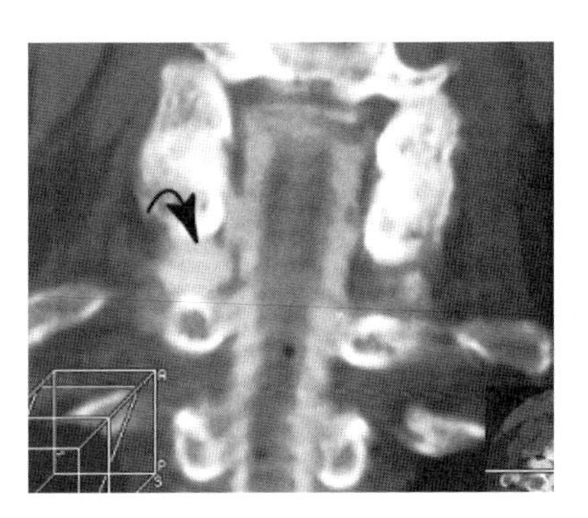

Figure 6.23.3.

Findings. An oblique view from a cervical myelogram (Fig. 6.23.1) demonstrates no normal exiting nerve roots and an abnormal collection of contrast on the right at C7/T1 (*arrows*). Axial postmyelogram CT (Fig. 6.23.2) and coronal reformatted images (Fig. 6.23.3) better show the right-sided C7/T1 contrast collection (*curved arrow*).

Diagnosis. Right C8 nerve root avulsion with pseudomeningocele

Discussion. Nerve root avulsions occur secondary to severe traction on the exiting nerve roots. These are seen most commonly in the cervical spine in association with traction injuries of the arm but can occur in the lumbosacral region secondary to lumbosacral or pelvic fractures. The typical appearance on myelography, CT myelography, or MRI is that of an absent exiting nerve root at the level of the neural foramen (56, 57). The avulsed nerve root often retracts laterally, leaving a cerebrospinal fluid filled cavity or pseudomeningocele in the lateral aspect of the spinal canal extending into the neural foramen and occasionally extra-foraminally into the surrounding paraspinous soft tissues. Although pseudomeningoceles typically fill with contrast introduced into the subarachnoid space, they can occasionally become walled off and present as extradural cystic masses. Although many nerve root avulsions occur in association with motor vehicle accidents they also occur during birth from excessive traction on the shoulder (58).

Aunt Minnie's Pearls

- *Severe traction injuries of the arm can lead to nerve root avulsion and pseudomeningocele formation.*

Case 24

History. 5-year-old boy with a pulsatile mass of the left middle ear discovered during tympanostomy tube placement

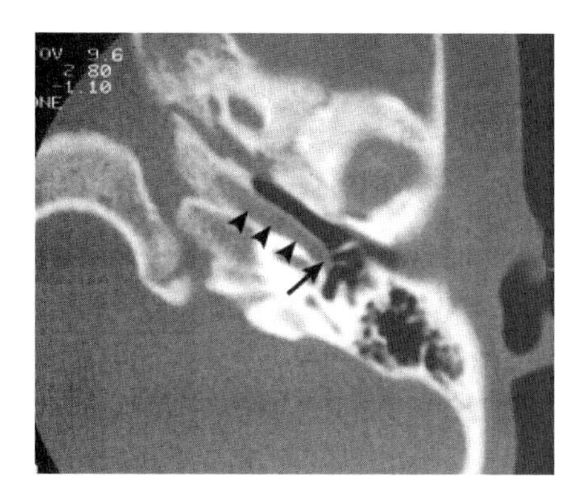

Figure 6.24.1.

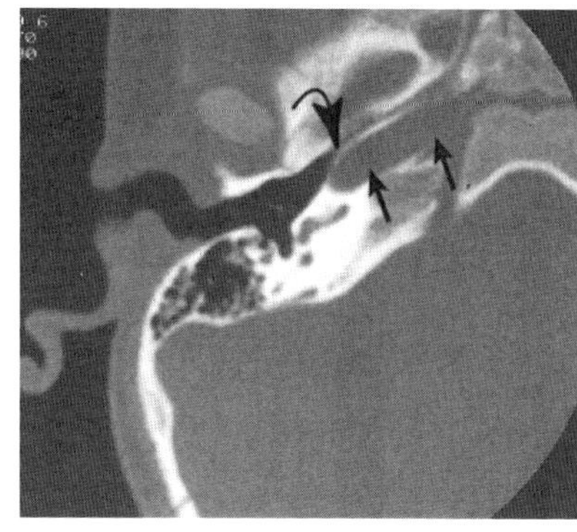

Figure 6.24.2.

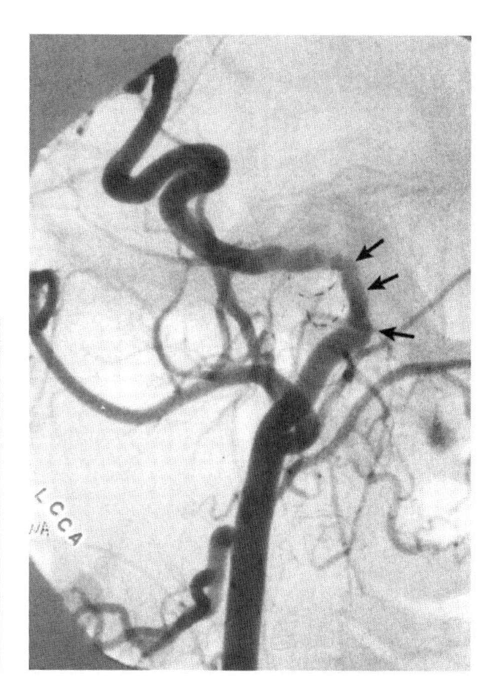

Figure 6.24.3.

Findings. An axial CT scan of the left temporal bone (Fig. 6.24.1) demonstrates a soft tissue mass on the cochlear promontory (*arrow*) contiguous with the carotid canal (*arrowheads*). Axial CT of the opposite temporal bone (Fig. 6.24.2) shows normal appearance of the carotid canal (*arrows*) with intact posterolateral bony wall (*curved arrow*). A lateral view from a left carotid arteriogram (Fig. 6.24.3) reveals an aberrant course of the petrous portion of the carotid artery that extends too far posteriorly (*arrows*).

Diagnosis. Aberrant internal carotid artery

Discussion. An aberrant internal carotid artery is an unusual anomaly that can present at any age. Symptoms are usually mild although pulsatile tinnitus can occur. On physical examination a pulsatile middle ear mass may be identified. This lesion can mimic a glomus tympanicum tumor clinically, and multiple cases have been reported of biopsy of this "mass," often with disastrous consequences (59). The CT appearance of this condition is diagnostic (60, 61). Catheter or MR angiography, although unnecessary in most cases, is confirmatory. The aberrant internal carotid artery is formed from anastomosis between the inferior tympanic artery and the caroticotympanic artery that occurs when the petrous segment of the internal carotid artery fails to develop normally (60). Every radiologist must know about this condition and inform the referring clinician when this diagnosis is made.

Aunt Minnie's Pearls

- *An aberrant internal carotid artery is an important cause of pulsatile tinnitus.*
- *Inform the referring clinician when this diagnosis is made, so a potentially disastrous biopsy can be avoided.*

CASE 25

History. 11-year-old boy with a swollen right eye

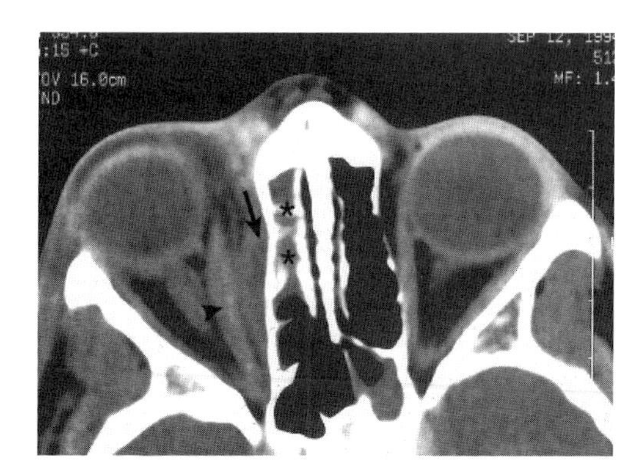

Figure 6.25.1.

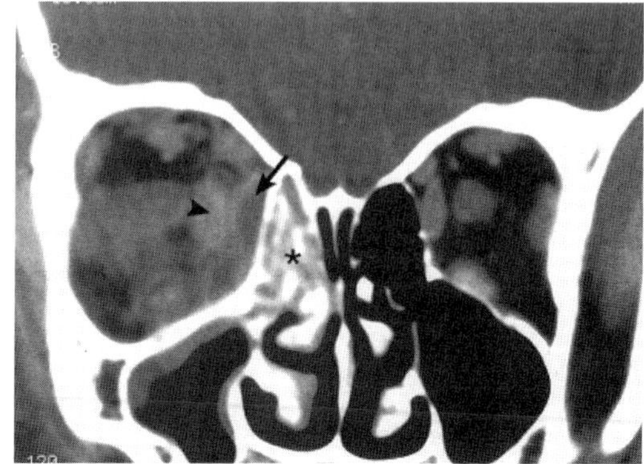

Figure 6.25.2.

Findings. Axial (Fig. 6.25.1) and coronal (Fig. 6.25.2) contrast-enhanced CT images through the midorbit demonstrate a low attenuation, peripherally enhancing extraconal fluid collection within the medial aspect of the right orbit (*arrow*). There is lateral displacement of an enlarged medial rectus muscle on this side (*arrowhead*) as well as opacification of the right ethmoid sinus (*asterisks*).

Diagnosis. Subperiosteal orbital abscess associated with ethmoid sinusitis

Discussion. Infections and inflammatory conditions commonly involve the orbit and periorbital regions in children (62). Preseptal cellulitis involving the eyelid and surrounding facial soft tissues can be successfully treated with antibiotics. Postseptal orbital cellulitis is a significantly more serious condition that often necessitates surgical drainage (63). This case demonstrates a typical subperiosteal abscess located along the medial orbital wall. This condition is usually associated with sinusitis. CT scanning is indicated whenever orbital cellulitis is clinically suspected (64, 65). Without prompt treatment further complications can result, including development of intracranial abnormalities such as subdural empyema or cavernous sinus thrombosis.

Aunt Minnie's Pearls

- *A subperiosteal abscess occurs in the postseptal extraconal space of the orbit and is usually associated with acute bacterial sinusitis.*
- *Surgical drainage is usually indicated to prevent severe sequelae such as subdural empyema or cavernous sinus thrombosis.*

Case 26

History. Teenage boy with epistaxis after contact during a football game

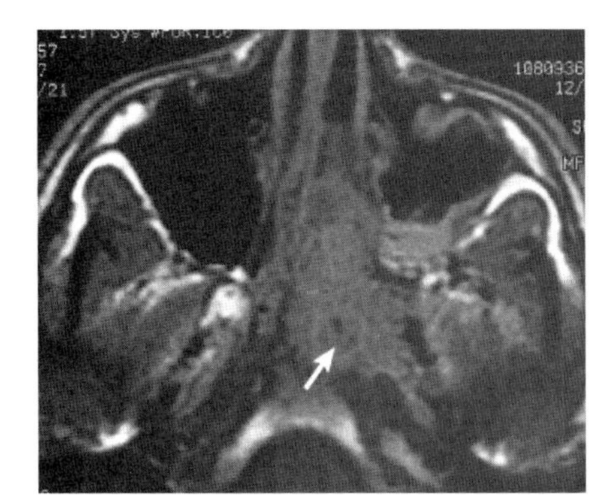

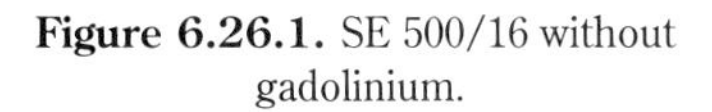

Figure 6.26.1. SE 500/16 without gadolinium.

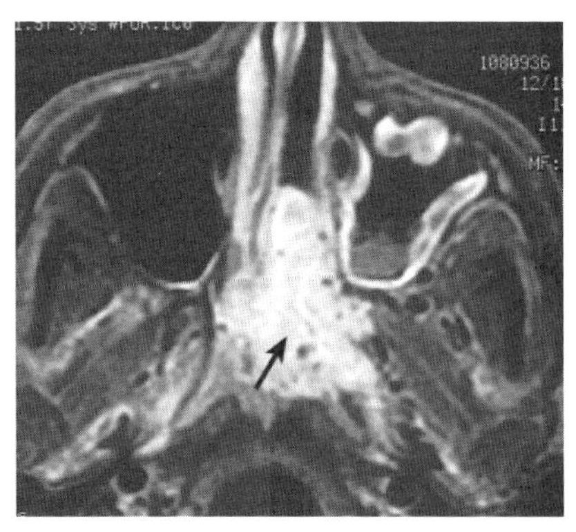

Figure 6.26.2. SE 600/15 without gadolinium.

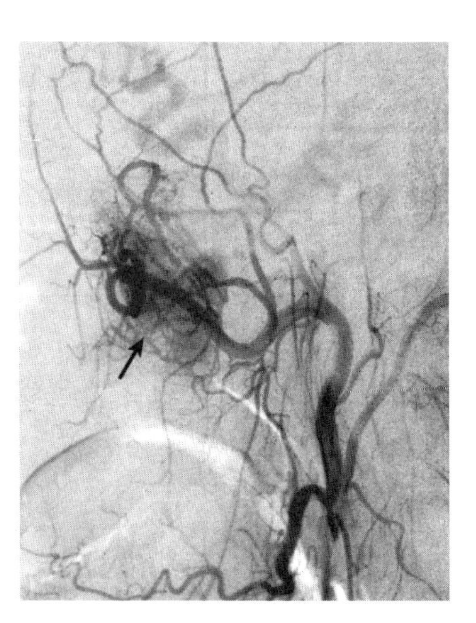

Figure 6.26.3.

Findings. Axial T1-weighted MR images before (Fig. 6.26.1) and after (Fig. 6.26.2) gadolinium administration demonstrate an enhancing soft tissue mass filling the nasopharynx and left posterior nasal cavity (*arrow*). The mass is isointense to muscle, demonstrates flow voids, and extends into the left pterygopalatine fossa. A lateral view from a left external carotid artery injection (Fig. 6.26.3) shows intense enhancement of this mass (*arrow*), which is fed primarily by branches of the internal maxillary artery.

Diagnosis. Juvenile angiofibroma

Discussion. Juvenile angiofibromas are benign vascular tumors that typically arise in the posterior nasal cavity (66). The classic history is that of a teenage boy with nasal stuffiness and a nosebleed. These tumors are quite vascular and demonstrate intense enhancement on CT, MRI, and at angiography. Prominent flow voids within juvenile angiofibromas often give them a "salt and pepper" appearance on MRI scans. Extension through the sphenopalatine foramen into the pterygopalatine fossa and occasionally through the pterygomaxillary fissure are classic spread patterns for this tumor (67, 68). Frequently there is associated bony remodeling with anterior displacement of the posterior wall of the maxillary sinus. Treatment is usually preoperative embolization to reduce blood loss followed by surgical resection.

Aunt Minnie's Pearls

- *Juvenile angiofibromas are benign vascular tumors that arise in the posterior nasal cavity and extend through the sphenopalatine foramen into the pterygopalatine fossa.*
- *These tumors are usually fed by branches of the internal maxillary artery.*

CASE 27

History. 5-year-old boy with bilateral hearing loss since birth

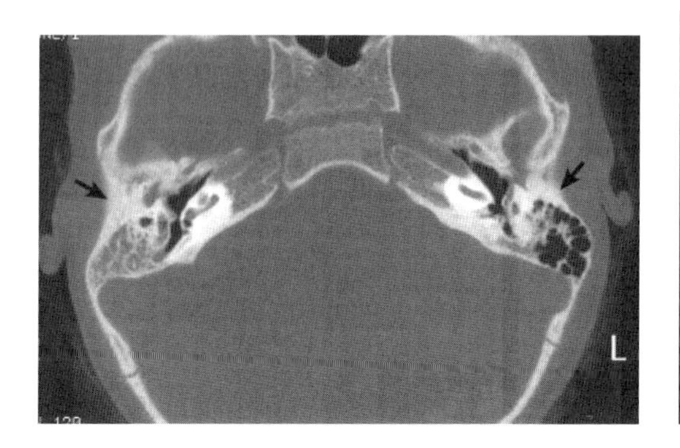

Figure 6.27.1.

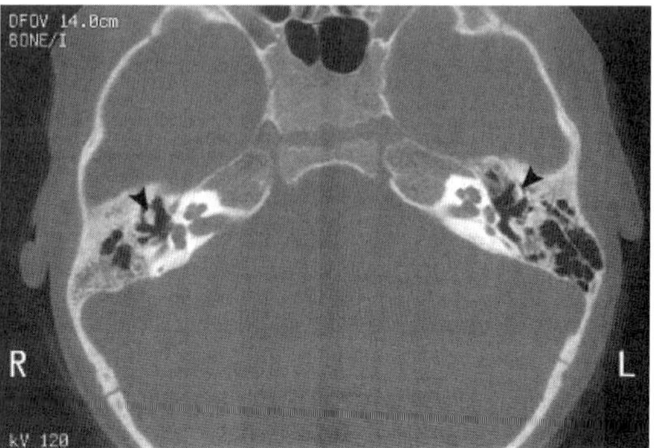

Figure 6.27.2.

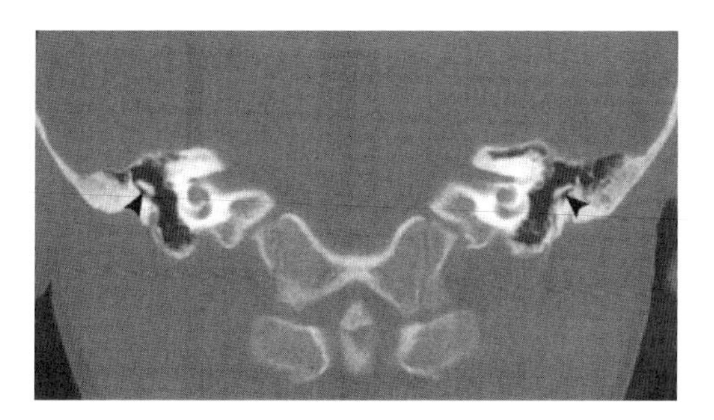

Figure 6.27.3.

Findings. Axial (Figs. 6.27.1 and 6.27.2) and coronal (Fig. 6.27.3) CT images through the temporal bones demonstrate lack of development of the external auditory canals bilaterally (*arrows*) with small middle ear cavities and an ossicular mass closely applied to the lateral walls of the epitympanic spaces (*arrowheads*). The inner ear structures are normal.

Diagnosis. Bilateral external auditory canal atresia

Discussion. External auditory canal atresia is one of the more common congenital anomalies affecting the temple bone (69). Patients with this condition typically have a malformed pinna and no visible external auditory canal. Atresia of the external auditory canal can be either bony or membranous, and occasionally there is stenosis or hypoplasia rather than a true atresia (70). The condition is bilateral in up to one-third of patients. External auditory canal atresia is associated with ossicular fusion abnormalities, most commonly fusion of the malleus and incus. The middle ear cavity is often small, and the facial nerve may have an anomalous course. The inner ear structures are usually normal. Bilateral external auditory canal atresia always requires surgery, usually at an early age (71). Unilateral atresia may not need to be surgically repaired until the teenage years if hearing in the opposite ear is normal.

Aunt Minnie's Pearls

- *Atresia or hypoplasia of the external auditory canal is associated with fusion anomalies of the ossicles and malformations of the pinna.*

Case 28

History. 50-year-old man with pulsatile right neck mass

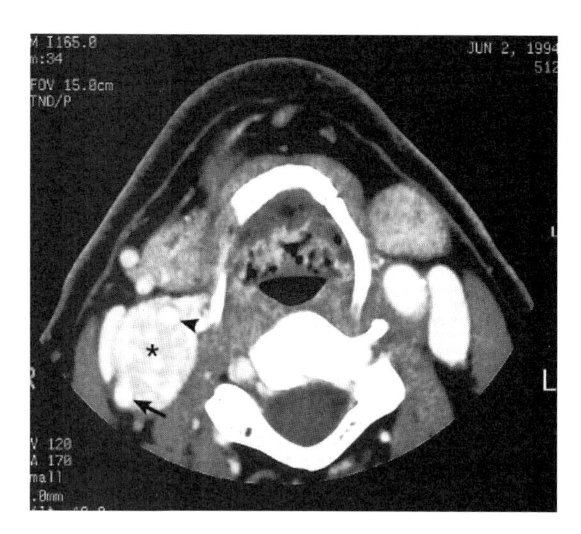

Figure 6.28.1.

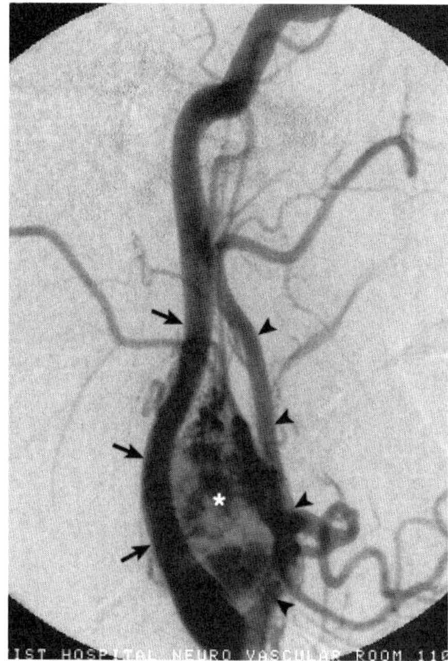

Figure 6.28.2.

Findings. An axial CT image (Fig. 6.28.1) demonstrates an intensely enhancing right carotid space mass (*asterisk*) that splays the internal (*arrow*) and external (*arrowhead*) carotid arteries. A lateral view of a right carotid arteriogram (Fig. 6.28.2) shows the intensely enhancing carotid bifurcation mass (*asterisk*) separating the internal (*arrows*) and external (*arrowheads*) carotid arteries.

Diagnosis. Carotid body paraganglioma

Discussion. Carotid body tumors are the most common extracranial head and neck paraganglioma. They arise from the carotid body, which is derived from neural crest tissue of the autonomic nervous system (72). Carotid body tumors typically splay the internal and external carotid arteries because they arise from tissue located at the carotid artery bifurcation. These tumors dramatically enhance on CT or MRI scans and demonstrate a persistent and intense vascular blush at arteriography (73, 74). The combination of intense enhancement and flow voids on MRI has often been described as "salt and pepper" appearance. Carotid body tumors are typically nonfunctional and are treated surgically, often after preoperative embolization. These tumors may be familial or multicentric and are malignant in 10% of cases. One unusual fact is that they are much more common in people living at high altitudes than at sea level (72).

Aunt Minnie's Pearls

- *Carotid body tumors occur in the carotid space and splay the internal and external carotid arteries.*
- *These tumors enhance intensely and cause a "salt and pepper" appearance on MRI.*

CASE 29

History. 15-year-old girl with a history of right maxillary sinusitis and right nasal obstruction

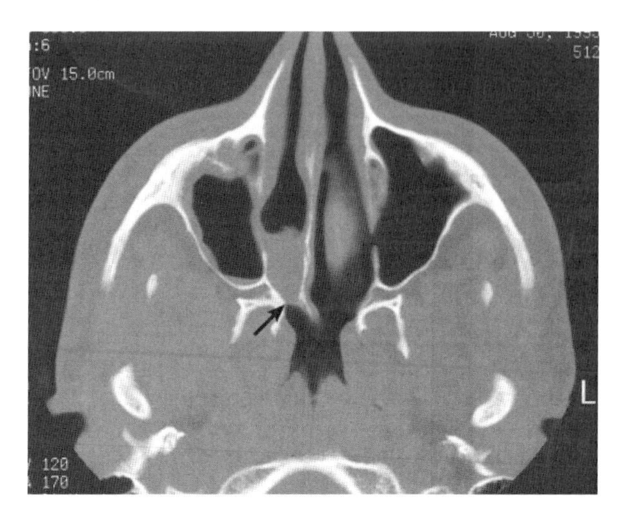

Figure 6.29.1.

Findings. An axial CT image through the lower nasal cavity (Fig. 6.29.1) demonstrates an air-fluid level within the right nasal cavity, which is occluded posteriorly by a thin, bony plate (*arrow*). Also present is mucoperiosteal thickening within the right maxillary sinus.

Diagnosis. Unilateral choanal atresia

Discussion. Choanal atresia is an unusual congenital anomaly in which there is obstruction of the posterior nasal cavity. There may be complete obstruction by either a bony (85%) or membranous (15%) plate or a partial obstruction from a posterior nasal cavity stenosis (75). Because infants are obligate nose breathers, babies with bilateral atresia will present shortly after birth with respiratory distress. Unilateral lesions often present later in childhood or even early adulthood; 50% of the cases are isolated, and the remaining are associated with other congenital anomalies (76). CT is the radiographic modality of choice in evaluating these patients. Axial images should be angled +15 degrees to the hard palate for optimal visualization of this anomaly (77). The treatment is surgical.

Aunt Minnie's Pearls

- *Bony or membranous obstruction of the posterior nasal cavity = choanal atresia.*
- *Babies with bilateral atresia will present with respiratory distress at birth.*

Case 30

History. 35-year-old woman with right true vocal cord paralysis after remote thyroid surgery, now with a left false vocal cord and neck "mass"

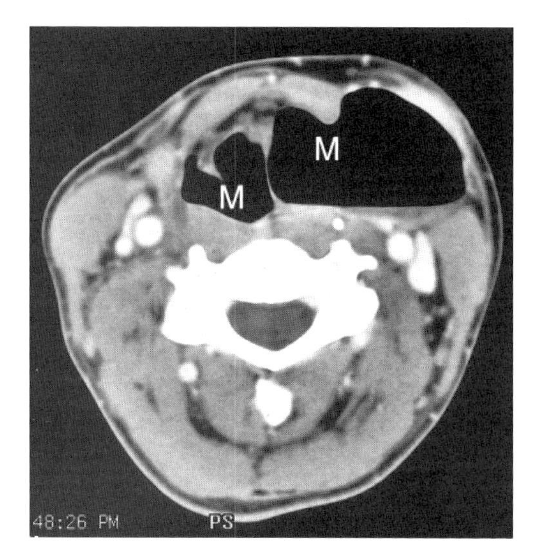

Figure 6.30.1.

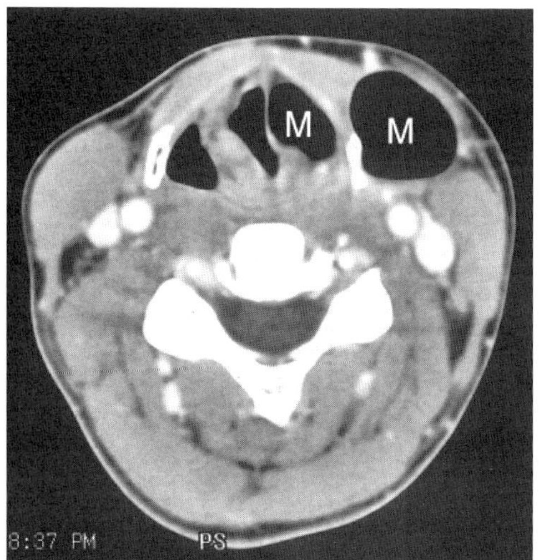

Figure 6.30.2.

Findings. Axial CT images through the larynx (Figs. 6.30.1 and 6.30.2) demonstrate a predominantly air-filled mass (M) within the left anterior cervical space and supraglottic larynx. The mass extends through the thyrohyoid membrane into the left periglottic space at the level of the false cord.

Diagnosis. Mixed laryngocele

Discussion. Laryngoceles are abnormal dilatations of the laryngeal ventricle or its more distal saccule (often referred to as the appendix of the ventricle) (78, 79). Most laryngoceles are acquired and develop when the laryngeal ventricle is obstructed either functionally or structurally. Functional obstructions develop from conditions associated with increased intraglottic pressure such as excessive coughing, playing a wind instrument, or glass blowing. Ventricular obstruction can also be from neoplasms or inflammatory masses that obstruct the opening of the laryngeal ventricle (80). Symptoms depend on location of the laryngocele. Internal or simple laryngoceles are confined to the paraglottic space of the supraglottic larynx (usually medial to the thyroid cartilage), whereas mixed or external laryngoceles begin as internal laryngoceles but enlarge and extend through the thyrohyoid membrane into the anterior cervical or submandibular spaces of the neck. Laryngoceles are located superficial to the strap muscles, whereas thyroglossal duct cysts are usually embedded within them. Surgery is required for large or symptomatic laryngoceles. Adults who develop laryngoceles should be closely evaluated to make sure that an obstructing cancer is not in the region of the laryngeal ventricle (80). Interestingly, this anomaly is a common finding in gorillas.

Aunt Minnie's Pearls

- *Laryngoceles originate at the laryngeal ventricle.*
- *Be sure that a mass is not the etiologic agent of the obstruction that leads to laryngocele formation.*

CASE 31

History. Asymptomatic 3-year-old boy

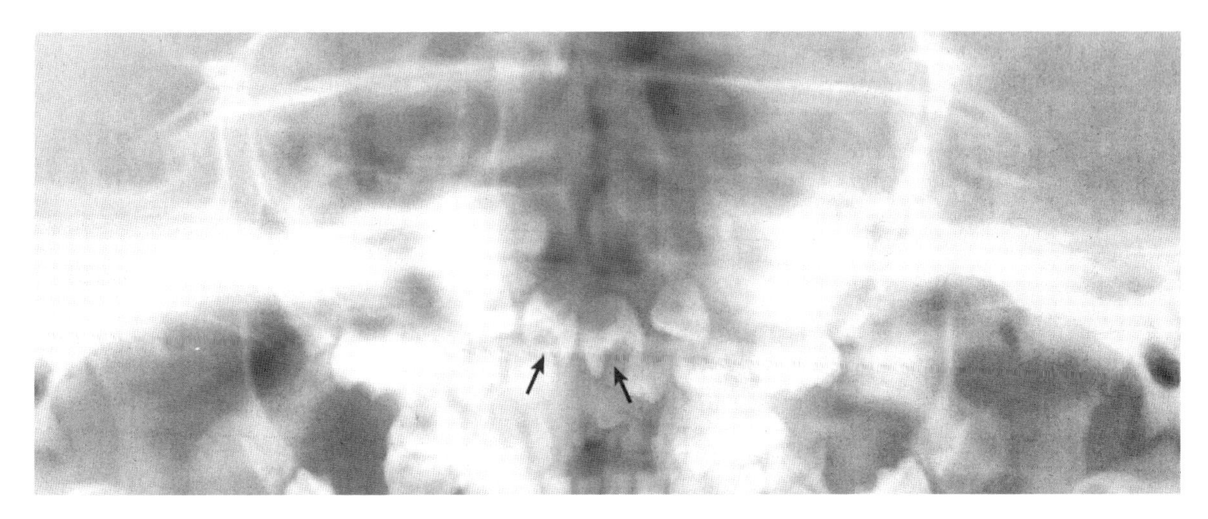

Figure 6.31.1.

Findings. A panoramic dental radiograph (Fig. 6.31.1) demonstrates notching of the unerupted maxillary central incisors (*arrows*).

Diagnosis. Congenital syphilis

Discussion. Congenital syphilis can result in Hutchinson's triad: interstitial keratitis, deafness, and abnormal teeth (81). The cusps of the permanent molars are dysplastic and resemble the surface of a mulberry. The permanent central incisors are notched. This characteristic notching is termed Hutchinson's teeth and is virtually pathognomonic of congenital syphilis. The primary teeth are rarely affected. The maxillary central incisors do not erupt until age 6. The diagnosis of congenital syphilis can be established on the basis of the characteristic radiographic appearance of the unerupted teeth before the other stigmata appear.

Aunt Minnie's Pearls

- *Notched permanent central incisors indicate congenital syphilis.*

REFERENCES

1. Guner M, Shaw MDM, Turner JW, Steven JL. Computed tomography in the diagnosis of colloid cyst. Surg Neurol 1976;6:345–348.
2. Maeder PP, Holtås SL, Basibüyük LN, Salford LG, Tapper UAS, Brun A. Colloid cysts of the third ventricle: correlation of MR and CT findings with histology and chemical analysis. AJR 1990;155:135–141.
3. Wilms G, Marchal G, Van Hecke P, et al. Colloid cysts of the third ventricle: MR findings. J Comput Assist Tomogr 1990;14:527–531.
4. Adams RD, Victor M. Principles of neurology, 3rd ed. New York: McGraw-Hill, 1985:415.
5. Smirniotopoulos JG, Murphy FM. The phakomatoses. AJNR 1992;13:725–746.
6. Pont MS, Elster AD. Lesions of skin and brain: modern imaging of the neurocutaneous syndromes. AJR 1992;158:1193–1203.
7. Elster AD, Chen MYM. MR imaging of Sturge-Weber syndrome: role of gadopentetate dimeglumine and gradient-echo techniques. AJNR 1990;11:685–689.
8. Naidich TP, McLone DG, Mutleur S. A new understanding of dorsal dysraphism with lipoma (lipomyeloschisis): radiological evaluation and surgical correction. AJNR 1983;4:103–116.
9. Brophy JD, Sutton LN, Zimmerman RA, Bury E, Schut L. Magnetic resonance imaging of lipomyelomeningocele and tethered cord. Neurosurgery 1989;25:336–340.
10. Elster AD. Radiologic screening in the neurocutaneous syndromes: strategies and controversies. AJNR 1992;13:1078–1082.
11. Egelhoff JC, Bates DJ, Ross JS, Rothner AD, Cohen BH. Spinal MR findings in neurofibromatosis types 1 and 2. AJNR 1992;13:1071–1077.
12. Elster AD. Modern imaging of the pituitary. Radiology 1993;187:1–14.
13. Friedman L, Patel VH. Normal variation in MRI of the brain. Semin Ultrasound CT MR 1995;16:175–185.
14. Kelly WM, Kucharczyk W, Kucharczyk J, et al. Posterior pituitary ectopia: an MR feature of pituitary dwarfism. AJNR 1988;9:453–460.
15. Chiari H. Über Veränderungen des Kleinhirns infolge von Hydrocephalie des Grosshirns. Dtsch Med Wochenschr 1891;17:1172–1175.
16. Elster AD, Chen MYM. Chiari I malformations: clinical and radiologic reappraisal. Radiology 1992:183:347–353.
17. Joubert M, Eisenring J-J, Robb JP, Andermann F. Familial agenesis of the cerebellar vermis: a syndrome of episodic hyperpnea, abnormal eye movements, ataxia, and retardation. Neurology 1969;19:813–825.
18. Kendall B, Kingsley D, Lambert SR, Taylor D, Finn P. Joubert syndrome: a clinico-radiological study. Neuroradiology 1990;31:502–506.
19. Truwit CL, Barkovich AJ. Pathogenesis of intracranial lipoma: an MR study in 42 patients. AJNR 1990;11:665–674.
20. Tart RP, Quisling RG. Curvilinear and tubulonodular varieties of lipoma of the corpus callosum: an MR and CT study. J Comput Assist Tomogr 1991;15:805–810.
21. Dean B, Drayer BP, Beresini DC, Bird CR. MR imaging of pericallosal lipoma. AJNR 1988;9:929–931.
22. Osborn AG. Disorders of diverticulation and cleavage, sulcation and cellular migration. In: Osborn AG, Diagnostic neuroradiology. St. Louis: Mosby-Year Book, 1994:52–55.
23. Barkovich AJ, Gressens P, Evrard P. Formation, maturation, and disorders of brain neocortex. AJNR 1992;13:423–446.
24. Barkovich AJ, Kjos BO. Gray matter heterotopias: MR characteristics and correlation with developmental and neurologic manifestations. Radiology 1992:182:493–499.
25. Byrd SE, Osborn RE, Radkowski MA, McArdle CB, Prenger EC, Naidich TP. Disorders of midline structures: holoprosencephaly, absence of corpus callosum, and Chiari malformations. Semin Ultrasound CT MR 1988;9:201–215.
26. Demyer W. Holoprosencephaly. In: Vinken PI, Bruyn GW, eds: Handbook of clinical neurology. Amsterdam: Elsevier/North-Holland, 1977;30:431–478.
27. Raybaud C. Cystic malformations of the posterior fossa: abnormalities associated with the development of the roof of the fourth ventricle and adjacent meningeal structures. J Neuroradiol 1982;9:103–133.
28. Hart MN, Malamud N, Ellis WG. The Dandy-Walker syndrome: a clinicopathological study based on 28 cases. Neurology 1972;22:771–780.
29. Zimmerman RA, Bilaniuk LT. Computed tomographic staging of traumatic epidural bleeding. Radiology 1982;144:809–812.
30. Kim KS, Walczak TS. Computed tomography of deep cerebral venous thrombosis. J Comput Assist Tomogr 1986;10:386–390.
31. Brown JIM, Coyne TJ, Hurlbert RJ, Fehlings MG, Ter Brugge KG. Deep cerebral venous system thrombosis: case report. Neurosurgery 1993;33:911–913.
32. Naidich TP, Altman NR, Braffman BH, McLone DG, Zimmerman RA. Cephaloceles and related malformations. AJNR 1992;13:655–690.
33. Diebler C, Dulac O. Cephaloceles: clinical and neuroradiological appearance. Associated cerebral malformations. Neuroradiology 1983;25:199–216.
34. Curnes JT, Oakes WJ. Parietal cephaloceles: radiographic and magnetic resonance imaging evaluation. Pediatr Neurosci 1988;14:71–76.
35. Fearnley JM, Stevens JM, Rudge P. Superficial siderosis of the central nervous system. Brain 1995;118:1051–1066.
36. Koeppen AH, Dickson AC, Chu RC, Thach RE. The pathogenesis of superficial siderosis of the central nervous system. Ann Neurol 1993;34:646–653.
37. Willeit S, Aichner F, Felber S, et al. Superficial siderosis of the central nervous system: report of three cases and review of the literature. J Neurol Sci 1992;111:20–25.

38. Bracchi M, Savoiardo M, Triulzi F, et al. Superficial siderosis of the CNS: MR diagnosis and clinical findings. AJNR 1993;14:227–236.
39. Adam RU, Lee SH, Truex RC Jr. Computer tomography in primary craniosynostosis. J Comput Tomogr 1980;4:125–131.
40. Parisi M, Mehdizadeh HM, Hunter JC, Finch IJ. Evaluation of craniosynostosis with three-dimensional CT imaging. J Comput Assist Tomogr 1989;13:1006–1012.
41. Vannier MW, Pilgram TK, Marsh JL, et al. Craniosynostosis: diagnostic imaging with three-dimensional CT presentation. AJNR 1994;15:1861–1869.
42. Elster AD, Arthur DW. Intracranial hemangioblastomas: CT and MR findings. J Comput Assist Tomogr 1988;12:736–769
43. Burro BL and Fiandaca MS. Carotid cavernous sinus fistulas: anatomical considerations, diagnosis and management—part one. Contemp Neurosurg 1988;10:1–5.
44. Debrun GM, Lacour P, Fox AJ, et al. Traumatic carotid-cavernous fistulas: etiology, clinical presentation, diagnosis, treatments, results. Semin Interventional Radiol 1987;4:242–248.
45. Ahmadi J, Teal JS, Segall HD, et al. Computed tomography of carotid-cavernous fistula. AJNR 1983;4:131–136.
46. Elster AD, Chen MYM, Richardson DN, Yeatts PR. Dilated intercavernous sinuses: an MR sign of carotid-cavernous and carotid-dural fistulas. AJNR 1991;12:641–645.
47. Hilal SK, Marton D, Pollack E. Diastematomyelia in children: radiographic study of 34 cases. Radiology 1974;112:609–621.
48. Byrd SE, Darling CF, McLone DG. Developmental disorders of the pediatric spine. Radiol Clin North Am 1991;29:711–752.
49. Naidich TP, McLone DG. Congenital pathology of the spine and spinal cord. In: Taveris JM, Ferrucci JT, eds. Radiology: diagnosis-imaging-intervention. Philadelphia: Lippincott, 1993;103:1–28.
50. Barkovich AJ. Congenital anomalies of the spine. In Barkovich AJ. Pediatric neuroimaging, 2nd ed. New York: Raven, 1995:477–540.
51. Barkovich AJ, Raghavan N, Chuang S, Peck WW. The wedge-shaped cord terminus: a radiographic sign of caudal regression. AJNR 1989;10:1223–1231.
52. Nievelstein RAJ, Valk J, Smit ME, Vermeij-Keers C. MR of the caudal regression syndrome: embryologic implications. AJNR 1994;15:1021–1029.
53. Anson JA, Spetzler RF. Classification of spinal arteriovenous malformations and implications for treatment. Barrow Neurol Inst Q 1992;8:2–8.
54. Osborn AG. Nonneoplastic disorders of the spine and spinal cord. In: Osborn AG. Diagnostic neuroradiology. St. Louis: Mosby 1994:820–875.
55. Nichols DA, Rufenacht DA, Jack DR Jr., Forbes GA. Embolization of spinal dural arteriovenous fistula with polyvinyl alcohol particles: experience in 14 patients. AJNR 1992;13:933–940.
56. Pétras A, Sobel DF, Mani JR, Lucas PR. CT myelography in cervical nerve root avulsion. J Comput Assist Tomogr 1985;9:275–279.
57. Hashimoto T, Mitoma M, Hirabuki N, et al. Nerve root avulsion of birth palsy: comparison of myelography with CT myelography and somatosensory potential. Radiology 1991;178:841–845.
58. Miller SF, Glasier CM, Griebel ML, Boop FA. Brachial plexopathy in infants after traumatic delivery: evaluation with MR imaging. Radiology 1993;189:481–484.
59. Reilly JJ, Caparosa RJ, Latchaw RE, et al. Aberrant carotid artery injured at myringotomy: control of hemorrhage by a balloon catheter. JAMA 1983;249:1473–1475.
60. Lo WWM, Solti-Bohman LG, McElveen JT. Aberrant carotid artery: radiologic diagnosis with emphasis on high-resolution computed tomography. RadioGraphics 1985;5:985–993.
61. Swartz JD, Bazarnic ML, Naidich TP, et al. Aberrant internal carotid artery lying within the middle ear: high resolution CT diagnosis and differential diagnosis. Neuroradiology 1985;27:322–326.
62. Weber et al. Inflammatory disorders of the periorbital sinuses and their complications. Radiol Clin North Am 1987;25:615–630.
63. Williams BJ, Harrison HC. Subperiosteal abscesses of the orbit due to sinusitis in childhood. Aust N Z J Ophthalmol 1991;19:29–36.
64. Towbin R, Han BK, Kaufman RA, Burke M. Post-septal cellulitis: CT in diagnosis and management. Radiology 1986;158:735–737.
65. Handler LC, Davey IC, Hill JC, Lauryssen C. The acute orbit: differentiation of orbital cellulitis from subperiosteal abscess by computerized tomography. Neuroradiology 1991;33:15–18.
66. Hyams VJ, Batsakis JG, Michaels L. Angiofibroma. In: Hyams VJ, Batsakis JG, Michaels L, eds. Tumor of the upper respiratory tract and ear. Washington DC. Armed Forces Institute of Pathology 1988:130–134 (fascicle 27, 2nd series).
67. Bryan RN, Sessions RB, Horowitz BL. Radiographic management of juvenile angiofibroma. AJNR 1981;2:157–166.
68. Mehra YN, Mann SB, Dubey SP, et al. Computed tomography for determining pathways of extension and a staging and treatment system for juvenile angiofibromas. Ear Nose Throat J 1989;68:576–589.
69. Eelkema EA, Curtin HD. Congenital anomalies of the temporal bone. Semin Ultrasound CT MR 1989;10:195–212.
70. Swartz JD, Wolfson RJ, Marlow FI, et al. External auditory canal dysplasia: CT evaluation. Laryngoscope 1985;95:841–845.
71. Swartz JD, Faerber EN. Congenital malformations of the external and middle ear: high resolution CT findings of surgical import. AJR 1985;144:501–506.
72. Wenig BM. Neoplasms of the oral cavity, nasopharynx, tonsils and neck. In: Wenig BM. Atlas of head and neck pathology. Philadelphia: Saunders, 1993;9:143–199.
73. Vogl T, Brüning R, Schedel H et al. Paragangliomas of the jugular bulb and carotid body: MR imaging with short sequences and Gd-DTPA enhancement. AJR 1989;153:583–587.
74. Olsen WL, Dillon WP, Kelly W, et al. MR imaging of paragangliomas. AJR 1987;148:201–204.
75. Slovis PL, Renfrow B, Watts FB, et al. Choanal atresia: precise CT evaluation. Radiology 1985;155:345–348.
76. Tadmor R, Rivad M, Millet DM, Leventon G. Computed tomographic demonstration of choanal atresia. AJNR 1984;5:743–745.

77. Chinwuba C, Wallman J, Strand R. Nasal airway obstruction: CT assessment. Radiology 1986;159:503–506.
78. Glazer HS, Mauro MM, Aronberg DJ, et al. Computed tomography of laryngoceles. AJR 1983;140:549–552.
79. Hubbard C. Laryngocele—a study of five cases with reference to radiologic features. Clin Radiol 1987;38:639.
80. Celin SE, Johnson J, Curtin H, Barnes L. The association of laryngoceles with squamous cell carcinoma of the larynx. Laryngoscope 1991;101:529–536.
81. Cotran RS, Kumar V, Robbins SL. Robbins pathologic basis of disease, 5th ed. Philadelphia: Saunders, 1994:345–346.

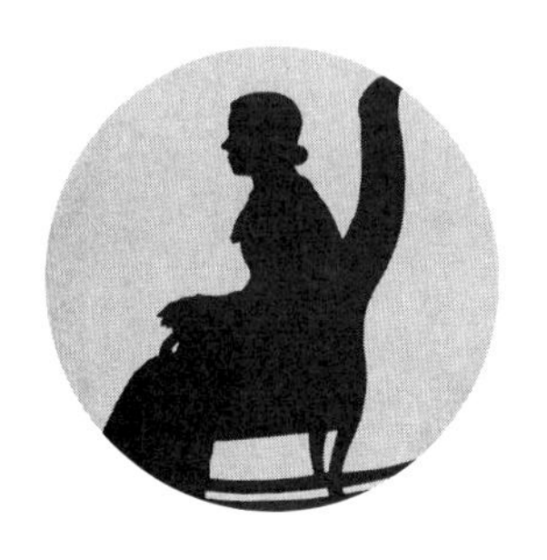

chapter 7

THORACIC RADIOLOGY

CAROLINE CHILES

CASE 1

History. 45-year-old woman with recurrent respiratory infections

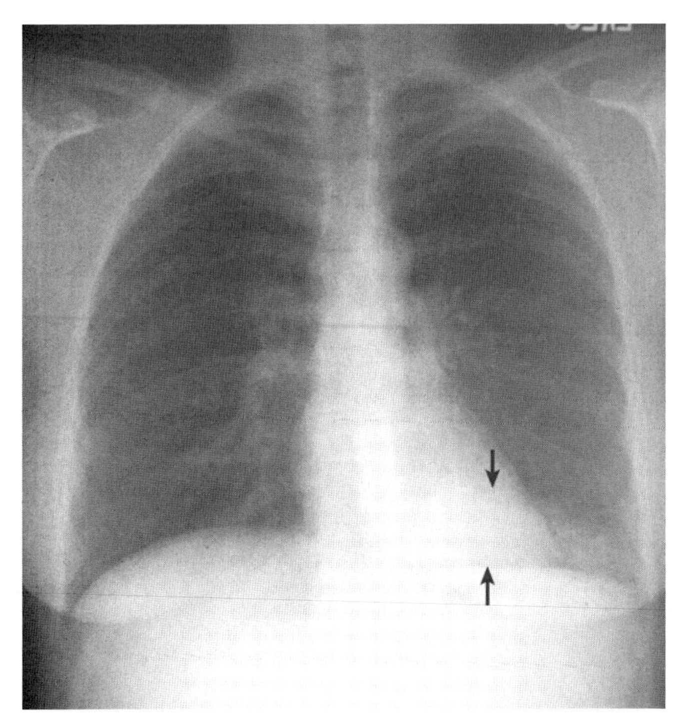

Figure 7.1.1.

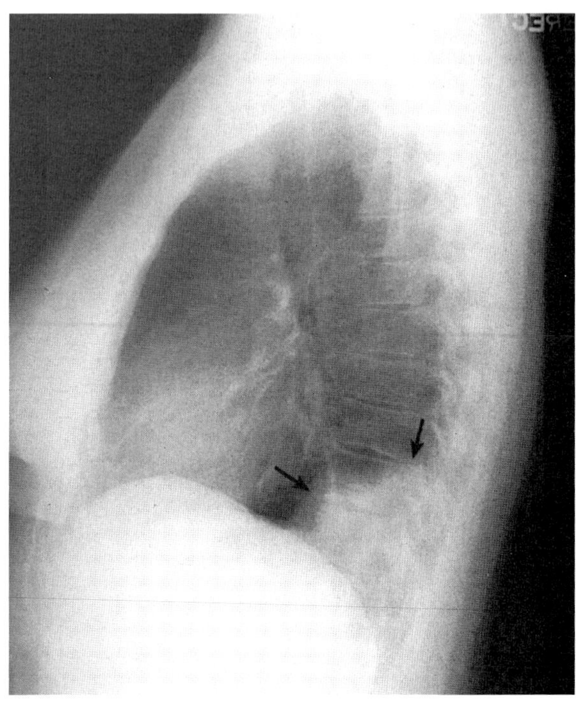

Figure 7.1.2.

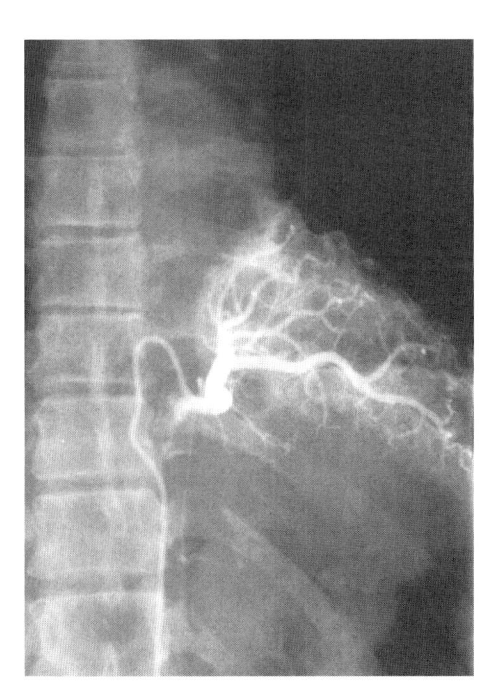

Figure 7.1.3.

Findings. A mass-like opacity is visible in the posterior basal segment of the left lower lobe (*arrows*) on the posteroanterior (Fig. 7.1.1) and lateral (Fig. 7.1.2) views of the chest. No air bronchograms are visible within the mass. A selective arteriogram (Fig. 7.1.3) shows systemic arterial supply to the mass from an anomalous vessel originating from the thoracic aorta.

Diagnosis. Bronchopulmonary sequestration (intralobar)

Discussion. Bronchopulmonary sequestration is a rare congenital anomaly in which a portion of lung is set apart from the remainder of the lung and receives systemic arterial supply. Sequestration has been divided into two categories, intralobar and extralobar. Characteristics of intralobar sequestration include systemic arterial supply and pulmonary venous drainage from a portion of lung with no connection to the tracheobronchial tree (1). It most commonly occurs in a paravertebral location in the posterior basal segments of the lower lobes; 60% occur on the left side. An extralobar sequestration is more truly sequestered from the remainder of the lung by its separate pleural covering. It is related to the left hemidiaphragm (above, below, or within) in 90% of cases. The systemic arterial supply often consists of multiple small aortic branches rather than the single large artery seen in intralobar sequestration. Drainage is usually via the systemic venous system, including the inferior vena cava, azygous or hemizygous veins, or portal veins (2, 3).

Infection of an intralobar sequestration can result in communication with the bronchial tree so that the solid mass is converted to an air-containing cystic mass, with or without air-fluid levels (4). This is less likely to occur in an extralobar sequestration because of its separate pleural investment.

Aunt Minnie's Pearls

- *Intralobar bronchopulmonary sequestration has systemic arterial supply and pulmonary venous drainage and may become infected.*
- *Extralobar bronchopulmonary sequestration has a pleural covering, systemic arterial supply, and systemic venous drainage; usually in left lower lobe.*

CASE 2

History. Withheld

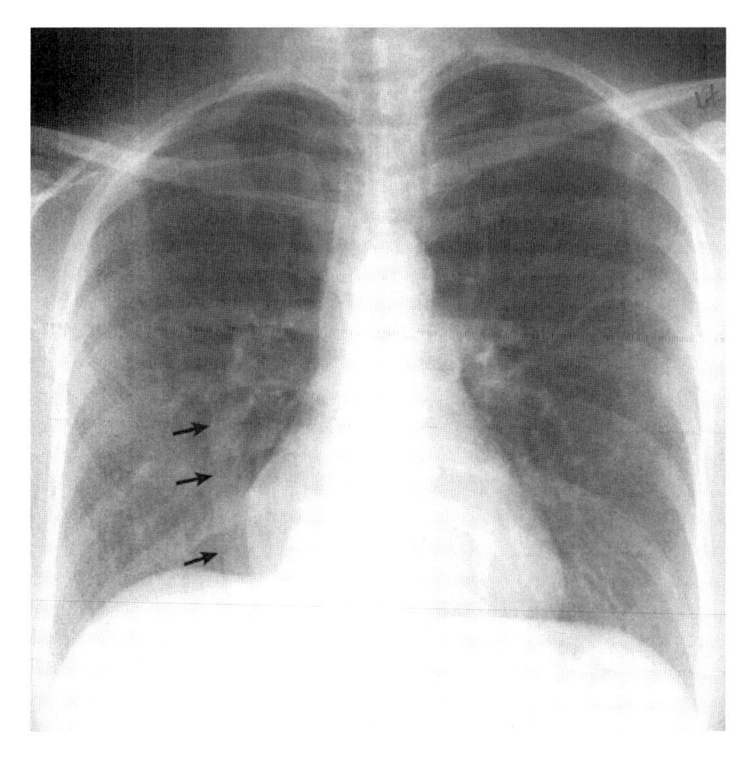

Figure 7.2.1.

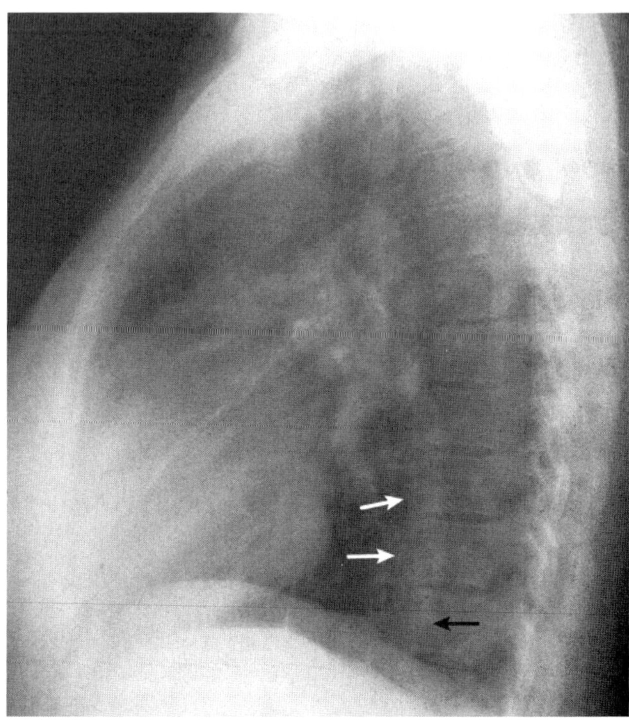

Figure 7.2.2.

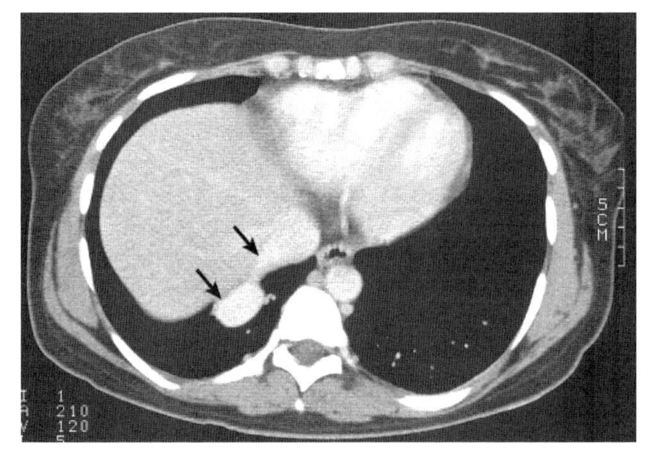

Figure 7.2.3.

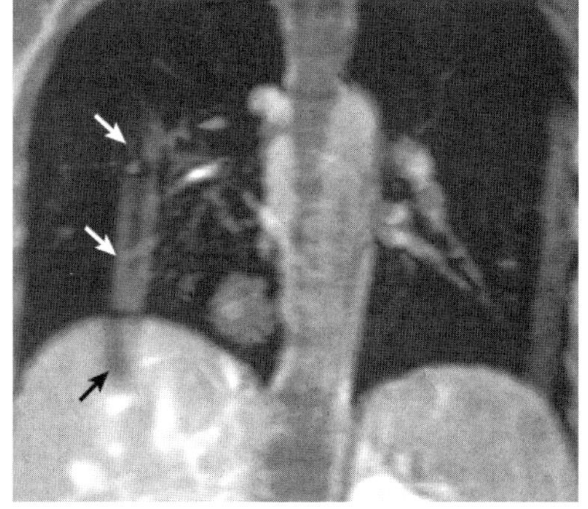

Figure 7.2.4. FLASH 2D 150/4.

Findings. Posteroanterior and lateral views of the chest (Figs. 7.2.1 and 7.2.2) show that the right lung and right hemithorax are smaller than the left lung and left hemithorax. Adjacent to the heart, a large blood vessel is seen draining toward the right hemidiaphragm (*arrows*). A contrast enhanced axial CT through the lower chest (Fig. 7.2.3) confirms the large vessel and reveals its connection to the inferior vena cava (*arrows*). Finally, a coronal MR image (Fig. 7.2.4) also demonstrates the large anomalous vessel coursing from the right hilar region to below the hemidiaphragm (*arrows*).

Diagnosis. Congenital venolobar syndrome

Discussion. The congenital venolobar syndrome, or scimitar syndrome, is a form of partial anomalous pulmonary venous return. The syndrome includes an anomalous pulmonary vein draining the right lower lobe, or sometimes the entire right lung, to the inferior vena cava (5, 6). The right lung is usually hypoplastic so that the heart and mediastinum are shifted into the right hemithorax (cardiac dextroposition). The right lung may have morphological features like those of the left lung, including a hyparterial bronchus and absence of the minor fissure. The right pulmonary artery is usually small; there may be systemic arterial supply to the right lung as well, arising from the abdominal aorta or descending thoracic aorta. About 25% of patients will also have a congenital heart defect, most commonly an atrial septal defect.

Aunt Minnie's Pearls

- *Congenital venolobar syndrome = hypoplastic right lung and right pulmonary artery, partial anomalous pulmonary venous return into inferior vena cava, cardiac dextroposition, and bilateral "left-sided" lungs.*

CASE 3

History. 50-year-old woman with recurrent respiratory infections

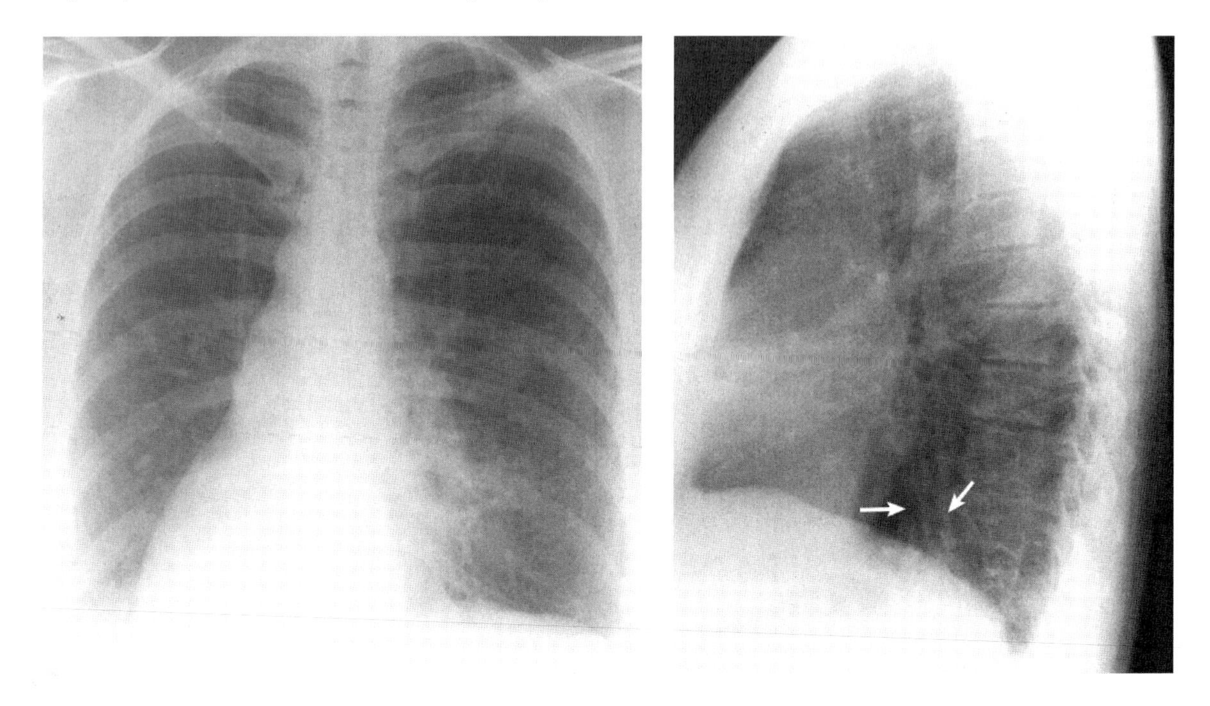

Figure 7.3.1.

Figure 7.3.2.

Figure 7.3.3.

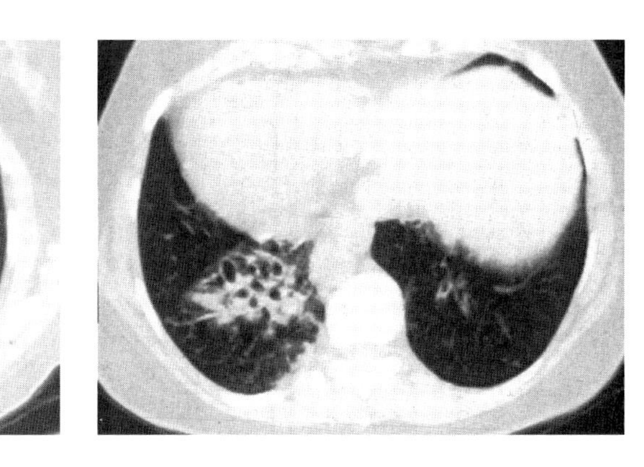

Figure 7.3.4.

Findings. Posteroanterior (Fig. 7.3.1) and lateral (Fig. 7.3.2) views of the chest show situs inversus and coarse tubular opacities at both lung bases (*arrows*). The CT study confirms varicose and cystic bronchiectasis within the left middle (Fig. 7.3.3) and right lower lobes (Fig. 7.3.4).

Diagnosis. Kartagener's syndrome

Discussion. Kartagener's syndrome describes a triad of bronchiectasis, sinusitis, and situs inversus (7). The bronchiectasis is attributed to dyskinetic, or immotile, cilia. Of patients with immotile cilia syndrome, 50% will have situs inversus and the diagnosis of Kartagener's syndrome. Of patients with situs inversus, 15% will have complete Kartagener's syndrome.

Aunt Minnie's Pearls

- *Kartagener's syndrome = situs inversus, bronchiectasis, and sinusitis.*

CASE 4

History. Withheld

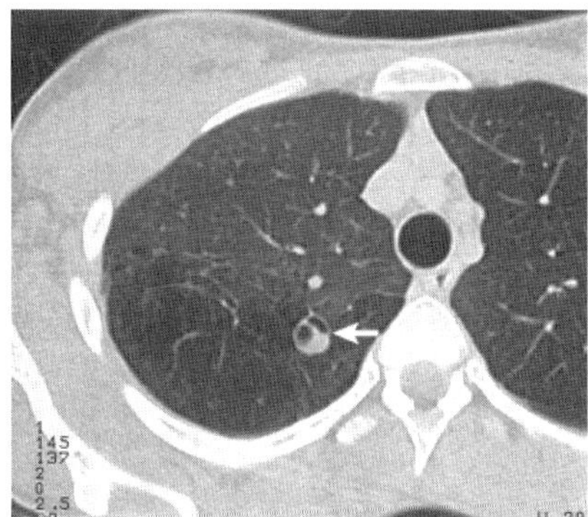

Figure 7.4.2.

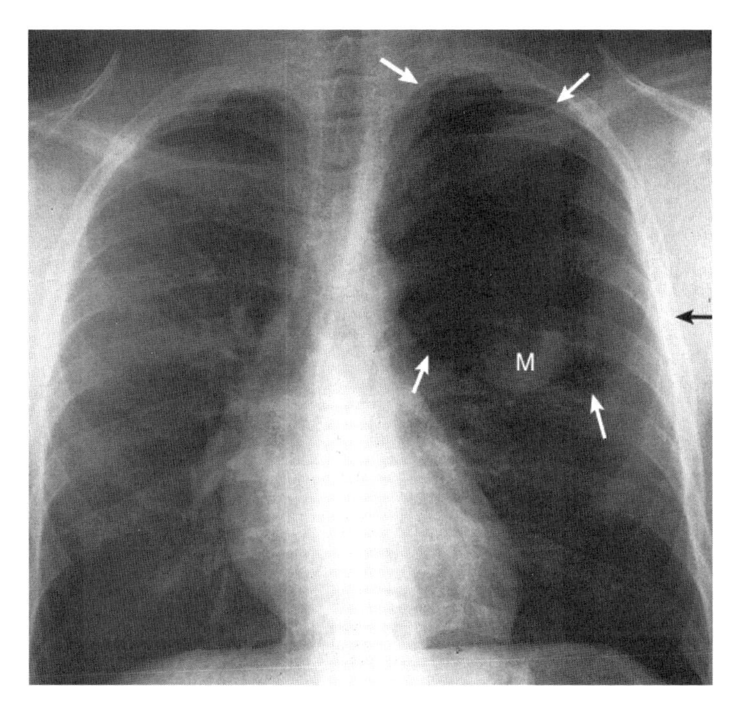

Figure 7.4.1.

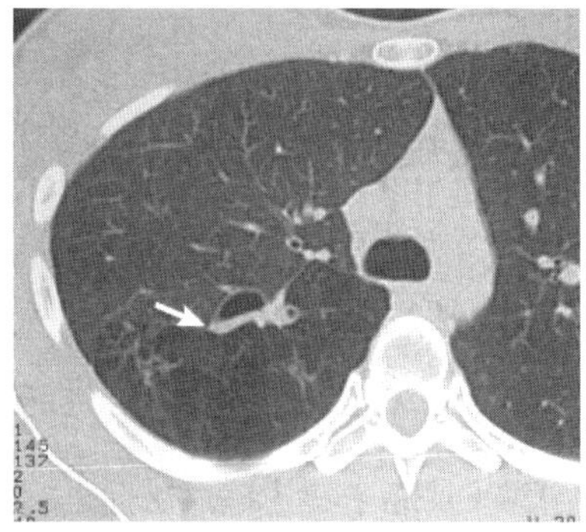

Figure 7.4.3.

Findings. Left upper lobe is hyperlucent and hyperexpanded on posteroanterior view of the chest (Fig. 7.4.1, *arrows*). A lobular mass lies adjacent to the left hilum (M). High resolution CT images in a different patient (Figs. 7.4.2 and 7.4.3) again reveal the presence of a dilated bronchus that contains a plug of soft tissue floating within it (*arrows*). The lung peripheral to the abnormal bronchus is emphysematous. The lungs elsewhere were normal.

Diagnosis. Bronchial atresia with mucoid impaction

Discussion. Bronchial atresia is an uncommon congenital anomaly that is usually detected as an incidental finding in adults (8). Some cases may actually be acquired as a result of trauma or inflammation postnatally (9). The apicoposterior segment of the left upper lobe is most commonly affected. The lung develops normally in a position distal to the atretic bronchus and is ventilated by collateral air drift (10). Airways distal to the atretic segmental bronchus continue to produce mucus, which leads to mucoid impaction or mucocele formation within the bronchus. The affected lobe appears hyperaerated and is both oligemic and hyperlucent (11).

Aunt Minnie's Pearls

- *Bronchial atresia = mucoid impaction distal to atretic bronchus and hyperexpanded lobe; usually apicoposterior segment of left upper lobe.*

CASE 5

History. Routine chest radiograph in an asymptomatic 37-year-old woman

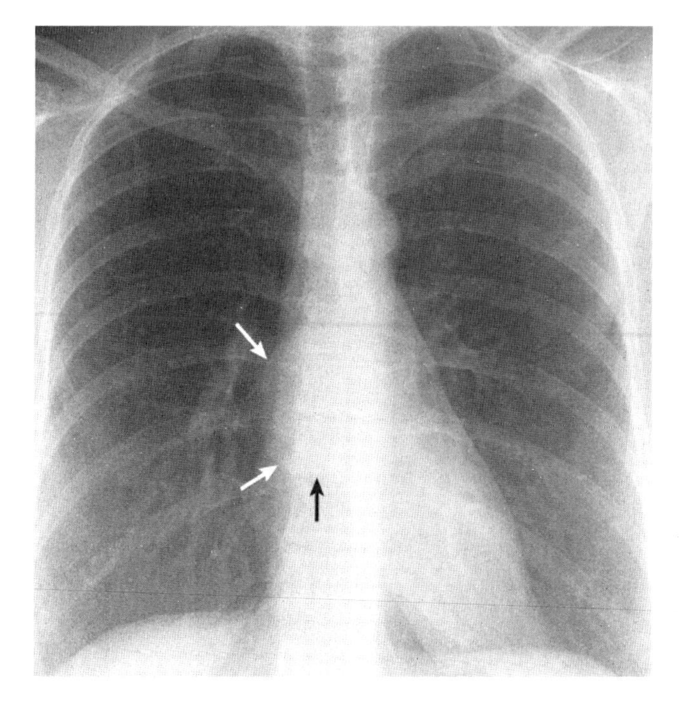

Figure 7.5.1.

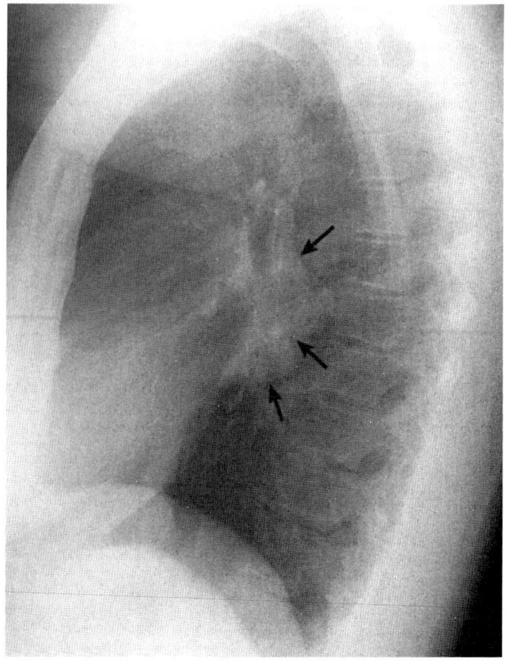

Figure 7.5.2.

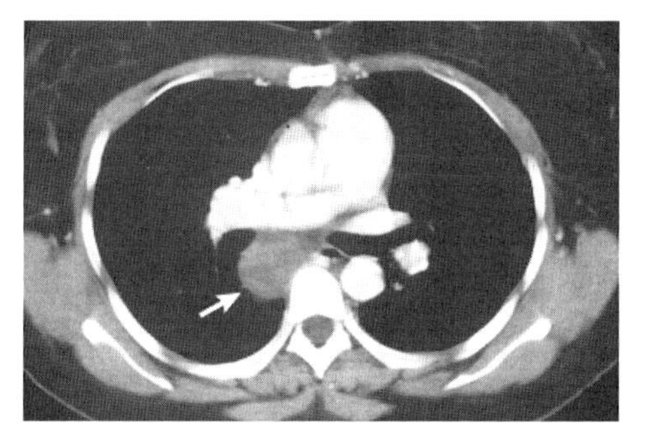

Figure 7.5.3.

Findings. Posteroanterior and lateral views of the chest (Figs. 7.5.1 and 7.5.2) show a 4-cm, sharply marginated subcarinal mass (*arrows*). Contrast enhanced CT scan reveals that the mass (Fig. 7.5.3, *arrow*) is of homogeneous fluid attenuation.

Diagnosis. Mediastinal bronchogenic cyst

Discussion. A bronchogenic cyst is a mass of nonfunctioning pulmonary tissue that has cartilage in its wall, is lined by columnar epithelium, and is filled with either clear serous or thick mucoid material. Although most bronchogenic cysts are often asymptomatic and incidentally discovered on routine chest radiographs, intrapulmonary bronchogenic cysts may become infected, resulting in a cough or fever. Large bronchogenic cysts within the mediastinum can create symptoms related to compression of the trachea and esophagus, including dyspnea and dysphagia. Most series report a greater percentage of mediastinal bronchogenic cysts, although intrapulmonary bronchogenic cysts predominated in some series (12–14). Mediastinal bronchogenic cysts are usually round or ovoid masses near the carina. Intrapulmonary bronchogenic cysts have a predilection for the lower lobes. In an infected intrapulmonary bronchogenic cyst, a fistulous communication with the tracheobronchial tree may develop; the cyst may then contain an air-fluid level or may appear cavitary.

On CT images, bronchogenic cysts typically appear as homogeneous water-attenuation masses. When the fluid contains calcium oxalate, proteinaceous material, or hemorrhage, the contents of the cysts may have higher attenuation and may mimic soft tissue masses (15–17). On T1-weighted MR images, the bronchogenic cyst may have low signal intensity, or it may have high signal intensity if the contents of the cysts are proteinaceous. On T2-weighted images, the cyst has homogeneously high attenuation.

Bronchogenic cysts are often treated by surgical excision to relieve or avoid symptoms of compression or infection. An alternative to surgery is needle aspiration of the mediastinal cyst (18).

Aunt Minnie's Pearls

- *Bronchogenic cysts are most often subcarinal and may be water attenuation or higher on CT.*

CASE 6

History. 17-year-old girl with a history of recurrent pneumonia in childhood

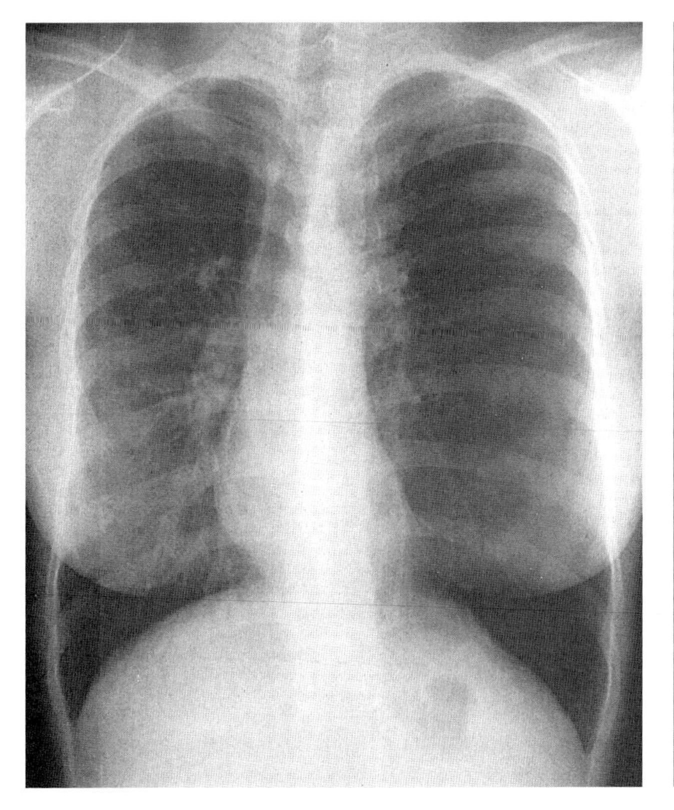

Figure 7.6.1.

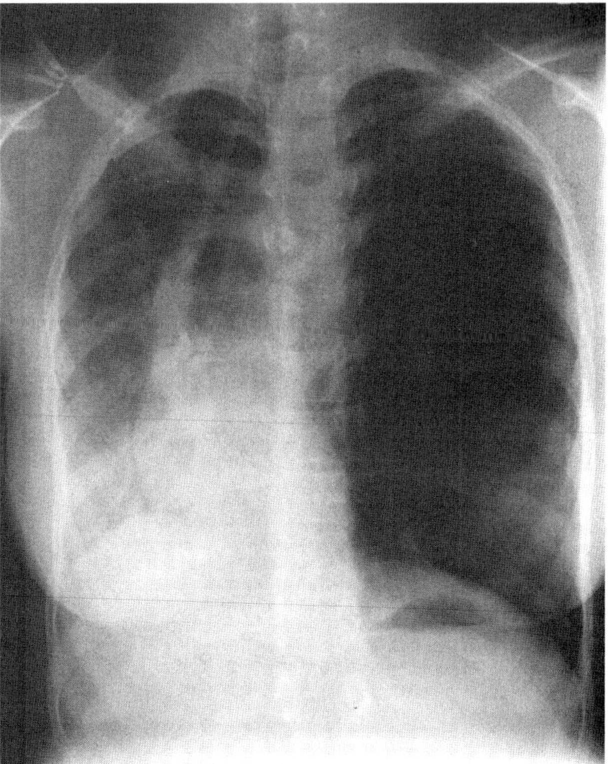

Figure 7.6.2.

Findings. Inspiratory and expiratory views of the chest (Figs. 7.6.1 and 7.6.2) show a hyperlucent left lung, with shift of the mediastinum away from the hyperlucent lung on expiration.

Diagnosis. Swyer-James syndrome

Discussion. Swyer-James, or Macleod's, syndrome is an uncommon form of bronchiolitis obliterans resulting from adenovirus pulmonary infection in childhood (19). The diagnosis is usually based on radiologic and clinical findings, including unilateral hyperlucency with evidence of air trapping on expiration. The hyperlucent lung may be either smaller than the contralateral lung or abnormally large (20). The presence of air trapping on expiration helps exclude other causes of a hyperlucent lung, e.g., pulmonary hypoplasia. However, other causes of air trapping, including obstructive tumor or foreign body, must be excluded.

Aunt Minnie's Pearls

- *Swyer-James syndrome is thought to be due to bronchiolitis obliterans resulting from adenovirus infection.*
- *Unilateral hyperlucent lung with air trapping is seen on chest films.*

CASE 7

History. 75-year-old woman with respiratory distress

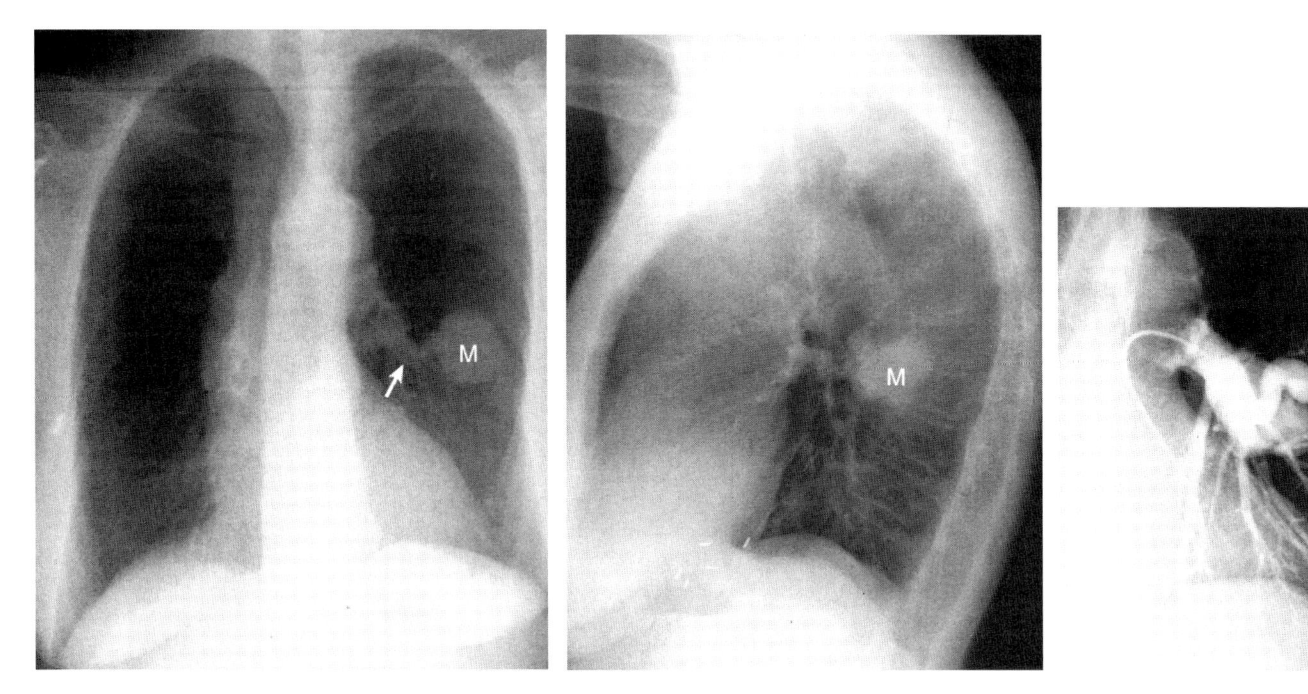

Figure 7.7.1. **Figure 7.7.2.** **Figure 7.7.3.**

Findings. A rounded, lobular mass (M) is present within the superior segment of the left lower lobe on the posteroanterior and lateral chest radiographs (Figs. 7.7.1 and 7.7.2). The mass appears to be connected to the hilum by a tubular vessel (*arrow*). Selective injection of the left pulmonary artery (Fig. 7.7.3) shows a dilated, tortuous vessel supplying the vascular mass.

Diagnosis. Pulmonary arteriovenous malformation

Discussion. A pulmonary arteriovenous malformation (PAVM) is a congenital lesion resulting from persistent fetal capillaries. A dilated vascular sac is supplied by a distended pulmonary artery and drained by a distended pulmonary vein. White et al. (21) divide PAVMs into two types. Simple PAVM is a single pulmonary artery to pulmonary vein communication, which is usually aneurysmal and nonseptate. Complex PAVM has multiple feeding arteries and draining veins, usually with a septate aneurysmal communication between arteries and veins (21). The distinction between simple and complex PAVM is of significance when embolotherapy is contemplated. The angioarchitecture of PAVMs may be confirmed by angiography or, more recently, by three-dimensional helical CT (22).

Approximately 30–50% of patients with PAVM have hereditary hemorrhagic telangiectasia, also known as Osler-Weber-Rendu syndrome (23). The association is even higher when multiple PAVMs are present. Patients with hereditary hemorrhagic telangiectasia have arteriovenous malformations elsewhere, including the skin, mucous membranes, and other organs and may present with epistaxis or hematuria. Because the normal pulmonary capillary bed is bypassed, untreated arteriovenous malformations may cause dyspnea and cyanosis as a result of the pulmonary to systemic shunt and cerebrovascular ischemia and infarction, as well as brain abscess, as a result of the passing of emboli and bacteria directly into the systemic circulation (23, 24).

Aunt Minnie's Pearls

- *30–50% of patients with a PAVM have hereditary hemorrhagic telangiectasia.*
- *The simple form has single artery and vein.*
- *The complex form has multiple feeding arteries and veins.*

CASE 8

History. 61-year-old woman with cough and dyspnea

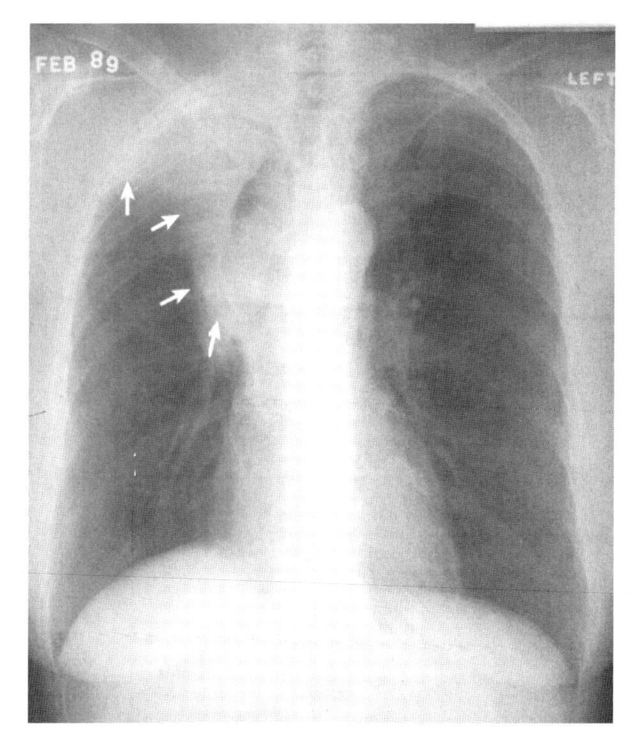

Figure 7.8.1.

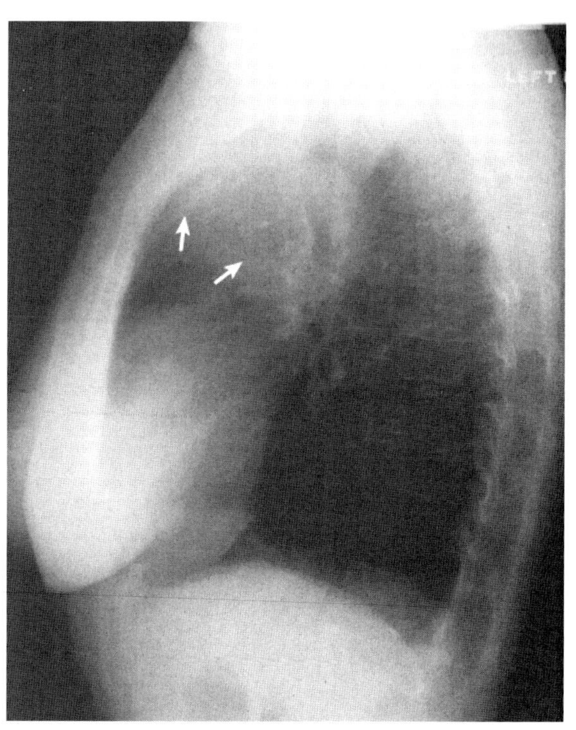

Figure 7.8.2.

Findings. On the frontal chest radiograph (Fig. 7.8.1), there is superior retraction of the right hilum and minor fissure, which assumes a reverse-S configuration (*arrows*). The right hemidiaphragm is elevated; the trachea is shifted to the right. On the lateral view (Fig. 7.8.2), the sharp margin of the lateral aspect of the minor fissure is visible at the lung apex (*arrows*), and there is increased opacity anterior to the trachea.

Diagnosis. Right upper lobe collapse caused by bronchogenic carcinoma—"S sign of Golden"

Discussion. In 1925, Golden (25) described the orientation of the minor fissure in patients with upper lobe collapse caused by a central mass (25). The medial aspect of the minor fissure outlines the inferior margin of the mass; the lateral aspect of the minor fissure moves superiorly as the right upper lobe collapses, producing a reverse-S appearance. Additional signs of volume loss in the right upper lobe include rightward shift of the trachea and mediastinum, elevation of the right hemidiaphragm, a juxtaphrenic peak, splaying of pulmonary vessels in the hyperexpanded right middle and lower lobes, and crowding of the ribs (26–28). In this patient, the hyperexpanded superior segment of the right lower lobe produces radiolucency in the right paratracheal region.

Lobar collapse in an adult should always prompt consideration of an endobronchial lesion, e.g., bronchogenic carcinoma or carcinoid. Collapse may also occur as a result of extrinsic compression of the bronchus by enlarged lymph nodes. The S sign of Golden suggests collapse because of a central mass, which may be either endobronchial or extrinsic to the bronchus, compressing the bronchus. Lobar collapse extending to the hilum in a patient with bronchogenic carcinoma is considered T2 disease (TNM staging).

Aunt Minnie's Pearls

- *The S sign of Golden indicates right upper lobe collapse caused by central neoplasm and implies T2 disease.*

CASE 9

History. 57-year-old woman with a history of breast carcinoma

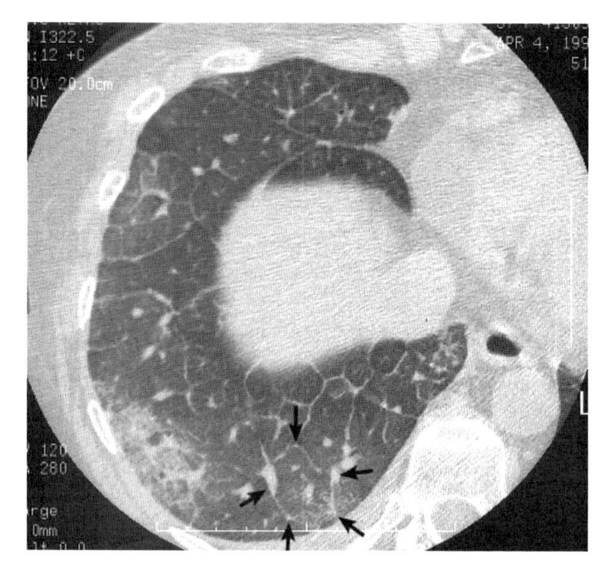

Figure 7.9.1.

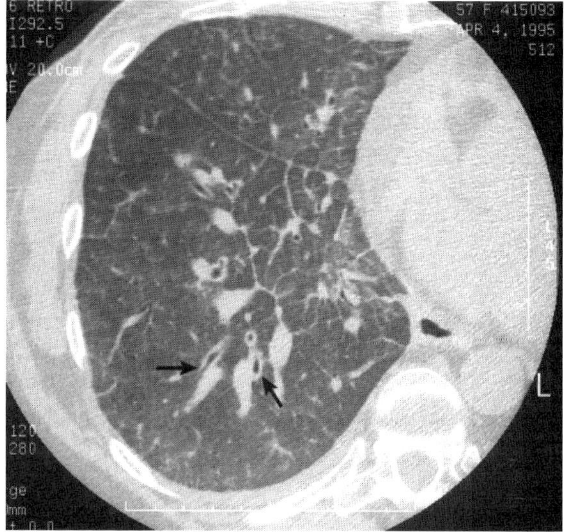

Figure 7.9.2.

Findings. Axial high resolution CT images of right lung (1-mm collimation, high spatial frequency algorithm, targeted image) show thickening of the interlobular septa throughout the right lung. Polygonal structures represent secondary pulmonary lobules outlined by thickened septa (Fig. 7.9.1, *arrows*). The bronchovascular bundles seen tangentially and in cross-section are thickened (Fig. 7.9.2, *arrows*).

Diagnosis. Lymphangitic carcinomatosis

Discussion. Lymphangitic spread of tumor in the lung is often due to adenocarcinoma; stomach, lung, and breast are the typical sites of the primary tumor (29). Infiltration of tumor cells into lymphatic vessels produces thickening of the interlobular septa and peribronchovascular interstitium (30). Pulmonary sarcoidosis may closely mimic this radiographic appearance, but the patient's clinical presentation and past medical history should allow the radiologist to differentiate sarcoidosis from lymphangitic carcinomatosis. Lymphangitic carcinomatosis is the most common cause of unilateral interstitial pulmonary disease (31). When treated with modern chemotherapy, a pattern of lymphangitic carcinomatosis may be stable or may slowly progress over months and, in some cases, years (32).

Aunt Minnie's Pearls

- *Lymphangitic carcinomatosis is often unilateral.*
- *Look for thickened interlobular septa and bronchovascular bundles on high resolution CT.*

CASE 10

History. 35-year-old woman with cough

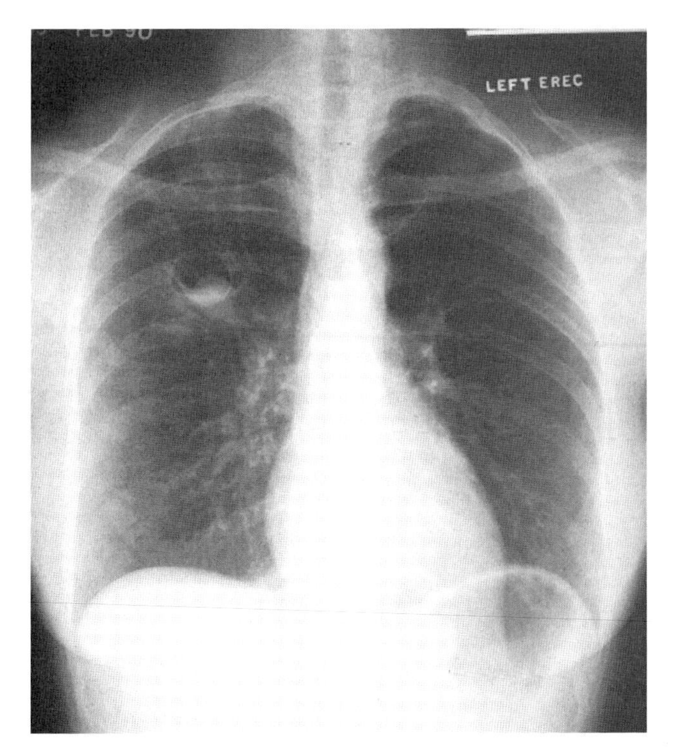

Figure 7.10.1.

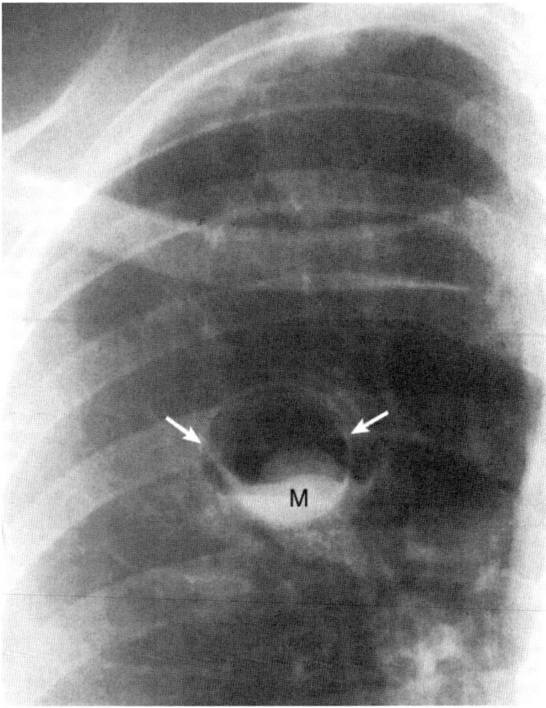

Figure 7.10.2.

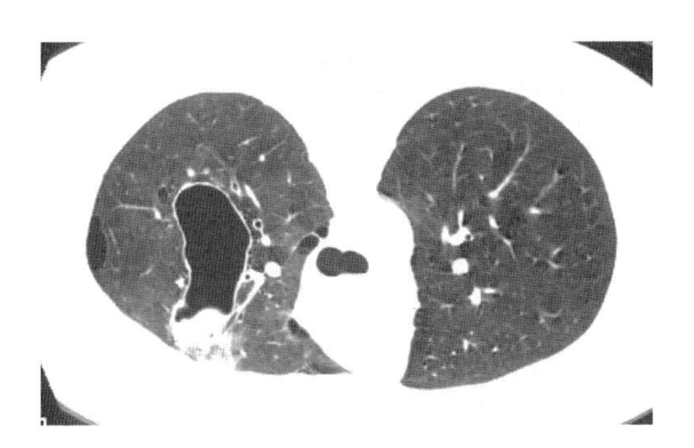

Figure 7.10.3.

Findings. A frontal chest radiograph (Fig. 7.10.1) shows thin-walled bullae within both upper lobes. A detail of the right upper lobe reveals a rounded mass (M) and an air-fluid level within a bulla (Fig. 7.10.2, *arrows*). Axial CT study with the patient in a prone position (Fig. 7.10.3) demonstrates that the mass is mobile, dropping to a dependent position within the bulla.

Diagnosis. Mycetoma

Discussion. The response of the lungs to infection with the fungus *Aspergillus fumigatus* is largely dependent on the patient's underlying pulmonary and immune status (33, 34). In this patient with normal immune status and preexisting pulmonary cavities, mycetomas represent saprophytic infection. Cavities of prior tuberculosis are the most common sites, but cysts and cavities from sarcoidosis, chronic infection, bronchiectasis, and bullae may also become infected. The patient may have a chronic productive cough or hemoptysis. Pleural thickening adjacent to the cavity may precede visualization of the fungus ball (35). Decubitus films may demonstrate the mobile nature of the mycetoma and may help to distinguish it from tumor.

Alterations of the patient's immune status lead to different forms of *Aspergillus* infection. In the patient with hypersensitivity, inhalation of *Aspergillus* spores produces allergic bronchopulmonary aspergillosis with mucoid impaction of bronchi and central bronchiectasis. In the granulocytopenic patient, invasive *Aspergillus* is characterized by pulmonary vascular invasion and pulmonary parenchymal infarction. Less commonly, *Aspergillus* can produce vascular invasion in a patient who is only mildly immunocompromised, as with malnutrition, diabetes mellitus, or alcoholism. This form has been called semiinvasive.

Aunt Minnie's Pearls

- *The saprophytic form of* Aspergillus *infection is recognized as a fungus ball (aspergilloma) within a preexisting cavity.*
- *Common causes of the preexisting cavity include tuberculosis, sarcoidosis, and emphysema.*

CASE 11

History. 28-year-old asymptomatic man, routine chest radiograph

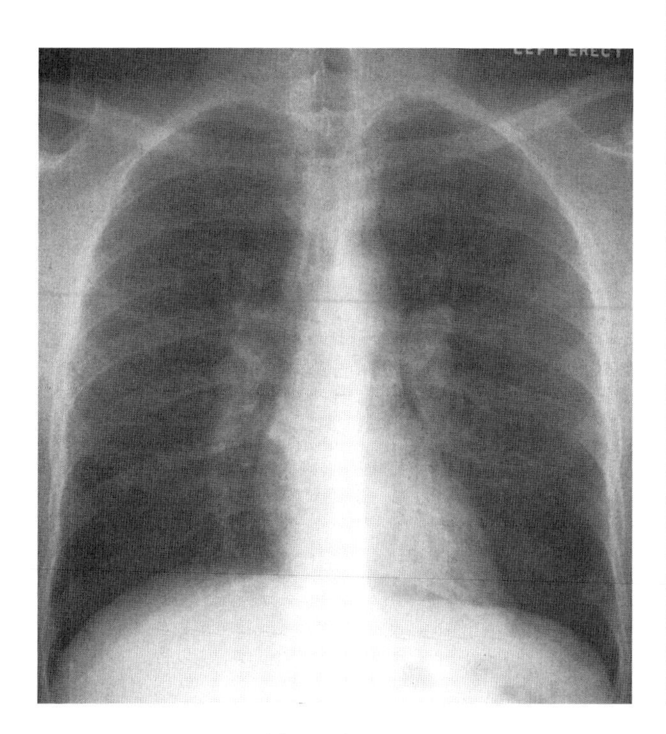

Figure 7.11.1.

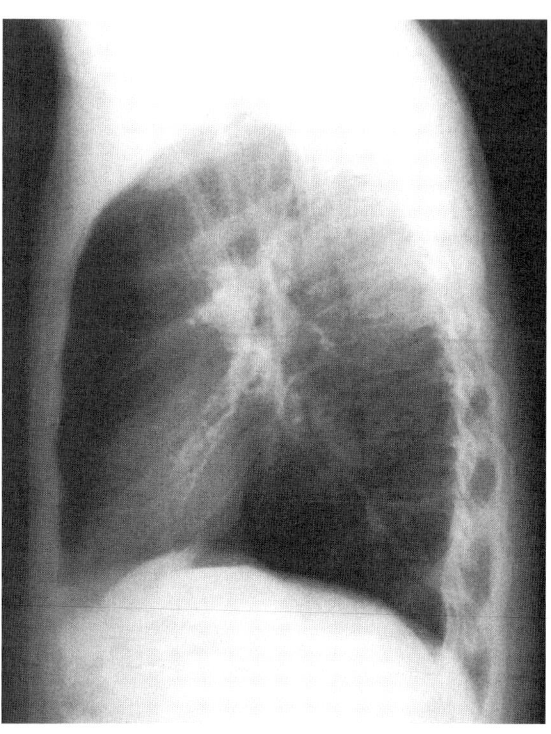

Figure 7.11.2.

Findings. Bilateral hilar, bilateral paratracheal, and aortopulmonary window lymphadenopathy are present on posteroanterior and lateral views of the chest (Figs. 7.11.1 and 7.11.2). The lungs are clear.

Diagnosis. Sarcoidosis

Discussion. Sarcoidosis is a systemic disease of unknown etiology characterized by formation of noncaseating epithelioid granulomata within lymph nodes, lungs, liver, and other organs (36). Cardiac involvement may cause arrhythmias, ventricular aneurysms, or even sudden death (37).

The clinical and radiological manifestations of sarcoidosis are predominantly related to pulmonary involvement. The most common radiographic finding in sarcoidosis is bilateral hilar and right paratracheal lymphadenopathy (1-2-3 sign or Garland's triad) (38). CT often reveals enlarged lymph nodes within the aorticopulmonary window and left paratracheal region as well. Pulmonary parenchymal involvement includes alveolitis and interstitial granulomata. The radiographic pattern is often reticulonodular. CT shows small nodules located along bronchovascular bundles (39). The pulmonary involvement may also appear alveolar or miliary. With chronic pulmonary disease, fibrosis and bullae may be visible in the radiographic picture of end-stage lung disease.

Sarcoidosis is staged radiographically as stage I (disease limited to mediastinal nodes), stage II (lung and lymph node involvement), stage III (lung involvement only), and stage IV (pulmonary fibrosis). Some authors believe that the clinical progression of sarcoidosis will follow this radiographic continuum and that the prognosis worsens as the patient progresses to higher stages of radiographic disease.

Aunt Minnie's Pearls

- *Sarcoidosis produces symmetric, bilateral hilar, paratracheal, and anteroposterior window nodes.*
- *Pulmonary involvement includes peribronchial granulomata, alveolitis, and interstitial fibrosis.*

CASE 12

History. 40-year-old man with fever

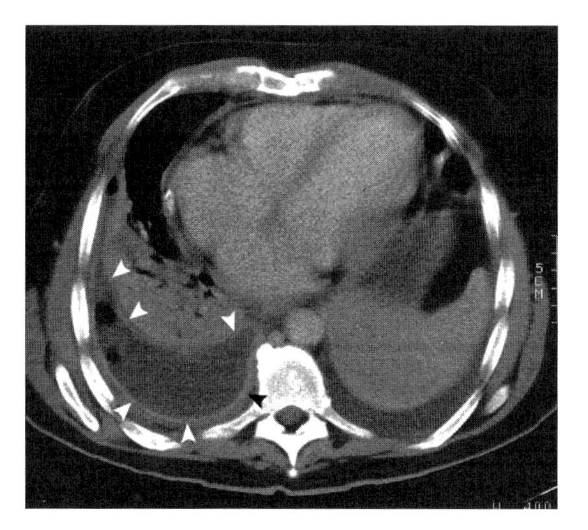

Figure 7.12.1.

Findings. Axial contrast enhanced chest CT (Fig. 7.12.1) shows a fluid collection in the periphery of the right thorax, which is adjacent to a pulmonary infiltrate. Thin enhancing pleural lines that are seen on both sides of the collection (*arrowheads*) place it in the pleural space (i.e., between the enhancing visceral and parietal pleura). Air is also identified within the fluid, raising the possibility of a bronchopleural fistula. The pleural effusion in the left hemithorax does not contain air and is not surrounded by enhancing pleura.

Diagnosis. Empyema on the right, demonstrating the split pleura sign, and simple pleural effusion on the left

Discussion. A parapneumonic effusion is a pleural effusion that occurs in association with pulmonary infection, including pneumonia, lung abscess, or bronchiectasis. An empyema is a parapneumonic pleural effusion with positive pleural fluid bacterial cultures (40). CT is helpful in the differentiation of lung abscess from parapneumonic effusion or empyema. A lung abscess is spherical, has thick irregular walls, forms acute angles with the chest wall, and replaces lung parenchyma (41). An empyema is lenticular and has thin smooth walls. It forms obtuse angles with the chest wall and compresses and displaces adjacent lung tissue. An empyema separates thickened visceral and parietal pleura, which, in contrast to a transudative pleural effusion, is more likely to enhance after administration of intravenous contrast material (split pleura sign) (42, 43). Extrapleural fat adjacent to the empyema may also be thickened and of increased attenuation (44).

The presence of air in the pleural space suggests, in the absence of recent intervention, bronchopleural fistula formation. Although a parapneumonic effusion may resolve with antibiotic therapy, an empyema generally requires chest tube drainage.

Aunt Minnie's Pearls

- *Empyemas are lenticular shaped and have enhancing, thickened pleura on CT.*
- *Empyemas generally require chest tube drainage.*

CASE 13

History. 72-year-old man with a history of recurrent ventricular tachycardia, now with exertional dyspnea and nonproductive cough

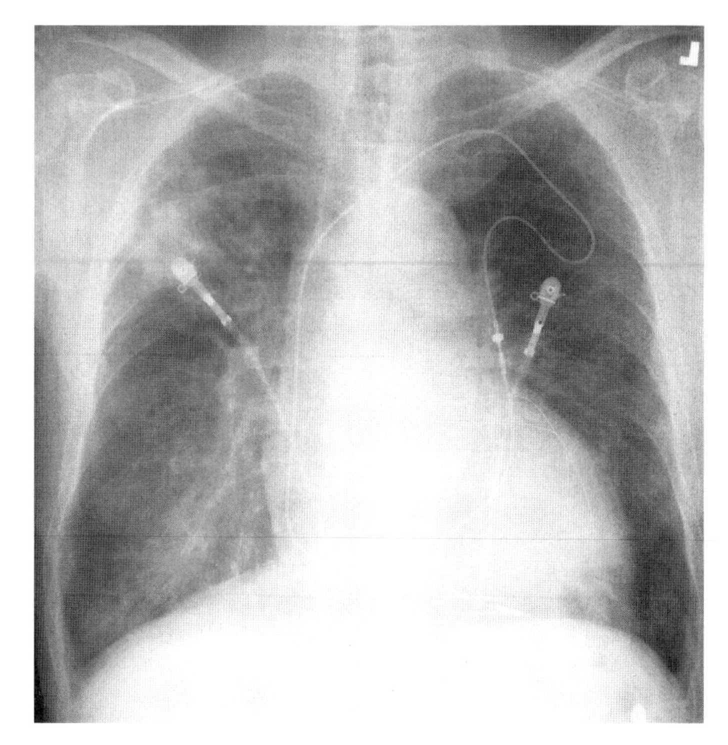

Figure 7.13.1.

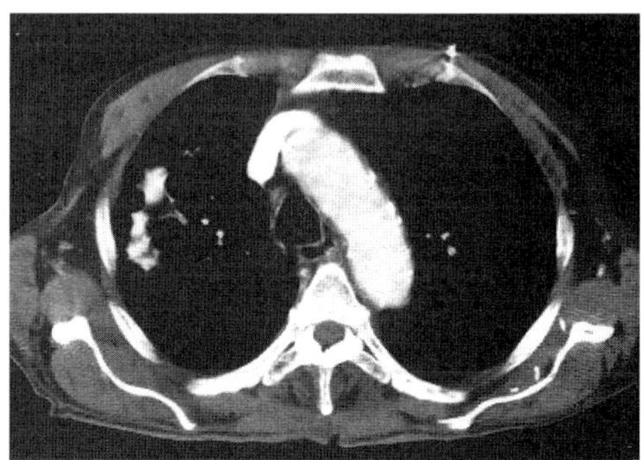

Figure 7.13.2. Soft tissue window.

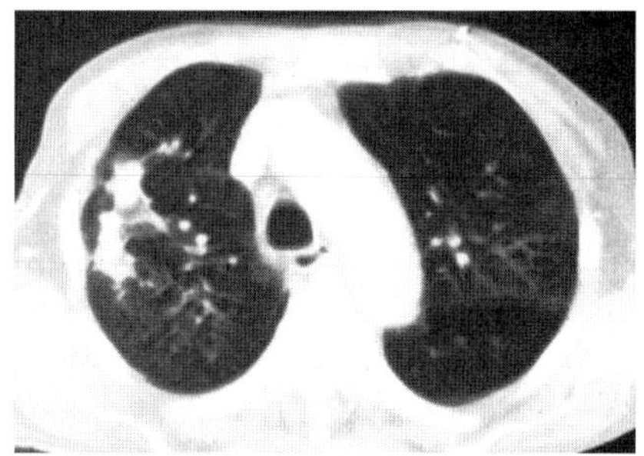

Figure 7.13.3. Lung window.

Findings. Chest radiograph (Fig. 7.13.1) shows cardiomegaly and a transvenous pacemaker, as well as automatic implantable cardioverter defibrillator (AICD) patches. Focal areas of increased opacity in the right upper lobe are better seen on the CT images (Figs. 7.13.2 and 7.13.3) as areas of high attenuation (almost as high as the contrast enhanced aorta).

Diagnosis. Amiodarone pulmonary toxicity

Discussion. Amiodarone is an antiarrhythmic agent that can cause pulmonary toxicity. Patients may present with a subacute course of dyspnea and nonproductive cough or with a more acute onset that mimics pulmonary infection. Physiologic studies show a decrease in carbon monoxide diffusing capacity (D_LCO). Chest radiographs may show focal areas of interstitial disease or dense areas of alveolar consolidation (45).

The CT appearance of high attenuation alveolar consolidation is thought to be related to the high iodine content (37% by weight) of amiodarone and its prolonged half-life within the lung (46). Attenuation of the liver and spleen is also often increased. Amiodarone pneumonitis is less likely to occur with dosages of ≤400 mg/day; it is treated by withdrawal of the drug, with or without corticosteroid therapy (47).

Aunt Minnie's Pearls

- *Amiodarone pulmonary toxicity is dose related and produces high attenuation lung consolidation on CT.*

CASE 14

History. 54-year-old woman with dyspnea and right-sided pleuritic chest pain

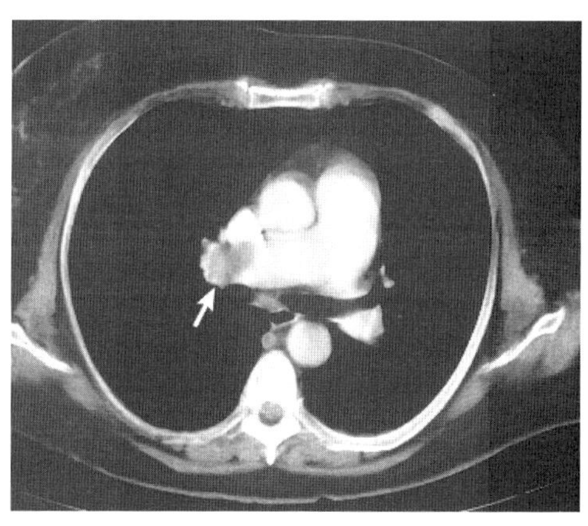

Figure 7.14.2. Soft tissue window.

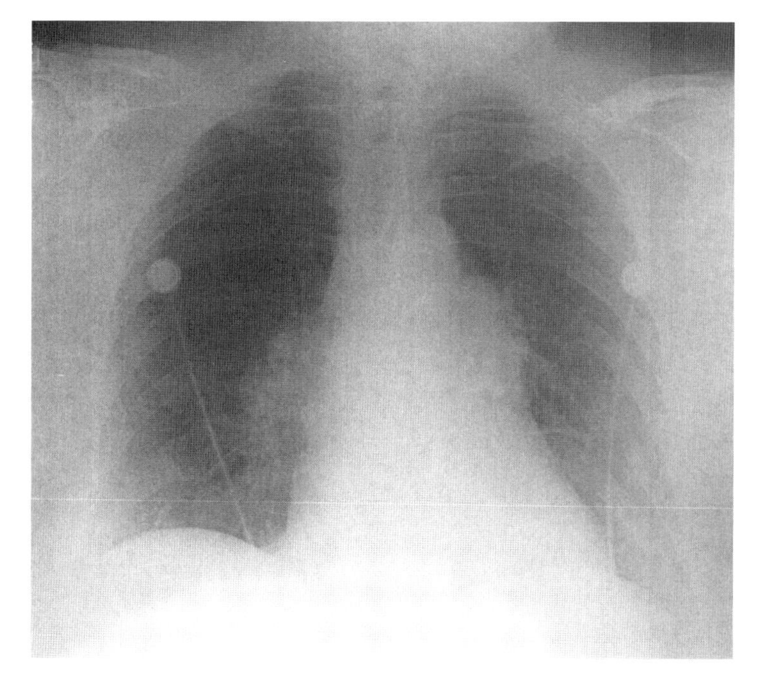

Figure 7.14.1.

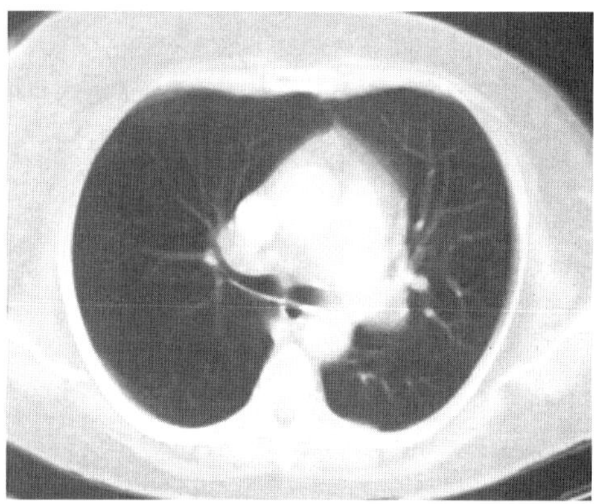

Figure 7.14.3. Lung window.

Findings. On the chest radiograph (Fig. 7.14.1), the right lung appears oligemic, and the central right pulmonary artery is prominent. On a contrast enhanced CT image, a filling defect is present in the right main pulmonary artery (Fig. 7.14.2, *arrow*). Windowing the CT image for lung detail (Fig. 7.14.3) clearly shows oligemia in the right lung.

Diagnosis. Acute pulmonary embolism

Discussion. Pulmonary emboli are most often the result of thrombi dislodged from the deep veins of the legs. Risk factors for pulmonary embolism include advanced age, malignant disease, pelvic or abdominal surgery, orthopedic surgery in the lower limbs, prolonged immobilization, obesity, congestive heart failure, and trauma. Dyspnea and chest pain, often pleuritic in nature, are the only symptoms reported by more than 50% of patients with pulmonary embolism.

In the prospective investigation of pulmonary embolism diagnosis (PIOPED), chest radiograph results were normal in 12% of patients with pulmonary embolism. A prominent central pulmonary artery (Fleischner's sign) was seen in 20%; a pleural-based area of increased opacity (Hampton's hump) was seen in 22%; and oligemia (Westermark's sign) was seen in 14% of patients with pulmonary embolism. Pleural effusion was present in 35% of patients with pulmonary embolism. Of the radiographic abnormalities, oligemia had the highest positive predictive value for pulmonary embolism (48).

With contrast enhanced CT, thrombi may be seen within central pulmonary arteries, allowing a specific diagnosis of pulmonary embolism. Fast CT techniques may also demonstrate thrombi in second- to fourth-order branches. The lung parenchyma distal to the thrombus may be oligemic, visible as a decrease in number and caliber of vessels, decrease in lung attenuation, or both (49). Both CT and MR imaging are under investigation as possible noninvasive alternatives to pulmonary angiography.

Aunt Minnie's Pearls

- *Westermark's sign = oligemia.*
- *Hampton's hump = wedge-shaped pulmonary infarction.*
- *Fleischner's sign = prominent pulmonary artery.*

CASE 15

History. 70-year-old man with dyspnea who has worked as a concrete driller for many years

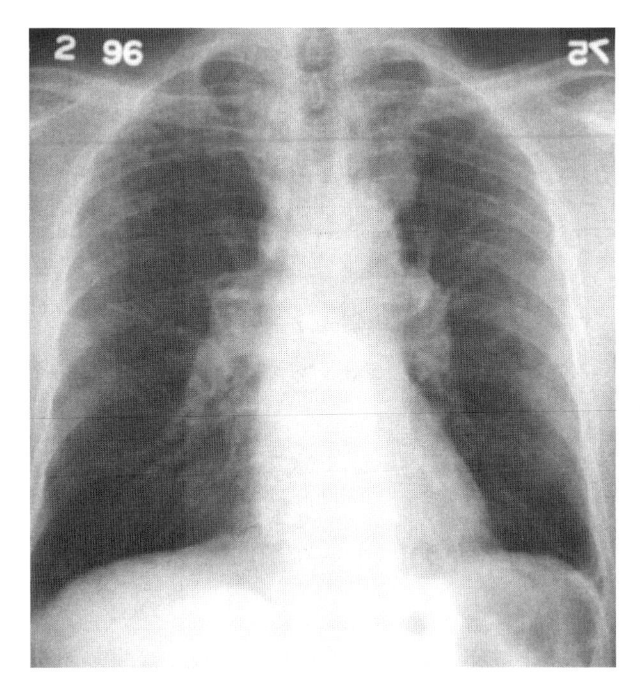

Figure 7.15.1.

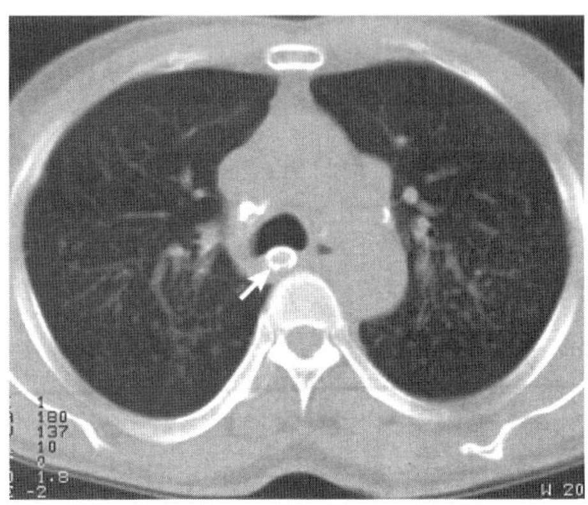

Figure 7.15.2.

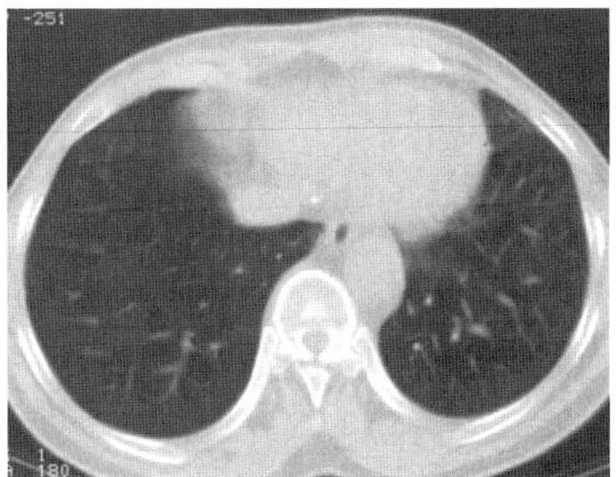

Figure 7.15.3.

Findings. A posteroanterior view of the chest (Fig. 7.15.1) shows small, well-defined interstitial nodules in the upper lobes and calcified mediastinal lymph nodes. A single view from a chest CT confirms the presence of upper lobe interstitial nodules and also shows calcified eggshell lymph nodes (Fig. 7.15.2, *arrow*). Another CT image through the lower lobes (Fig. 7.15.3) demonstrates no abnormality.

Diagnosis. Silicosis

Discussion. Pneumoconiosis develops when the dust-cleaning mechanisms of the lung are overwhelmed (50). In concrete, the mixed dust contains silica, which produces silicosis. Exposure to free silica also occurs in sandblasters, quarry workers, and miners. Coal miners are also exposed to a mixed dust, including silica dust as well as coal dust. There is tremendous overlap between the radiographic pictures of coal workers' pneumoconiosis and silicosis.

Both diseases have simple and complicated forms. Simple coal workers' pneumoconiosis and simple silicosis consist of small, rounded opacities (p, q, and r type) with predominant upper lobe involvement (51). Complicated silicosis, or progressive massive fibrosis, describes coalescence of these small, rounded opacities or nodules into masses at least 1 cm in diameter. Lesions are often flat; smaller dimensions are more evident on the lateral view than on the frontal view. Coalescent or large opacities (types A, B, and C) are more readily recognized on CT than on chest radiographs (52). These large opacities are often surrounded by emphysematous lung or small nodules.

Although most common in silicosis, eggshell (peripheral) calcification of hilar and mediastinal lymph nodes may also be present in patients with coal workers' pneumoconiosis, sarcoidosis, and postirradiation Hodgkin's disease (53).

Aunt Minnie's Pearls

- *Silicosis causes upper lobe nodules and conglomerate masses.*
- *Eggshell calcification of lymph nodes is usually caused by silicosis.*

CASE 16

History. 72-year-old World War II veteran with abnormal chest radiography results

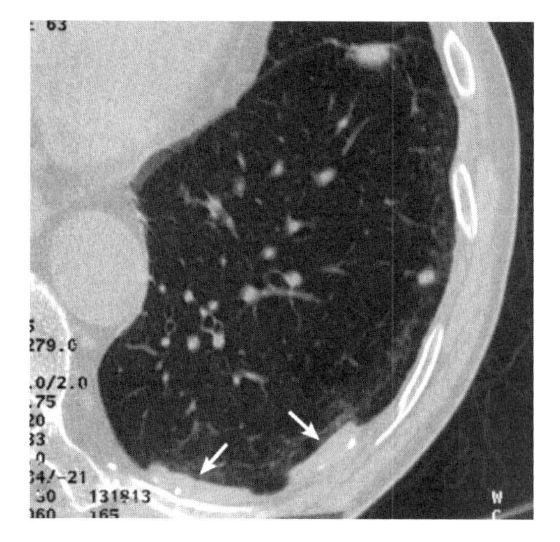

Figure 7.16.1.

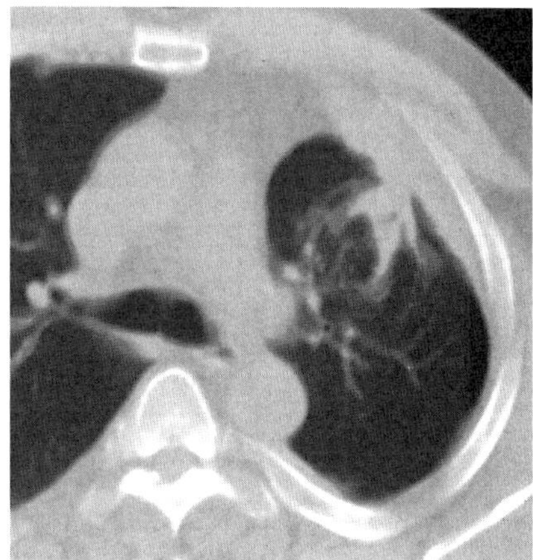

Figure 7.16.2.

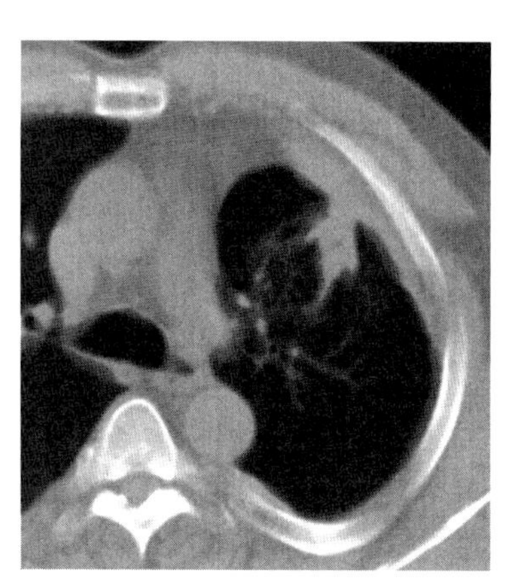

Figure 7.16.3.

Findings. A high resolution CT image shows pleural thickening and partially calcified pleural plaques (Fig. 7.16.1, *arrows*). Subpleural arcuate and short lines are faintly seen. Two CT images separated by 3 years (Figs. 7.16.2 and 7.16.3) show bronchi and vessels spiraling toward a mass in the left upper lobe. The mass is subtended by thickened pleura. No change in size or shape of the mass is seen over the 3 years.

Diagnosis. Asbestosis and rounded atelectasis

Discussion. Asbestos exposure has been associated with the development of three diseases: asbestosis, bronchogenic carcinoma, and mesothelioma. Construction workers and shipyard workers are among those who are occupationally exposed to asbestos. The clinical diagnosis of asbestosis requires a history of exposure and an appropriate time since exposure (at least 15 years). In asbestos-exposed individuals, pleural abnormalities include calcified and noncalcified pleural plaques, diffuse pleural thickening, and pleural effusion. Pulmonary parenchymal abnormalities are required for the diagnosis of asbestosis and include curvilinear subpleural lines, parenchymal bands 2–5 cm long that traverse the lung at angles inconsistent with vessels, thickened short peripheral lines, and honeycombing (54).

Rounded atelectasis occurs when an area of thickened pleura envelops adjacent lung. Owing to the increased incidence of bronchogenic carcinoma, the diagnosis of rounded atelectasis should be made with extreme caution. CT characteristics of rounded atelectasis include a mass contiguous with an area of pleural thickening, with evidence of volume loss in the adjacent lung and a comet tail appearance of vessels and bronchi sweeping into the margin of the mass (55).

Aunt Minnie's Pearls

- *Rounded atelectasis = rounded mass adjacent to thickened pleura, usually in a patient with asbestos exposure.*
- *Volume loss in the involved lobe and comet tail appearance of vessels and bronchi around the mass are classic for rounded atelectasis.*

CASE 17

History. 69-year-old woman with dyspnea

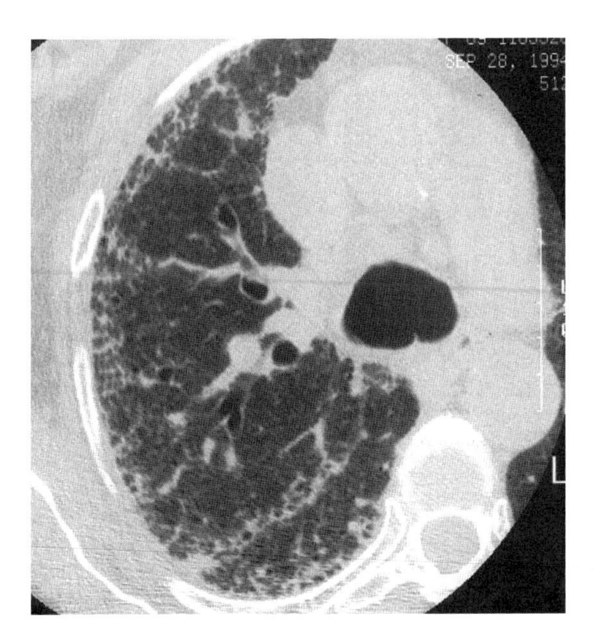

Figure 7.17.1.

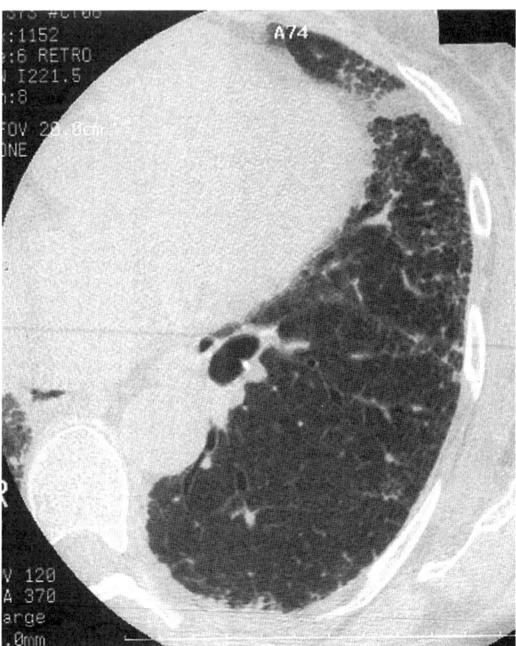

Figure 7.17.2.

Findings. CT images with 1-mm collimation (high spatial frequency algorithm, targeted image) show a peripheral, basal distribution of short lines, thickened and distorted interlobular septa, and subpleural cysts (Figs. 7.17.1 and 7.17.2). Although the disease is more severe on the right, bilateral involvement is evident.

Diagnosis. Idiopathic pulmonary fibrosis

Discussion. Idiopathic pulmonary fibrosis is a progressive fibrosing disease of the lungs, characterized by the gradual onset of dyspnea and restrictive lung disease with reduction in carbon monoxide diffusing capacity (D_LCO). The disease is also known as cryptogenic fibrosing alveolitis or usual interstitial pneumonia (56). The reticular pattern seen on CT correlates with histologic findings of fibrosis. The subpleural cysts communicate with the airways and produce a honeycomb appearance that represents irreversible disease. As the disease progresses, the reticular pattern becomes coarser; loss of lung volume progresses; and the peripheral, basal predominance may become less evident (57).

Aunt Minnie's Pearls

- *CT shows basal distribution of subpleural cysts and short peripheral lines in idiopathic pulmonary fibrosis.*

CASE 18

History. Withheld

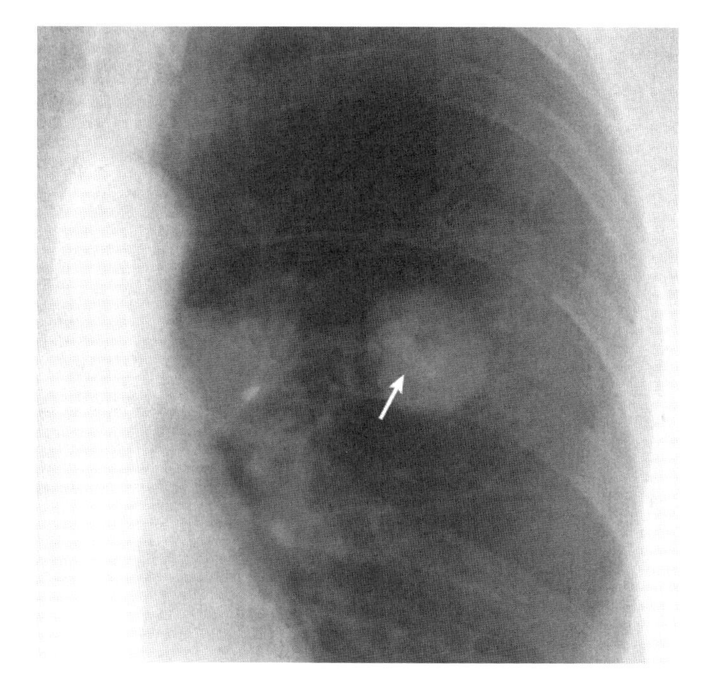

Figure 7.18.1.

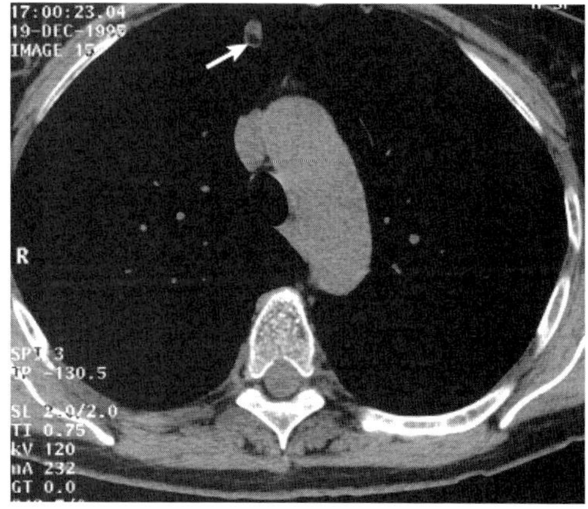

Figure 7.18.2.

Findings. A frontal view of the chest (Fig. 7.18.1) shows a well-defined round mass in the left upper lobe. The mass contains internal calcification that is in the shape of a kernel of popcorn (*arrow*). A CT image of a solitary pulmonary nodule in a different patient reveals fat attenuation in the center of the mass (Fig. 7.18.2, *arrow*).

Diagnosis. Pulmonary hamartoma

Discussion. A hamartoma is a mass that contains tissues that are normally found in the organ of origin. The tissues that make up the mass, however, are disorganized and in abnormal amounts. Because pulmonary hamartomas are actually of mesenchymal origin, consisting mainly of fat and cartilage, they may not fit the true definition of a hamartoma. These benign masses tend to occur in patients at least 30 years old and are typically round. The presence of characteristic "popcorn" calcification within the mass, such as in the index case, allows a highly specific plain-film diagnosis. Unfortunately, less than one-third of these masses will show calcification on plain films. The observation of fat and calcium on thin section CT images within a smoothly marginated mass less than 2.5 cm in size virtually excludes other neoplastic possibilities (58). These masses may grow slowly on follow-up chest radiographs, and therefore management of these patients may still require surgical excision. The proper identification of a pulmonary hamartoma preoperatively, however, may allow conservative nonoperative management or wedge resection of the mass.

Aunt Minnie's Pearls

- *Popcorn calcification on plain films = pulmonary hamartoma.*
- *The observation of fat and calcium on thin section CT images within a smoothly marginated mass less than 2.5 cm in size virtually excludes other neoplastic possibilities.*

CASE 19

History. Relatively asymptomatic middle-aged man

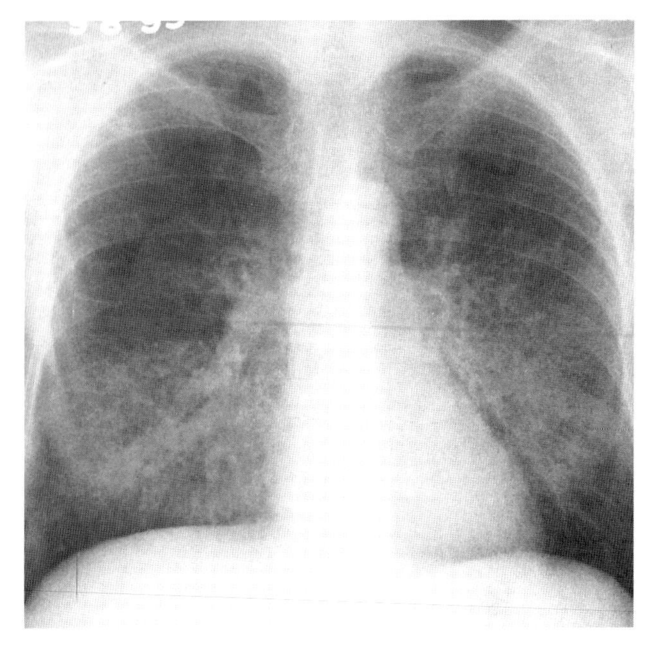

Figure 7.19.1.

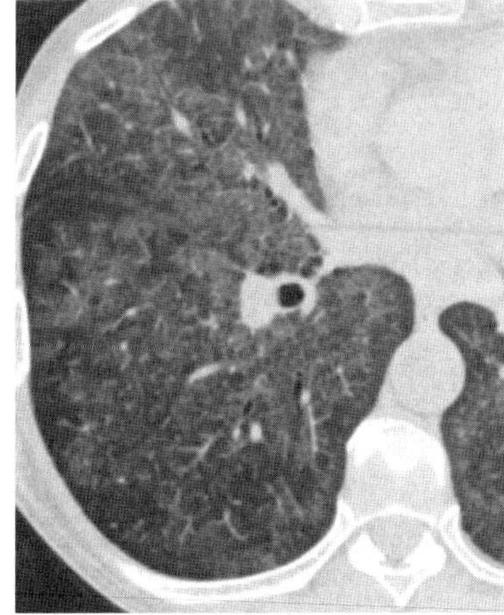

Figure 7.19.2.

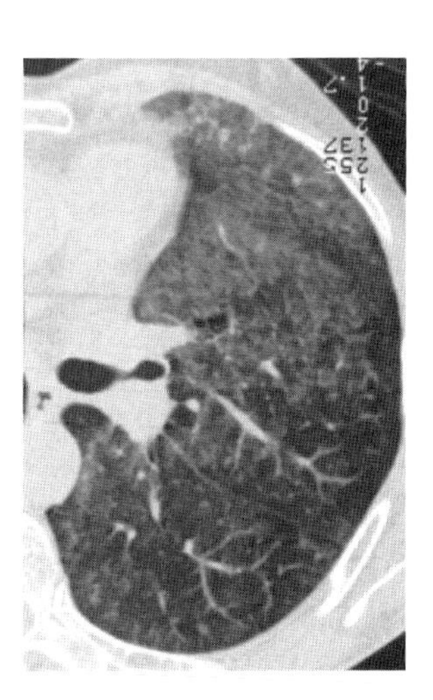

Figure 7.19.3.

Findings. Posteroanterior view of the chest (Fig. 7.19.1) reveals small ill-defined opacities that approximate the size of a pulmonary acinus (6–10 mm). Kerley B lines are faintly seen in the periphery of the lung, and subpleural edema is identified as thickening of the minor fissure. Two views from a high resolution CT scan of the lungs (Figs. 7.19.2 and 7.19.3) show ground glass opacification of the secondary pulmonary lobule, which is outlined by smooth, mild thickening of the interlobular septa.

Diagnosis. Alveolar proteinosis

Discussion. Pulmonary alveolar proteinosis (PAP) is a condition in which PAS + phospholipoproteinaceous material accumulates in the end air spaces. Although the pathogenesis of PAP is incompletely understood, the close resemblance of the secretions to surfactant has led to the hypothesis that dysfunction of type II pneumocytes leads to the disease. PAP most commonly affects middle-aged males, who may present with mild symptoms of dyspnea, cough, and fatigue. Chest radiographs reveal ill-defined acinar opacities with relative sparing of the extreme lung periphery. High resolution CT is helpful in establishing the diagnosis by demonstrating a characteristic patchwork quilt or "crazy paving" pattern, which consists of ground glass opacity of the secondary pulmonary lobule surrounded by smooth thickening of the interlobular septa (caused by superimposed edema) that border the lobule (59). The final diagnosis is confirmed by lung biopsy.

Patients are treated by pulmonary lavage under general anesthesia. This procedure is curative in some patients; other patients will experience relapse and progressive worsening of the disease. PAP carries an increased risk of pulmonary infections, especially by nocardia.

Aunt Minnie's Pearls

- *Tiny ill-defined acinar opacities in a middle-aged male may indicate PAP.*
- *The patchwork quilt or crazy paving appearance of the secondary pulmonary lobule on high resolution CT is very characteristic of PAP.*

REFERENCES

1. Savic B, Birtel FJ, Tholen W, Funke HD, Knoche R. Lung sequestration: report of seven cases and review of 540 published cases. Thorax 1979;34:96–101.
2. Felker RE, Tonkin ILD. Imaging of pulmonary sequestration. AJR 1990;154:241–249.
3. Rosado-de-Christenson ML, Frazier AA, Stocker JT, Templeton PA. Extralobar sequestration: radiologic-pathologic correlation. RadioGraphics 1993;13:425–441.
4. Stern EJ, Webb WR, Warnock ML, Salmon CJ. Bronchopulmonary sequestration: dynamic, ultrafast, high-resolution CT evidence of air trapping. AJR 1991;157:947–949.
5. Godwin JD, Tarver RD. Scimitar syndrome: four new cases examined with CT. Radiology 1986;159:15–20.
6. Woodring JH, Howard TA, Kanga JF. Congenital pulmonary venolobar syndrome revisited. RadioGraphics 1994;14:349–369.
7. Winer-Muram HT. Adult presentation of heterotaxic syndromes and related complexes. J Thorac Imaging 1995;10:43–57.
8. Rappaport DC, Herman SJ, Weisbrod GL. Congenital bronchopulmonary diseases in adults: CT findings. AJR 1994;162:1295–1299.
9. Keslar P, Newman B, Oh KS. Radiographic manifestations of anomalies of the lung. Radiol Clin North Am 1991;29:255–270.
10. Cohen AM, Solomon EH, Alfidi RJ. Computed tomography in bronchial atresia. AJR 1980;135:1097–1099.
11. Felson B. Mucoid impaction (inspissated secretions) in segmental bronchial obstruction. Radiology 1979;133:9–16.
12. Di Lorenzo M, Collin PP, Vaillancourt R, Duranceau A. Bronchogenic cysts. J Pediatr Surg 1989;24:988–991.
13. Reed JC, Sobonya RE. Morphologic analysis of foregut cysts in the thorax. AJR 1974;120:851–860.
14. Rogers LF, Osmer JC. Bronchogenic cyst: a review of 46 cases. AJR 1964;91:273–283.
15. Nakata H, Sato Y, Nakayama T, Yoshimatsu H, Kobayashi T. Bronchogenic cyst with high CT number: analysis of contents. J Comput Assist Tomogr 1986;10:360.
16. Yernault J-C, Kuhn G, Dumortier P, Rocmans P, Ketelbant P, De Vuyst P. "Solid" mediastinal bronchogenic cyst: mineralogic analysis. AJR 1986;146:73–74.
17. Nakata H, Nakayama C, Kimoto T, et al. Computed tomography of mediastinal bronchogenic cysts. J Comput Assist Tomogr 1982;6:733–738.
18. Kuhlman JE, Fishman EK, Wang KP, Zerhouni EA, Seigelman SS. Mediastinal cysts: diagnosis by CT and needle aspiration. AJR 1988;150:75–78.
19. Swyer PR, James GCW. A case of unilateral pulmonary emphysema. Thorax 1953;8:133–136.
20. Moore ADA, Godwin JD, Dietrich PA, Verschakelen JA, Henderson WR Jr. Swyer-James syndrome: CT findings in eight patients. AJR 1992;158:1211–1215.
21. White RI Jr, Mitchell SE, Barth KH, et al. Angioarchitecture of pulmonary arteriovenous malformations: an important consideration before embolotherapy. AJR 1983;140:681–686.
22. Remy J, Remy-Jardin M, Giraud F, Wattinne L. Angioarchitecture of pulmonary arteriovenous malformations: clinical utility of three-dimensional helical CT. Radiology 1994;191:657–664.
23. Burke CM, Safai C, Nelson DP, Raffin TA. Pulmonary arteriovenous malformations: a critical update. Am Rev Respir Dis 1986;134:334–339.
24. White RI Jr, Lynch-Nyhan A, Terry P, et al. Pulmonary arteriovenous malformations: techniques and long-term outcome of embolotherapy. Radiology 1988;169:663–669.
25. Golden R. The effect of bronchostenosis upon the roentgen ray shadows in carcinoma of the bronchus. AJR 1925;13:21–30.
26. Proto AV, Tocino I. Radiographic manifestations of lobar collapse. Semin Roentgenol 1980;15:117–173.
27. Don C, Desmarais R. Peripheral upper lobe collapse in adults. Radiology 1989;170:657–659.
28. Kattan KR, Eyler WR, Felson B. The juxtaphrenic peak in upper lobe collapse. Radiology 1980;134:763–765.
29. Yang SP, Lin C. Lymphangitic carcinomatosis of the lungs: the clinical significance of its roentgenologic classification. Chest 1972;62:179–187.
30. Stein MG, Mayo J, Müller N, Aberle DR, Webb WR, Gamsu G. Pulmonary lymphangitic spread of carcinoma: appearance on CT scans. Radiology 1987;162:371–375.
31. Youngberg AS. Unilateral diffuse lung opacity: differential diagnosis with emphasis on lymphangitic spread of cancer. Radiology 1977;123:277–281.
32. Ikezoe J, Godwin JD, Hunt KJ, Marglin SI. Pulmonary lymphangitic carcinomatosis: chronicity of radiographic findings in long-term survivors. AJR 1995;165:49–52.
33. Thompson BH, Stanford W, Galvin JR, Kurihara Y. Varied radiographic appearances of pulmonary aspergillosis. RadioGraphics 1995;15:1273–1284.
34. Greene R. The pulmonary aspergilloses: three distinct entities or a spectrum of disease. Radiology 1981;140:527–530.
35. Libshitz HI, Atkinson GW, Israel HL. Pleural thickening as a manifestation of *Aspergillus* superinfection. AJR 1974;120:883–886.
36. Miller BH, Rosado-de-Christenson ML, McAdams HP, Fishback NF. Thoracic sarcoidosis: radiologic-pathologic correlation. RadioGraphics 1995;15:421–437.
37. Chiles C, Adams GW, Ravin CE. Radiographic manifestations of cardiac sarcoid. AJR 1985;145:711–714.
38. Bein ME, Putman CE, McLoud TC, Mink JH. A reevaluation of intrathoracic lymphadenopathy in sarcoidosis. AJR 1978;131:409–415.
39. Nishimura K, Itoh H, Kitaichi M, Nagai S, Izumi T. Pulmonary sarcoidosis: correlation of CT and histopathologic findings. Radiology 1993;189:105–109.

40. Light RW. Parapneumonic effusions and empyema. Clin Chest Med 1985;6:55–62.
41. Williford ME, Godwin JD. Computed tomography of lung abscess and empyema. Radiol Clin North Am 1983;21:575–583.
42. Stark DD, Federle MP, Goodman PC, Podrasky AE, Webb WR. Differentiating lung abscess and empyema: radiography and computed tomography. AJR 1983;141:163–167.
43. Waite RJ, Carbonneau RJ, Balikian JP, Umali CB, Pezzella AT, Nash G. Parietal pleural changes in empyema: appearances at CT. Radiology 1990;175:145–150.
44. Aquino SL, Webb WR, Gushiken BJ. Pleural exudates and transudates: diagnosis with contrast-enhanced CT. Radiology 1994;192:803–808.
45. Olson LK, Forrest JV, Friedman PJ, Kiser PE, Henschke CI. Pneumonitis after amiodarone therapy. Radiology 1984;150:327–330.
46. Kuhlman JE, Teigen C, Ren H, Hruban RH, Hutchins GM, Fishman EK. Amiodarone pulmonary toxicity: CT findings in symptomatic patients. Radiology 1990;177:121–125.
47. Adams GD, Kehoe R, Lesch M, Glassroth J. Amiodarone-induced pneumonitis: assessment of risk factors and possible risk reduction. Chest 1988;93:254–263.
48. Worsley DF, Alavi A, Aronchik JM, Chen JTT, Greenspan RH, Ravin CE. Chest radiographic findings in patients with acute pulmonary embolism: observations from the PIOPED study. Radiology 1993;189:133–136.
49. Greaves SM, Hart EM, Brown K, Young DA, Batra P, Aberle DR. Pulmonary thromboembolism: spectrum of findings on CT. AJR 1995;165:1359–1363.
50. Heitzman ER. The lung: radiologic-pathologic correlations. St. Louis: Mosby, 1984:321.
51. International Labor Office/University of Cincinnati. International classification of radiographs of pneumoconiosis 1980, 22 revised, Occupational Safety and Health Series. Geneva: International Labor Office, 1980.
52. Bégin R, Bergeron D, Samson L, Boctor M, Cantin A. CT assessment of silicosis in exposed workers. AJR 1987;148:509–514.
53. Jacobson G, Felson B, Pendergrass EP, Flinn RH, Lainhart WS. Eggshell calcifications in coal and metal miners. Semin Roentgenol 1967;2:276–282.
54. Aberle DR, Gamsu G, Ray CS. High-resolution CT of benign asbestos-related diseases: clinical and radiographic correlation. AJR 1988;151:883–891.
55. Lynch DA, Gamsu G, Ray CS, Aberle DR. Asbestos-related focal lung masses: manifestations on conventional and high-resolution CT scans. Radiology 1988;169:603–607.
56. Müller NL, Miller RR, Webb MR, Evans KG, Ostrow DN. Fibrosing alveolitis: CT-pathologic correlation. Radiology 1986;160:585–588.
57. Akira M, Sakatani M, Ueda F. Idiopathic pulmonary fibrosis: progression of honeycombing at thin-section CT. Radiology 1993;189:687–691.
58. Siegelman SS, Khouri NF, Scott Jr. WW, et al. Pulmonary hamartoma: CT findings. Radiology 1986;160:313–317.
59. Godwin JD, Müller NL, Takasugi JE. Pulmonary alveolar proteinosis: CT findings. Radiology 1988;169:609–613.

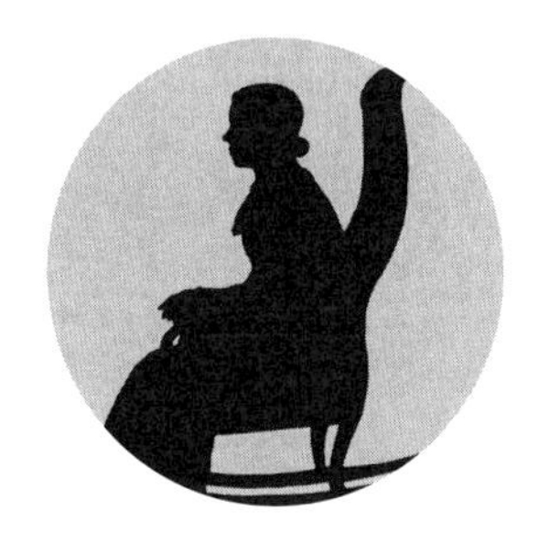

chapter 8

MAMMOGRAPHY

RITA L. FREIMANIS

CASE 1

History. Withheld

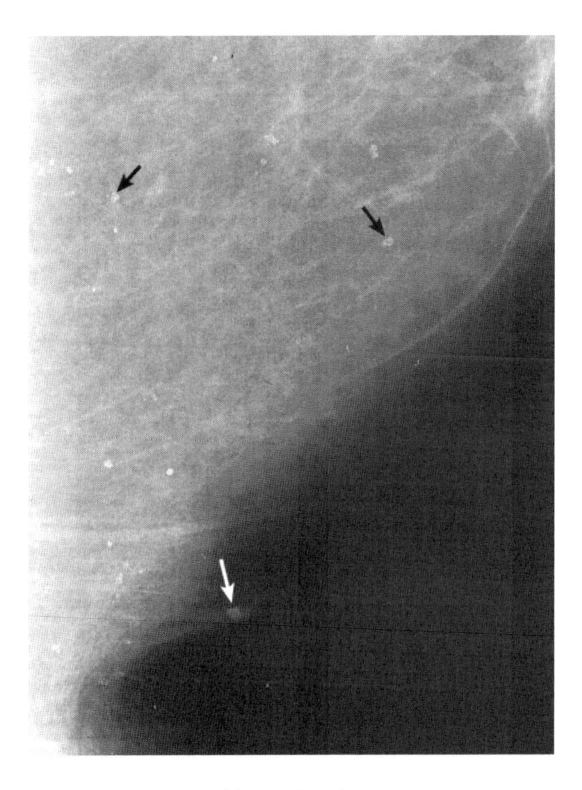

Figure 8.1.1.

Findings. There are numerous, scattered, ring-shaped calcifications (*arrows*) measuring 0.5–1 mm on the craniocaudal view of the medial right breast (Fig. 8.1.1). Their superficial location is best appreciated in the cleavage area in this case. The calcifications are mostly single, but some are clustered. Their centers are low-density or lucent. The distinguishing feature is the less-than-perfect shape of the calcified ring, which often has a flattened side, giving it a polygonal appearance.

Diagnosis. Dermal calcification (sebaceous glands)

Discussion. Sebaceous glands occur in the skin in association with hair follicles. When calcified, they are differentiated from fat necrosis by the location in the skin and by their polygonal shape. Their size corresponds to that of skin pores, whereas fat necrosis may have larger rings. Typical dermal calcifications are always benign and do not require biopsy (1). If the classic features are not present, however, the suspected location in the skin can be confirmed with tangential views, thereby avoiding biopsy of atypical skin calcifications that may mimic carcinoma (2).

Aunt Minnie's Pearls

- *Polygonal calcified rings in a superficial location = sebaceous glands.*
- *Tangential views will confirm the diagnosis.*

CASE 2

History. 45-year-old woman with a vaguely palpable soft mass in breast tail that has been unchanged for several years

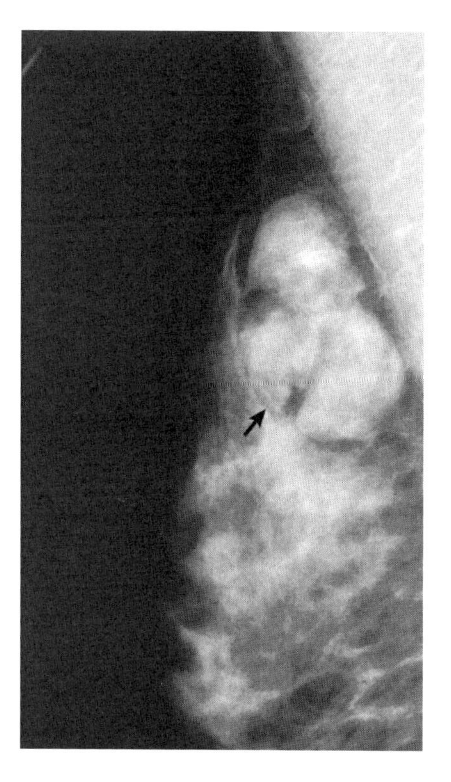

Figure 8.2.1.

Findings. Mediolateral oblique view of the right breast (Fig. 8.2.1) reveals a 5-cm complex mass in the breast tail with densities of both fat and water. The mass appears encapsulated (*arrow*). Other than slight adjacent soft tissue displacement, no architectural distortion or other effect on the surrounding tissue is seen.

Diagnosis. Fibroadenolipoma

Discussion. Fibroadenolipoma is an uncommon benign entity composed of encapsulated fat and lobulations of fibroglandular tissue. When palpable, it is mobile and smooth. A pseudocapsule demarcates this round or oval lesion from the surrounding breast tissue. The term hamartoma has been used, because it simulates a "breast within a breast" histologically. Size varies greatly, from 1 cm to a lesion that occupies most of the breast (3–5).

This classic appearance indicates a benign lesion, and additional studies or biopsy are unnecessary. Although one sarcoma mimicking this appearance has been reported, the lack of suspicious change on physical examination or mammograms permits fibroadenolipomas to be followed on a routine screening schedule (6).

Aunt Minnie's Pearls

- *Encapsulated fat and fibroglandular tissue = fibroadenolipoma.*

CASE 3

History. Patient A: 78-year-old woman who recently underwent excisional biopsy (benign); patient B: 47-year-old asymptomatic woman

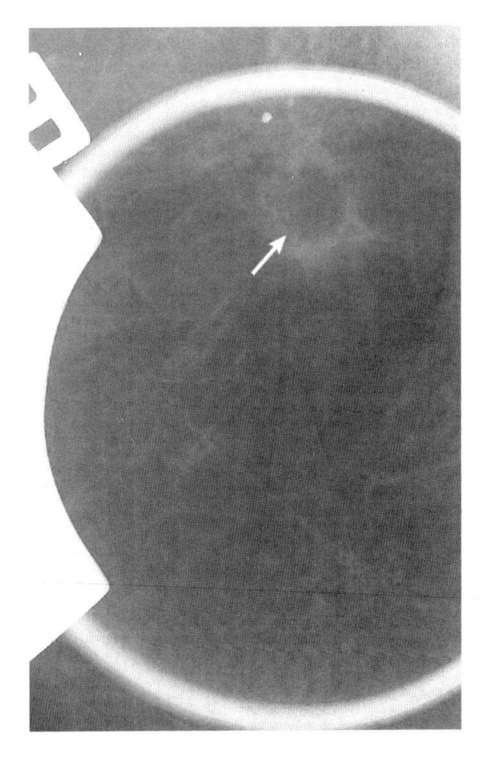

Figure 8.3.1. Patient A.

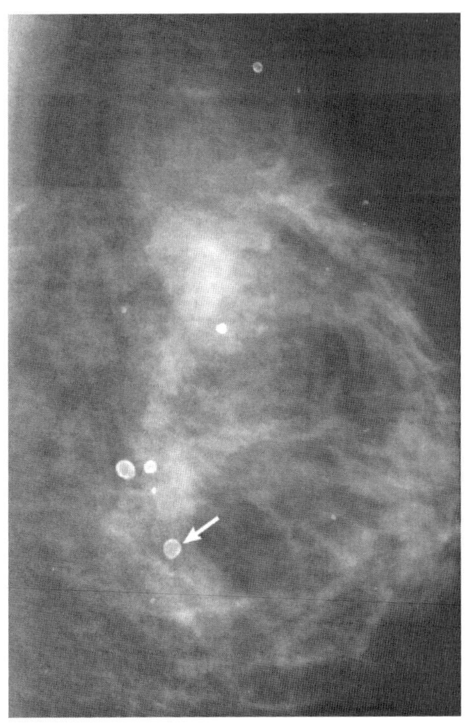

Figure 8.3.2. Patient B.

Findings. Craniocaudal spot film of the right breast in patient A (Fig. 8.3.1) shows a uniformly lucent 1-cm lesion (*arrow*) with a smooth wall that demarcates it from the surrounding tissue. A small rim of irregular soft tissue opacity represents resolving postsurgical change. Mediolateral oblique view of the left breast in patient B (Fig. 8.3.2) reveals multiple calcified spherical structures with lucent centers (*arrow*) scattered throughout the breast. Sizes range from 0.5 to 3 mm.

Diagnosis. Two types of fat necrosis: patient A, posttraumatic oil cyst; patient B, liponecrosis microcystica calcificans

Discussion. Fat necrosis is thought to result from trauma, although the traumatic event may be remote in time or even forgotten (7). Both types shown here have fat-density centers, indicating benignity (8). The type shown in patient A ranges in size from 3 mm to 5 cm (9), is characteristically solitary but may be multiple, and is typically seen after breast surgery (10). When this type calcifies, it may be called liponecrosis macrocystica calcificans because of its larger size. The smaller multiple calcified oil cysts seen in patient B are less often associated with a definite, remembered traumatic event. These are seen more often in large, pendulous, fatty breasts (10). Both types of oil cysts typically have thin rims.

Aunt Minnie's Pearls

- *Small lucent lesion with smooth rim (calcified or not) = oil cyst of fat necrosis.*

CASE 4

History. Withheld

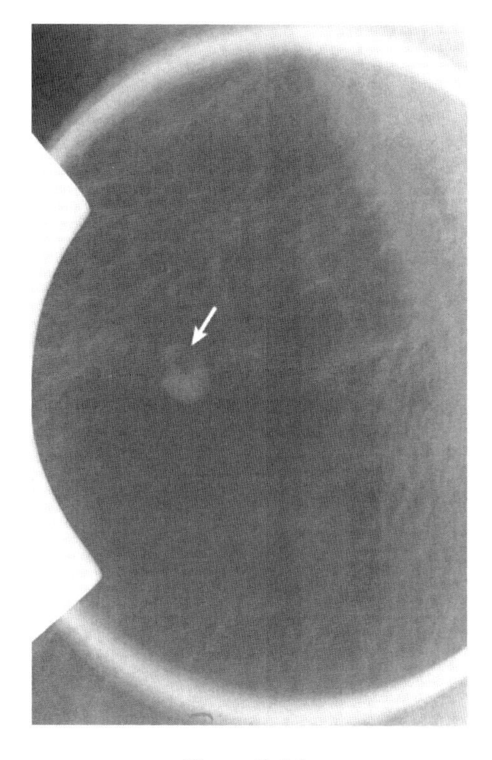

Figure 8.4.1.

Findings. Mediolateral oblique view of the right breast (Fig. 8.4.1) demonstrates an 8-mm oval soft tissue opacity in the breast tail that has smooth margins and a lucent notch or hilum (*arrow*).

Diagnosis. Intramammary lymph node

Discussion. The fatty notch or hilum in a circumscribed mass of soft tissue density identifies this as a lymph node (11). The location in the breast tail, clustered around the vessels, is also typical of intramammary lymph nodes. Histologically, lymph nodes occur anywhere in the breast, but there is disagreement regarding whether they may be seen outside the peripheral upper outer quadrant mammographically (12). The fatty hilum may be seen en face and therefore centrally, rather than peripherally, if the lymph node is rotated. Other descriptions of their shape are reniform and horseshoe-shaped. Typically, lymph nodes are 1.5 cm or smaller, have sharp margins, and contain no calcification (13). Axillary lymph nodes may be much larger but usually are largely fat-replaced. Lymph nodes that become larger, denser, or irregular are worrisome because the findings may indicate involvement of the node with tumor.

Aunt Minnie's Pearls

- *Smooth, small mass with fatty hilum = intramammary lymph node.*
- *Increased density in lymph node or loss of fatty hilum = possible tumor involvement.*

CASE 5

History. 83-year-old woman with "knotty" breasts for more than 60 years

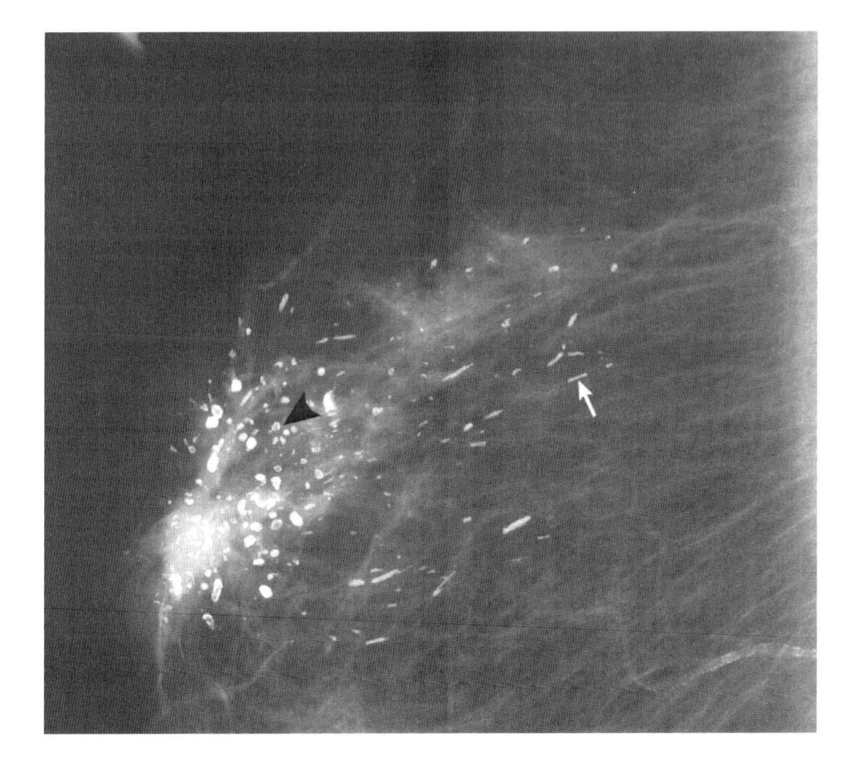

Figure 8.5.1.

Findings. Mediolateral oblique view of the right breast (Fig. 8.5.1) shows multiple rod-shaped (*arrow*), ring-shaped (*arrowhead*), spherical, and tubular coarse calcifications arranged in a radiating pattern in a large area of the upper breast. Poorly defined patchy densities are seen in roughly the same area. The nipple is retracted. All these findings have been stable for years.

Diagnosis. Secretory disease with plasma-cell mastitis

Discussion. With duct ectasia, secretions accumulate in the mammary ducts, and an aseptic inflammatory condition may result from leakage of antigenic proteins and fat through the duct wall. Histologically, there is a lymphocytic or plasmocytic infiltration in the periductal tissues. This process results in heavy calcification of intraductal secretions and duct walls, as well as fat necrosis, giving rise to the distinguishing shapes of calcifications. The radial pattern reflects the anatomic distribution of the involved ductal system (14). The rounded calcifications are a form of fat necrosis, and the linear calcifications are secretions within the ducts (15).

When the linear calcifications are seen alone, the term secretory disease is usually applied. These calcifications are distinguished by their smooth edges, uniform density, and nonbranching shapes. They are usually long, bilateral, and symmetric and are oriented toward the nipple (16). The term plasma-cell mastitis is generally reserved for the clinicopathologic condition that includes secretory disease, periductal plasma-cell infiltration and inflammation, which may cause palpable masses, nipple retraction, and mammographic soft tissue opacities and calcifications.

Aunt Minnie's Pearls

- *Smooth, uniform, calcified rods oriented toward nipple = secretory disease.*
- *Secretory disease with fat necrosis-type calcifications, soft tissue opacities, and nipple retraction = plasma-cell mastitis.*

CASE 6

History. Withheld

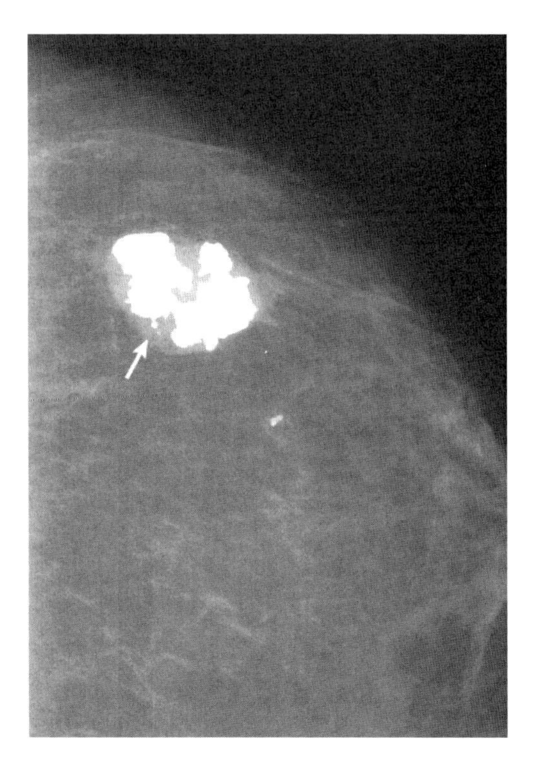

Figure 8.6.1.

Findings. A 2-cm mass is seen in the lateral aspect of the left breast on this craniocaudal mammogram (Fig. 8.6.1, *arrow*). It is smoothly marginated and has medium density, except for the large, sharply outlined high-density calcification involving much of the mass. The calcification is coarse and irregular.

Diagnosis. Hyalinized fibroadenoma with characteristic popcorn calcification

Discussion. Fibroadenoma is a common benign entity, usually developing in young women. The "young" fibroadenoma is usually smooth, rubbery, and mobile clinically and cannot be reliably distinguished from a circumscribed carcinoma on the first mammogram. The absence of growth over several years is typical, and then with advancing age and during menopause, the fibroadenoma usually degenerates and may shrink. Degeneration also causes the margins to become irregular, a suspicious characteristic in the absence of a sequence of mammograms demonstrating this evolution. As the fibroadenoma involutes further, calcifications may develop. Two patterns of calcification reflect the hyalinization that occurs in myxoid degeneration: (*a*) coarse central popcorn type and (*b*) coarse subcapsular plaque-like shell type. A third pattern results from one of several causes and consists of peripheral or central speckled calcifications (17). The latter may mimic carcinoma, but the first two patterns are pathognomonic, if the lesion is solid. Carcinomas arising within fibroadenomas have been reported (18), but such reports are rare. If malignant features (e.g., microcalcifications or irregular borders) develop within a benign-appearing mass, biopsy should be considered.

Aunt Minnie's Pearls

- *Popcorn or coarse, shell-like calcifications in a solid mass = hyalinized fibroadenoma.*

CASE 7

History. Withheld

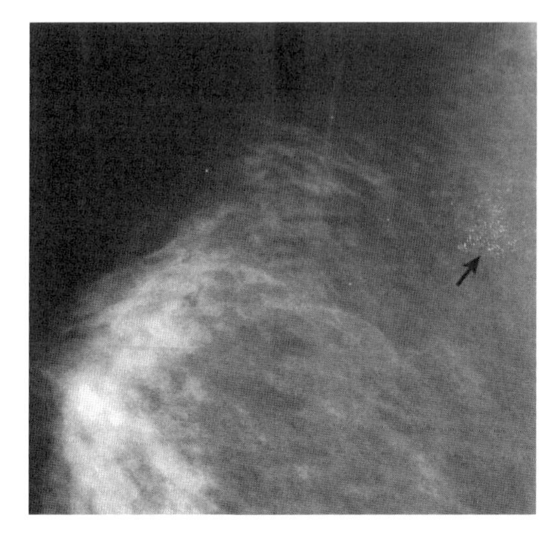

Figure 8.7.1.

Findings. Mediolateral oblique view of the left breast (Fig. 8.7.1) shows a group of very-high-density small marks arranged in a pattern of parallel curved lines, some of which are continuous and others of which are broken (*arrow*). There is no effect on the surrounding tissue.

Diagnosis. Fingerprint artifact

Discussion. Many artifacts can degrade image quality, but few cause false-positive mammograms. A fingerprint may mimic microcalcifications of tumor and, if not recognized as such, may result in a false-positive diagnosis. Fingerprint film artifacts are due to improper handling of the film (19). Mishandling before exposure results in a white print; mishandling after exposure produces a black print (20). If only random portions of the fingerprint are visible, it may be difficult to recognize. Such a finding on a single film of a routine mammographic study suggests the possibility of an artifact. The view should be repeated if there is any question that an artifact may be present.

Aunt Minnie's Pearls

- *A fingerprint artifact may mimic microcalcifications of tumor.*

CASE 8

History. 60-year-old woman who underwent breast-conserving surgery with radiation for carcinoma 2 years before the mammogram shown in Figure 8.8.1.

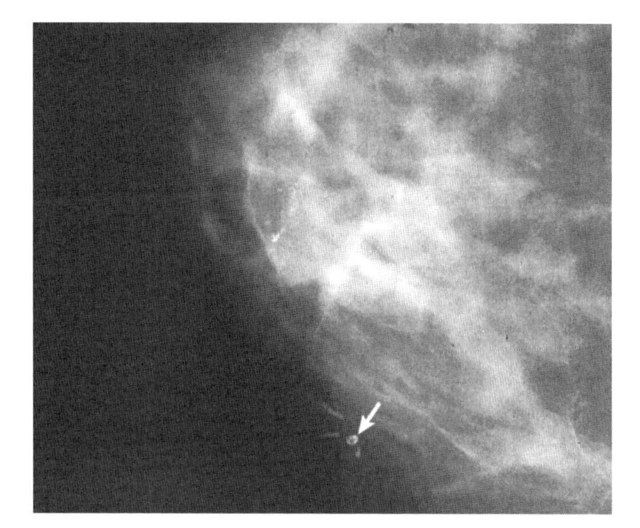

Figure 8.8.1.

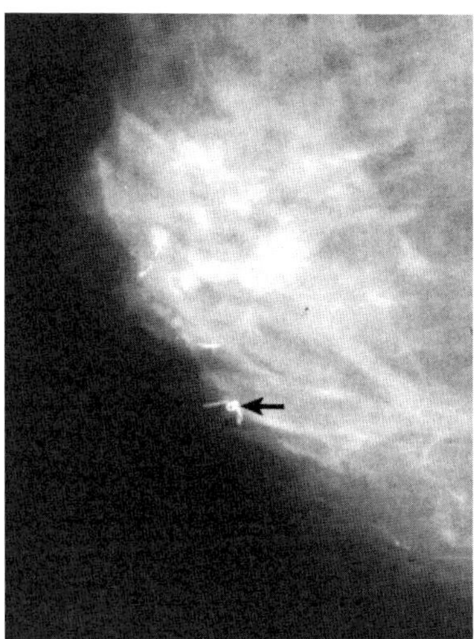

Figure 8.8.2.

Findings. Craniocaudal view of the right breast (Fig. 8.8.1) shows thin, linear calcifications in close proximity to a ring-shaped calcification (*arrow*); 1 year later (Fig. 8.8.2) the calcifications have progressed and have become one continuous structure with a knotted configuration (*arrow*).

Diagnosis. Sutural calcifications

Discussion. Sutures within the breast may rarely calcify. Calcification is more likely if the patient has undergone radiation therapy, which is known to promote soft tissue calcification (21). The knotted configuration is the distinguishing feature. Location within the surgical bed should be confirmed, however, before making this diagnosis.

Aunt Minnie's Pearls

- *Thin, linear, knotted calcifications in surgical bed = sutural calcification.*

CASE 9

History. 49-year-old woman who underwent a procedure on her breasts many years ago and more recently had breast implants placed

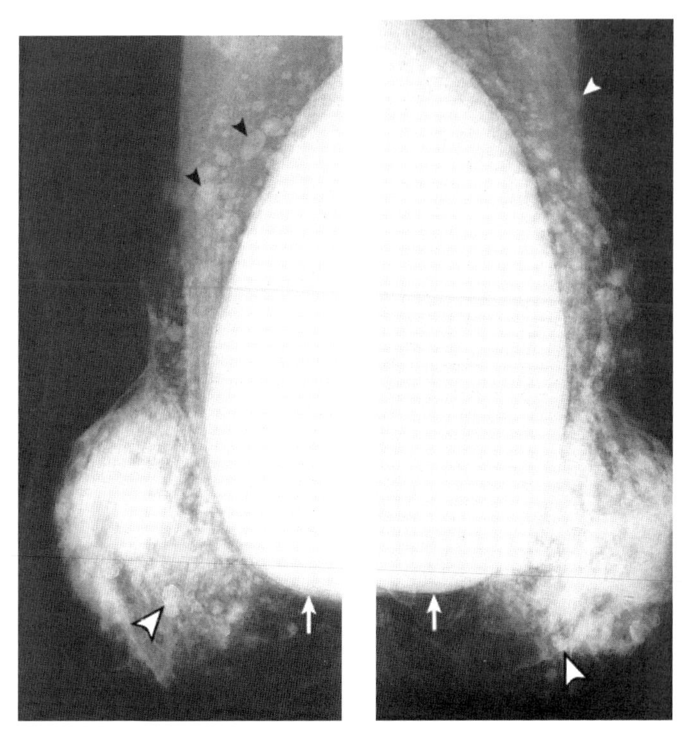

Figure 8.9.1. **Figure 8.9.2.**

Findings. Bilateral mediolateral oblique views (Figs. 8.9.1 and 8.9.2) reveal bilateral subpectoral implants (*arrows*) as well as innumerable oval-to-rounded opacities ranging in size from 1 mm to 1 cm that are distributed fairly evenly throughout both breasts and into the axillae (*solid arrowheads*). Most are of rather uniform medium density, although some have calcified rims (*open arrowheads*).

Diagnosis. Free silicone injected into both breasts. The bilateral implants were placed later and were unrelated to the silicone injections.

Discussion. Injection of free silicone into the breasts was practiced primarily outside this country (it is now illegal), particularly in southeast Asia, as a form of augmentation (22, 23). The silicone is immiscible with body fluids and remains in globular form after injection (24). Some of these deposits calcify, and granulomas result from the body's reaction to the foreign material (25). Streaky opacities may also form when the silicone is absorbed by the lymphatic system—see case 16 (26).

The sheer number and random distribution of the globules, bearing little relationship to the glandular tissue, indicates silicone injection. The fact that the calcified nodules do not have lucent centers indicates that this is not due to fat necrosis alone, although there may be necrosis associated with the regions that contain silicone.

Aunt Minnie's Pearls

- *Innumerable nodules of medium density, some with rim calcifications, in a random distribution = injected silicone.*

CASE 10

History. Withheld

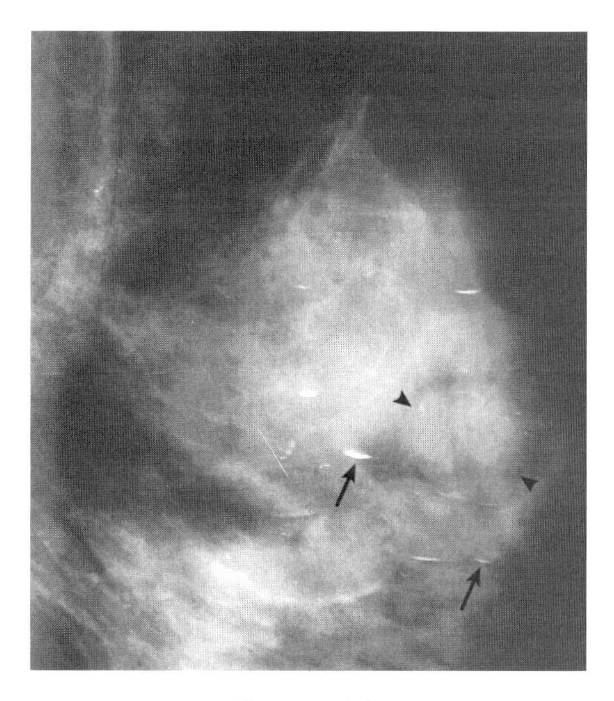

Figure 8.10.1.

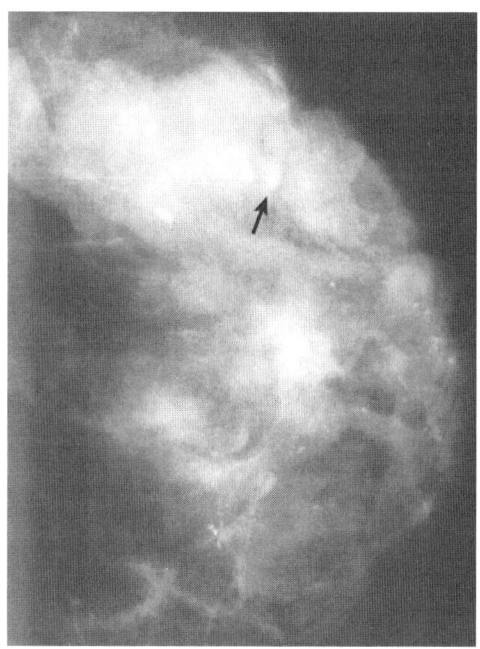

Figure 8.10.2.

Findings. On the mediolateral oblique view (Fig. 8.10.1) there are several high-density crescentic structures, all with an orientation parallel to the floor (*arrows*). They vary in size, but some correspond with a medium-density rounded mass-like opacity (*arrowheads*). On the craniocaudal view (Fig. 8.10.2), the crescents are absent, being replaced by lower density, smudgy, rounded opacities with indistinct, fading margins (*arrow*).

Diagnosis. Milk of calcium

Discussion. Milk of calcium is a benign entity caused by tiny calcium fragments that layer within the dependent portions of a cyst, appearing meniscoid in shape on the lateral view and as a thin-edged disc en face on the craniocaudal view (27). This classic appearance was first described by Lanyi in 1977 and is known as the teacup sign (27). Occasionally, as in this case, the teacups can be seen on the mediolateral oblique view, but often a straight lateral view is needed to demonstrate this feature of milk of calcium. Therefore, when evaluating calcifications that may be milk of calcium, one mammographic projection should be a straight lateral view to avoid missing this obviously benign diagnosis.

Aunt Minnie's Pearls

- *Teacup calcifications = milk of calcium.*
- *Confirm diagnosis with a straight lateral projection.*

CASE 11

History. Withheld

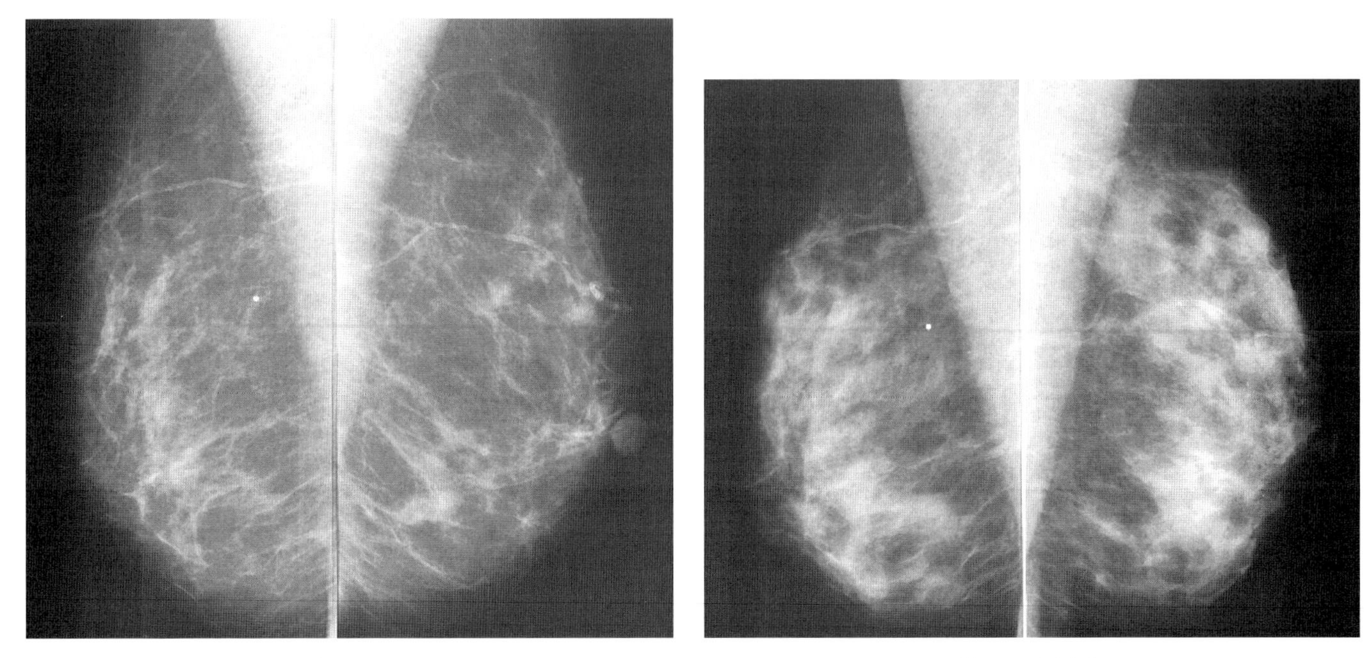

Figure 8.11.1. Figure 8.11.2.

Findings. Bilateral mediolateral oblique view of the breasts (Fig. 8.11.1) shows fat-replaced breasts. A repeat mammogram 2 years later (Fig. 8.11.2) demonstrates marked bilateral diffuse increase in breast density. The increased density takes the form of indistinct wispy and cloud-like opacities that are interspersed with fat and trabeculae; i.e. it has characteristics of normal fibroglandular tissue. Although it is asymmetric, there are no suspicious features.

Diagnosis. Estrogen effect

Discussion. The interval proliferation of normal bilateral breast tissue as shown here is commonly seen after institution of estrogen replacement therapy (28). This response is poorly understood and idiosyncratic, with some women responding dramatically and others showing no response at all (29). A similar hormone effect may also be detected by mammography in some perimenopausal women who experience an endogenous estrogen flare as luteal activity wanes (30). If the patient is not on estrogen replacement, then the radiologist should consider the possibility that the patient may have a source of endogenous estrogen production, e.g., an ovarian mass. Biopsy is not warranted in the absence of other specific signs of carcinoma if the breast physical examination is normal.

Aunt Minnie's Pearls

- *Interval diffuse increase in breast density with fibroglandular character in a patient with changing hormonal status = estrogen effect.*
- *If the patient is not on estrogen replacement, then the radiologist should consider the possibility that the patient may have a source of endogenous estrogen production, e.g., an ovarian mass.*

CASE 12

History. Withheld

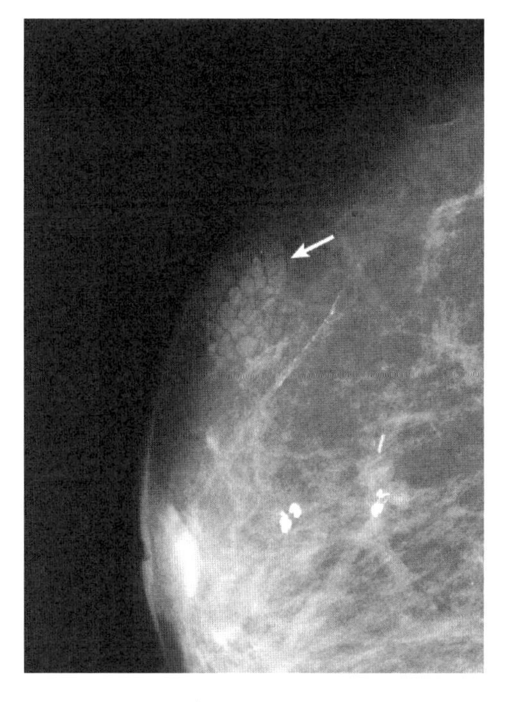

Figure 8.12.1.

Findings. There is a well-defined yet irregular ovoid lesion with a verrucous pattern projected over the upper portion of the breast on this mediolateral oblique view of the right breast (Fig. 8.12.1, *arrow*).

Diagnosis. Seborrheic keratosis

Discussion. Seborrheic keratosis is the most common skin lesion encountered on mammography. Although simple moles are more common, most are not raised enough to be visible on the mammogram. The horny proliferation of the thicker keratosis causes the characteristic verrucous or reticular surface pattern produced by the air-skin interface of the thin interstices between the scaly surface projections. Localization in the skin, using tangential views if necessary, confirms the presence and benign nature of this entity.

Rarely, the interstices may trap materials (e.g., deodorant or talc), and their appearance may mimic that of malignant microcalcifications. Therefore, careful correlation to eliminate a deeper carcinoma fortuitously superimposed on a benign skin lesion may be required (31).

Aunt Minnie's Pearls

- *Verrucous skin lesion = seborrheic keratosis.*

CASE 13

History. 50-year-old woman with a palpable mass at the 1 o'clock position in the left breast

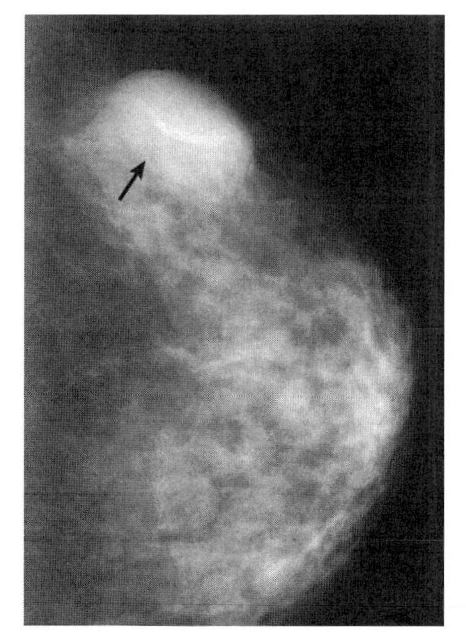

Figure 8.13.1.

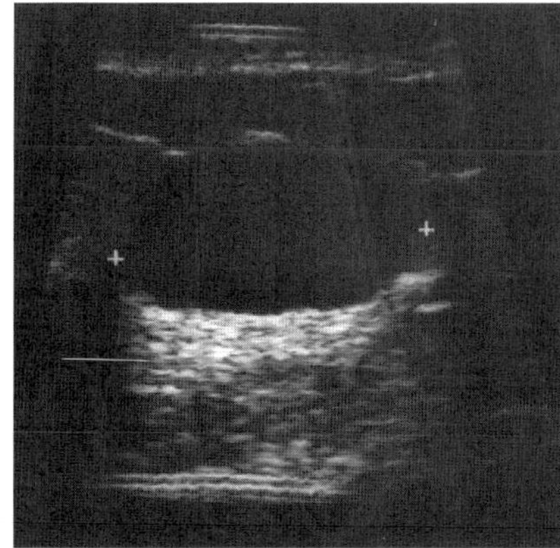

Figure 8.13.2.

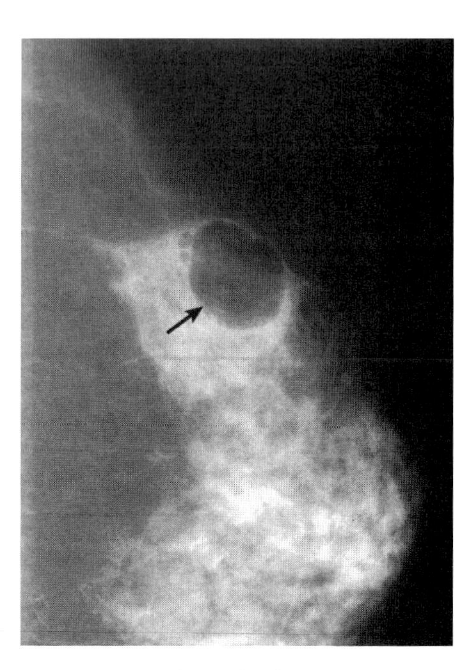

Figure 8.13.3.

Findings. Craniocaudal view of the left breast (Fig. 8.13.1) shows a 3.5-cm oval mass in the lateral breast with well-circumscribed margins (*arrow*). Structures are visible "through" the lesion, indicating that it is a low-density radiopaque mass. Breast sonography (Fig. 8.13.2) shows a completely anechoic, smooth-walled structure with a sharp back wall and enhanced through-transmission (between cursors). Postaspiration pneumocystogram (Fig. 8.13.3) reveals a well demarcated air-filled structure with a smooth inner wall (*arrow*).

Diagnosis. Simple cyst

Discussion. Cysts are some of the commonly encountered abnormalities on mammography. Usually seen in the fourth through sixth decades, they may be solitary or multiple. Patients may present because of palpable cysts, prompting the clinician to request mammography. Generally, the definitive diagnosis requires both mammography and ultrasonography. Only when all criteria exhibited in Fig. 8.13.2 are met can a simple cyst be diagnosed with confidence (32). When ultrasonography is unavailable, pneumocystography can also demonstrate a smooth inner wall by utilizing air as the contrast medium. This procedure is performed mainly to exclude an intracystic mass, a rare cause of cyst formation (33).

Aunt Minnie's Pearls

- *Smooth-walled, fluid-filled mass = simple cyst.*
- *Ultrasound will show a round lesion that is anechoic with a well-defined posterior wall and enhanced through-transmission.*

CASE 14

History. Patient A: 53-year-old woman with bloody discharge from nipple; patient B: 60-year-old woman with palpable mass and no other pertinent history

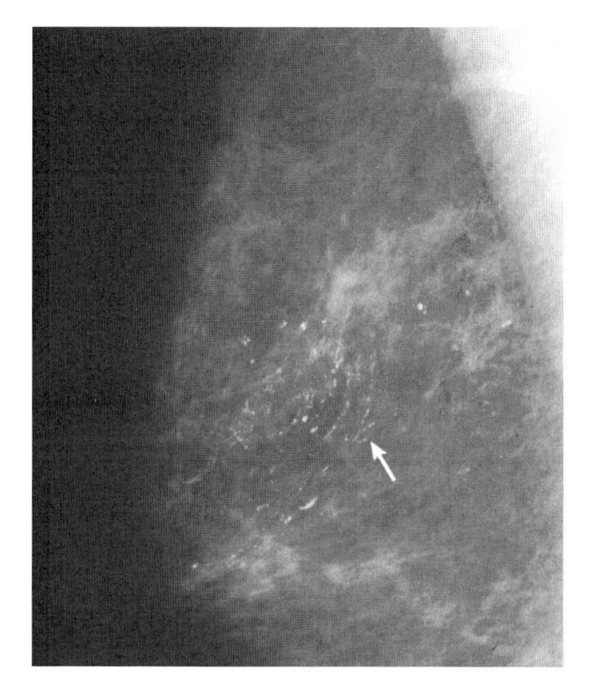

Figure 8.14.1. Patient A.

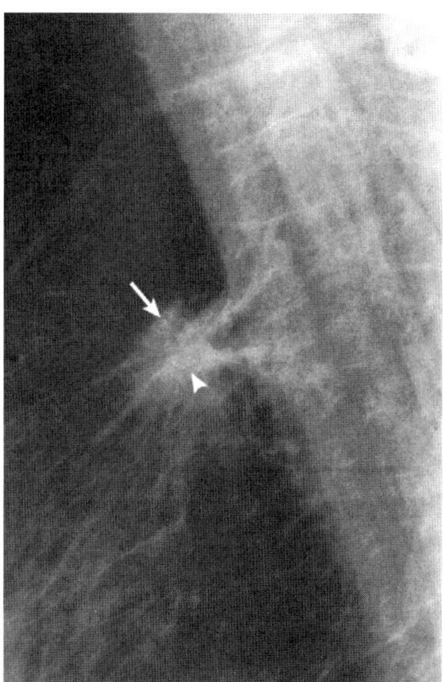

Figure 8.14.2. Patient B.

Findings. Mediolateral view of the right breast in patient A (Fig. 8.14.1) shows "casting" calcifications involving a large part of the breast extending to the nipple. The calcifications are nonuniform, irregular, and branched (*arrow*), and they form a dot-dash linear pattern. They are aligned with the ductal system. Mediolateral view of the right breast in patient B (Fig. 8.14.2) reveals a spiculated mass (*arrow*) with architectural distortion. Within the center of the mass there are irregular (pleomorphic) microcalcifications (*arrowhead*).

Diagnosis. Patient A: carcinoma (largely ductal carcinoma-in-situ, of comedo type); patient B: carcinoma (invasive ductal, not otherwise specified)

Discussion. There are no truly pathognomonic signs of carcinoma of the breast, but the two patterns above approach this standard so closely that it would be remiss not to include them in this chapter. The classic casting calcifications of comedocarcinoma (Fig. 8.14.1) are differentiated from secretory disease by their irregular margins and nonuniform density (34, 35). Secretory calcifications seldom branch (see case 5), although this feature is common in comedocarcinoma. The history of bloody discharge further increases the likelihood of carcinoma (remember that the most common cause of a bloody nipple discharge is actually an intraductal papilloma).

A spiculated mass like that seen in Figure 8.14.2 may indeed be caused by trauma, infection, or radial scar, but the lack of an appropriate history essentially excludes the first two causes. Radial scars are not associated with palpable masses. The pleomorphic calcifications further raise the positive predictive value. Last, the findings had increased over time, yielding the mammographic diagnosis "carcinoma until proven otherwise." The spiculations and architecture distortion usually indicate adjacent soft tissue invasion by the tumor (35).

Aunt Minnie's Pearls

- *Irregular casting calcifications = comedocarcinoma until proven otherwise.*
- *Spiculated mass with pleomorphic microcalcifications = invasive carcinoma until proven otherwise.*

CASE 15

History. Young woman with bilateral silicone breast implants

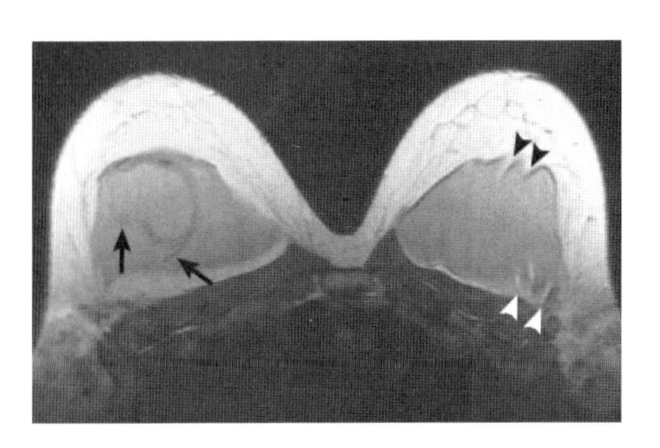

Figure 8.15.1. SE 2680/20.

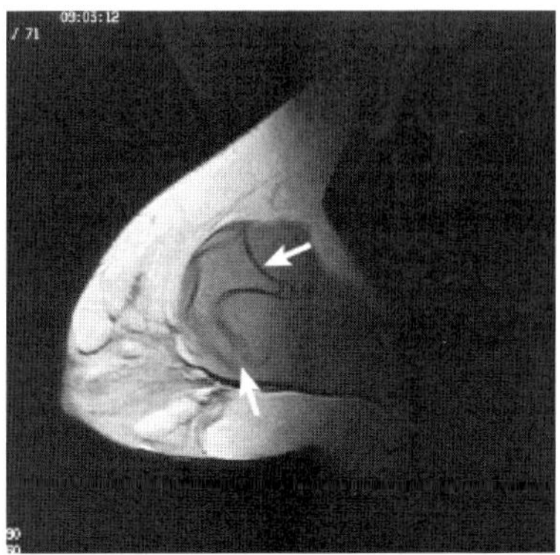

Figure 8.15.2. SE 2680/20.

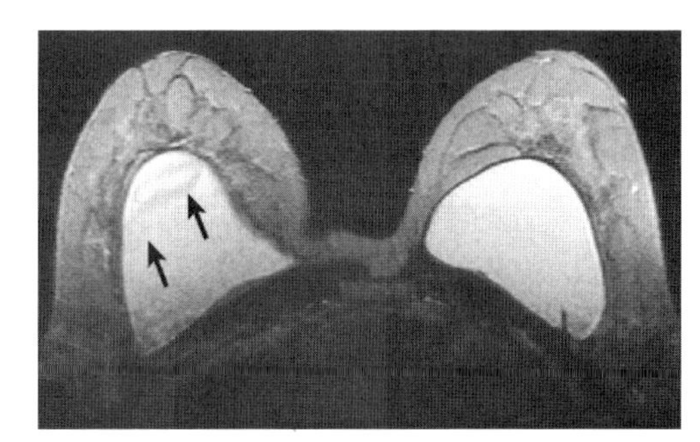

Figure 8.15.3. SE 2680/20.

Findings. An axial MR image of both breasts (Fig. 8.15.1) shows curvilinear low intensity lines in the right breast (*arrows*) floating freely within the medium signal intensity silicone. No silicone is seen outside the implant region. A sagittal MR image (Fig. 8.15.2) also shows the low intensity linear structures (*arrows*) that give the appearance of a collapsed implant shell. Finally, an axial MR image of both breasts obtained slightly more inferiorly (Fig. 8.15.3) reveals a portion of the collapsed implant shell crumpled in the inferior portion of the implant (*arrows*).

Diagnosis. Intracapsular rupture of silicone implant with linguine sign

Discussion. Breast implants become surrounded by a reactive fibrous capsule as the body attempts to isolate the foreign body. The covering that the manufacturer uses to contain the silicone is called the shell. When the shell ruptures and the silicone remains contained within the capsule, the rupture is termed intracapsular (36). This type of rupture may result in no mammographic findings. The collapsed ruptured shell, however, is seen on MR images as linear hypointensities "floating" within the silicone. This appearance has been described as the linguine sign (37). If the linguine sign is present, the shell has ruptured. If no silicone is outside the capsule and the capsule appears intact, the diagnosis is intracapsular rupture. The radiologist should exercise caution in making this diagnosis when the findings are not as obvious as in this case, because normal radial folds in the periphery of the shell (Fig. 8.15.1, *arrowheads*) may closely mimic intracapsular implant rupture.

Aunt Minnie's Pearls

- *Linguine sign = implant shell rupture.*
- *Intact capsule = intracapsular rupture.*

CASE 16

History. Patient with breast implants who noticed a change in the shape and feel of her breast

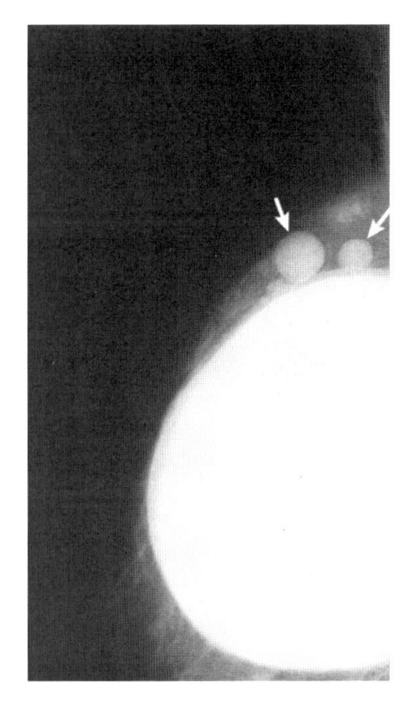

Figure 8.16.1.

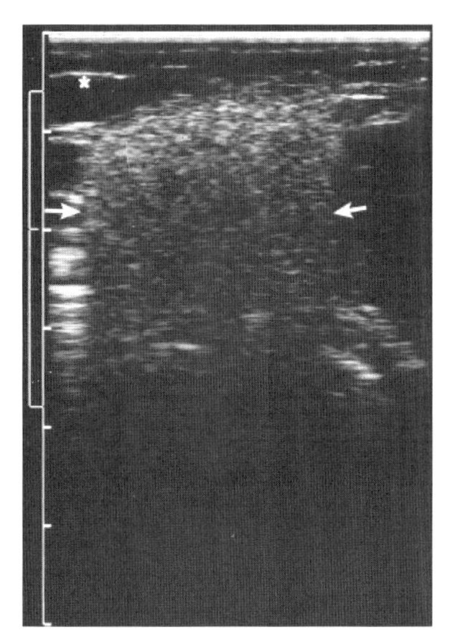

Figure 8.16.2.

Findings. Mediolateral oblique view of the right breast (Fig. 8.16.1) shows two rounded high-density opacities in the breast tail (*arrows*), along with surrounding smaller, less well-defined abnormal opacities. These separate collections of high-density silicone are outside the main portion of the implant and are clearly outside the expected location of the fibrous capsule. The material appears to be extruded into the breast tissue.

A breast sonogram (Fig. 8.16.2) shows a somewhat poorly marginated, intensely hyperechoic collection (*between arrows*) with distal acoustic shadowing. This material is between the subcutaneous tissues and the chest wall and is adjacent to both breast tissue and implant.

Diagnosis. Extracapsular implant rupture with extrusion of silicone

Discussion. When silicone is extruded beyond both the ruptured implant shell and ruptured fibrous capsule, it may appear mammographically as distinct from the main portion of the implant. Streaking of silicone may then be seen in the lymphatics as the material migrates and is cleared lymphatically (Fig. 8.16.1, *arrowhead*). It retains the high-density characteristic of silicone.

Silicone within an intact implant is anechoic at sonography. Free silicone in the breast, however, adopts a hyperechoic texture called the snowstorm pattern (38). The presence of this echogenic material outside an implant capsule has also been termed echogenic confusion because normal structures in the area are obliterated. This phenomenon is likely due to a phase aberration phenomenon (39).

Aunt Minnie's Pearls

- *A collection of silicone separate from an implant on mammography or a snowstorm pattern on ultrasound = extracapsular silicone implant rupture or extrusion.*

CASE 17

History. Withheld

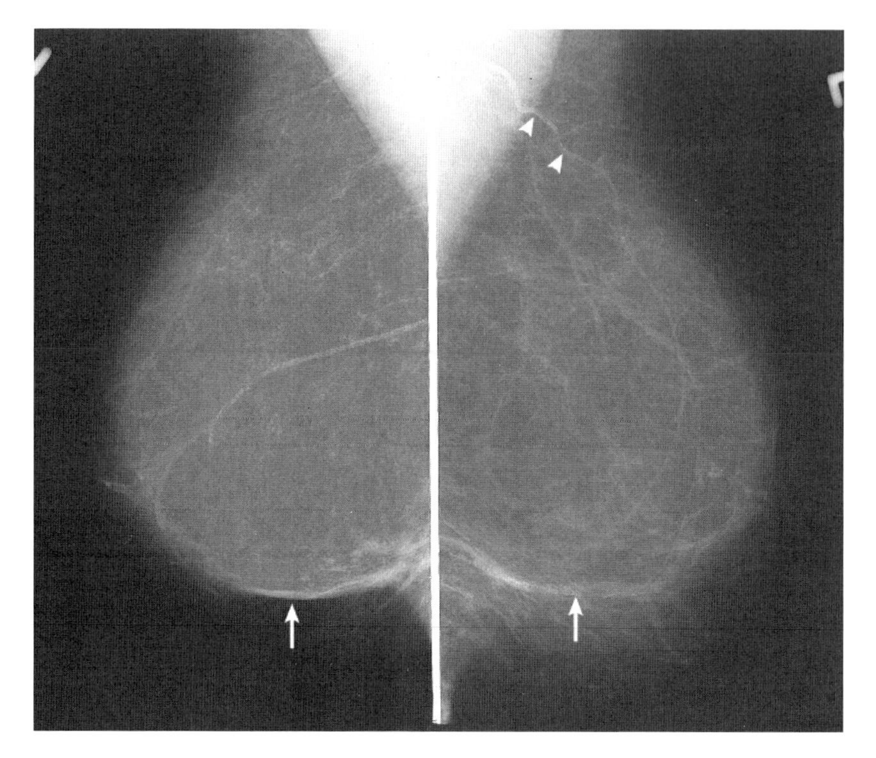

Figure 8.17.1.

Findings. Bilateral mediolateral oblique views of the breasts (Fig. 8.17.1) show curvilinear opacities coursing across the inferior portions of both breasts (*arrows*). Also, no glandular tissue is identified above the level of the nipple. Incidental note is made of characteristic vascular calcifications that are tubular in shape (*arrowheads*).

Diagnosis. Bilateral reduction mammoplasty

Discussion. Reduction mammoplasty is a common surgical procedure that often manifests characteristic changes on mammography. The surgical procedure involves an inframammary incision that is connected to a circumareolar incision by a third vertical incision. Glandular tissue and fat are removed from the breast in the regions of these incisions. This causes the remaining breast tissue to redistribute into the infraareolar portion of the breast on the mediolateral oblique view. Nonanatomic curvilinear bands, often accompanied by dystrophic calcifications, are seen in the inferior breast as in the index case. This combination of findings should allow the radiologist to recognize that the patient has undergone this surgical procedure (40).

Aunt Minnie's Pearls

- *Curvilinear bands and calcifications in the lower breasts, with no glandular tissue seen superior to the nipple = reduction mammoplasty.*

REFERENCES

1. Homer MJ. Imaging features and management of characteristically benign and probably benign breast lesions. Radiol Clin North Am 1987;25:939–951.
2. Berkowitz JE, Gatewood OMB, Donovan GB, Gayler BW. Dermal breast calcifications: localization with template-guided placement of skin marker. Radiology 1987;163:282.
3. Hessler C, Schnyder P, Ozzello L. Hamartoma of the breast: diagnostic observation of 16 cases. Radiology 1978;126:95–98.
4. Riveros M, Cubilla A, Perotta F, Solalinde V. Hamartoma of the breast. J Surg Oncol 1989;42:197–200.
5. Helvie MA, Adler DD, Rebner M, Oberman HA. Breast hamartomas: variable mammographic appearance. Radiology 1989;170:417–421.
6. Kopans D. Breast imaging. Philadelphia: Lippincott, 1989:284.
7. Meyer JE, Silverman P, Gandbhir L. Fat necrosis of the breast. Arch Surg 1978;113:801–805.
8. Evers K, Troupin RH. Lipid cyst: classic and atypical appearances. AJR 1991;157:271–273.
9. Morgan CL, Trought WS, Peete W. Xeromammographic and ultrasonic diagnosis of a traumatic oil cyst. AJR 1978;130:1189–1190.
10. Tabár L, Dean PB. Teaching atlas of mammography. New York: Thieme-Stratton, 1985:172.
11. Homer MJ, Pile-Spellman ER. Marchant DJ, Smith TJ. The normal intramammary lymph node: mammographic appearance and management. Appl Radiol 1985;14:115–122.
12. Kopans DB. Breast imaging. Philadelphia: Lippincott, 1989:105.
13. Egan RL, McSweeney MB. Intramammary lymph nodes. Cancer 1983;51:1838–1842.
14. Lanyi M. Diagnosis and differential diagnosis of breast calcifications. Berlin: Springer-Verlag, 1988:131.
15. Lanyi M. Diagnosis and differential diagnosis of breast calcifications. Berlin: Springer-Verlag, 1988:159.
16. Sickles EA. Breast calcifications: mammographic evaluation. Radiology 1986;160:289–293.
17. Lanyi M. Diagnosis and differential diagnosis of breast calcifications. Berlin: Springer-Verlag, 1988:146.
18. Baker KS, Monsees BS, Diaz NM, Destouet JM, McDivitt RW. Carcinoma within fibroadenomas: mammographic features. Radiology 1990;176:371–374.
19. Wentz G. Mammography for radiologic technologists. New York: McGraw-Hill, 1992:28.
20. Powell DE, Stelling CB. The diagnosis and detection of breast disease. St. Louis: Mosby, 1994:30.
21. Davis SP, Stomper PC, Weidner N, Meyer JE. Suture calcification mimicking recurrence in the irradiated breast: a potential pitfall in mammographic evaluation. Radiology 1989;172:247–248.
22. Steinbach BG, Hardt NS, Abbitt PL, Lanier L, Caffee HH. Breast implants, common complications, and concurrent breast disease. RadioGraphics 1993;13:95–118.
23. Letterman G, Schurter M. History of aesthetic breast surgery. In: Lewis JR, ed. The art of aesthetic plastic surgery. Boston: Little, Brown, 1989;1:24–27.
24. Minagi H, Youker JE, Knudson HW. The roentgen appearance of injected silicone in the breast. Radiology 1968;90:57–61.
25. Koide T, Katayama H. Calcification in augmentation mammoplasty. Radiology 1979;130:337–340.
26. Ganott MA, Harris KM, Ilkhanipour ZS, Costa-Greco MA. Augmentation mammoplasty: normal and abnormal findings with mammography and US. RadioGraphics 1992;12:281–295.
27. Sickles EA, Abele JS. Milk of calcium within tiny benign breast cysts. Radiology 1981;141:655–658.
28. Berkowitz JE, Gatewood OMB, Goldblum LE, Gayler BW. Hormonal replacement therapy: mammographic manifestations. Radiology 1990;174:199–201.
29. Stomper PC, Van Voorhis BJ, Ravnikar VA, Meyer JE. Mammographic changes associated with postmenopausal hormone replacement therapy: a longitudinal study. Radiology 1990;174:487–490.
30. Korenman SG. The endocrinology of breast cancer. Cancer 1980;46:874–878.
31. Kopans DB. Breast imaging. Philadelphia: Lippincott, 1989.
32. Sickles EA. Breast masses: mammographic evaluation. Radiology 1989;173;297–303.
33. Tabár L, Pentek Z, Dean PB. The diagnostic and therapeutic value of breast cyst puncture and pneumocystography. Radiology 1981;141:659–663.
34. Hassler O. Microradiographic investigations of calcifications of the female breast. Cancer 1969;23:1103–1109.
35. Tabár L, Dean P. Teaching atlas of mammography. New York: Thieme-Stratton, 1985:88–89, 138.
36. Dowden RV. Definition of terms for describing loss of gel from breast implants. AJR 1993;160:1360 (letter).
37. Gorczyca DP, Sinha S, Ahn CY, et al. Silicone breast implants in vivo: MR imaging. Radiology 1992;185:407–410.
38. Harris KM, Ganott MA, Shestak KC, Losken HW, Tobon H. Silicone implant rupture: detection with US. Radiology 1993;187:761–768.
39. Rosculet KA, Ikeda DM, Forrest ME, et al. Ruptured gel-filled silicone breast implants: sonographic findings in 19 cases. AJR 1992;159:711–716.
40. Mendelson EB. Evaluation of the postoperative breast. Radiol Clin North Am 1992;30:134–135.

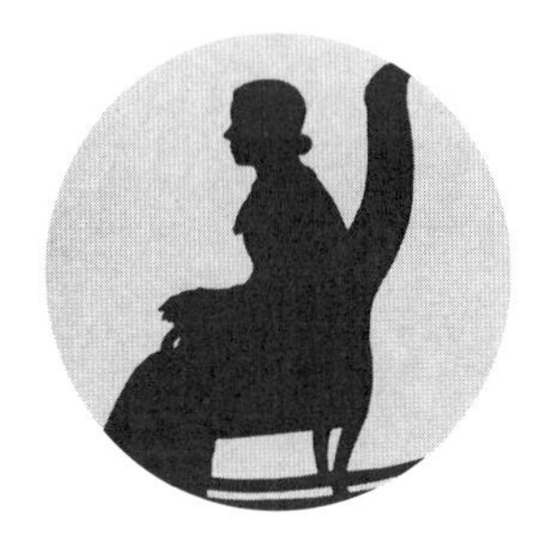

chapter 9

GASTROINTESTINAL RADIOLOGY

ROGER Y. SHIFRIN, ROBERT BECHTOLD, AND DAVID W. GELFAND

CASE 1

History. 56-year-old man with a long history of heartburn

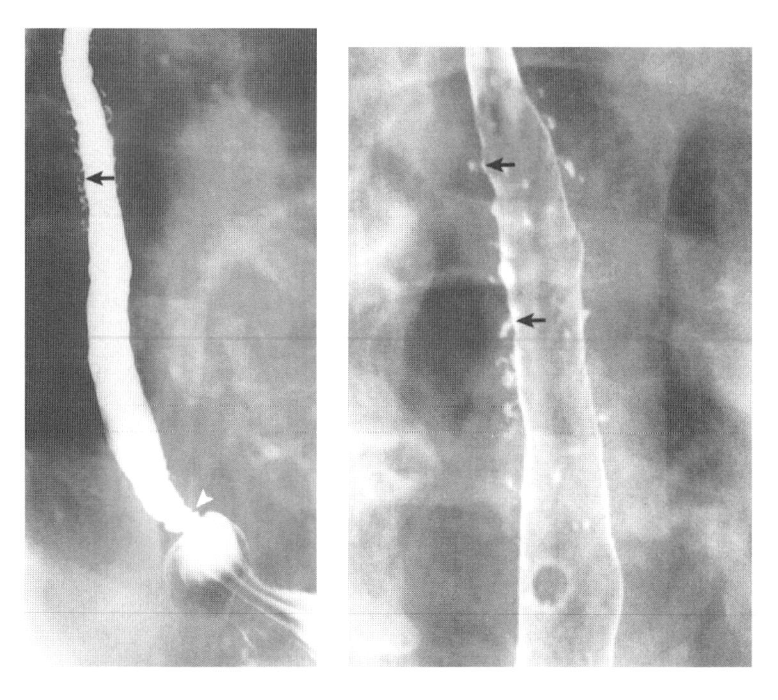

Figure 9.1.1. Figure 9.1.2.

Findings. Single- (Fig. 9.1.1) and double-contrast (Fig. 9.1.2) esophagrams demonstrate innumerable small flask-shaped outpouchings projecting off the esophageal lumen (*arrows*). These outpouchings measure several millimeters in length and width and have tiny ostia connecting them to the lumen of the esophagus. The distribution of the outpouchings is confined primarily to the midportion of the esophagus, although several are also seen in the distal esophagus. Also demonstrated is a sliding hiatal hernia with a stricture (Fig. 9.1.1, *arrowhead*) at the esophagogastric junction.

Diagnosis. Esophageal intramural pseudodiverticulosis with hiatal hernia and peptic stricture

Discussion. Esophageal intramural pseudodiverticulosis is a rare entity in which there is dilatation of the excretory ducts of submucosal mucous glands (1, 2). Approximately 90% of patients have a long history of reflux esophagitis, and most have peptic strictures at the time of diagnosis. The condition is usually diagnosed by means of barium swallow, which reveals the numerous dilated excretory ducts. The distribution of pseudodiverticula may be diffuse or segmental. Although *Candida albicans* has been cultured from the esophagus in about half of affected patients, it is not thought to play any causal role in the development of pseudodiverticula and is likely just a secondary saprophyte. The condition itself is benign, and treatment should be directed toward the underlying reflux disease and stricture.

Aunt Minnie's Pearls

- *Numerous tiny flask-shaped outpouchings from the esophagus = intramural pseudodiverticulosis.*
- *This entity is associated with chronic esophagitis and peptic strictures.*

CASE 2

History. Dysphagia and halitosis

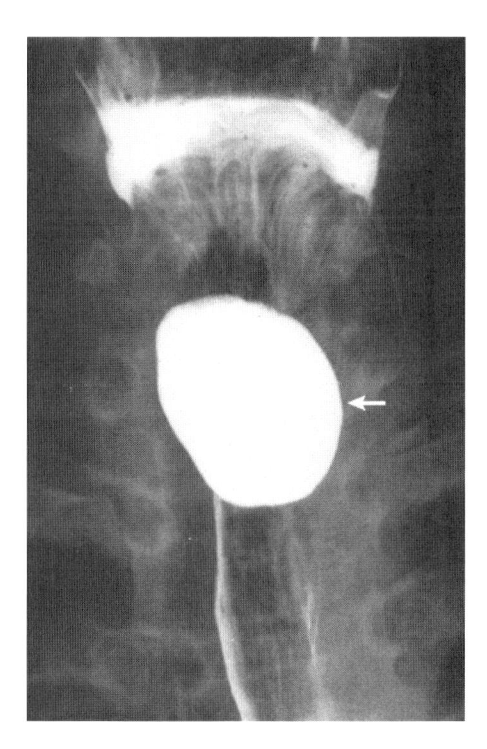

Figure 9.2.1.

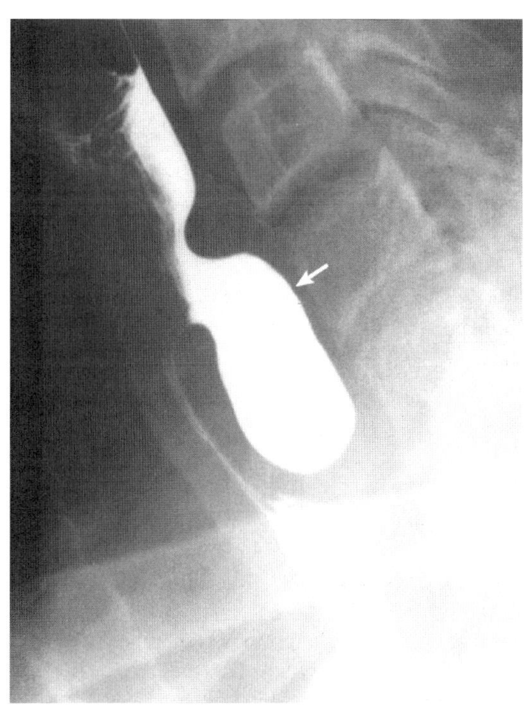

Figure 9.2.2.

Findings. Anteroposterior (Fig. 9.2.1) and lateral (Fig. 9.2.2) views of the neck obtained during a barium swallow study demonstrate a contrast-filled pouch (*arrow*) emanating from the posterior aspect of the esophagus just at the level of the pharyngoesophageal junction. The internal wall of the pouch is smooth, and the proximal esophageal folds are unremarkable. The proximal cervical esophagus is displaced anteriorly by the contrast-filled pouch.

Diagnosis. Zenker's diverticulum

Discussion. A Zenker's diverticulum is a pulsion pseudodiverticulum of the pharyngoesophageal junction. It arises as a result of uncoordinated relaxation of the upper esophageal sphincter (primarily the cricopharyngeus muscle) as a food bolus is delivered from the pharynx (3, 4). This produces elevated pressure in the hypopharynx and eventually leads to herniation of mucosa through a triangular defect in the posterior aspect of the inferior pharyngeal constrictor muscle known as Killian's dehiscence. These "diverticula" may become large, and patients frequently present with dysphagia, regurgitation, aspiration, pneumonia, weight loss, and halitosis.

Aunt Minnie's Pearls

- *A Zenker's diverticulum is a pulsion pseudodiverticulum that occurs through Killian's dehiscence.*

CASE 3

History. Epigastric pain

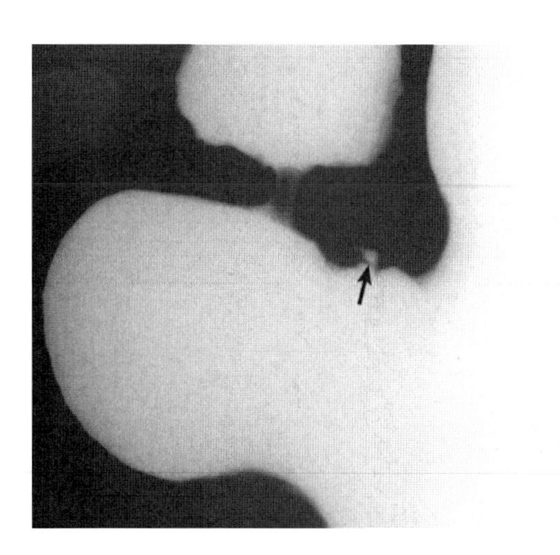

Figure 9.3.1.

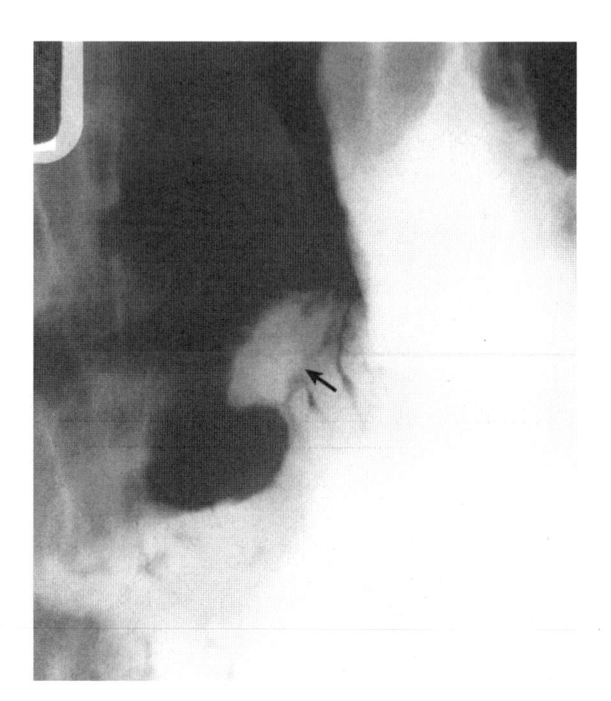

Figure 9.3.2.

Findings. A view from a barium upper gastrointestinal series in two different patients (Figs. 9.3.1 and 9.3.2) demonstrates a small collection of contrast material along the lesser curvature of the stomach, consistent with gastric ulcers. At the base of each ulcer crater, a thin radiolucent line is seen separating the ulcers from the gastric lumen (*arrows*).

Diagnosis. Benign gastric ulcers, each with a Hampton's line

Discussion. Numerous radiographic signs have been reported in the literature to establish benignity of gastric ulcers (5). Smooth mucosal folds that extend to the edge of the ulcer crater are a reliable indicator of benignity. The smooth nature of the folds must be seen with certainty, because nodular radiating folds may indicate an ulcerated malignancy. Other signs of a benign gastric ulcer are the ulcer collar, Hampton's line, and the penetration sign. The ulcer collar represents a rim of mucosa along the margin of the ulcer crater that is lifted by submucosal edema. An etiologically related sign, the Hampton's line, is an extremely narrow radiolucent line (1–2 mm) that separates the ulcer crater from the gastric lumen. This sign is rarely seen but virtually assures the benign nature of the ulcer, because a tumor mass would not be expected to preserve a thin band of normal mucosa at its margin. The penetration sign is seen when the ulcer crater, viewed in profile, projects beyond the gastric lumen. The single best sign of a benign ulcer is complete healing after a course of conservative medical therapy.

Aunt Minnie's Pearls

- *Signs of a benign gastric ulcer include smooth radiating mucosal folds, penetration sign, ulcer collar, and especially a Hampton's line.*
- *Complete ulcer healing with medical therapy is the best sign of benignity.*

CASE 4

History. No acute complaints and no history of surgery

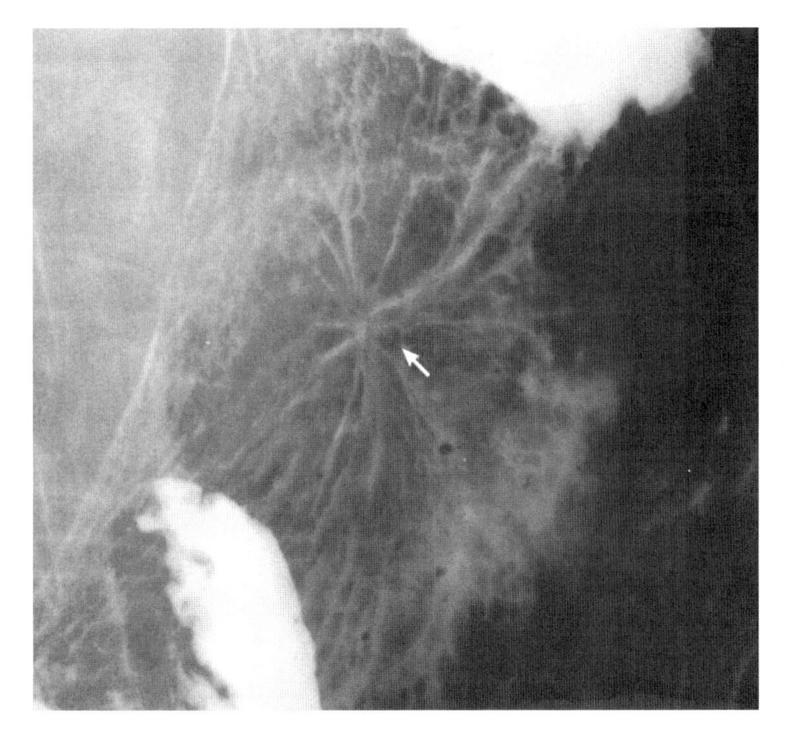

Figure 9.4.1.

Findings. An air-contrast spot film of the stomach (Fig. 9.4.1) shows a stellate pattern of smooth, thin radiating folds along the lesser curvature of the stomach (*arrow*).

Diagnosis. Healed ulcer scar

Discussion. Several reports in the literature have described the appearance of the stomach after partial or complete healing of a benign gastric ulcer (6). The appearance of the so-called ulcer scar is variable. The four most common appearances of the ulcer scar are (*a*) smooth, converging folds that may meet at the center, (*b*) converging folds with a central pit or depression, (*c*) converging folds with a linear center, and (*d*) a residual pit or depression without radiating folds. Deformity of the stomach, usually in the antrum, may also be seen with healed ulcers. Demonstration of the ulcer scar requires the application of surface tension to a portion of the stomach that is nondistensible as a result of fibrosis. This may be accomplished by distending the stomach with air and barium. However, if barium alone is used to distend the stomach, the underlying scar is rendered inconspicuous. Therefore, the gastric ulcer scar is usually only seen on air-contrast upper gastrointestinal series.

Aunt Minnie's Pearls

- *Smooth, thin radiating folds, with or without central depression or central linear scar, indicate a healed gastric ulcer.*
- *Ulcer scars are seen only on air-contrast upper gastrointestinal series.*

CASE 5

History. Epigastric pain

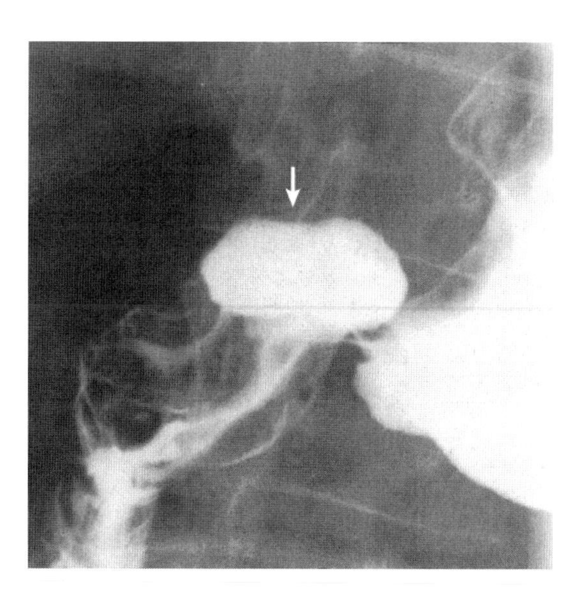

Figure 9.5.1.

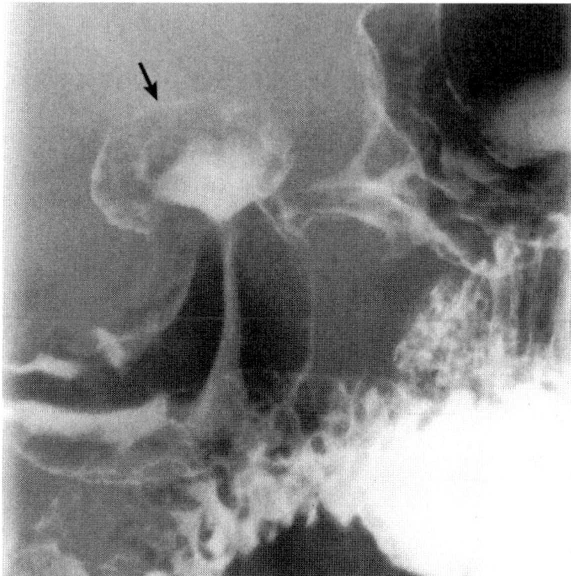

Figure 9.5.2.

Findings. A spot film from an upper gastrointestinal series (Fig. 9.5.1) demonstrates a large ovoid collection of barium (*arrow*) that replaces the proximal duodenal bulb and is surrounded by thickened mucosal folds. In the next image, the barium collection has evacuated, and the cavity is demonstrated in air-contrast (Fig. 9.5.2, *arrow*). The shape of the cavity is constant on the two films, and no normal duodenal bulb is seen.

Diagnosis. Giant duodenal ulcer

Discussion. A giant duodenal ulcer is simply a peptic ulcer of the duodenal bulb in which the ulcer crater occupies a considerable fraction of the total size of the duodenal bulb. Various measurements have been reported in the literature, and a meaningful figure to aid in the diagnosis of this entity is the ulcer-to-bulb ratio proposed by Eisenberg and colleagues (7). This ratio is the longest diameter of the ulcer, divided by the longest diameter of the bulb including the ulcer. If this measurement is 0.8 or greater, a diagnosis of giant duodenal ulcer can be made with confidence. The relevance of the giant duodenal ulcer and the impetus for its consideration as a separate entity is because there is a much higher incidence of hemorrhage and perforation caused by the greater area of ulceration involved. In the past, patients were often brought swiftly to surgery after diagnosis of giant duodenal ulcer. However, with the availability of H_2 receptor antagonists and other antiacid therapy, patients are usually observed during a course of conservative medical therapy.

Aunt Minnie's Pearls

- *A giant duodenal ulcer is present when the ulcer-to-bulb ratio is ≥0.8.*
- *Giant duodenal ulcers carry an increased risk of hemorrhage and perforation.*

CASE 6

History. 37-year-old immunocompromised man with odynophagia

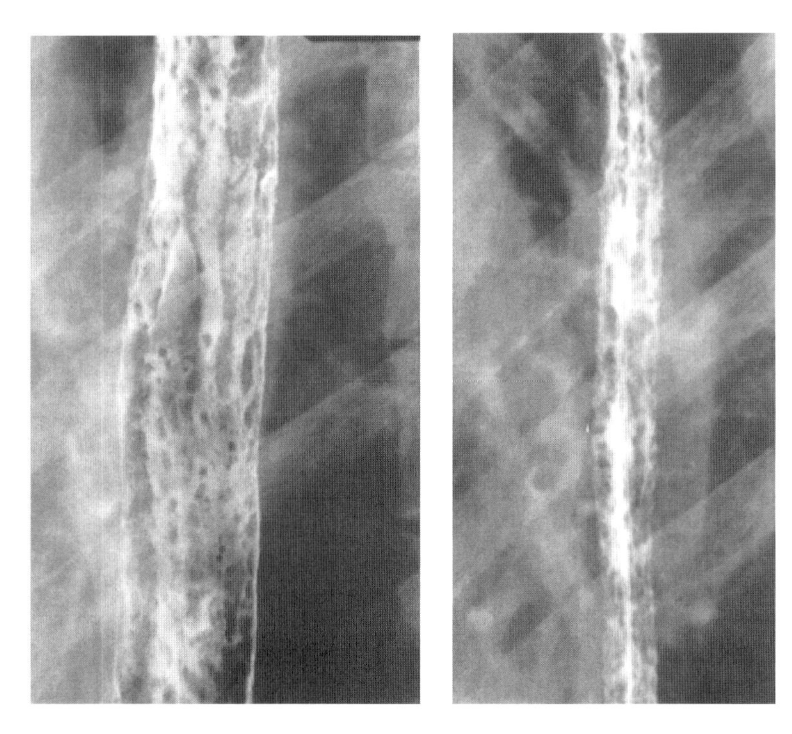

Figure 9.6.1. Figure 9.6.2.

Findings. Double-contrast (Fig. 9.6.1) and mucosal-relief (Fig. 9.6.2) esophagrams reveal diffuse and irregular plaque-like filling defects.

Diagnosis. Esophageal candidiasis

Discussion. Infectious esophagitis is an increasingly common problem in patients with the human immunodeficiency virus, malignancy, chronic immunosuppression for organ transplantation, or other illnesses that compromise the patient's immune status. Although various etiologic agents may be implicated in infectious esophagitis, the most common offending organism is *Candida albicans*. Affected patients typically present with dysphagia, odynophagia, or chest pain. The roentgenographic appearance of *Candida* esophagitis is that of irregular plaque-like filling defects that tend to be oriented along the long axis of the esophagus. With severe involvement, the plaques become coalescent and produce a "shaggy esophagus" (8). Although this appearance is characteristic of *Candida* esophagitis, advanced herpetic esophagitis may have a similar appearance. Furthermore, the compromised immune status of these patients places them at increased risk for other infections that may be superimposed on the *Candida* esophagitis.

Aunt Minnie's Pearls

- *Plaque-like filling defects = esophageal candidiasis.*
- *Esophageal candidiasis is usually seen in immunocompromised patients.*

CASE 7

History. 14-year-old Korean boy with abdominal pain

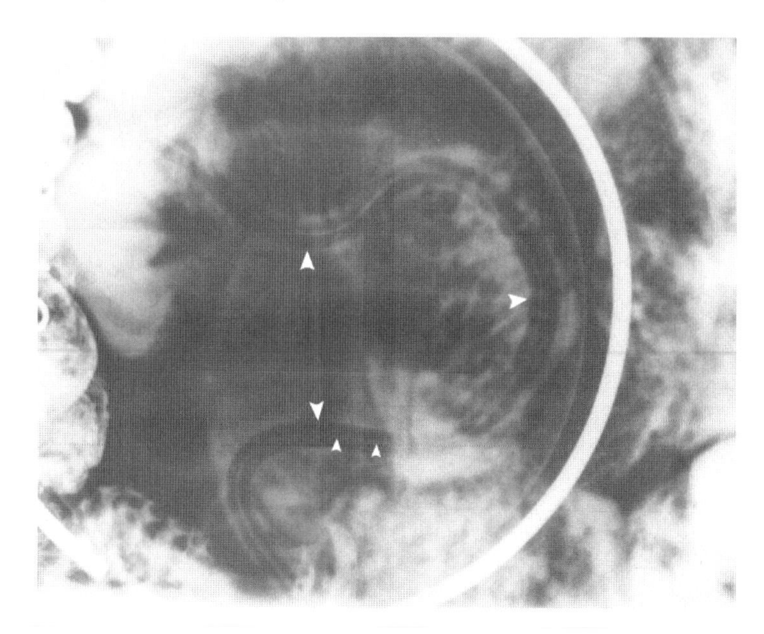

Figure 9.7.1.

Findings. A fluoroscopic spot film obtained during a small bowel follow-through (Fig. 9.7.1) shows a tubular radiolucent filling defect (*large arrowheads*) within the lumen of the small bowel. A thin opaque line (*small arrowheads*) is seen coursing through the center of the tubular filling defect.

Diagnosis. Enteric ascariasis

Discussion. Infection with *Ascaris lumbricoides* is one of the most common parasitic infections worldwide. The condition is endemic in the tropics and subtropics, and sporadic cases appear throughout the world. Human infection begins with the ingestion of food contaminated with ova from the feces of infected hosts. The developing larvae penetrate the intestinal wall and migrate through the portal venous system, liver, heart, and lungs where they penetrate the pulmonary alveolar capillaries and migrate up the tracheobronchial tree. Upon reaching the glottis, the developing larvae are swallowed and again begin their descent down the alimentary tract. The larvae reach sexual maturity after approximately 10 weeks in the intestines. After copulation, the adult female deposits about 200,000 ova per day! These ova are eliminated in the excreta, and the life cycle begins again. Human infection is often without significant morbidity. The pulmonary phase may be accompanied by mild, nonspecific complaints including cough and fever and possibly patchy alveolar infiltrates on chest radiographs. The intestinal phase may be clinically silent, although massive infestation may produce abdominal pain related to obstruction (vermicular ileus). Malnutrition and biliary obstruction may also occur (9). Barium small bowel examination reveals the adult worms as radiolucent filling defects in the lumen of the intestine, with a characteristic thin column of barium in the alimentary tract of the adult worm.

Aunt Minnie's Pearls

- *Ascariasis is endemic in the tropics and subtropics.*
- *Barium within the alimentary tract of the adult worm is characteristic.*

CASE 8

History. Withheld

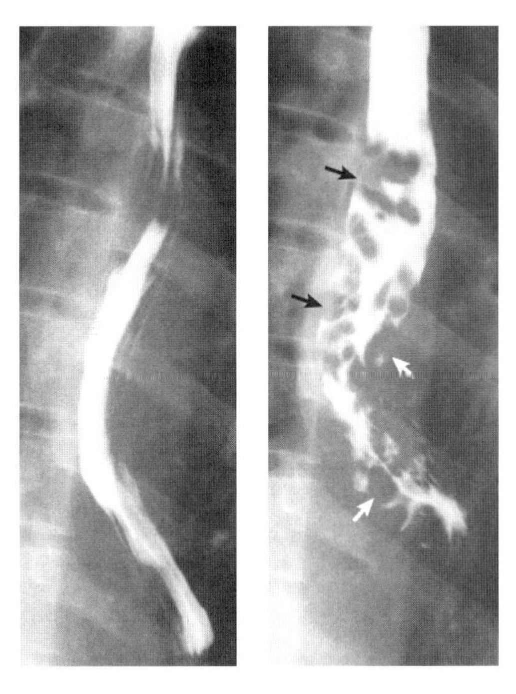

Figure 9.8.1. Figure 9.8.2.

Findings. The initial upright oblique full column esophagram film (Fig. 9.8.1) is unremarkable. The following film (Fig. 9.8.2) obtained with the patient in the recumbent position demonstrates serpiginous, nodular filling defects (*arrows*).

Diagnosis. Esophageal varices

Discussion. Esophageal varices represent portal-systemic venous collateral pathways. They occur most commonly in the setting of portal hypertension in which venous blood from the splanchnic system is shunted through the esophageal/paraesophageal venous plexus into the azygous system and superior vena cava. Because of the cephalad direction of flow through the varices, these are referred to as "uphill" varices. Esophageal varices develop less commonly in the setting of superior vena cava obstruction, in which venous blood from the head, upper extremities, and trunk is shunted through the esophageal/paraesophageal venous plexus and into the portal or azygous systems. These collaterals are referred to as "downhill" varices (10). The clinical relevance of esophageal varices lies in their tendency for rupture with potentially severe upper gastrointestinal bleeding.

Varices may appear as nodular, serpiginous filling defects on barium esophagography. It is important to recognize the changing character of the filling defects during fluoroscopy, because fixed defects may be encountered with varicoid carcinoma. Because the varices may be intermittently decompressed as a result of esophageal peristalsis and changing perfusion pressure during the exam, various provocative maneuvers have been proposed to increase the visualization of the varices. Common maneuvers used in radiology include prone and upright patient positioning and performance of Valsalva and Müller maneuvers (11).

Aunt Minnie's Pearls

- *Changing, serpiginous filling defects in the esophagus = varices.*
- *"Uphill" varices are due to portal hypertension.*
- *"Downhill" varices are due to superior vena cava obstruction.*

CASE 9

History. 43-year-old woman with a history of a malignant skin lesion

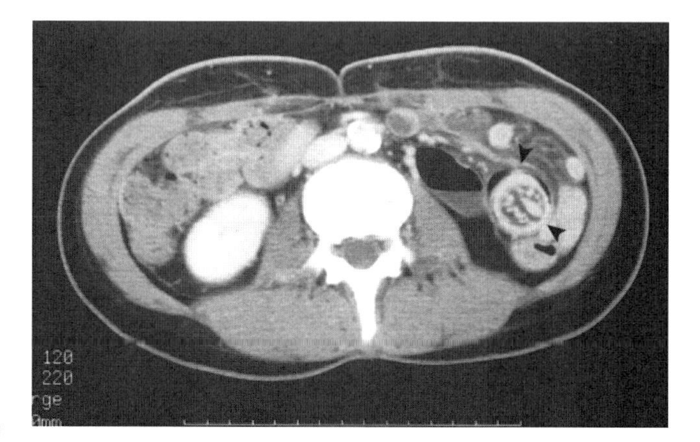

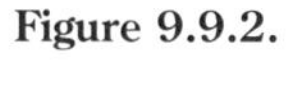

Figure 9.9.2.

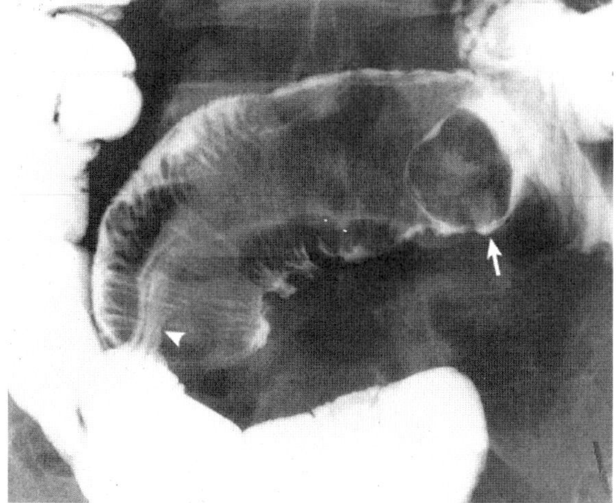

Figure 9.9.1.

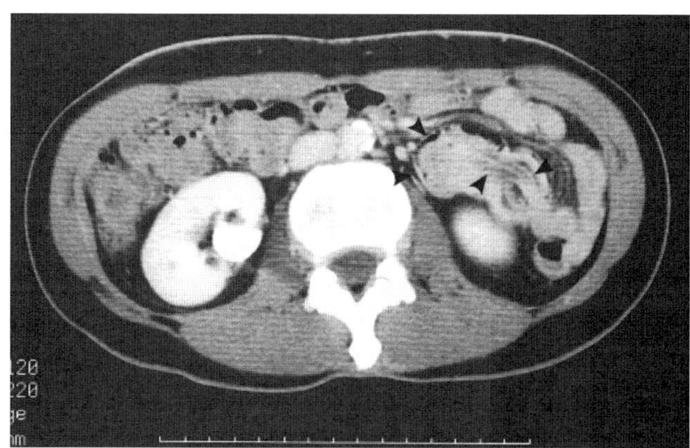

Figure 9.9.3.

Findings. A single view from a peroral small bowel follow-through examination (Fig. 9.9.1) demonstrates a filling defect within the small bowel, surrounded by a "coiled spring" pattern of mucosal folds. The leading edge of the filling defect looks like a mass (*arrow*). Barium extends into the central portion of the mass (*arrowhead*), which is a distinguishing feature of this case. CT confirms the abnormality and shows a filling defect in the small bowel, which has concentric bands of high and low attenuation (Figs. 9.9.2 and 9.9.3, *arrowheads*).

Diagnosis. Small-bowel intussusception secondary to metastatic melanoma

Discussion. Idiopathic intussusception is a disease of the young. When intussusception is encountered in older individuals or neonates, a pathologic lead point is a primary consideration. In this case, the melanoma metastasis is seen leading the intussusceptum into the intussuscipiens. Peutz-Jeghers syndrome, lymphoma, lipomas, or Meckel's diverticula may also present as lead masses. Causes of transient intussusception include scleroderma, sprue, and cystic fibrosis. The "coiled-spring" (12, 13) appearance is due to projection of inflamed and engorged mucosa into a barium pool that has retrogradely filled the lumen of the intussuscipiens. The alternating bands of high and low attenuation demonstrated by CT are due to intussuscepted mesenteric fat contrasted with mucosal-muscular interfaces (14).

Aunt Minnie's Pearls

- *"Coiled-spring" appearance on small bowel follow-through = intussusception.*
- *Suspect a lead point in neonates, older children, and adults.*

CASE 10

History. 37-year-old woman with epigastric pain

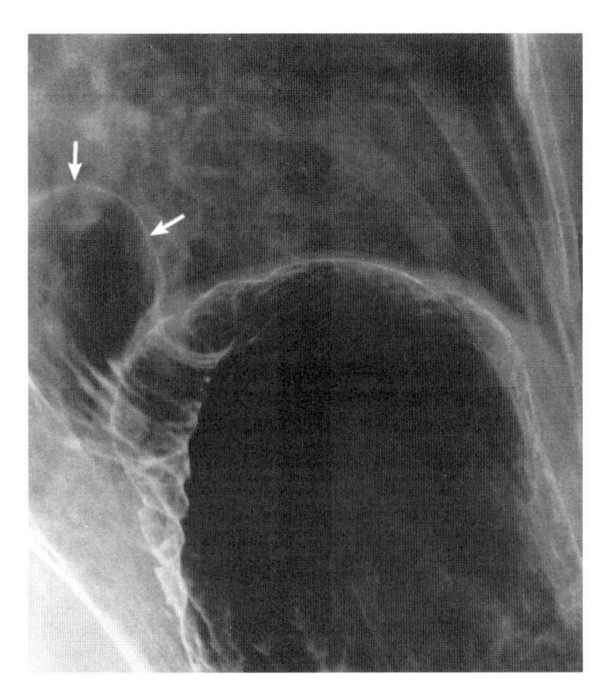

Figure 9.10.1.

Findings. A fluoroscopic spot film from air-contrast upper gastrointestinal series (Fig. 9.10.1) shows the esophagogastric junction to be in its normal anatomic position. A small portion of the gastric fundus is seen above the diaphragm alongside the distal esophagus (*arrows*).

Diagnosis. Paraesophageal hiatal hernia

Discussion. Hernias of the esophagogastric junction through the esophageal diaphragmatic hiatus are a relatively common entity. Based on anatomic considerations, various classification schemes have been proposed for these hernias. The most widely used classification system includes the "sliding" hiatal hernia, the paraesophageal or "rolling" hiatal hernia, or a mixture of these two. The most common type of hiatal hernia is the simple sliding hernia (not pictured) (15). It is thought that this is caused by a defect in the phrenoesophageal membrane, which allows cephalad migration of the esophagogastric junction through the esophageal hiatus. There is a high incidence of gastroesophageal reflux associated with the sliding hiatal hernia. The rolling or paraesophageal hiatal hernia, in contrast to the sliding hernia, maintains a normal position of the esophagogastric junction relative to the esophageal diaphragmatic hiatus. However, a portion of the gastric fundus or cardia herniates through a defect in the diaphragm or phrenoesophageal membrane and is located alongside the normally positioned distal esophagus. The clinical significance of this entity is the potential for incarceration of the hernia sac with compromise of the vascular supply and subsequent gastric infarction and perforation (10).

Aunt Minnie's Pearls

- *A sliding hernia is associated with gastroesophageal reflux.*
- *A paraesophageal hernia has potential for incarceration and strangulation.*

CASE 11

History. 46-year-old woman with dysphagia

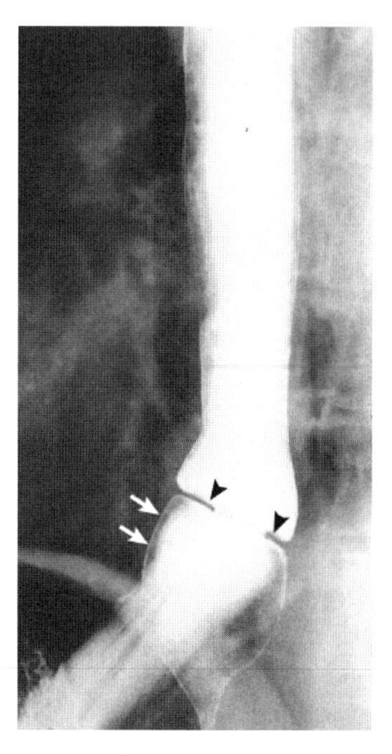

Figure 9.11.1.

Findings. A single contrast prone-oblique barium esophagram (Fig. 9.11.1) shows a "sliding" type hiatal hernia (*arrows*) with a 13-mm annular narrowing (*arrowheads*) at the junction of the hernia sac with the inferior aspect of the esophageal vestibule. This narrowing remained fixed on multiple views, as well as during real time fluoroscopy.

Diagnosis. Lower esophageal mucosal ring or Schatzki's ring

Discussion. The lower esophageal mucosal ring represents a thin, annular narrowing of the esophageal lumen located at the gastroesophageal junction (B line). The term lower esophageal ring was introduced by Schatzki and Gary in 1953, and this entity is still sometimes referred to as the Schatzki's ring (16). Note, however, that Schatzki described patients with mucosal rings and with dysphagia particularly for solid food. Although some mucosal rings produce dysphagia (especially if the internal diameter of the ring is ≤13 mm), many wide-aperture rings are asymptomatic. Therefore, the preferred term for this entity is lower esophageal mucosal ring. Various theories regarding the pathogenesis of the mucosal ring have been proposed, including congenital and acquired causes. The absence of rings in young patients argues against a congenital origin, and the weight of evidence supports the origin of the ring as a thin peptic stricture in patients with chronic reflux esophagitis (16).

Aunt Minnie's Pearls

- *A lower esophageal mucosal ring is a thin, fixed annular narrowing at the gastroesophageal junction.*
- *Solid food dysphagia occurs if ring aperture is small (≤13 mm).*

CASE 12

History. 69-year-old man with suspected abdominal injury after a motor vehicle accident

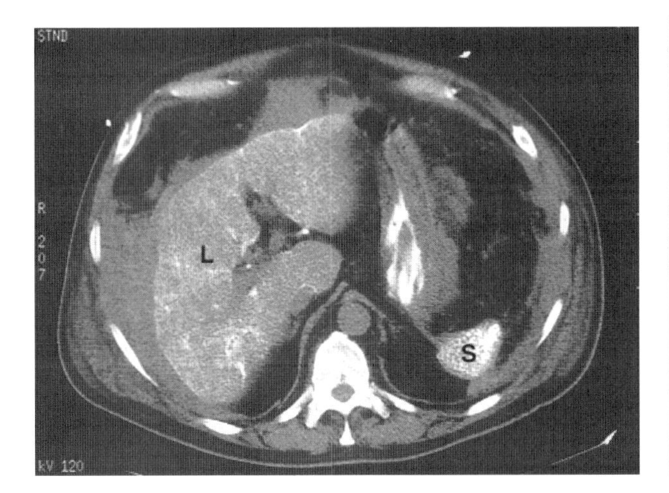

Figure 9.12.1.

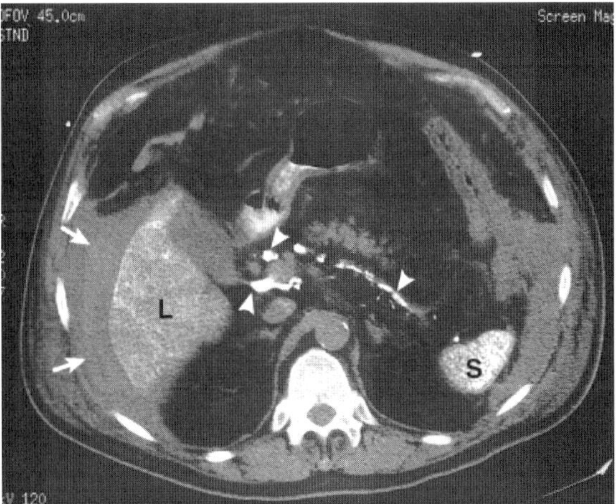

Figure 9.12.2.

Findings. The examination is performed without intravascular contrast (normally a contrast enhanced CT is performed on trauma patients). Two axial CT images through the midabdomen (Figs. 9.12.1 and 9.12.2) reveal irregular reticular densities in the liver parenchyma (L) and dense opacification of the spleen (S). Additionally, there is confluent opacification of numerous peripancreatic, periportal, and portocaval lymph nodes (*arrowheads*). The presence of perihepatic and perisplenic fluid collections with hyperdense components (*arrows*) is diagnostic of acute hemoperitoneum.

Diagnosis. (*a*) Previous Thorotrast exposure; (*b*) acute hemoperitoneum

Discussion. Thorotrast (20% thorium dioxide or thorium-232) was widely used as a radiographic contrast material from the late 1920s through the early 1950s. After administration, Thorotrast is absorbed and concentrated by the reticuloendothelial system. Thorium is a radioactive material (alpha-particle emitter) with a biologic half-life of approximately 400 years. The use of Thorotrast was discontinued in the 1950s because of the concern for long-term radiation effects. Indeed it has been shown that people exposed to Thorotrast have an increased incidence of primary hepatic and splenic malignancies, especially angiosarcoma. Other carcinomas that occur with increased frequency in patients with this exposure history include cholangiocarcinomas, hepatocellular carcinomas, and even transitional cell carcinomas of the genitourinary tract. The characteristic CT manifestations of Thorotrast exposure include a reticular opacification of the liver as well as dense opacification of the spleen and peripancreatic and periportal lymph nodes (17). Dense opacification of the spleen may also be seen with sickle cell anemia, but this can be differentiated from Thorotrast exposure by the absence of liver opacities and the patient's age.

Aunt Minnie's Pearls

- *Thorotrast exposure causes dense opacification of the reticuloendothelial system.*
- *This alpha-particle emitter places the patient at increased risk for various carcinomas and is therefore no longer in use.*

CASE 13

History. Withheld

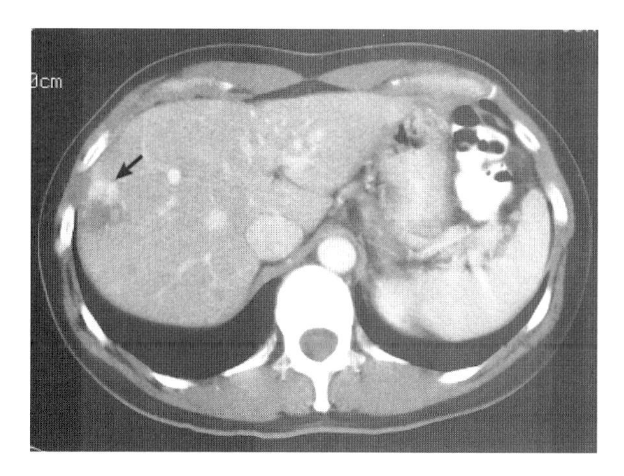

Figure 9.13.1. During bolus contrast infusion

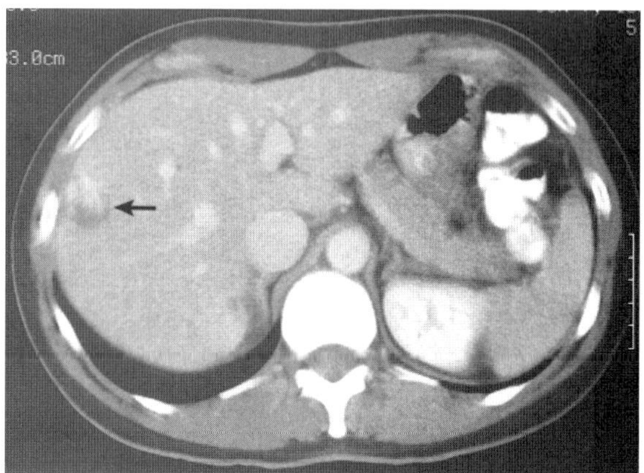

Figure 9.13.2. 1 minute after infusion.

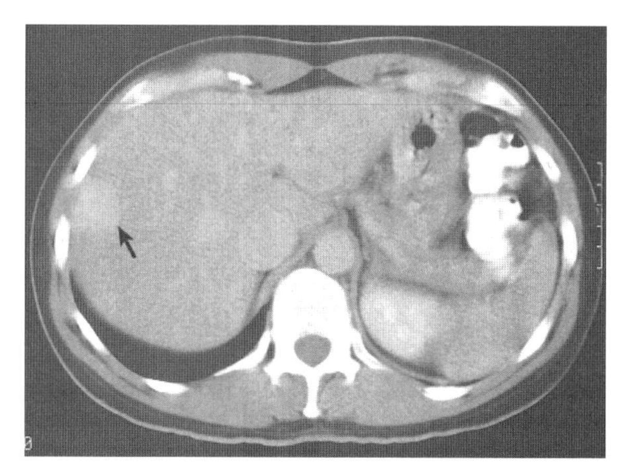

Figure 9.13.3. 10 minutes after infusion.

Findings. Three serial dynamic CT scans of the liver after bolus contrast infusion demonstrate enhancement of a lesion that is initially peripheral and nodular in nature (Fig. 9.13.1, *arrow*). The enhancement progresses in a centripetal fashion until the lesion "fills in" and is homogeneously hyperdense (Figs. 9.13.2 and 9.13.3, *arrows*) relative to the surrounding liver parenchyma.

Diagnosis. Hepatic cavernous hemangioma

Discussion. Cavernous hemangioma is the most common benign tumor of the liver. The lesion is composed of a complex interconnecting network of vascular spaces lined by endothelial cells. This lesion is often readily diagnosable by CT, MRI, nuclear medicine and even sonography. The CT appearance after bolus contrast infusion demonstrates early peripheral and nodular enhancement that is isodense to the aorta and that progresses in a centripetal fashion until homogeneous "fill-in" of contrast occurs (18). Two important points should be remembered regarding the CT appearance of hepatic cavernous hemangiomas: (*a*) the criteria listed above that are requisite for a high specificity necessarily lower the sensitivity so that only about 55% of hemangiomas display this pattern and (*b*) although some hepatic metastases may demonstrate some features characteristic of cavernous hemangioma, if all of the above criteria are met no metastasis should be misdiagnosed as a hemangioma. Hemangiomas may also display imaging specific features on MRI where they are exquisitely bright on T2-weighted images, with the degree of brightness only increasing as the TE values are increased. Lesions larger than 2 cm may also be studied effectively with nuclear medicine.

Aunt Minnie's Pearls

- *Hemangiomas are the most common benign tumors of the liver.*
- *Contrast enhancement on CT is peripheral and nodular, with centripetal progression and homogeneous "fill-in."*

CASE 14

History. Withheld

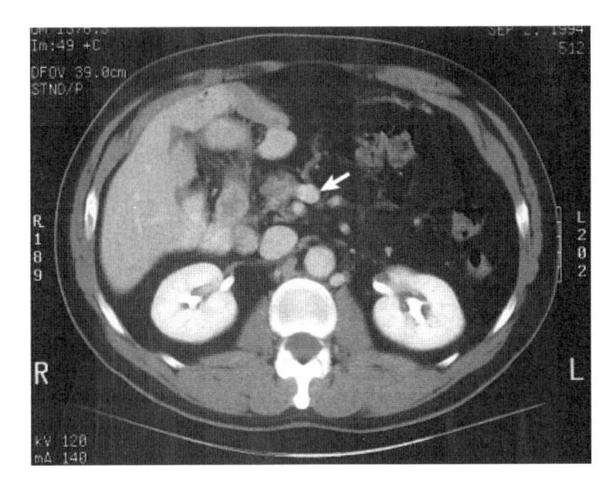

Figure 9.14.1.

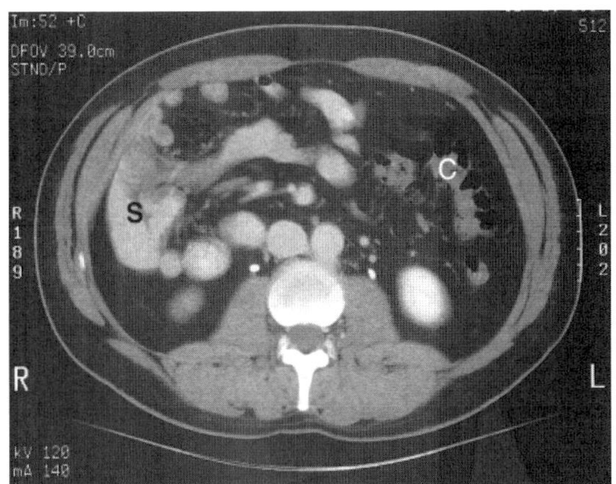

Figure 9.14.2.

Findings. A view from a contrast enhanced CT of the abdomen (Fig. 9.14.1) shows the normal orientation of the superior mesenteric artery and vein is reversed with the larger vein (*arrow*) lying to the left of the artery. On an additional image (Fig. 9.14.2) the colon (C) is seen to lie only on the left side of the abdomen and the small intestine (S) only on the right.

Diagnosis. Midgut malrotation (nonrotation)

Discussion. The normal embryologic development of the intestines involves a complex sequence of events that results in the fixation of the cecum in the right lower quadrant of the abdomen and the duodenojejunal flexure in the left upper quadrant (19). Between these two points, the small intestine is anchored by the attachment of its mesentery. When abnormalities in this process occur, it may result in an abnormal fixation of the small bowel mesentery and predispose the midgut to volvulus. Patients with midgut malrotation also have an increased risk of small-bowel obstruction caused by peritoneal (Ladd's) bands. Nonrotation of the bowel may also occur and is diagnosed when the large intestine is located in the left hemiabdomen and the small bowel in the right hemiabdomen as in the index case. On cross-sectional imaging studies, a reversal of the normal orientation of the superior mesenteric artery and vein is frequently seen in cases of midgut malrotation and nonrotation (20, 21).

Aunt Minnie's Pearls

- *Reversal of superior mesenteric artery and vein orientation on CT is seen in malrotation/nonrotation of the bowel.*
- *Large intestine on left and small intestine on right = nonrotation.*
- *There is an increased risk of midgut volvulus and small bowel obstruction.*

CASE 15

History. Withheld

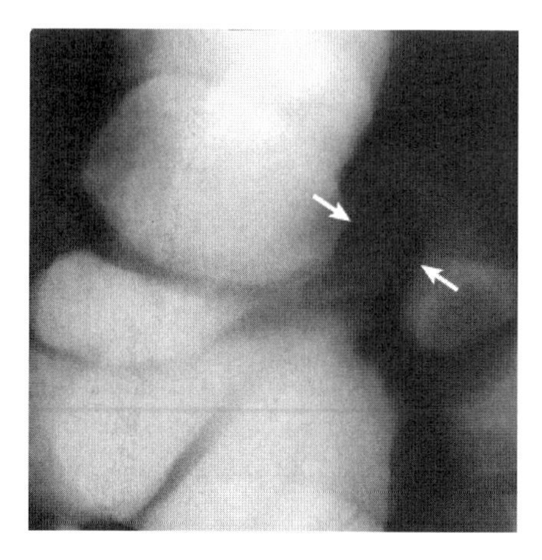

Figure 9.15.1.

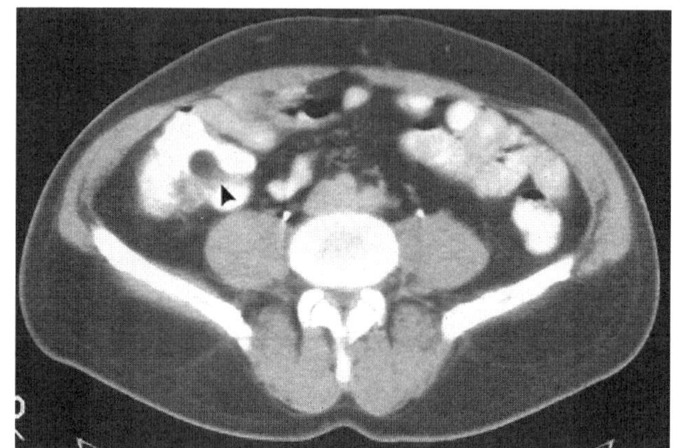

Figure 9.15.2.

Findings. A fluoroscopic spot film of the ileocecal valve during a single contrast barium enema demonstrates a smooth polypoid filling defect in the region of the ileocecal valve (Fig. 9.15.1, *arrows*). An axial CT image through the same area reveals homogeneous fatty density of the enlarged ileocecal valve (Fig. 9.15.2, *arrowhead*).

Diagnosis. Lipohyperplasia of the ileocecal valve

Discussion. Lipohyperplasia of the ileocecal valve refers to a diffuse infiltration and replacement of the valve by fatty tissue. Although this lesion is not rare, it has received little attention in the literature. It has been variously referred to as a lipoma of the ileocecal valve or as ileocecal valve lipomatosis. Recognize, however, that the lesion is not a true encapsulated lipoma (although true lipomas of the ileocecal valve rarely occur) but rather a proliferation of fatty tissue found normally in the ileocecal valve (22). This entity is usually silent from a clinical standpoint, although the lesion may occasionally bleed or produce mechanical small bowel obstruction. In the past, laparotomy was required for definitive diagnosis. This is no longer the case because the lesion is readily diagnosed with modern noninvasive cross-sectional imaging techniques that allow direct visualization of the fatty valve (23).

Aunt Minnie's Pearls
- *Lipohyperplasia of the ileocecal valve = diffuse infiltration and replacement of the valve by fatty tissue.*
- *This entity is not a true lipoma.*

CASE 16

History. Elderly diabetic woman with abdominal pain and fever

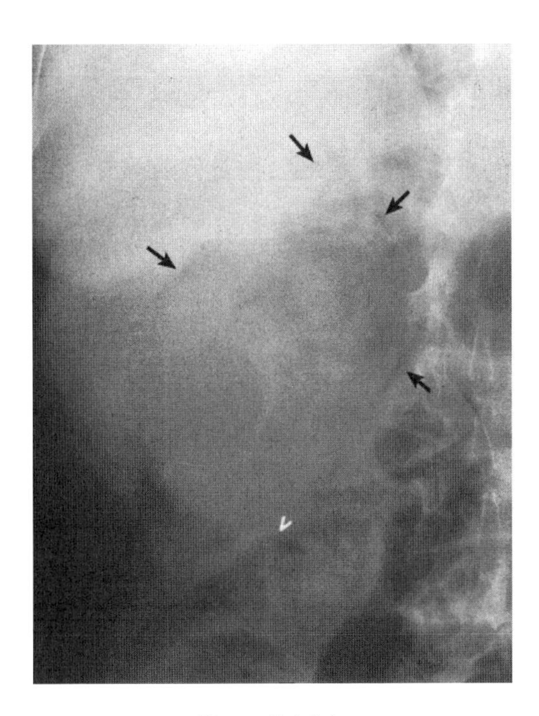

Figure 9.16.1.

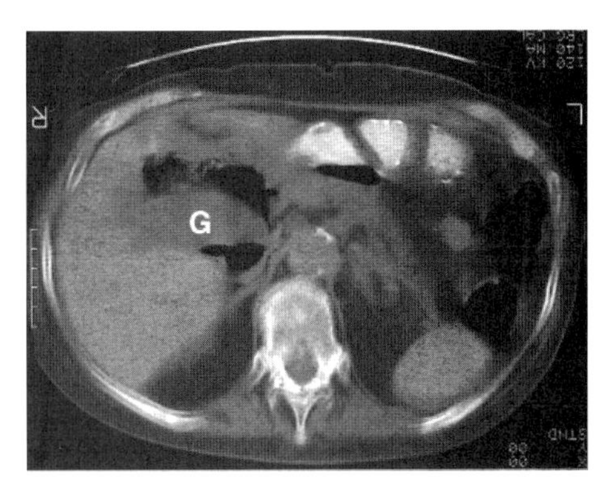

Figure 9.16.2.

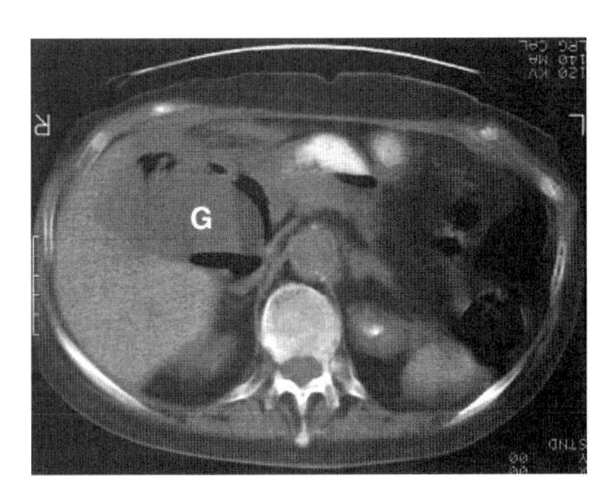

Figure 9.16.3.

Findings. A plain film of the abdomen (Fig. 9.16.1) reveals abnormal collections of air in the expected location of the gallbladder (*arrows*). Two axial CT images of the upper abdomen performed with the patient prone (Figs. 9.16.2 and 9.16.3) confirm that gas is present in the wall of the gallbladder (G) and in the gallbladder fossa.

Diagnosis. Emphysematous cholecystitis

Discussion. Emphysematous cholecystitis is a severe form of acute cholecystitis in which cystic duct obstruction is followed by infection of the gallbladder by gas-producing organisms, usually *Escherichia coli*, *Clostridium* sp., or both. The condition is seen most frequently in diabetic patients and, unlike nonemphysematous acute cholecystitis, it is more frequent in men than in women (male:female ~3:1). Emphysematous cholecystitis must be diagnosed early in its course, because it has a high incidence of perforation and a high mortality rate. Percutaneous cholecystostomy is often performed as a temporizing measure until the patient is stable enough to undergo cholecystectomy. CT readily demonstrates air, which may be confined to the gallbladder lumen or may extend intramurally or into the pericholecystic space (24).

Aunt Minnie's Pearls

- *Emphysematous cholecystitis is due to secondary infection by gas-producing organisms.*
- *Emphysematous cholecystitis is more common in diabetics and in men.*
- *There is a high risk of perforation and high mortality.*

CASE 17

History. Abdominal distention

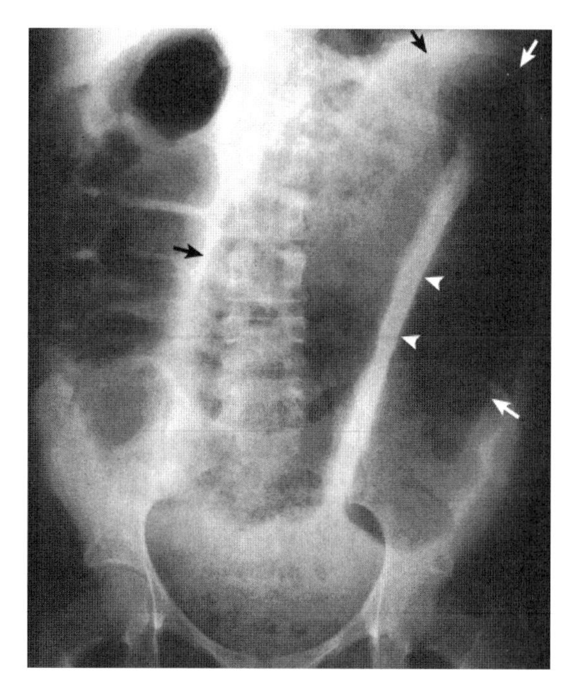

Figure 9.17.1.

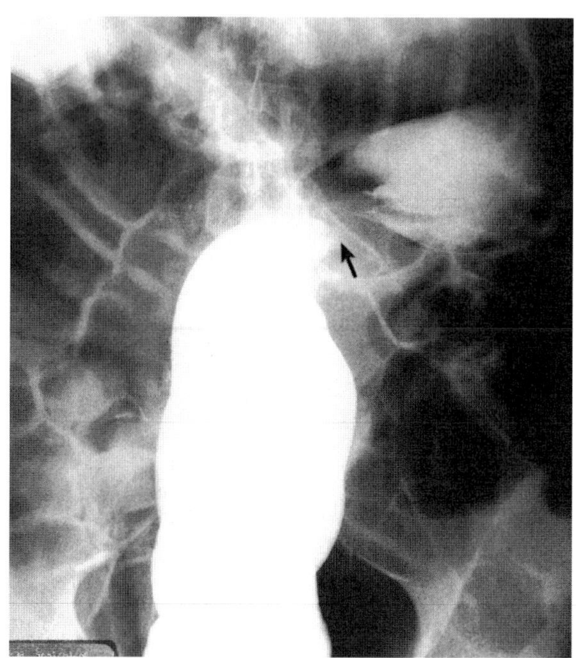

Figure 9.17.2.

Findings. A plain radiograph of the abdomen (Fig. 9.17.1) demonstrates a markedly distended loop of colon that projects superiorly from the pelvis to the level of the left hemidiaphragm (*white arrows*). A prominent stripe (*arrowheads*) is seen in the middle of the distended loop, which makes the loop mimic the appearance of a coffee bean. A fluoroscopic spot film from a contrast enema demonstrates tapered narrowing of the rectum at the rectosigmoid junction with a "bird's beak" deformity (Fig. 9.17.2, *arrow*). A small amount of contrast material is seen traversing the narrowed segment.

Diagnosis. Sigmoid volvulus

Discussion. Colonic volvulus is the third most common form of large intestine obstruction, after carcinoma and diverticulitis. A requisite condition for volvulus is the presence of a relatively redundant and mobile segment of bowel. The segments of the colon that are prone to volvulus include the sigmoid colon, cecum, and transverse colon. Sigmoid volvulus is more common in elderly patients and in populations that consume high-residue diets. Several findings on plain abdominal radiographs have been described with sigmoid volvulus, and some have been reported to be specific such as the "coffee bean" sign (dilated sigmoid loops with opposed walls that converge toward the lower left abdomen) (25). A more specific sign of sigmoid volvulus is the characteristic "bird's beak" deformity demonstrated on contrast enema near the rectosigmoid junction at the actual site of the volvulus. In some cases, the enema may actually reduce the volvulus, although sigmoidoscopy or tube decompression is usually the preferred treatment.

Aunt Minnie's Pearls

- *Sigmoid volvulus occurs in patients with a redundant sigmoid colon.*
- *Look for the "coffee bean" sign on plain films and the "bird's beak" deformity on contrast enemas.*

CASE 18

History. Chronic abdominal pain

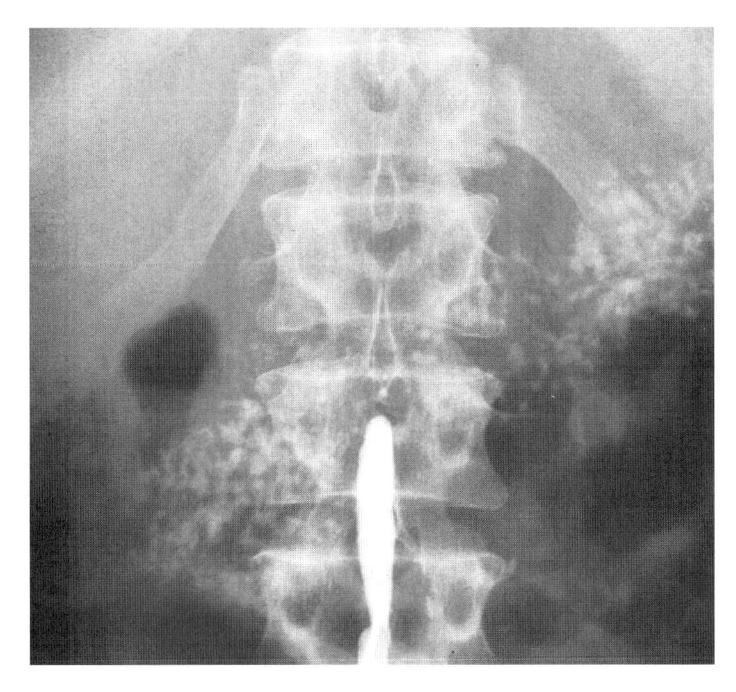

Figure 9.18.1.

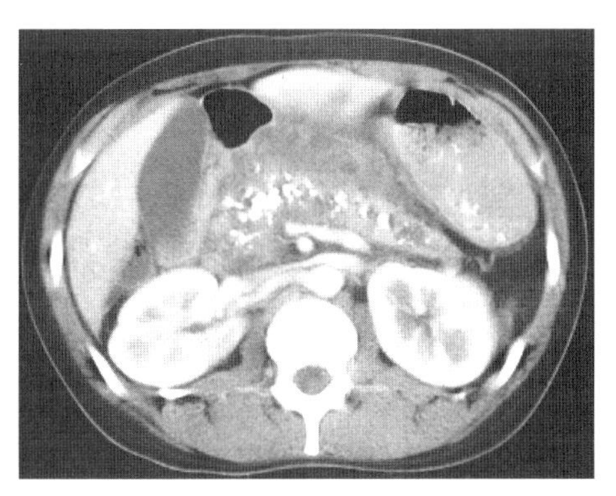

Figure 9.18.2.

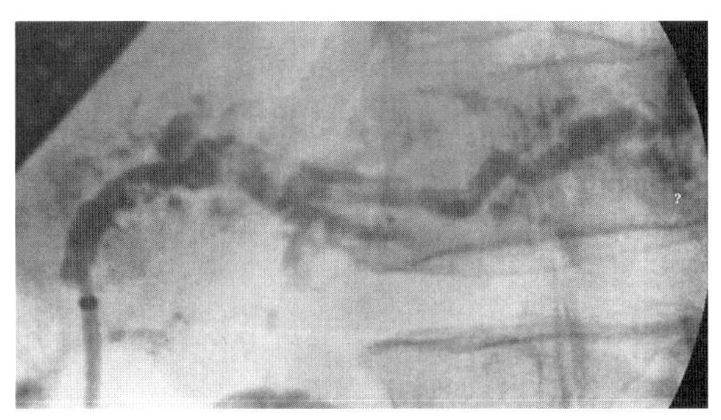

Figure 9.18.3.

Findings. A plain radiograph of the abdomen (Fig. 9.18.1) shows coarse calcification oriented obliquely in the upper abdomen in the expected position of the pancreas. Incidental note is made of retained myelographic contrast material. An axial CT image through the upper abdomen (Fig. 9.18.2) demonstrates calcification scattered diffusely throughout the pancreas, along with peripancreatic inflammatory changes.

Diagnosis. Chronic calcific pancreatitis with superimposed acute pancreatitis

Discussion. Although most cases of acute pancreatitis resolve without residual functional impairment or morphologic alteration, some patients go on to have recurrent episodes of acute pancreatitis. This is particularly true with alcohol induced pancreatitis. These repeated episodes of pancreatitis result in progressive fibroinflammatory changes with reduction in the exocrine and endocrine function of the pancreas (26). Morphologic alterations include diffuse or focal enlargement of the gland, pseudocyst or abscess formation, intraductal calcification, parenchymal atrophy, and ductal dilatation (27). The intraductal calcifications form by apposition of calcium carbonate onto intraductal proteinaceous concretions. In advanced cases, these calcifications are easily seen on plain abdominal radiographs and are virtually pathognomonic of chronic calcific pancreatitis. With less advanced cases, the calcifications may not be evident by plain film but are easily seen by CT.

A specific appearance of chronic pancreatitis may also be seen on ERCP, as in Fig. 9.18.3, where the main duct looks dilated and irregular and marked dilatation of side branches or "side branch ectasia" occurs.

Aunt Minnie's Pearls

- *Calcification of intraductal proteinaceous pancreatoliths = calcific pancreatitis.*
- *There is an increased incidence of chronic calcific pancreatitis with alcohol abuse.*

CASE 19

History. 58-year-old man with history of pancreatitis

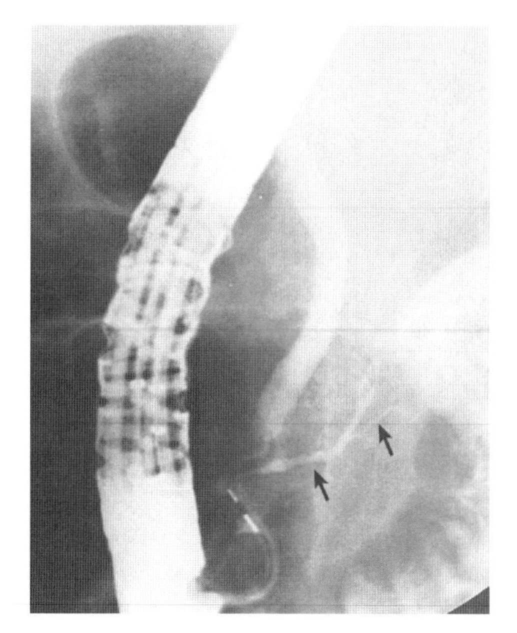

Figure 9.19.1.

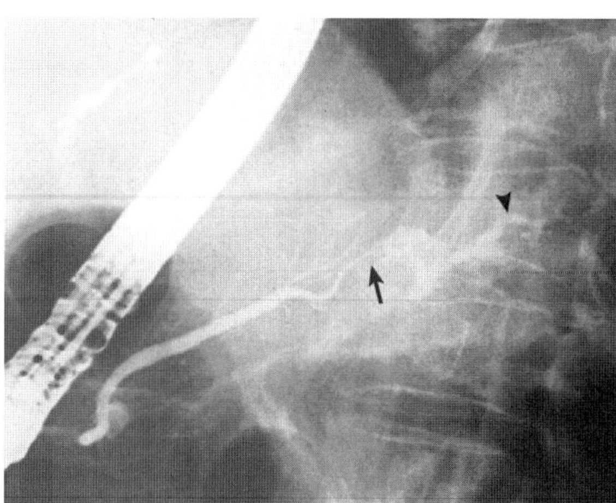

Figure 9.19.2.

Findings. An initial fluoroscopic ERCP spot film obtained during injection of major papilla (Fig. 9.19.1) demonstrates filling of the ventral bud of the pancreas (*arrow*) and the common bile duct. The remainder of the pancreatic duct in the dorsal pancreas is seen after injection of the minor papilla (Fig. 9.19.2). Incidentally noted are a stricture (*arrow*) and duct enlargement with side branch ectasia in the tail (*arrowhead*).

Diagnosis. Pancreas divisum with changes of chronic pancreatitis in the dorsal pancreas

Discussion. The normal pancreas is derived embryologically from the fusion of two distinct pancreatic buds: the ventral and dorsal pancreatic anlage. The major pancreatic duct of Wirsung supplies most of the pancreatic head, uncinate process, body, and tail and is drained by the major pancreatic papilla. The minor pancreatic duct of Santorini is formed by that portion of the dorsal pancreatic duct that does not fuse with the ventral duct, and supplies a portion of the pancreatic head, and is drained through the accessory or minor pancreatic papilla. Pancreas divisum results when the ventral anlage fails to fuse with the dorsal anlage (28). In this case, the dorsal duct supplies the entirety of the pancreatic tail and body and a portion of the head and is drained through the accessory papilla. The ventral duct then supplies a portion of the pancreatic head and is drained through the major papilla. It has been proposed that patients with pancreas divisum have an increased risk for developing pancreatitis, especially in the dorsal pancreas, because the minor papilla cannot accommodate the normal volume of secretions from the major duct, resulting in stasis and inflammation.

Aunt Minnie's Pearls

- *Nonfusion of ventral and dorsal pancreatic anlage = pancreas divisum.*
- *There is an increased risk of pancreatitis, especially in the dorsal pancreas.*

Case 20

History. Intermittent abdominal pain

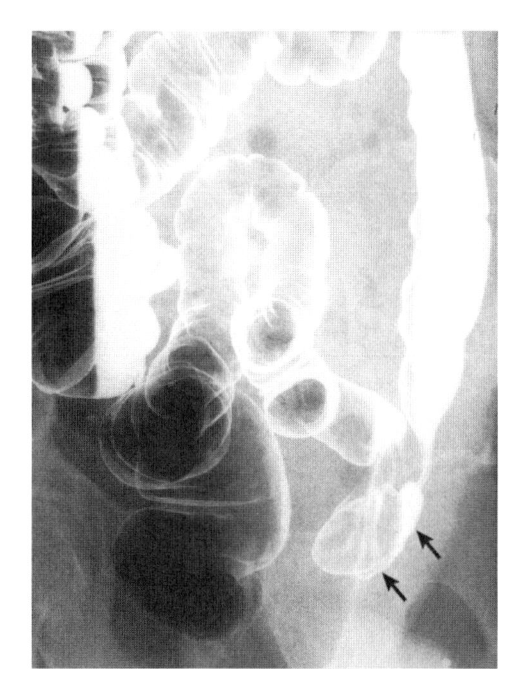

Figure 9.20.1.

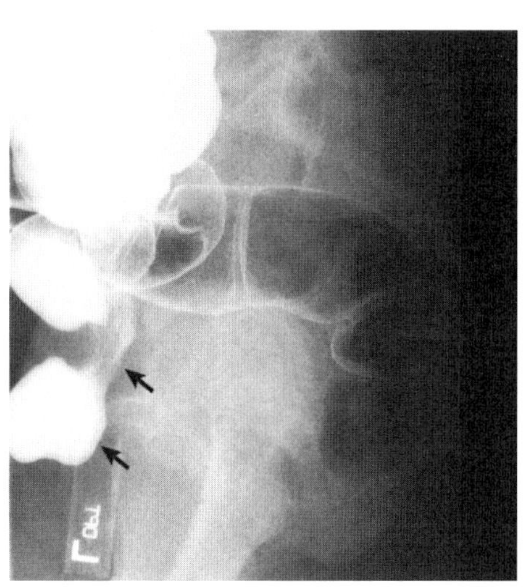

Figure 9.20.2.

Findings. Frontal (Fig. 9.20.1) and lateral (Fig. 9.20.2) views of the abdomen taken during a double-contrast barium enema show a hairpin loop of colon (*arrows*) extending inferiorly and anteriorly from its normal anatomic position. An extrinsic and smooth impression is seen along the neck of hairpin loop.

Diagnosis. Inguinal hernia

Discussion. A hernia is defined as the protrusion of a structure through an abnormal opening. Groin hernias are classified as indirect inguinal hernia, direct inguinal hernia, or femoral hernia. The indirect hernia is the most common groin hernia in men and women of all ages. It is thought to be a congenital lesion related to persistent patency of the processus vaginalis. The patent processus vaginalis allows for herniation of abdominal contents (usually mesenteric fat and/or small or large intestine) through the internal inguinal ring into the inguinal canal. Herniation may be intermittent and may be aggravated by coughing, lifting heavy objects, or other maneuvers that increase intraabdominal pressure. However, the hernia sac may become edematous and incarcerated, in which case strangulation and bowel infarction may occur. The direct inguinal hernia is thought to be an acquired lesion that results from traumatic herniation of abdominal contents through a weakness in the posterior wall of the inguinal canal (Hesselbach's triangle) (29).

Aunt Minnie's Pearls

- *Indirect inguinal hernia = congenital; patent processus vaginalis = most common.*
- *Direct inguinal hernia = acquired herniation through Hesselbach's triangle.*

CASE 21

History. Intermittent right upper quadrant pain and recent weight loss

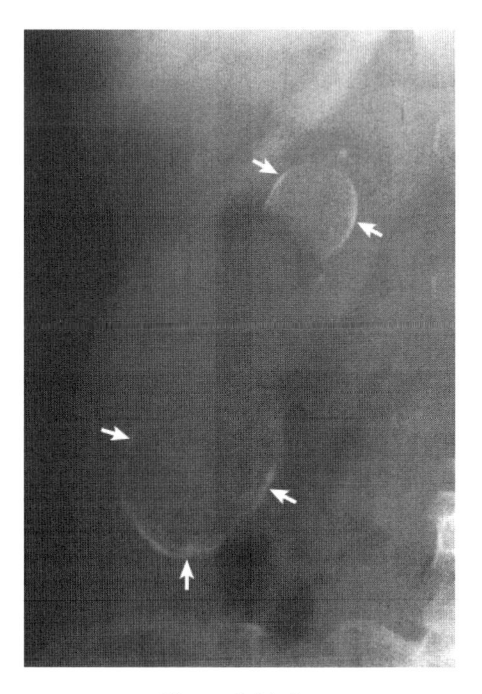

Figure 9.21.1.

Findings. A plain radiograph of the abdomen (Fig. 9.21.1) shows a thin curvilinear calcification (*arrows*) that conforms to the expected shape of the gallbladder. The continuity of the calcification is disrupted abruptly, and a homogeneous soft tissue mass spans the interval between the two calcifications.

Diagnosis. Porcelain gallbladder with gallbladder carcinoma

Discussion. The term porcelain gallbladder is derived from the appearance and texture of the gallbladder by gross pathologic examination (30). The affected gallbladder will usually manifest a blue discoloration and brittle consistency. Roentgenographic examination demonstrates calcification of the gallbladder wall that may be extensive or patchy in distribution. The mural calcification may also be demonstrated by CT or ultrasound. Cholelithiasis is present in most cases. Numerous theories have been proposed with respect to the pathogenesis of porcelain gallbladder including chronic low-grade inflammation, intramural hemorrhage, and disorders of calcium metabolism. Most authorities believe the condition represents a form of chronic cholecystitis. The entity is important from a clinical standpoint because of the association between porcelain gallbladder and gallbladder carcinoma. This occurs with sufficient frequency to warrant prophylactic cholecystectomy.

Aunt Minnie's Pearls

- *There is an association between porcelain gallbladder and gallbladder carcinoma.*

Case 22

History. Right upper quadrant pain

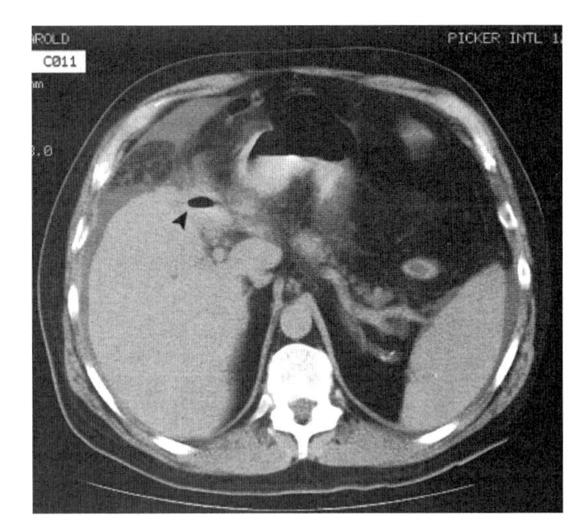

Figure 9.22.2.

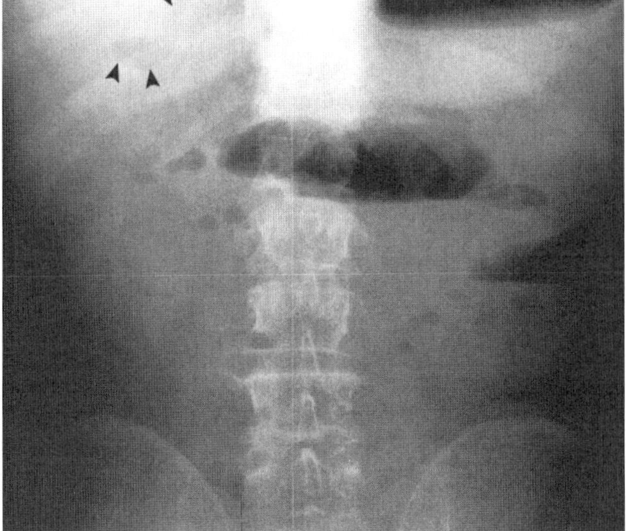

Figure 9.22.1.

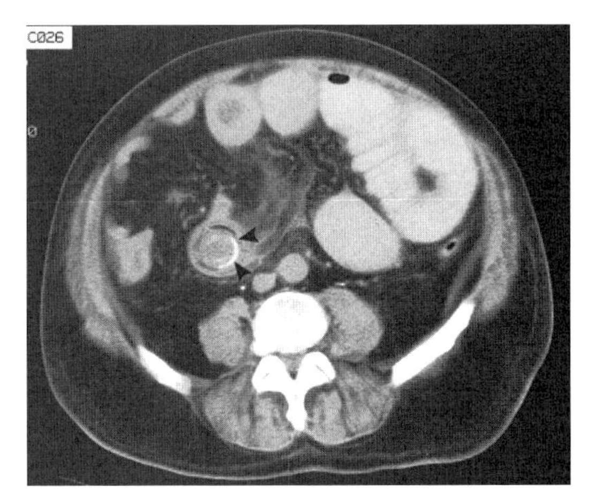

Figure 9.22.3.

Findings. An upright plain radiograph of the abdomen (Fig. 9.22.1) shows a collection of air (*large arrowheads*) over the liver as well as air-filled, branching tubular structures (*small arrowhead*) in the liver. Also demonstrated are numerous dilated loops of small intestine with air-fluid levels and other signs of small-bowel obstruction. A CT scan through the upper abdomen reveals mild interstitial infiltration of the pericholecystic fat as well as air within the gallbladder (Fig. 9.22.2, *arrowhead*). An additional CT image through the lower abdomen demonstrates dilated loops of small intestine and a peripherally calcified structure (Fig. 9.22.3, *arrowheads*) contained within the lumen of the small intestine, consistent with an ectopic gallstone.

Diagnosis. Gallstone ileus

Discussion. Gallstone ileus develops after the erosion of a gallstone through the gallbladder wall and into a portion of the gastrointestinal tract. The fistulous tract usually forms between the gallbladder and duodenum, although fistulas to the stomach or colon may also occur. Small stones usually pass through the alimentary tract without consequence. Larger stones usually become impacted in the distal ileum, resulting in a mechanical small-bowel obstruction. The classic plain-film findings of pneumobilia, dilated small bowel, and an ectopic calcified gallstone (Rigler's triad) are considered pathognomonic of gallstone ileus. However, the complete triad is not seen on plain film in most cases (31).

Aunt Minnie's Pearls

- *Rigler's triad of gallstone ileus includes pneumobilia, dilated small bowel, and an ectopic calcified gallstone.*

CASE 23

History. 55-year-old man with increasing abdominal pain and intermittent flushing episodes

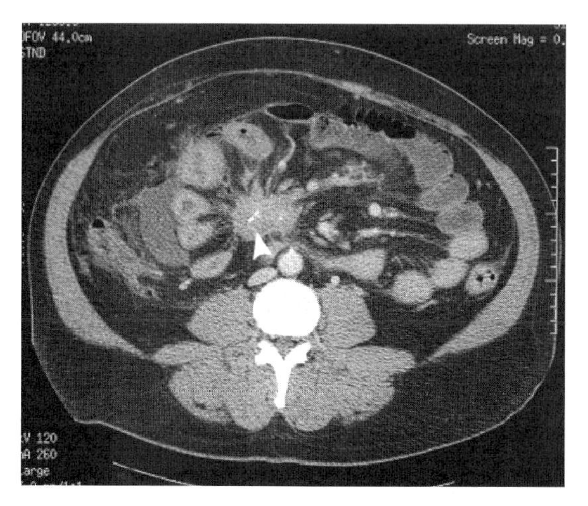

Figure 9.23.1.

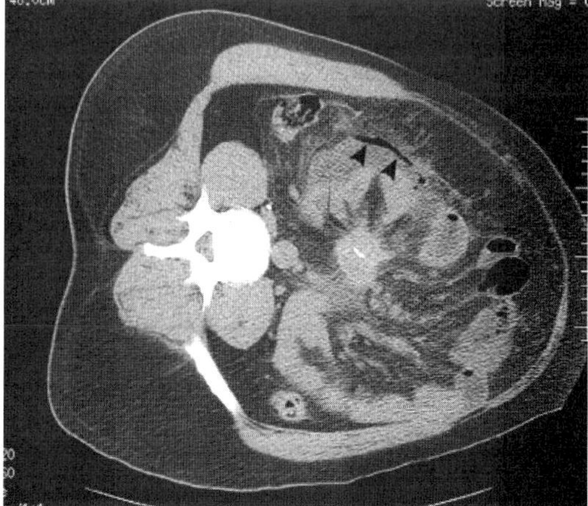

Figure 9.23.2.

Findings. An axial CT image through the midabdomen (Fig. 9.23.1) demonstrates a partially calcified mesenteric soft tissue mass (*arrowhead*). Thickened mesenteric vessels are seen radiating away from the mass toward nearby small intestinal loops, which have thickened walls. An axial CT image through the midabdomen with patient in left lateral decubitus position (Fig. 9.23.2) shows free air (*arrowheads*) and fluid adjacent to the thick-walled loops of intestine.

Diagnosis. Midgut carcinoid tumor with mesenteric metastasis producing small bowel ischemia with perforation

Discussion. Carcinoids are neuroendocrine tumors that arise from enterochromaffin cells at the base of the crypts of Lieberkühn. Most carcinoid tumors arise in the gastrointestinal tract, and most of these arise in the appendix or the ileum. All carcinoids are thought to have malignant potential, although their biologic behavior is widely disparate and depends on their site of origin. This diagnosis may be made on CT scans by recognizing the characteristic appearance of the carcinoid mesenteric metastasis—a partially calcified, solitary mesenteric mass with radiating mesenteric vessels. The appearance of the thickened, radiating mesenteric vessels is attributed to the intense desmoplastic response that the tumor incites. The thickened bowel is related to ischemia engendered by perivascular tumor infiltration as well as an intrinsic vasculopathy (elastic vascular sclerosis) that is believed to be caused by humoral factors liberated by the tumor. Patients with gastrointestinal carcinoid tumors usually manifest symptoms of the carcinoid syndrome (e.g., flushing, vasomotor instability, etc.) only if hepatic metastases are present. In the absence of hepatic metastases, the liver can metabolize the vasoactive mediators (principally serotonin) responsible for the carcinoid syndrome (32).

Aunt Minnie's Pearls

- *A solitary, calcified, mesenteric mass with radiating mesenteric vessels = carcinoid tumor.*
- *Carcinoid syndrome occurs only if hepatic metastases are present.*

Case 24

History. Recent stab wound to the chest

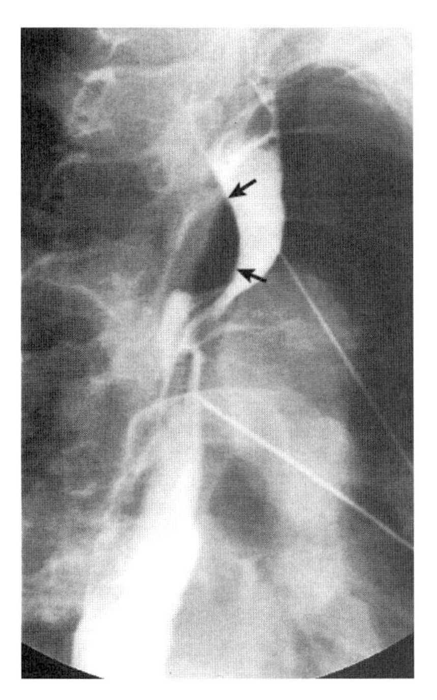

Figure 9.24.1.

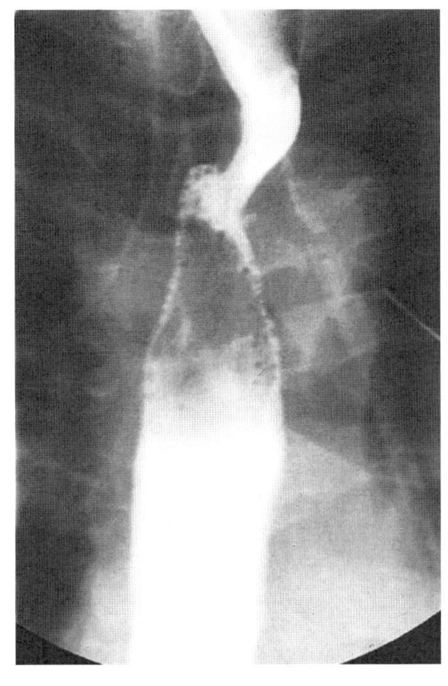

Figure 9.24.2.

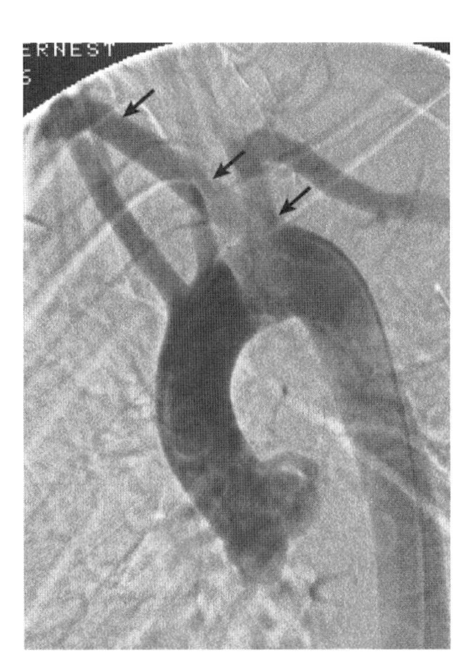

Figure 9.24.3.

Findings. An oblique image from a full column barium esophagram reveals a smooth extrinsic mass effect on the posterior esophagus (Fig. 9.24.1, *arrows*). On the anteroposterior view, the impression appears to course obliquely from the lower left to the upper right side of the patient (Fig. 9.24.2). An oblique view of a thoracic aortogram (Fig. 9.24.3) shows an anomalous vessel originating as the last branch of the aorta that courses obliquely across the mediastinum (*arrows*).

Diagnosis. Left aortic arch with an aberrant right subclavian artery

Discussion. As described in Chapter 3, the aberrant right subclavian artery represents the most common great vessel branching anomaly of the aortic arch, occurring in approximately 1% of the population. The anomalous vessel is always the last great vessel to originate from the aorta, and its carotid artery is always the first (the right subclavian is the last branch and the right common carotid the first, and the same rule applies to an aberrant left subclavian). The aberrant subclavian vessel will course obliquely across the mediastinum and produce a smooth extrinsic impression on the posterior esophagus (33). The radiologist can tell which arm will be supplied by the anomalous vessel by (*a*) noting the side of the aortic arch (the aberrant vessel will supply the opposite arm) or (*b*) noting the obliquity of the impression on the esophagus on the anteroposterior full column esophagram (an aberrant right subclavian will course from lower left to upper right and vice versa for an aberrant left subclavian).

Aunt Minnie's Pearls

- *An aberrant subclavian artery will produce a smooth, oblique, and extrinsic impression on the posterior esophagus.*

CASE 25

History. Recurrent bouts of abdominal pain

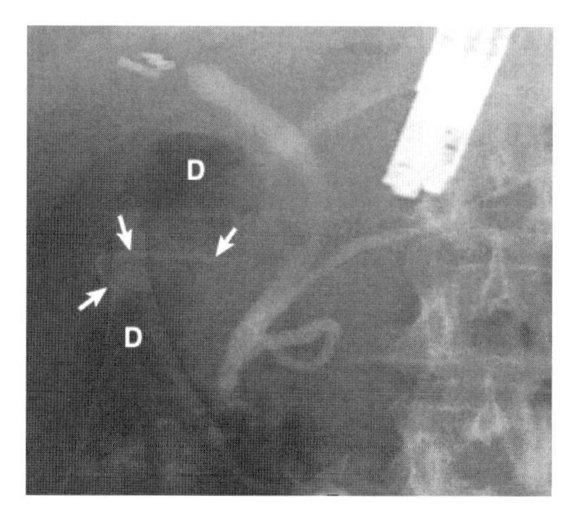

Figure 9.25.1.

Findings. A film from an ERCP obtained during injection of the major papilla (Fig. 9.25.1) shows a branch of the main pancreatic duct that courses toward the right side of the patient and encircles (*arrows*) the air-filled duodenum (D). Also seen is a smooth circumferential narrowing of the second portion of the air-filled duodenum.

Diagnosis. Annular pancreas

Discussion. Annular pancreas occurs when a thin band of pancreatic tissue encircles the second portion of the duodenum. In normal development of the pancreas, the gland is formed by fusion of the ventral and dorsal anlage, with the head and uncinate process arising from the former. If the ventral anlage becomes adherent to the duodenum, or if the left bud of the ventral anlage does not normally involute, the result is an annular pancreas. A characteristic smooth circumferential impression is seen on the second portion of the duodenum on upper gastrointestinal series, which may produce partial or complete duodenal obstruction. Many cases are associated with Down's syndrome, cardiac defects, and intestinal atresias. This disorder is also associated with an increased incidence of acute pancreatitis, chronic pancreatitis, and peptic ulcer disease.

CT or MRI can confirm the diagnosis by demonstrating the ventral pancreatic tissue surrounding the duodenum. During ERCP, injection of the major papilla usually opacifies the main duct in the body and tail of the esophagus and also fills a small duct in the pancreatic head that courses in a circular fashion around the duodenum (34). Symptomatic patients are treated with either gastrojejunostomy or duodenojejunostomy (35).

Aunt Minnie's Pearls

- *In annular pancreas, an anomalous ventral pancreas encircles the second stage of the duodenum.*
- *These patients have an increased risk of acute and chronic pancreatitis.*

REFERENCES

1. Mendl K, McKay JM, Tanner CH. Intramural diverticulosis of the oesophagus and Rokitansky-Aschoff sinuses in the gallbladder. Br J Radiol 1960;33:496–501.
2. Levine MS, Moolten DN, Herliger H, Laufer I. Esophageal intramural pseudodiverticulosis: a reevaluation. AJR 1986;147:1165–1170.
3. Lahey FH, Warren KW. Esophageal diverticula. Surg Gynecol Obstet 1954;98:1–28.
4. Ponzoli VA. Zenker's diverticulum: a review of pathogenesis and presentation of 25 cases. South Med J 1968;61:817–821.
5. Nelson SW. The discovery of gastric ulcers and the differential diagnosis between benignancy and malignancy. Radiol Clin North Am 1969;7:5–25.
6. Gelfand DW, Ott DJ. Gastric ulcer scars. Radiology 1981;140:37–43.
7. Eisenberg RL, Margulis AR, Moss AA. Giant duodenal ulcers. Gastrointest Radiol 1978;2:347–353.
8. Levine MS. Infectious esophagitis. Semin Roentgenol 1994;4:341–350.
9. Weatherly NF. Medical helminthology. In Joklik WK, Willett HP, Amos DB, Wilfert CM, eds. Zinsser microbiology, 19th ed. Norwalk: Appleton & Lange, 1988:976–977.
10. Levine MS. Radiology of the esophagus. Philadelphia: Saunders, 1989:193–203.
11. Cockerill EM, Miller RE, Chernish SM, McLaughlin GC III, Rodda BE. Optimal visualization of esophageal varices. AJR Radiat Therapy Nucl Med 1976;126:512–523.
12. Daneman A, Reilly BJ, de Silva M, Olutola P. Intussusception on small bowel examinations in children. AJR 1982;139:299–304.
13. Gourtsoyiannis NC, Papakonstantinou O, Bays D, Malamas M. Adult enteric intussusception: additional observations on enteroclysis. Abdom Imaging 1994;19:11–17.
14. Gelfand DW. Gastrointestinal radiology, New York: Churchill Livingstone, 1984:265.
15. Bockus HL. Diaphragmatic hernia, esophageal hiatus hernia, eventration and paralysis of the diaphragm. In: Bockus HL, ed., Gastroenterology. Philadelphia: Saunders, 1974:349–386.
16. Ott DJ, Gelfand DW, Wu WC, Castell DO. Esophagogastric region and its rings. AJR 1984;142:281–287.
17. Silverman PM, Ram PC, Korobkin M. CT appearance of abdominal thorotrast deposition and thorotrast-induced angiosarcoma of the liver. J Comput Assist Tomogr 1983;7:655–658.
18. Leslie DF, Johnson CD, Johnson CM, Ilstrup DM, Harmsen WS. Distinction between cavernous hemangiomas of the liver and hepatic metastases on CT: value of contrast enhancement patterns. AJR 1995;164:625–629.
19. Teele RL, Share JC. Diseases of the stomach and duodenum. In: Gore RM, Levine MS, Laufer I, eds. Textbook of gastrointestinal radiology. Philadelphia: Saunders, 1994:1443–1462.
20. Zerin JM, DiPietro MA. Mesenteric vascular anatomy at CT: normal and abnormal appearances. Radiology 1991;179:739–742.
21. Nichols DM, Li DK. Superior mesenteric vein rotation: a CT sign of midgut malrotation. AJR 1983;141:707–708.
22. Elliott GB, Sandy JTM, Elliott KA, Sherkat A. Lipohyperplasia of the ileocecal valve. Can J Surg 1968;11:179–187.
23. Heiken JP, Forde KA, Gold RP. Computed tomography as a definitive method for diagnosing gastrointestinal lipomas. Radiology 1982;142:409–414.
24. McMillin K. Computed tomography of emphysematous cholecystitis. J Comput Assist Tomogr 1985;9:330–332.
25. Burrell HC, Baker DM, Wardrop P, Evans AJ. Significant plain film findings in sigmoid volvulus. Clin Radiol 1994;49:317–319.
26. Radecki PD, Friedman AC, Dabezies MA. The pancreas: pancreatitis. In: Friedman AC, Dachman AH, eds. Radiology of the liver, biliary tract, and pancreas. St. Louis: Mosby, 1994:763–805.
27. Ferrucci JT, Wittenberg J, Black EB, Kirkpatrick RH, Hall DA. Computed body tomography in chronic pancreatitis. Radiology 1979;130:175–182.
28. Faerber EN, Friedman AC, Dabezies MA. The pancreas: anomalies and congenital disorders. In: Friedman AC, Dachman AH, eds. Radiology of the liver, biliary tract, and pancreas. St. Louis: Mosby, 1994:743–761.
29. Harrison LA, Keesling CA, Martin NL. Abdominal wall hernias: review of herniography and correlation with cross-sectional imaging. RadioGraphics 1995;15:315–332.
30. Berk RN, Armbuster TG, Saltzstein SL. Carcinoma in the porcelain gallbladder. Radiology 1973;106:29–31.
31. Friedman AC, Maurer AH. Cholelithiasis and cholecystitis. In: Friedman AC, Dachman AH, eds. Radiology of the liver, biliary tract, and pancreas. St. Louis: Mosby, 1994:445–538.
32. Buck JL, Sobin LH. Carcinoids of the gastrointestinal tract. RadioGraphics 1990;10:1081–1095.
33. Fernbach SK. Congenital and acquired lesions of the esophagus. In: Gore RM, Levine MS, Laufer I, eds. Textbook of gastrointestinal radiology. Philadelphia: Saunders, 1994;1:1427–1429..
34. Freeny PC, Lawson TL. Congenital and developmental abnormalities of the pancreas. In: Radiology of the pancreas. New York: Springer-Verlag, 1982:146–149.
35. Gore RM, Fernbach SK, Ghahremani GG. Anomalies and anatomic variants. In: Gore RM, Levine MS, Laufer I, eds. Textbook of gastrointestinal radiology. Philadelphia: Saunders, 1994:2126–2128.

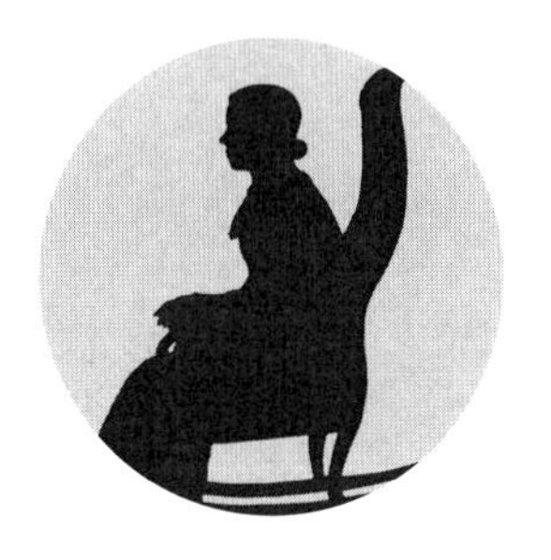

chapter 10

GENITOURINARY RADIOLOGY

H. STUART SAUNDERS AND RAYMOND B. DYER

CASE 1

History. 35-year-old man who underwent retrograde urethrography for evaluation of painful and difficult voiding as well as dribbling around his scrotum during urination

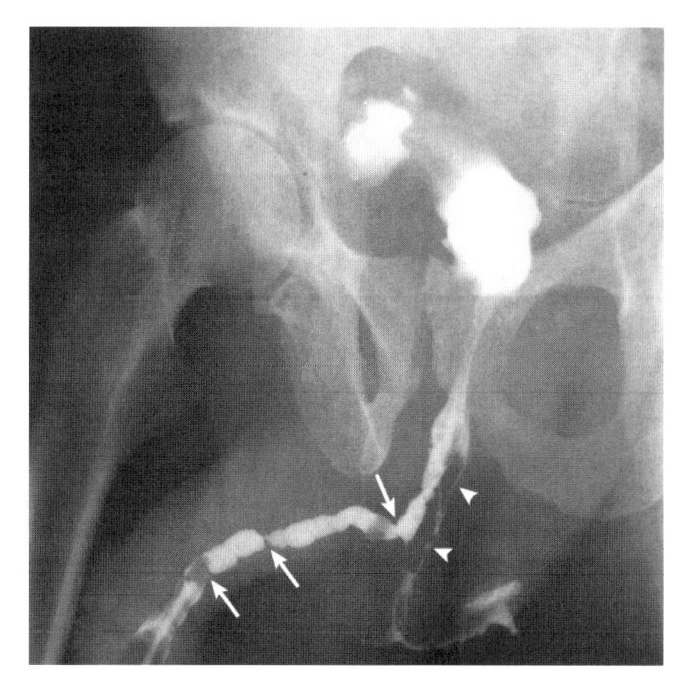

Figure 10.1.1.

Findings. A single film from a retrograde urethrogram demonstrates multiple strictures of the penile and bulbous urethra (Fig. 10.1.1, *arrows*). Multiple fistulae to the perineum are shown (*arrowheads*) with contrast medium collecting around the external surface of the scrotum.

Diagnosis. Multiple urethral strictures and perineal fistulae (watering can perineum)

Discussion. Strictures of the adult male urethra are usually the sequelae of previous urethral inflammation or trauma. Of the infectious organisms known to involve the urethra, one of the more common is *Neisseria gonorrhea*. This sexually transmitted bacterium initially lodges in the periurethral glands of Littré, which are most numerous in the bulbous portion of the anterior urethra. If treatment is inadequate, the infection spreads into submucosal tissues and the corpus spongiosum. Subsequent urethral fibrosis and scarring lead to the development of the characteristic urethral strictures, which may later result in the development of cutaneous perineal fistulae if resistance to voiding becomes excessively high (1). Similar findings can be seen with other infectious agents (e.g., tuberculosis), although this organism usually descends to involve the lower urinary tract after hematogenously seeding the kidney (2).

Aunt Minnie's Pearls

- *Urethral strictures are often related to previous urethral infection.*
- *High resistance to voiding can lead to fistula formation.*
- *Most infectious strictures occur in the bulbous urethra because the highest concentration of periurethral glands is within this segment.*

CASE 2

History. 38-year-old woman who was involved in a motor vehicle accident and afterward underwent cystography in the emergency department for evaluation of gross hematuria

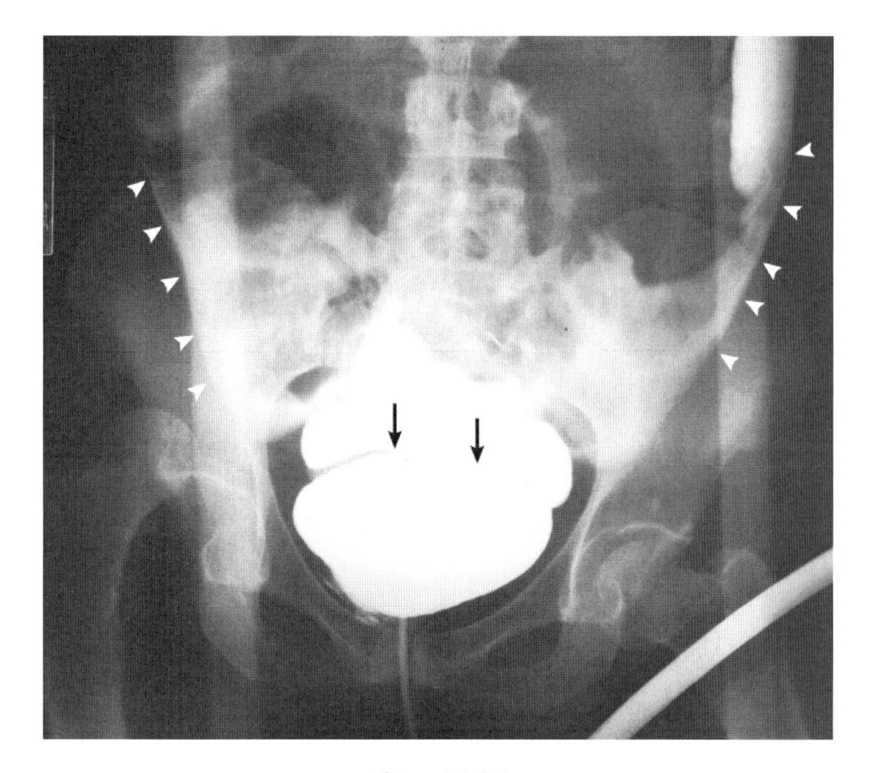

Figure 10.2.1.

Findings. This frontal film of the pelvis, obtained after catheterization of the bladder and instillation of contrast material, demonstrates extravasation along the superior aspect of the bladder (Fig. 10.2.1, *arrows*). Contrast medium outlines loops of bowel within the peritoneal space and fills the pericolic gutters (Fig. 10.2.1, *arrowheads*). Also note dislocation of the right femoral head.

Diagnosis. Intraperitoneal bladder rupture after blunt trauma to the pelvis

Discussion. The possibility of bladder injury should be considered in all patients who suffer blunt or penetrating pelvic trauma (especially in patients with gross hematuria or traumatic bony injuries of the pelvic ring). Intravenous urography is not sufficient to exclude an acute bladder injury in this setting, and retrograde cystography should be performed. Once the urethra has been fully evaluated and cleared of injury, the bladder can be catheterized safely and 300–400 ml dilute contrast material instilled to achieve adequate bladder distension. Lesser volumes of instilled contrast medium may lead to false-negative studies, because the intravesical pressure is insufficient to produce extravasation through the injured bladder wall (3). In the current case, acute compression of a full bladder resulted in a laceration along the bladder dome. The irritative effect of urine exposed to the large surface area of the peritoneum can cause rapid development of chemical peritonitis, which complicates the patient's clinical management. For this reason, intraperitoneal bladder rupture is generally considered a surgical emergency necessitating urgent primary repair of the bladder wall (4, 5).

Aunt Minnie's Pearls

- *In male patients, the urethra should be cleared of injury before the bladder is catheterized.*
- *Intraperitoneal bladder rupture is a surgical emergency.*

CASE 3

History. 28-year-old woman with vague left flank pain and multiple urinary tract infections in the past

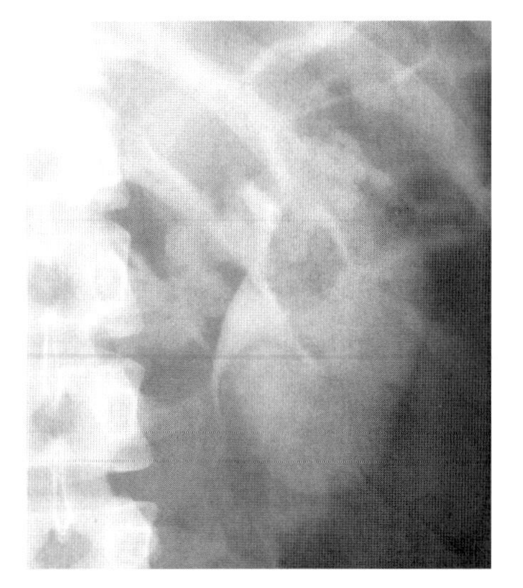

Figure 10.3.1.

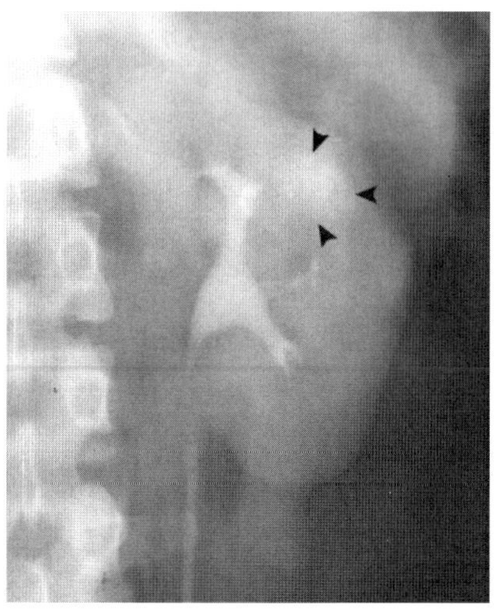

Figure 10.3.2.

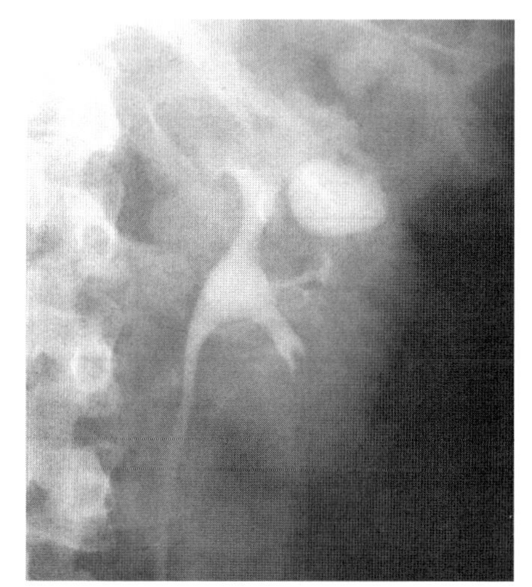

Figure 10.3.3.

Findings. A 1-minute film of the left kidney during intravenous urography (Fig. 10.3.1) shows no abnormality. A nephrotomogram obtained 3 minutes after contrast material injection (Fig. 10.3.2) reveals an ill-defined collection of contrast material at the junction of the middle and upper thirds of the left kidney (*arrowheads*). The third film obtained 10 minutes after contrast material injection (Fig. 10.3.3) demonstrates a well-defined 3.5-cm collection of contrast material immediately adjacent to the left upper pole collecting system, which appears to extend to the margin of the kidney.

Diagnosis. Caliceal diverticulum of the left upper pole collecting system

Discussion. A caliceal diverticulum is a cavity lined by transitional epithelium that is usually connected to the calyx by a narrow isthmus. Less commonly, the diverticulum may be connected directly to an infundibulum or to the renal pelvis where the term pyelogenic cyst is sometimes applied (6, 7). The incidence of caliceal diverticula in children and adults is similar, suggesting an embryologic etiology (6). A ureteral bud branch may fail to induce nephron development but maintain its connection to the collecting system (7). The resulting caliceal diverticulum must fill in a retrograde fashion after opacification of the collecting system (6). Thus, its filling is temporarily delayed as seen in this example. The narrow isthmus that connects the diverticulum to the collecting system may impede flow, creating stasis complications within the diverticulum such as stones (seen in 25–50% of diverticula), recurrent urinary tract infections, or hematuria (6, 7). The position of the diverticulum and the delayed temporal filling distinguish it from a hydrocalyx as a result of infundibular stenosis.

Aunt Minnie's Pearls

- *Caliceal diverticula fill in a delayed fashion on urography.*
- *Stasis occurs in the diverticulum, resulting in stones, infection, or hematuria.*

CASE 4

History. 45-year-old woman with vague left upper quadrant pain

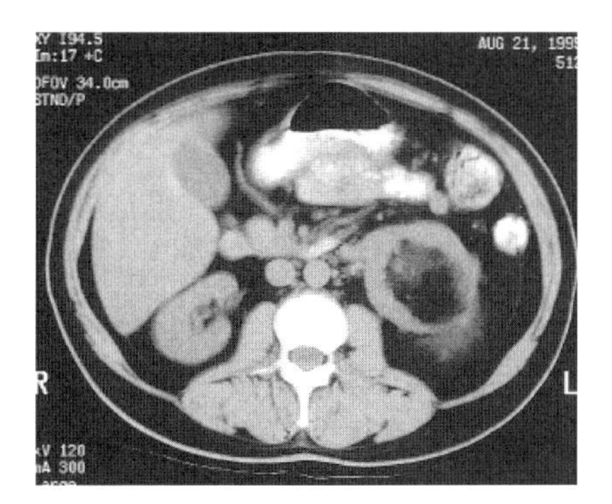

Figure 10.4.1.

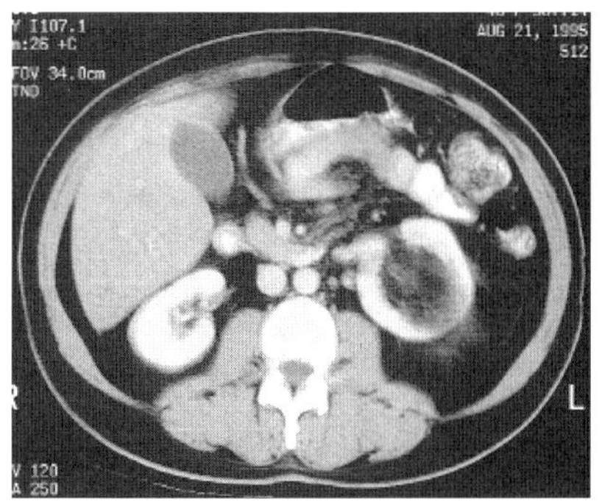

Figure 10.4.2.

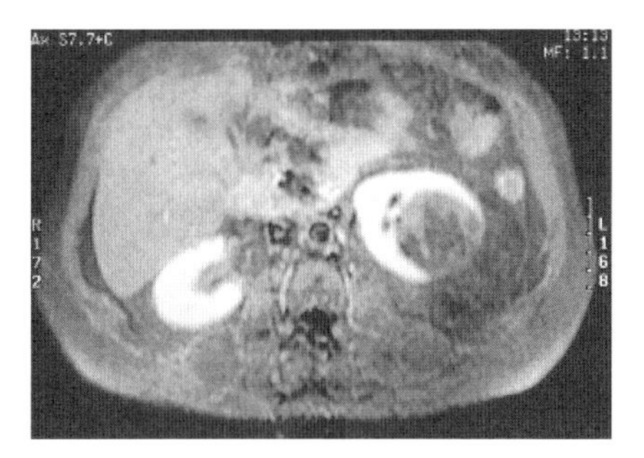

Figure 10.4.3. SE 600/15 with gadolinium with fat saturation.

Findings. On an unenhanced CT scan (Fig. 10.4.1), a mass lesion in the central portion of the left kidney is identified. A significant portion of the renal lesion is composed of tissue with attenuation characteristics similar to retroperitoneal and subcutaneous fat. There is mild stranding in the perirenal fat. On the enhanced CT study (Fig. 10.4.2) there is enhancement of some central elements within the mass. The gadolinium enhanced, T1-weighted MR image utilizing fat suppression technique (Fig. 10.4.3) shows the appearance of the mass lesion to be similar to subcutaneous fat.

Diagnosis. Renal angiomyolipoma

Discussion. The renal angiomyolipoma is a hamartoma composed of mature adipose tissue, thick-walled blood vessels that are prone to aneurysm formation, and smooth muscle in varying proportions. The angiomyolipoma occurs most commonly as an isolated lesion in women of childbearing age. Less commonly, multiple and bilateral lesions are seen with equal sex distribution in a younger age population in patients with tuberous sclerosis. The ability to confidently diagnose the fat within this renal lesion virtually assures the diagnosis of angiomyolipoma (8). This is best done with thin section CT using small regions of interest for density measurements. Low density areas within the renal lesion should be compared with retroperitoneal or subcutaneous fat and will generally measure less than –50 Hounsfield units (8). Fat suppression techniques available with MRI can also be used to confirm the fatty components of the tumor. There have been a few reports of more aggressive lesions engulfing sinus fat or containing small amounts of fat. In most instances, these lesions have had other features that are not characteristic of the angiomyolipoma (9).

Aunt Minnie's Pearls

- *A fat-containing lesion in the kidney is diagnostic of an angiomyolipoma.*

CASE 5

History. 47-year-old woman referred because painless hematuria was discovered on routine urinalysis

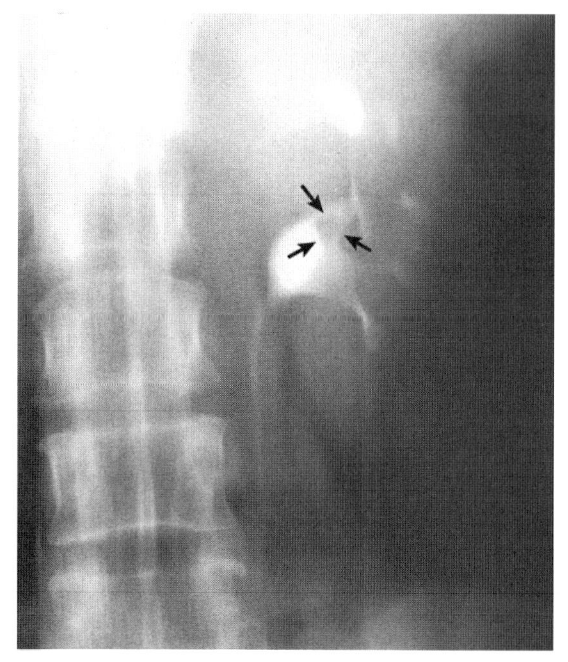

Figure 10.5.1.

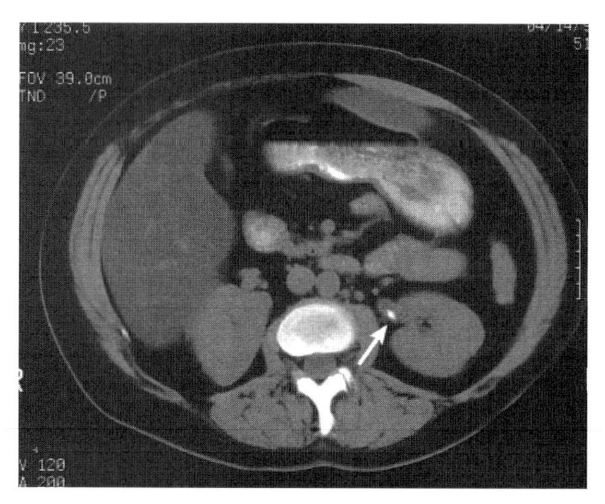

Figure 10.5.2.

Findings. A 4-minute postinjection nephrotomogram obtained during intravenous urography demonstrates an irregular filling defect in the major infundibulum of the left upper-pole collecting system (Fig. 10.5.1, *arrows*). Subsequent axial unenhanced CT image through this region demonstrates this lesion to be of uniform high attenuation (Fig. 10.5.2, *arrow*) compatible with a urinary tract calculus. Incidentally noted is an additional tiny calcification within the parenchyma of the left kidney and marked fatty infiltration of the liver.

Diagnosis. Nonobstructive, radiolucent left renal calculus

Discussion. The urographic differential diagnosis of radiolucent filling defects in the upper urinary tract includes nonopaque calculi, blood clots, transitional cell carcinoma, other benign and malignant neoplasms, air bubbles, infectious debris, and sloughed epithelium. Even though imaging features can suggest the diagnosis, confirmation is usually not possible with plain-film radiography. Because CT can demonstrate density differences of as little as 0.5%, even radiolucent stones appear much more dense than surrounding soft tissue structures on CT images. For this reason, a uric acid stone that is usually invisible on plain film becomes obvious because of its high attenuation (200–300 Hounsfield units) on CT studies. Other primary considerations in this differential diagnosis (i.e., tumors or blood clots) should have attenuation measurements in the range of 20–70 Hounsfield units. In this case, the CT scan allows confident diagnosis of a urinary tract calculus (10).

Aunt Minnie's Pearls

- *The differential diagnosis of a radiolucent filling defect is extensive.*
- *Virtually all urinary tract calculi have attenuation values of 200–300 Hounsfield units or higher on CT images.*
- *Blood clots or tumor measure approximately $\leq$70 Hounsfield units on CT images.*

CASE 6

History. 54-year-old woman with refractory hypertension

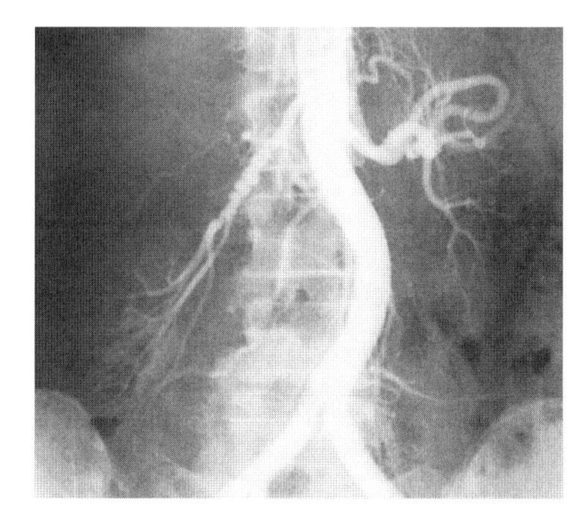

Figure 10.6.1.

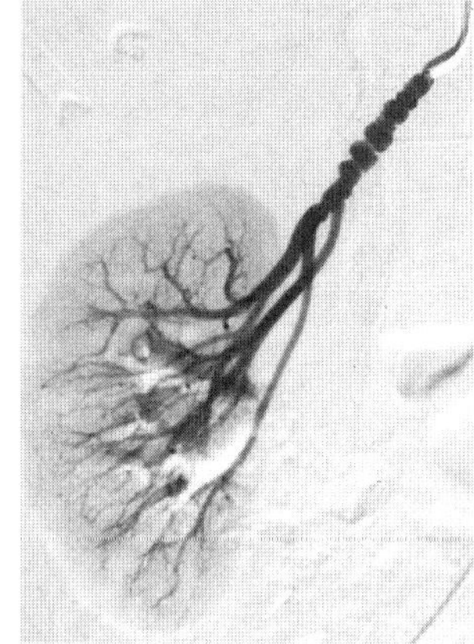

Figure 10.6.2.

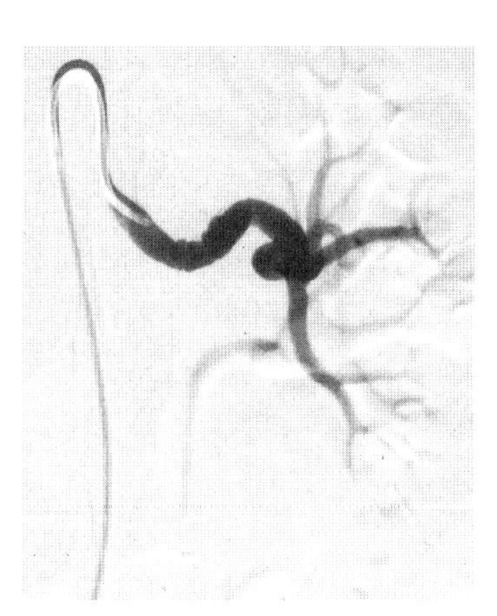

Figure 10.6.3.

Findings. Abdominal aortogram (Fig. 10.6.1) and bilateral selective renal arteriograms (Figs. 10.6.2 and 10.6.3) using intraarterial digital subtraction technique demonstrate areas of alternating stenosis and dilatation in the renal arteries bilaterally, more prominent on the right than the left. This imparts a "string-of-beads" appearance to the renal arteries.

Diagnosis. Fibromuscular dysplasia

Discussion. Fibromuscular dysplasia is the second most common cause of renovascular hypertension after atherosclerotic disease. Fibromuscular dysplasia is classified according to the portion of the arterial wall involved and includes intimal, medial, or adventitial types (11). In medial fibroplasia, the most common type encountered in the adult population, thickened stenotic fibromuscular ridges alternate with areas of arterial wall thinning and aneurysm formation. This leads to the classic string-of-beads appearance (12). In contrast to atherosclerotic lesions, fibromuscular disease is more frequently found in middle-aged females and involves the distal two-thirds of the main renal artery. It is frequently bilateral and may involve branch vessels. Fibromuscular dysplasia is responsive to percutaneous angioplasty, which is the treatment of choice for this abnormality.

Aunt Minnie's Pearls

- *String-of-beads sign in the renal artery = fibromuscular dysplasia.*
- *This lesion occurs in the distal two-thirds of the vessel, unlike atherosclerosis that usually involves the ostia of the artery.*

CASE 7

History. 38-year-old man with bilateral lower extremity swelling and microscopic hematuria

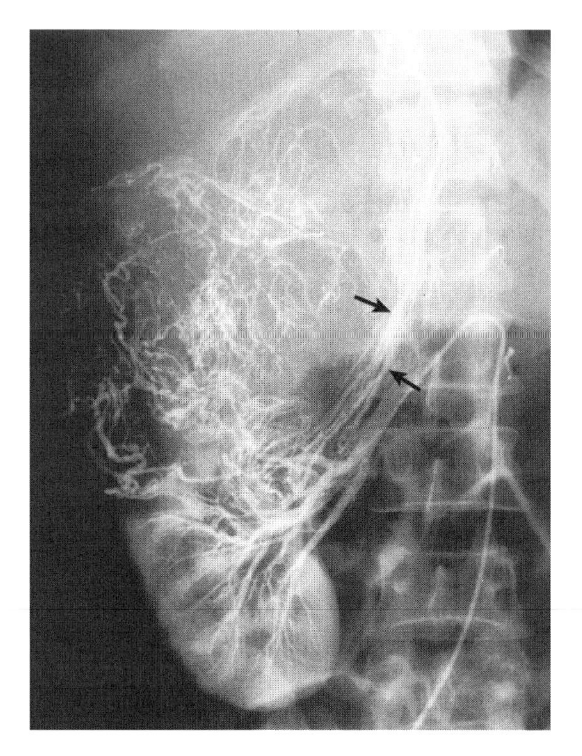

Figure 10.7.1.

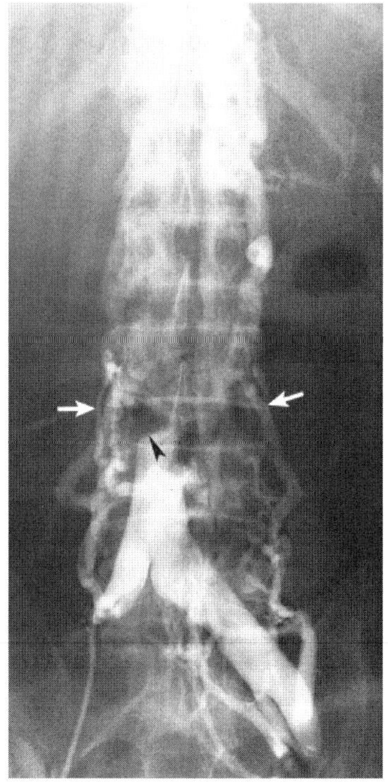

Figure 10.7.2.

Findings. The late arterial phase of a selective right renal arteriogram (Fig. 10.7.1) demonstrates a hypervascular mass in the upper pole of the right kidney with gross architectural distortion of nearby vessels. There is also a striated pattern of vessels (*arrows*) extending from the renal hilus along the course of the right renal vein into the inferior vena cava. Inferior venacavogram (Fig. 10.7.2) reveals occlusion of the inferior vena cava at the level of the upper margin of L4 (*arrowhead*) and collateral flow via the ascending lumbar and hemiazygos venous system (*arrows*).

Diagnosis. Renal cell carcinoma of the right upper renal pole with renal vein and inferior vena cava tumor extension

Discussion. Renal cell carcinoma is well-known for its propensity for venous extension. The striated pattern of vessels seen here represents vascularized tumor extending from the renal mass into the renal vein and inferior vena cava (13). Bland thrombosis has likely developed below the site of tumor thrombus, accounting for the caval obstruction at the level of L4. Intravenous tumor extension can occur in up to 20% of renal cell carcinomas. Extension of tumor into the inferior vena cava is more common on the right because of the shorter renal vein. The presence of venous extension does not preclude surgical extirpation of the tumor, but it is important to recognize preoperatively because it may alter the surgical approach (13, 14). The presence of tumor thrombus within the renal vein and inferior vena cava carries a better prognosis than metastatic lymphadenopathy, direct invasion of adjacent organs, or distant metastases (14).

Aunt Minnie's Pearls

- *Tumor thrombus in the renal vein or inferior vena cava can be diagnosed by the vascular nature of the thrombus.*
- *Vessel invasion carries a much better prognosis than regional adenopathy or metastasis.*

CASE 8

History. 72-year-old man with right flank pain and hematuria; a urogram was performed and showed no excretion from the right kidney; retrograde pyelogram was then performed

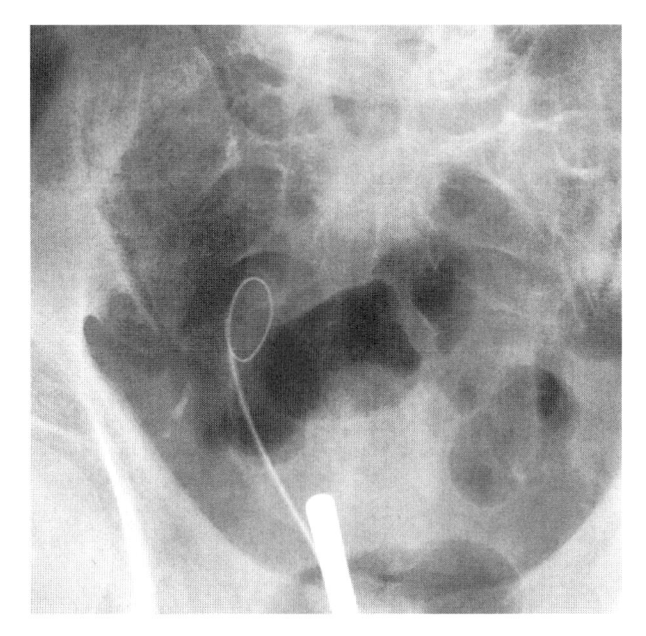

Figure 10.8.1.

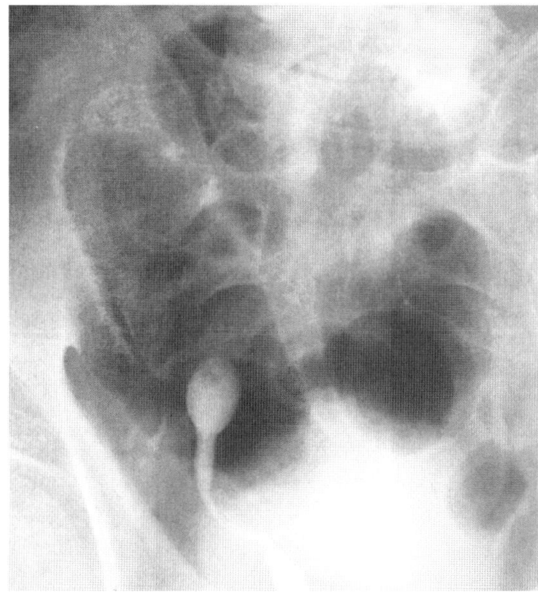

Figure 10.8.2.

Findings. A film obtained during cystoscopy after unsuccessful passage of a ureteral catheter and guide wire (Fig. 10.8.1) shows a cystoscope in place in the bladder and a catheter advanced into the distal right ureter. A guide wire is coiled in the ureter above the catheter. When passage of the catheter was unsuccessful, a retrograde ureterogram was performed (Fig. 10.8.2). This demonstrates complete obstruction of the ureter, with dilatation of the ureter below the obstruction.

Diagnosis. Ureteral transitional cell carcinoma exhibiting the coiled catheter sign and goblet sign

Discussion. Calculi and other causes of acute ureteral obstruction usually cause collapse of the ureter distal to the point of impaction. A transitional neoplasm, which slowly enlarges into the ureteral lumen, may cause dilatation of the ureter below the site of obstruction because of repeated prolapse of the tumor from ureteral peristalsis. A catheter or guide wire passed into the ureter may coil in the dilated ureter below the site of obstruction (coiled catheter sign). When contrast is injected into the ureter below the tumor, the dilated segment and the filling defect created by the tumor may create a goblet or champagne glass appearance of the ureter below the obstruction, as originally described by Bergman et al. (15). Although this appearance is most commonly seen with ureteral transitional cell neoplasms, the findings have also been described with metastatic lesions that traverse the ureteral wall or other processes that invade through the wall of the ureter such as endometriosis (16).

Aunt Minnie's Pearls

- *The coiled catheter sign or Bergman's goblet sign almost always imply ureteral transitional cell carcinoma.*

CASE 9

History. 29-year-old man referred for urography because of right flank pain and microscopic hematuria

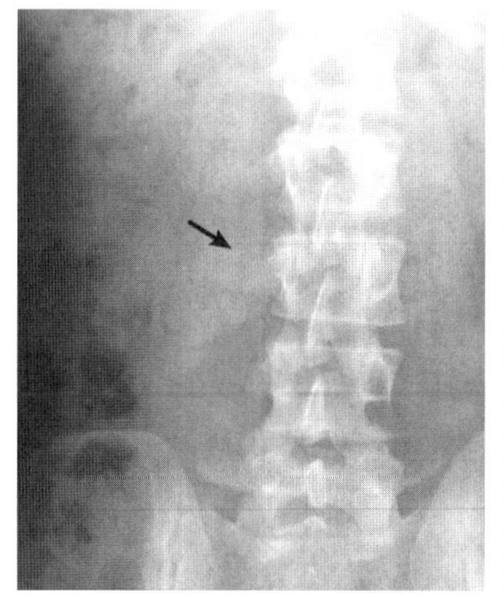

Figure 10.9.1.

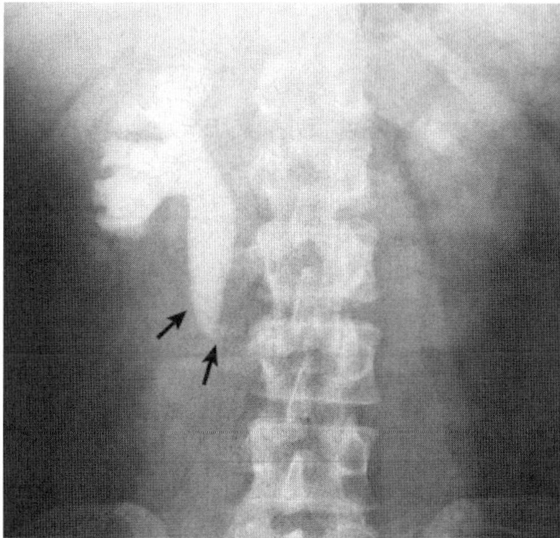

Figure 10.9.2.

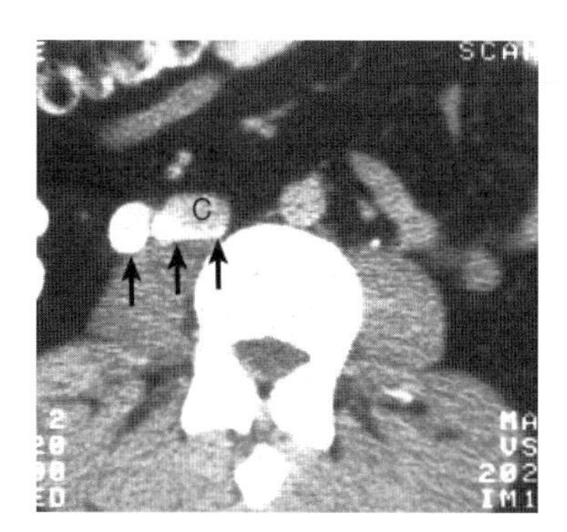

Figure 10.9.3.

Findings. Initial scout film from the intravenous urography demonstrates a 2-mm calcified stone projected just above the right transverse process of the L3 vertebra (Fig. 10.9.1, *arrow*). Delayed film obtained 4 hours after contrast material injection shows hydronephrosis on the right, with dilatation of the upper right ureter and unusual medial deviation of the upper ureteral segment (Fig. 10.9.2, *arrows*). Subsequent axial CT image confirms retrocaval course of the right ureter (Fig. 10.9.3, *arrows*). C, cava.

Diagnosis. Circumcaval right ureter with obstructing stone in upper ureteral segment

Discussion. Circumcaval ureter exists when the right ureter crosses posterior to the inferior vena cava and later descends medially and anteriorly to partially encircle this venous structure. This condition arises from anomalous development of the inferior vena cava rather than from abnormal development of the ureter itself. Normally, the infrarenal segment of the inferior vena cava is formed by the supracardinal vein, a medially located embryologic structure. In circumcaval ureter, the more laterally located embryologic right posterior cardinal vein persists to form the infrarenal inferior vena cava, which causes the ureter to pass posterior and medial to the cava (17). The findings of medial upper ureteral deviation on urography, although suggestive of circumcaval ureter, are not diagnostic; other processes (e.g., retroperitoneal mass, previous surgery, or possibly retroperitoneal fibrosis) can produce a similar appearance. Simultaneous visualization of both the inferior vena cava and the right ureter on CT scans provides a definitive diagnosis of circumcaval ureter. Mild ureteral obstruction independent of urinary tract calculi is a frequent finding in patients with circumcaval ureter (17).

Aunt Minnie's Pearls

- *Characteristic deviation of the upper right ureter medial to the L3 pedicle suggests circumcaval ureter.*
- *Circumcaval ureter arises when the right posterior cardinal vein persists to form the infrarenal inferior vena cava.*

CASE 10

History. 46-year-old man with a history of recurrent urinary tract stones

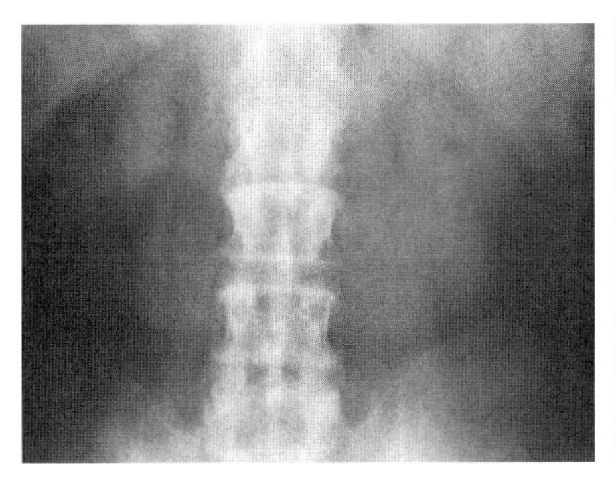

Figure 10.10.1.

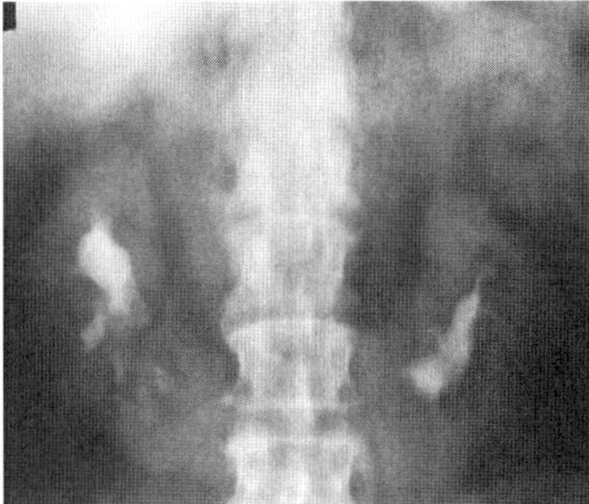

Figure 10.10.2.

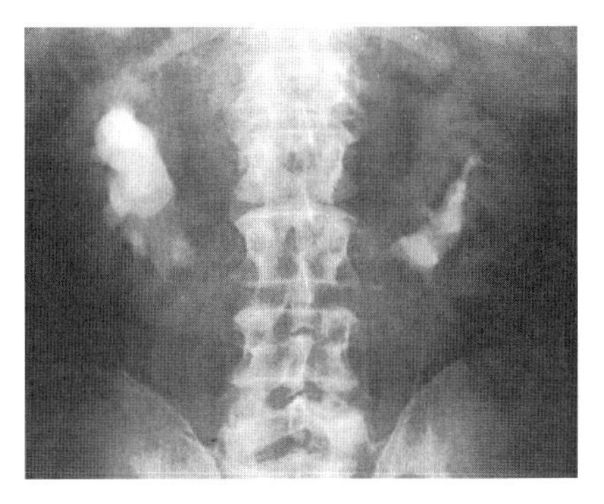

Figure 10.10.3.

Findings. A preliminary tomogram before contrast material injection for urography (Fig. 10.10.1) shows two small calcifications to the right of the L3–L4 disc space and renal outlines that are difficult to define. A nephrotomogram obtained 3 minutes after contrast material injection (Fig. 10.10.2) shows enhancing parenchyma crossing the midline below the pedicles of L3 and an abnormal axis of both kidneys. The 10-minute film from the urographic sequence (Fig. 10.10.3) shows fullness of the right collecting system, an abnormal axis of the collecting systems bilaterally, nonrotation of the collecting systems bilaterally, and an anterior location of the ureters, most notable on the left.

Diagnosis. Horseshoe kidney with mild right ureteropelvic junction obstruction complicated by calculi

Discussion. The horseshoe kidney is the most common fusion anomaly of the kidneys, occurring in approximately 1 in 400 births and showing a male predominance (18). The imaging features are a result of fusion of the inferior portion of the metanephric blastemas before their normal ascent and rotation. The fused tissue, referred to as the isthmus, may be a fibrous band or normally functioning parenchyma. The presence of the isthmus causes incomplete ascent of the kidneys as it impacts on the inferior mesenteric artery, a reversal of the normal axis of the kidneys, and absence of rotation that would normally bring the ureteropelvic junction from an anterior to a medial location (19). Because of the presence of the isthmus, and the rotation anomalies, drainage of the horseshoe kidney is often impaired. As a result, the patients may develop hydronephrosis and complications of stasis including recurrent urinary tract infections and renal calculi (18). It has also been suggested that the incidence of adenocarcinoma, Wilms tumor, and transitional cell carcinoma is probably increased in these patients (18). As with all congenital abnormalities of the urinary tract, there is an increased incidence of congenital anomalies elsewhere in the urinary tract and in other major organ systems including gastrointestinal, musculoskeletal, and cardiovascular systems.

Aunt Minnie's Pearls

- *Embryologic fusion of the inferomedial metanephric blastemas results in a horseshoe kidney.*
- *There is an increased risk of stones, infection, and tumor in a horseshoe kidney.*

CASE 11

History. 27-year-old woman presenting with renal colic as she has at least 50 times previously

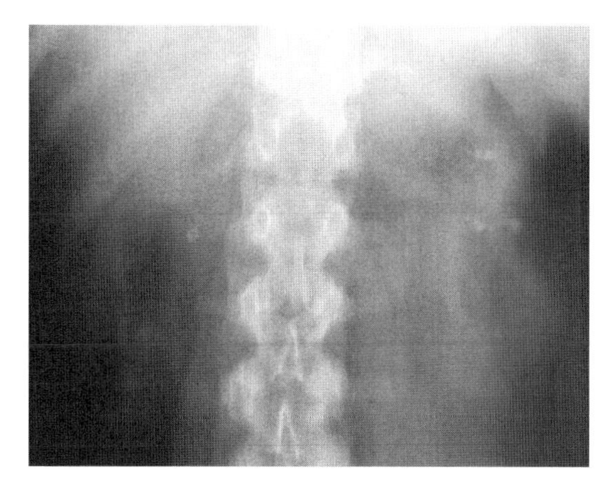

Figure 10.11.1.

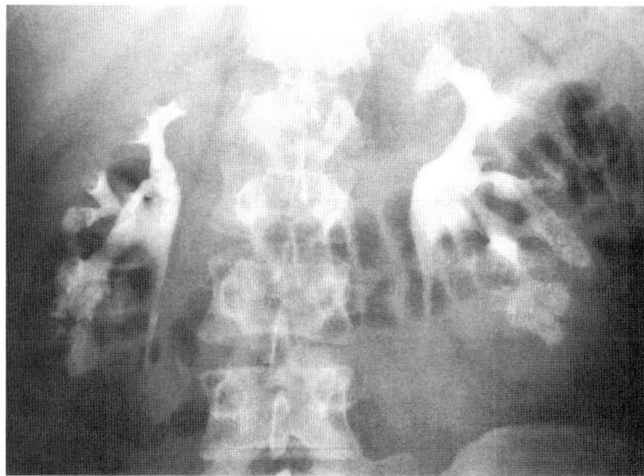

Figure 10.11.2.

Findings. The preliminary nephrotomogram (Fig. 10.11.1) shows multiple scattered calcifications overlying both kidneys. Note peripheral location of many of the calcifications. A 10-minute film from an excretory urogram (Fig. 10.11.2) demonstrates that the stones are contained within dilated cystic spaces in the medullary pyramids of the kidneys. In some areas (especially the left upper pole) the cystic spaces have become confluent and contain large stones. In addition, there are many cystic spaces that do not contain stones. Note that there are also some calyces that do not appear to be involved.

Diagnosis. Medullary nephrocalcinosis associated with medullary sponge kidney

Discussion. Nephrocalcinosis is defined as calcification occurring in the renal parenchyma. The presence of medullary nephrocalcinosis in association with the urographic demonstration of dilated cystic spaces in the medullary pyramids is diagnostic of medullary sponge kidney. As the foci of calcium within the pyramids become surrounded by contrast material in the dilated, ectatic tubules the stones may appear to enlarge. This has been described as the "growing calculus" sign during urography (20). The medullary pyramids may be involved diffusely (as seen on the left), or the condition may spare many papilla (as seen on the right). The calculi may be delivered from the pyramids into the collecting system and produce typical renal colic. Hematuria, flank pain, and dysuria are also common associated symptoms. The urographic demonstration of the dilated spaces in the renal pyramids associated with medullary nephrocalcinosis distinguishes medullary sponge kidney from the other common causes of medullary nephrocalcinosis (e.g., hyperparathyroidism and distal, type I renal tubular acidosis) (21).

Aunt Minnie's Pearls

- *Dilated, cystic spaces in the renal pyramids associated with medullary nephrocalcinosis = medullary sponge kidney.*

CASE 12

History. 61-year-old woman with a right adrenal mass discovered incidentally during renal sonography

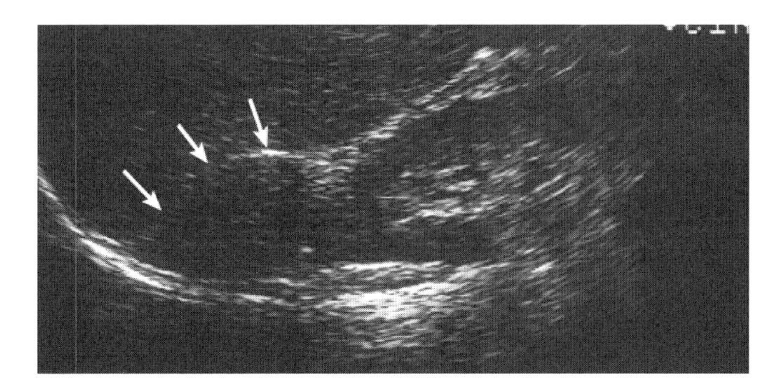

Figure 10.12.1.

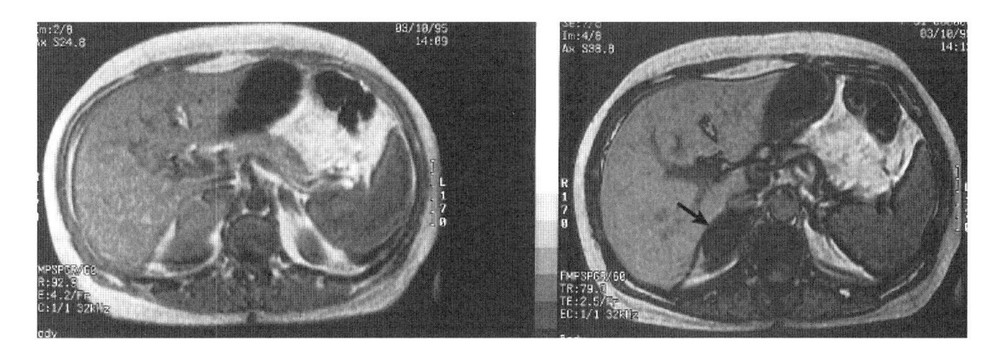

Figure 10.12.2.

Findings. Longitudinal sonographic image shows a solid mass lesion above the right kidney in the region of the right adrenal gland (Fig. 10.12.1, *arrows*). Abdominal MR image acquired with chemical-shift/opposed-phased technique (in-phase image on left, out-of-phase image on right) shows loss of signal intensity within the lesion on the out-of-phase pulse sequence (Fig. 10.12.2, *arrow*).

Diagnosis. Right adrenal adenoma

Discussion. Adrenal adenomas are common benign neoplastic lesions that are found in 2–8% of routine autopsy specimens (22). Adenomas tend to demonstrate various degrees of lipid accumulation, whereas primary and secondary adrenal malignancies generally do not; therefore, a method of detecting lipid within an adrenal mass has emerged as a means of differentiating between these common tumors (23). Chemical-shift/opposed-phase MR imaging is an important technique that relies on the difference between the resonance frequency of protons in water molecules and that of protons integrated into triglyceride molecules. By comparing the signal intensity of a lesion on in-phase breath-hold (fast multiplanar spoiled gradient-recalled) images with its intensity on similar opposed-phase images, the observer can easily identify the global loss of signal intensity within a mass characteristic of an adrenal adenoma. This noninvasive method accurately identifies most adenomas, thereby preventing unnecessary biopsy or prolonged imaging follow-up in patients with indeterminate adrenal lesions (24).

Aunt Minnie's Pearls

- *Adrenal adenomas tend to accumulate lipid.*
- *Loss of signal on out-of-phase MR imaging sequence is compatible with adenoma.*
- *Chemical-shift/opposed-phase MR imaging provides a noninvasive method of differentiating adrenal masses.*

CASE 13

History. 63-year-old diabetic woman with a 7-day history of nausea, vomiting, and fever and on physical examination severe left upper quadrant tenderness; subsequent urinalysis demonstrated 4+ glycosuria, pyuria, and numerous bacteria

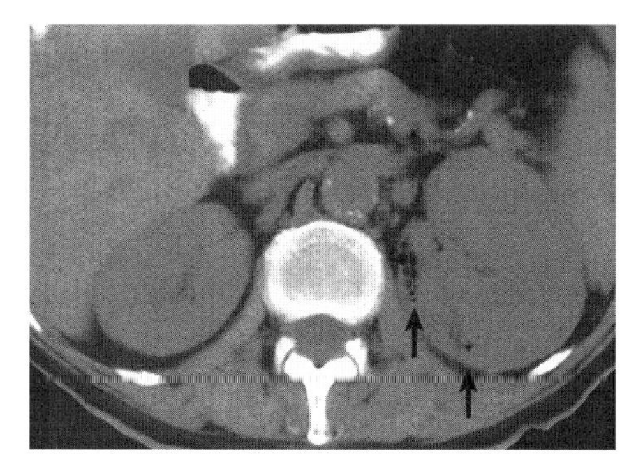

Figure 10.13.1.

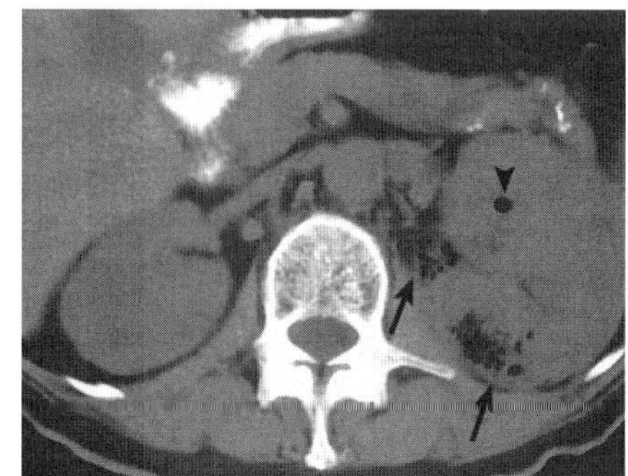

Figure 10.13.2.

Findings. Two axial images from an abdominal CT scan performed without contrast demonstrate gas within the parenchyma of the enlarged left kidney (Figs. 10.13.1 and 10.13.2, *arrows*) as well as a tiny amount of gas within the left intrarenal collecting system (Fig. 10.13.2, *arrowhead*).

Diagnosis. Emphysematous pyelonephritis and emphysematous pyelitis of the left kidney

Discussion. Emphysematous pyelonephritis is an unusual life-threatening form of renal infection characterized by the presence of gas-forming organisms within the renal parenchyma. Emphysematous pyelitis, in contrast, is characterized by gas that is limited to the renal collecting system. Approximately 90% of patients with emphysematous pyelonephritis have preexisting diabetes mellitus, and women are affected twice as commonly as men (25). Although the mechanism is poorly understood, one hypothesis suggests that gas formation is secondary to bacterial fermentation of glucose-rich substrate within the renal tissues. *Escherichia coli* is the causative organism in more than 70% of cases; *Klebsiella*, *Aerobacter*, and *Proteus* species are less frequently isolated (26). Several radiographic patterns of renal parenchymal involvement have been described. The earliest changes include mottling of the renal parenchyma, with gas bubbles extending radially along the renal pyramids. Further extension may lead to a crescentic gas collection within Gerota's fascia followed by erosion through this layer into the retroperitoneum (27). Prompt diagnosis of this condition is critical for early medical and surgical intervention, because mortality rates are high.

Aunt Minnie's Pearls

- *Gas within the renal parenchyma is diagnostic of emphysematous pyelonephritis.*
- *Ninety percent of patients with this disorder have underlying diabetes mellitus, and* E. coli is *the most common causative organism.*

CASE 14

History. Withheld

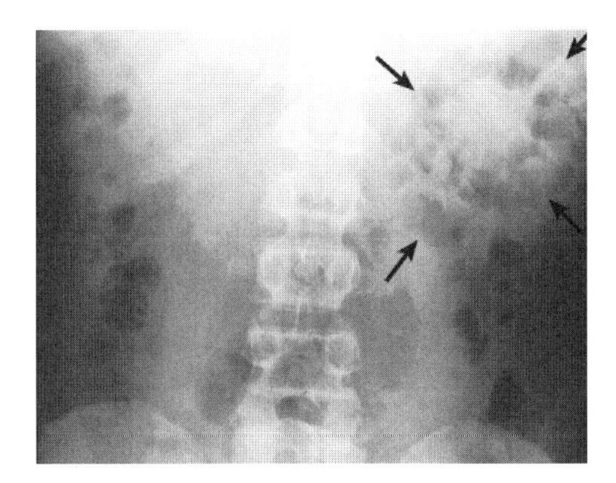

Figure 10.14.1.

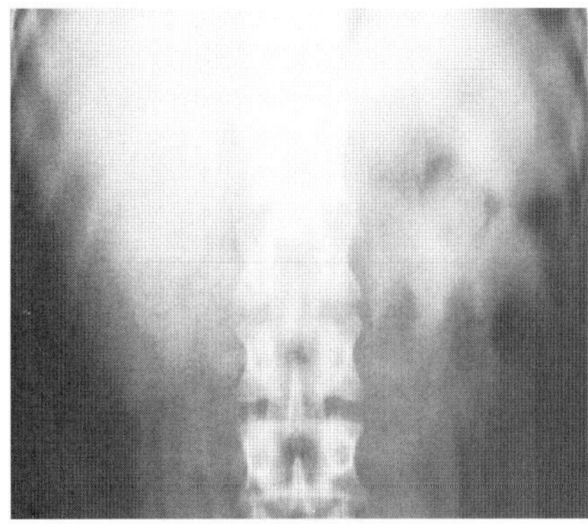

Figure 10.14.2.

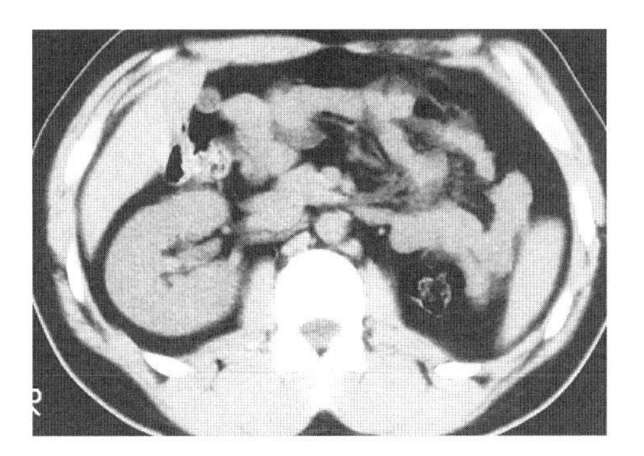

Figure 10.14.3.

Findings. On the abdominal film, as one traces the colon, one can see gas in the transverse colon extending to the lateral aspect of the abdomen and a peculiar looping configuration of the splenic flexure in the left upper quadrant (Fig. 10.14.1, *arrows*). The nephrotomogram (Fig. 10.14.2) shows the right kidney is enlarged, and a left renal outline is not seen. In fact, the only structures in focus on the left are gas containing bowel loops. Because of this finding, an unenhanced CT was obtained a few days later to confirm the diagnosis (Fig. 10.14.3).

Diagnosis. Malposition of the colon (loop-to-loop colon) in left renal agenesis, with right-sided compensatory renal hypertrophy

Discussion. In patients who have never undergone extensive anterior abdominal surgery, the presence of bowel in the renal fossa on conventional tomography or CT usually indicates that the kidney is embryologically absent (28). On the left, when the kidney is not present in the renal fossa, the lack of perirenal fascia allows the colon to occupy this space. As a result, the transverse colon usually extends to the lateral aspect of the abdomen, and the splenic flexure and proximal descending colon slip medially to occupy the fossa. The resulting loop-to-loop appearance may be seen (29). This appearance may be present in agenesis or ectopia of the kidney. When agenesis occurs on the right, the descending duodenum or proximal jejunum may occupy the area of the renal bed, projecting posteriorly over the lumbar spine (28). Hypoplasia or agenesis of the vas deferens and testicle and hypospadias are also seen as associated anomalies in males. In females uterine and vaginal anomalies may be seen in association with renal agenesis (19).

Aunt Minnie's Pearls

- *Loop-to-loop left colon = renal agenesis or ectopia.*

CASE 15

History. 42-year-old man was referred for urography after a traffic accident because of a palpable right-sided abdominal mass and microscopic hematuria on urinalysis

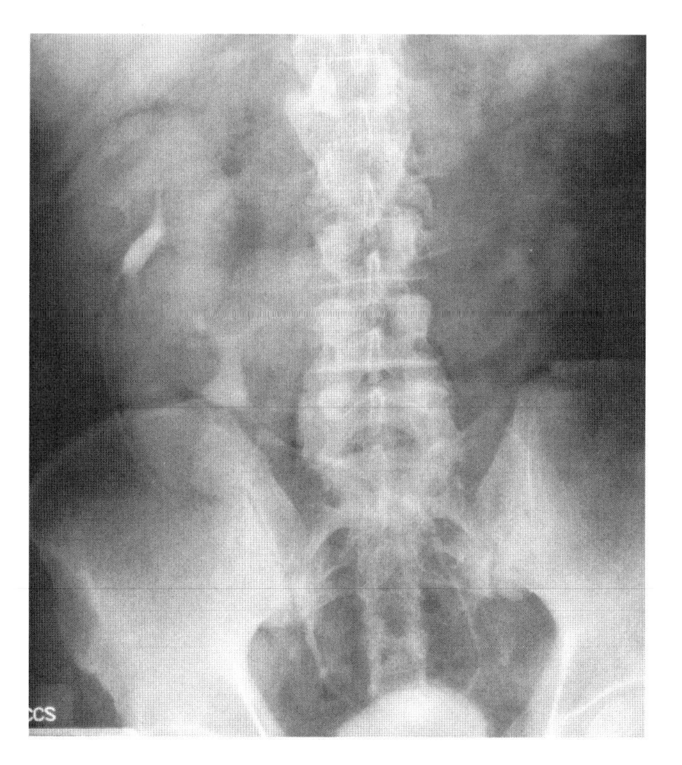

Figure 10.15.1.

Findings. The 5-minute film from the urographic sequence (Fig. 10.15.1) demonstrates two separate renal pelves, both in the right abdomen. The ureter from the upper renal pelvis extends to the right side of the bladder, and the ureter from the lower renal pelvis extends to the left-side of the bladder. There are several transverse process fractures on the right.

Diagnosis. Left to right crossed fused renal ectopia

Discussion. Ectopia refers to a kidney in a congenitally abnormal location. Crossed ectopy refers to a kidney located on the opposite side of its ureteral orifice. As in this case, the condition is more commonly seen in males and more commonly involves the left kidney migrating to the right. The kidney that crosses the midline usually lies inferior to the contralateral kidney. In its most common form, as illustrated here, the two renal moieties fuse. Less commonly, they may remain independent (19, 30). As with the horseshoe kidney, the fusion of the renal parenchyma may lead to abnormalities of rotation, producing stasis complications such as calculus formation, infection, and reflux. Other associated urinary tract anomalies include megaureter, hypospadias, cryptorchidism, urethral valves, and multicystic dysplasia. As with any genitourinary abnormality, there is an increased incidence of other nonurinary tract congenital abnormalities.

Aunt Minnie's Pearls

- *Crossed ectopia refers to a kidney that is on the opposite side of the body relative to its ureteral orifice.*
- *Ectopia is associated with other urinary tract anomalies.*

CASE 16

History. Elderly man with a history of claudication in the right leg, referred for angiography of the abdominal aorta and lower extremities

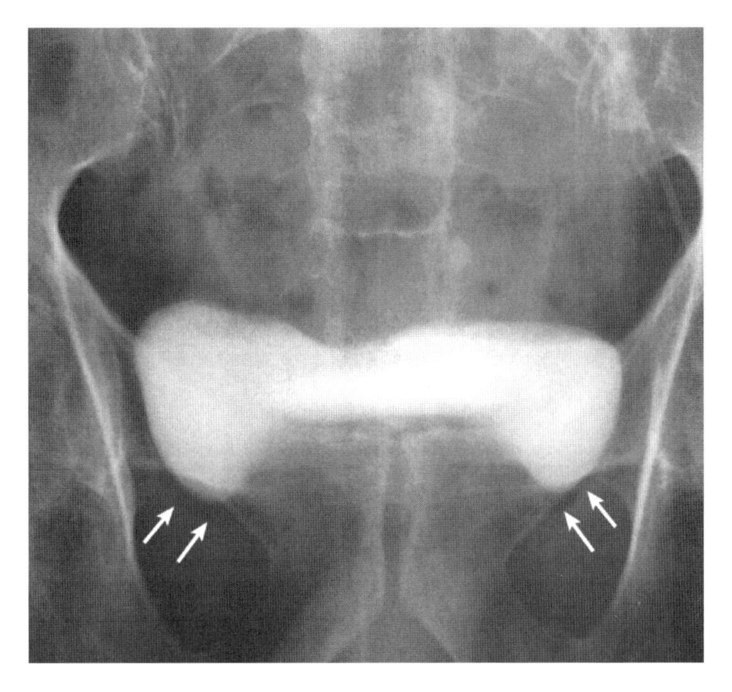

Figure 10.16.1.

Findings. Bilateral outpouchings at the inferior bladder base (Fig. 10.16.1, *arrows*) are incidentally noted during an angiographic procedure.

Diagnosis. Bladder herniation into bilateral inguinal hernias

Discussion. Bladder herniation is most commonly seen in conjunction with inguinal and femoral hernias, although the distended bladder has been documented to herniate into any pelvic or abdominal opening within its reach. Less common sites for herniation include the obturator canal, suprapubic space, and ischiorectal fossa. Herniations of the bladder are classified according to their relationship with the peritoneum as paraperitoneal, intraparaperitoneal, or extraperitoneal. The most common type is the paraperitoneal variety, in which the involved portion of the bladder remains medial to the herniated peritoneal sac. Intraperitoneal herniation occurs when the bladder is present within the hernia sac and is completely covered by peritoneal membrane. The least common form, extraperitoneal herniation, occurs when the bladder alone herniates, and the peritoneum remains within the confines of the pelvis. Bladder hernias are best detected when patients are evaluated in the upright position so that gravity generates sufficient intraluminal pressure to opacify the herniated segment. Because urography is usually performed with the patient in the supine position, only one-third of all bladder hernias are demonstrated with this technique (31). Most cases are mild and are seen radiographically as outpouchings of the inferior bladder margin near the inguinal or femoral canals. Moderate hernias are characterized by a length of herniated lumen of at least 2.5 cm; in more severe cases the hernia may extend caudally into the scrotum (31).

Aunt Minnie's Pearls

- *Bladder hernias are usually seen in conjunction with inguinal or femoral hernias.*
- *Paraperitoneal bladder herniation is the most common type.*
- *Only one-third of bladder hernias are demonstrated with supine cystography technique.*

CASE 17

History. 58-year-old diabetic woman with a 5-day history of worsening abdominal pain and dysuria; gross hematuria and bacteriuria were noted on urinalysis

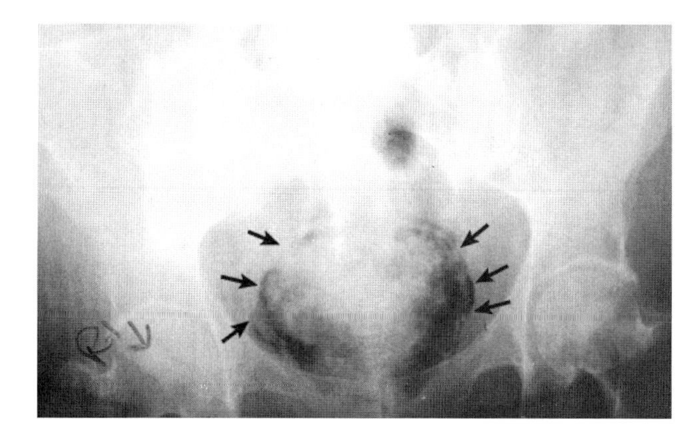

Figure 10.17.1.

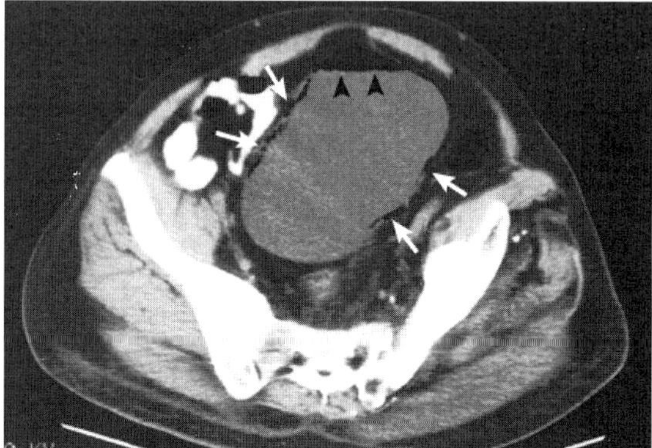

Figure 10.17.2.

Findings. Plain film of the abdomen demonstrates curvilinear mottled lucencies conforming to the outline of the bladder wall (Fig. 10.17.1, *arrows*). Axial unenhanced CT image from another patient with the same condition demonstrates gas within the bladder wall (Fig. 10.17.2, *arrows*) as well as a free gas collection in the nondependent portion of the bladder lumen (Fig. 10.17.2, *arrowheads*).

Diagnosis. Emphysematous cystitis

Discussion. Emphysematous cystitis is an unusual inflammatory condition characterized by the bacterial production of gas within layers of the bladder wall and bladder lumen. Like emphysematous pyelonephritis, this condition is seen most frequently in diabetic women infected with *Escherichia coli* (32). Unlike emphysematous pyelonephritis, this condition is not associated with significant morbidity and generally responds to appropriate antibiotic therapy. Plain films of the abdomen and pelvis often demonstrate the early characteristic findings, with multiple lucencies in a circular pattern conforming to the region of the bladder wall. CT allows confirmation of the anatomic location of the gas-filled vesicles within the lamina propria and muscular layer of the bladder wall (33). Although gas within the bladder lumen can be due to multiple causes (prior instrumentation, fistula formation, trauma, or infection), gas within the bladder *wall* is pathognomonic of infection with gas-forming organisms.

Aunt Minnie's Pearls

- *Gas within the bladder wall is diagnostic of emphysematous cystitis.*
- *Emphysematous cystitis is more common in women and diabetics.*
- *It usually responds to antibiotic therapy alone.*
- *It is associated with much less morbidity than is emphysematous pyelonephritis.*

CASE 18

History. 30-year-old woman in the third trimester of pregnancy with increasing right flank pain and microscopic hematuria. Because urinary tract stones were a clinical consideration in this patient, a limited intravenous urography was performed consisting of a scout view and a 20-minute postinjection film.

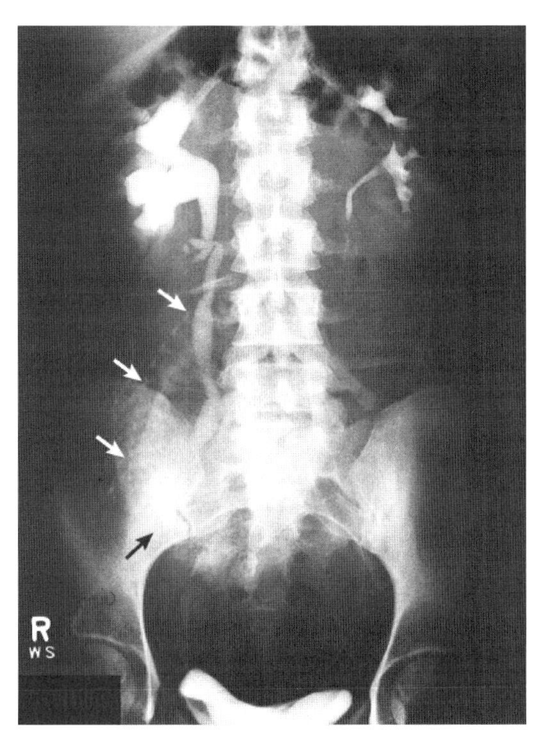

Figure 10.18.1.

Findings. The 20-minute delayed film (Fig. 10.18.1) shows the fetus (*arrows* mark fetal spine) as well as significant dilatation of the right intrarenal collecting system and right ureter extending caudally to the level of the pelvic brim. The characteristic abrupt transition of ureteral caliber usually seen with impacted calculi was not demonstrated, nor was there evidence of a filling defect on close inspection. The left collecting system was grossly normal.

Diagnosis. Hydroureteronephrosis of pregnancy

Discussion. Because the third trimester fetus is less sensitive to radiation injury, limited urography can be performed safely during late pregnancy to exclude the possibility of obstructive calculi. Should a stone be present, therapy would be determined by the size and location of the calculus, degree of obstruction, presence or absence of infection, and overall condition of the patient (34). In this case, the appearance of right-sided dilatation was attributed to hydronephrosis of pregnancy. During pregnancy, the renal collecting systems undergo a variable degree of dilatation, usually more pronounced on the right (35). The characteristic appearance is dilatation (right greater than left) of the collecting systems extending caudally to the level of the pelvic brim, with normal ureteral caliber more inferiorly (36). Regression of dilatation usually occurs several weeks to months postpartum. The most accepted theory for this phenomena is mechanical compression of the right ureter by the gravid uterus; the left ureter is somewhat protected by the cushioning effect of the sigmoid colon. Progesterone-related muscular relaxation, once thought to explain this condition, appears less likely given the lack of distal ureteral involvement (37).

Aunt Minnie's Pearls

- *Hydroureteronephrosis of pregnancy does not extend into the distal ureter.*
- *The left ureter is somewhat protected by the sigmoid colon.*

CASE 19

History. Views of the left kidney from three different patients show different urographic manifestations of the same disease process. For each patient, similar findings were also evident in the right kidney.

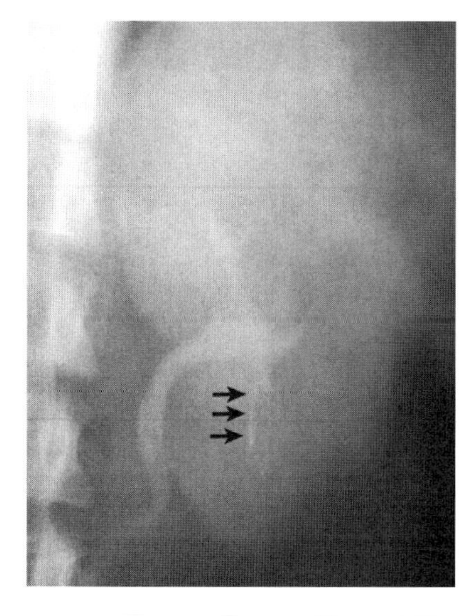

Figure 10.19.1. Lobster claw appearance.

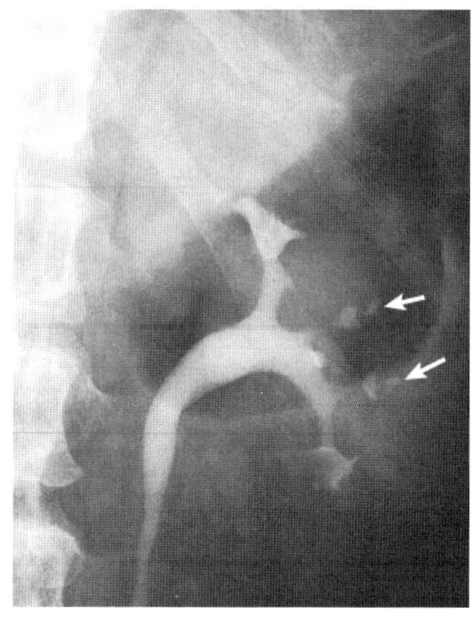

Figure 10.19.2. Ball-on-tee appearance.

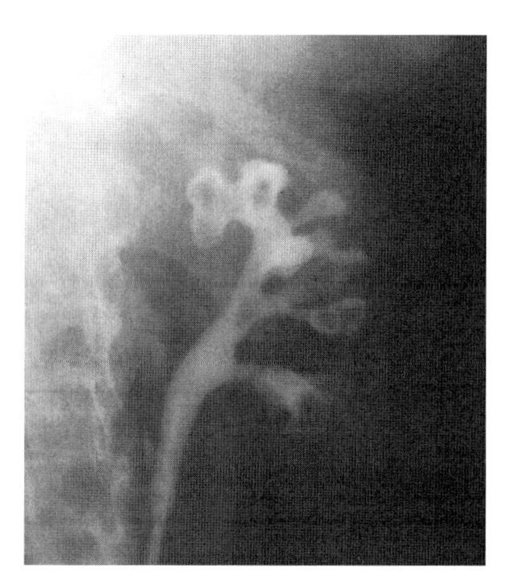

Figure 10.19.3. Signet ring appearance.

Findings. In Figure 10.19.1, there is a long extension of contrast material into the parenchyma along the right side of the enlarged and swollen lower pole papilla (*arrows*) and to a lesser degree along the left side of the papilla (lobster claw appearance). In Figure 10.19.2, the calyces of the midportion of the kidney show collections of contrast material in the central portion of the papillary tip (ball-on-tee appearance). Finally, in Figure 10.19.3, contrast material surrounds a filling defect, which represents a sloughed papillary tip in situ in virtually every calyx of the kidney (signet ring appearance).

Diagnosis. Renal papillary necrosis

Discussion. Papillary necrosis results from several disease processes that affect the renal medullary vasculature and produce focal ischemia in the papillary portions of the medullary pyramids. The radiologic findings will vary with the severity and chronicity of the insult (38–40). Acutely, swelling of the papilla and extension of the calyceal forniceal lines into the renal parenchyma occur. Central cavitation within the papillary tip may allow contrast to accumulate in the ball-on-tee pattern. With extensive necrosis, the entire papillary tip may separate and if held in situ will result in the signet ring appearance (39). If the tissue is passed from the collecting system, diffuse clubbing of the calyces often associated with a "wavy" renal outline may result (40). Conditions commonly associated with papillary necrosis include pyelonephritis, obstruction, sickle cell hemoglobinopathy, tuberculosis, cirrhosis of the liver, analgesic abuse, renal vein thrombosis, and diabetes mellitus (note the acronym POSTCARD). Patterns identified radiographically are not specific for any disease process.

Aunt Minnie's Pearls

- *Lobster claw, ball-on-tee, and signet ring calyces = papillary necrosis.*

CASE 20

History. 17-year-old girl referred for urography after the discovery of microscopic hematuria

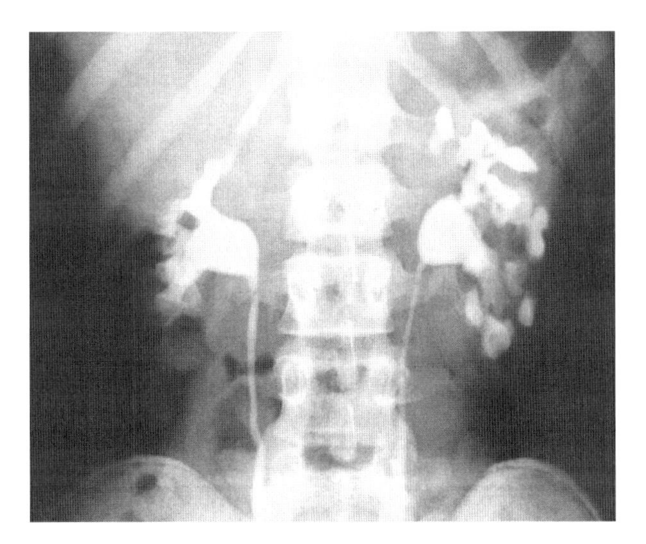

Figure 10.20.1.

Findings. A 10-minute film from an intravenous urogram (Fig. 10.20.1) shows a normal size kidney on the right with a normal intrarenal collecting system. On the left, the kidney is normal to slightly increased in size with an increased number of calyces, each having a faceted appearance. There is no evidence of dilatation of the renal pelvis or ureter on the left.

Diagnosis. Congenital megacalyces

Discussion. The term megacalyces refers to unilateral or bilateral nonobstructive enlargement of the calyces, associated with underdevelopment of the renal pyramids (41, 42). Mellins (43) has suggested that this is a result of calyceal development from a later generation of the ureteric bud than usual. As a result, the number of calyces may be increased to 20–25 compared with the usual 8–12. There is absence of the true papillary tip, giving the calyces a polygonal or faceted appearance. The infundibula are short and broad, but the renal pelvis and ureter are not dilated, indicating that obstruction has not been present (41, 42). As in the case illustrated, overall renal size is normal. Mild impairment of concentrating ability, stone formation, and hematuria after minor trauma may be encountered. Recognition of this condition is important so that differentiation from obstructive atrophy (with its more generalized dilatation of the ureter, renal pelvis, infundibula, and calyces), reflux injury, and papillary necrosis can be made. This finding may be seen in association with primary megaureter.

Aunt Minnie's Pearls

- *Increased number of abnormal, faceted calyces = congenital megacalyces.*

CASE 21

History. 22-year-old man had urography performed for flank pain

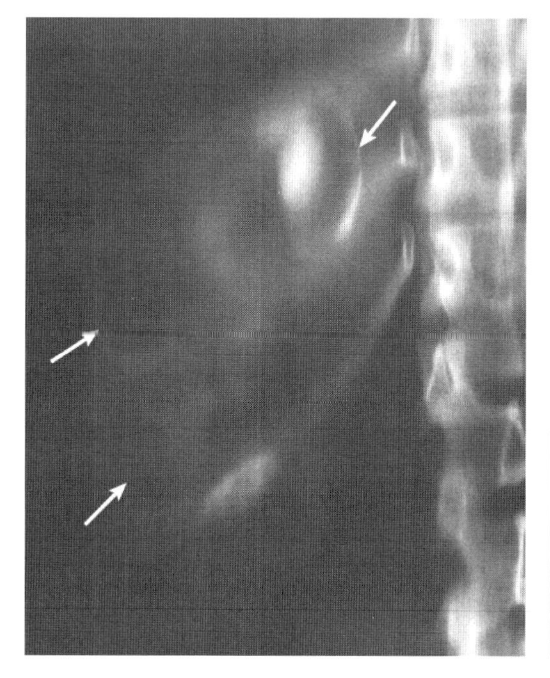

Figure 10.21.1.

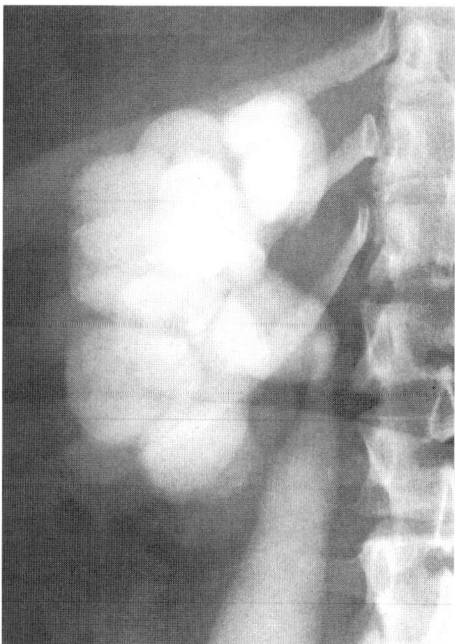

Figure 10.21.2.

Findings. A tomogram obtained 3 minutes after the injection of contrast material for urography (Fig. 10.21.1) shows an enlarged right kidney with thinned renal parenchyma. There are several thin, curvilinear collections of contrast material seen surrounding markedly dilated calyces (*arrows*). Faint ill-defined collections of contrast material are also seen more centrally over the kidney. This represents pooling of the heavier contrast laden urine within markedly dilated calyces. The second film, obtained 30 minutes after contrast material injection (Fig. 10.21.2), confirms marked dilatation of the intrarenal collecting system on the right as well as the renal pelvis and proximal ureter. These findings were the result of longstanding obstruction of the distal right ureter.

Diagnosis. Severe right hydronephrosis with calyceal or "Dunbar's" crescents

Discussion. Calyceal crescents represent contrast material in collecting tubules arranged parallel to the margin of a markedly dilated calyx (44, 45). The change in distal renal tubular orientation from vertical in the normal papillary tip to almost horizontal as seen here occurs in response to prolonged obstruction and dilatation of the collecting system (45). Urine laden with contrast material enters the dilated calyx with its higher specific gravity and accumulates in the dependent portion of these calyces, giving rise to ill-defined pools of contrast material. Early parenchymal opacification may surround the unopacified urine in the dilated collecting system, giving an appearance of a "negative pyelogram." As the dilated collecting system fills with contrast material, the calyceal crescents disappear. Delayed films usually allow opacification of the entire extent of the collecting system. Despite the degree of hydronephrosis and parenchymal loss, the presence of calyceal crescents implies significant residual concentrating ability in these kidneys.

Aunt Minnie's Pearls

- *Calyceal crescents are seen in chronic obstruction.*
- *Their presence implies significant residual concentrating ability in these kidneys.*

CASE 22

History. Patient A: multiple urinary tract stones; patient B: transitional cell carcinoma of the bladder.

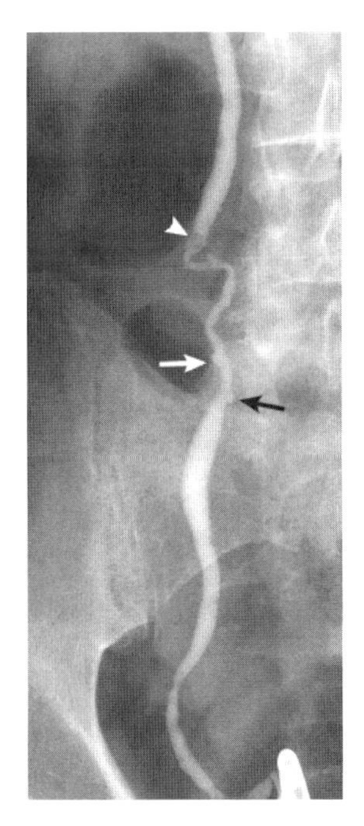

Figure 10.22.1. Patient A.

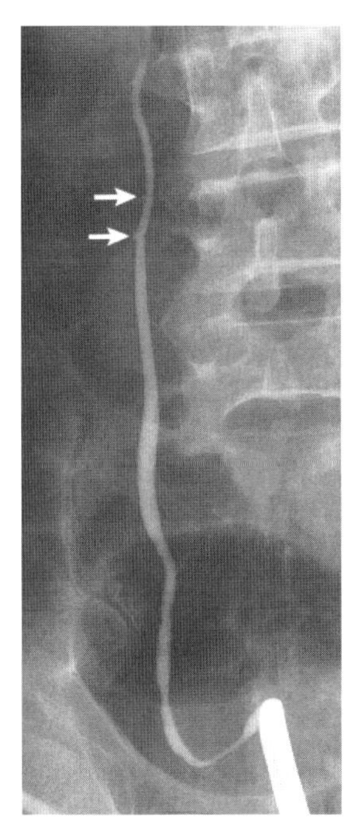

Figure 10.22.2. Patient B.

Findings. A stone creates a filling defect in the right ureter (Fig. 10.22.1, *arrowhead*) above an area of narrowing in the midureter. In the area of narrowing, there are several small contrast-filled outpouchings that project for a short distance into the ureteral wall (*arrows*). Several small contrast-filled outpouchings are seen in the midureter on this retrograde ureterogram in the second patient (Fig. 10.22.2, *arrows*).

Diagnosis. Ureteral pseudodiverticula

Discussion. Ureteral pseudodiverticula are small outpouchings of the ureteral lumen that are sharply demarcated and usually vary in size from 1 to 3 mm in both width and length (46, 47). As demonstrated in these cases, three to eight diverticula clustered over a distance of 2–6 cm in the midureter are commonly seen. The involved ureteral segment is often narrowed as illustrated in Figure 10.22.1 but is not usually obstructed. Bilateral ureteral involvement may be seen in up to 50% of cases. The outpouchings represent down-growth of the transitional epithelium into the ureteral wall, probably as a result of epithelial hyperplasia. Because the outpouchings do not contain all layers of the ureteral wall, they are pseudodiverticula (46, 47). The hyperplastic response has been associated with urinary stone disease and obstruction, infection, and transitional cell carcinoma especially in the urinary bladder (as occurred in the second patient). Patients with pseudodiverticula should therefore be monitored closely for the development of transitional cell neoplasms, especially in the bladder (48).

Aunt Minnie's Pearls

- *Small outpouchings of the ureter = pseudodiverticula.*
- *These patients should be monitored for the development of transitional cell carcinoma.*

CASE 23

History. 58-year-old man with a well-documented history of tuberculosis and recent complaints of painful urination and cloudy urine

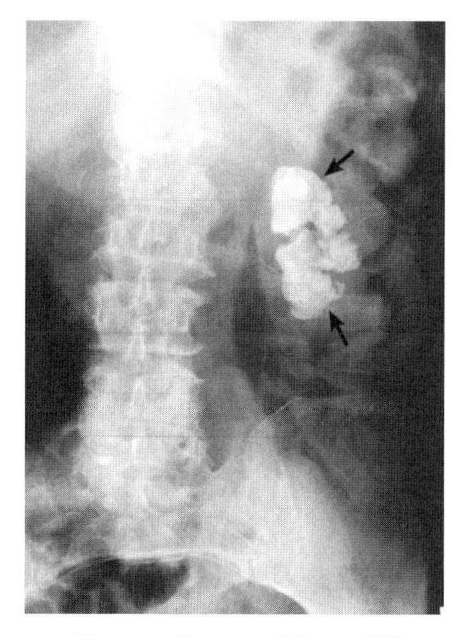

Figure 10.23.1.

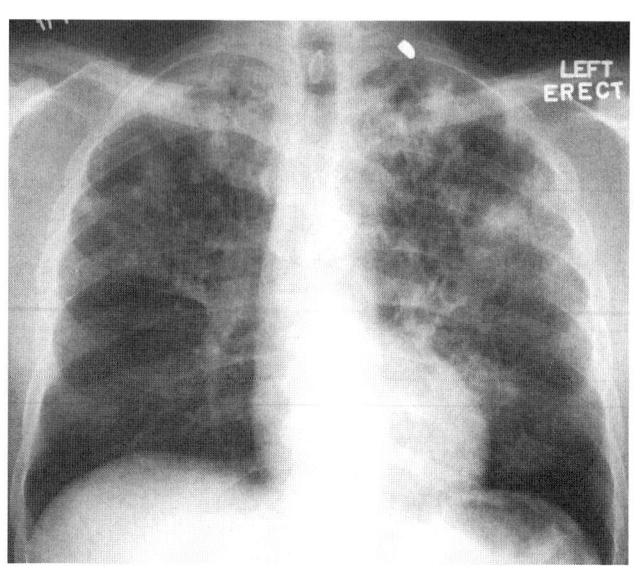

Figure 10.23.2.

Findings. Plain films of the abdomen obtained before urography demonstrate amorphous, putty-like parenchymal calcification within the left kidney (Fig. 10.23.1, *arrows*). Single frontal view of the chest obtained 10 years earlier (Fig. 10.23.2) demonstrates characteristic roentgenographic changes of active granulomatous infection with bilateral cavitary upper lobe infiltrates.

Diagnosis. Renal tuberculosis with "putty" kidney or "silent autonephrectomy"

Discussion. The number of documented tuberculous infections within the United States has been rising as a result of the influx of populations from underprivileged areas and the staggering increase in the number of patients with acquired immunodeficiency syndrome. Tuberculosis of the urinary tract has historically represented only 5% of all tuberculous infections (49). Primarily a disease of adults, tuberculosis affects more men than women. Renal involvement is rare before 20 years of age, and clinical signs and symptoms (dysuria, hematuria, and pyuria) are usually discovered in the third and fourth decades of life. Interestingly, less than 5% of patients with urinary tract tuberculosis have an active pulmonary infection, and less than 50% have any radiographic changes indicative of previous lung infection (49). Urinary tract tuberculosis is the result of hematogenous spread of tuberculous bacilli from the lungs and other primary sites of infection to the kidneys (50). Disease can spread along the urothelial submucosa and adjacent lymphatics to affect the pyelocaliceal system and eventually the ureters and bladder. Ironically, the healing phase of this infection can be the most damaging component of the disease process, because ulceration and caseation progress to severe fibrotic strictures and often irreversible scarring.

Aunt Minnie's Pearls

- *Radiographic changes associated with urinary tract tuberculosis are often unilateral or asymmetric (51).*
- *Urinary tract tuberculosis starts in the kidneys and spreads in an antegrade fashion.*
- *Amorphous unilateral renal parenchymal calcifications should raise the clinical suspicion of tuberculosis.*

CASE 24

History. 30-year-old man with abdominal pain

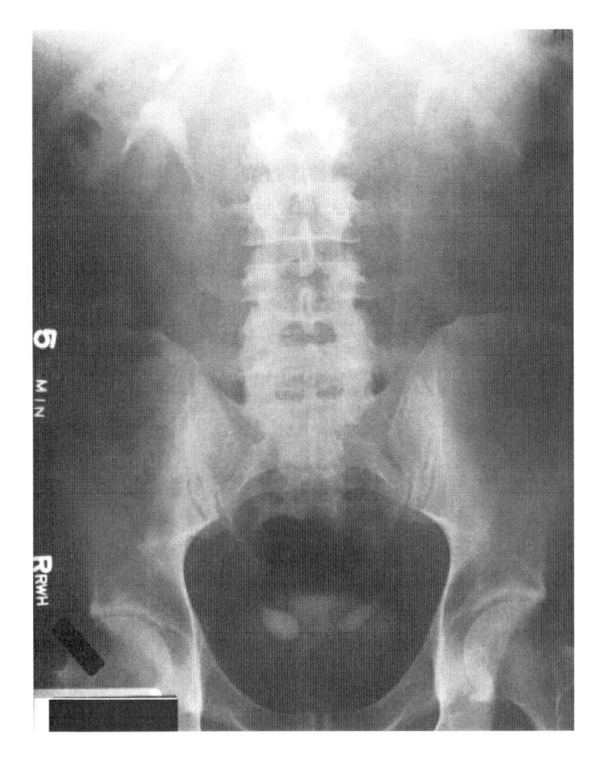

Figure 10.24.1.

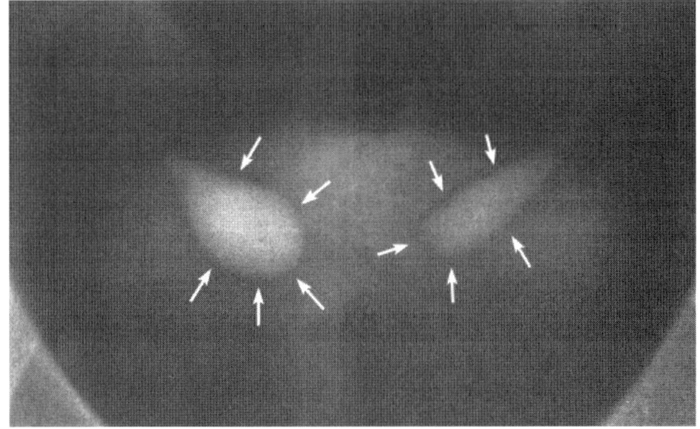

Figure 10.24.2.

Findings. 5-minute postinjection film from an intravenous urography demonstrates focal dilatation of the distal ureters bilaterally (Fig. 10.24.1). The distal ureters are protruding into the bladder and are surrounded by thin halos of lucency noted within the opacified bladder lumen (Fig. 10.24.2, *arrows*).

Diagnosis. Bilateral simple orthotopic ureteroceles

Discussion. The term ureterocele was coined by Stoeckel in the 1930s to describe focal dilatation of the submucosal portion of the distal ureter as it traverses the bladder wall. Since that time, ureteroceles have been subclassified into two varieties: orthotopic (occurring at the normal anatomic ureteral insertion site) and ectopic (occurring outside the normal trigonal entry site) (52). Of special note is the acquired orthotopic ureterocele, or pseudoureterocele, that results from incomplete distal ureteral obstruction secondary to an impacted urinary calculus or adjacent mucosal tumor. The radiographic appearance of this type of ureterocele mimics that of the congenital, or simple, orthotopic form of this lesion.

Simple orthotopic ureteroceles are often discovered incidentally during routine urographic examinations. The appearance of the distal ureter has been compared with a cobra head or spring onion. The thin halo of tissue often seen encircling the dilated ureteral segment represents the bladder mucosa outlined by contrast medium as it surrounds the protruding dilated ureter. Any thickening or irregularity of this surrounding lucent tissue, especially in older patients, should prompt suspicion of a pseudoureterocele. In questionable cases, cystoscopy may be necessary to evaluate the abnormality directly (53, 54).

Aunt Minnie's Pearls

- *Uncommonly, simple ureteroceles can cause obstruction, infection, or stone formation.*
- *Irregularity of the lucent halo should suggest an acquired lesion or pseudoureterocele.*
- *Ectopic ureteroceles are associated with duplicated collecting systems.*

CASE 25

History. 53-year-old man with a history of microscopic hematuria

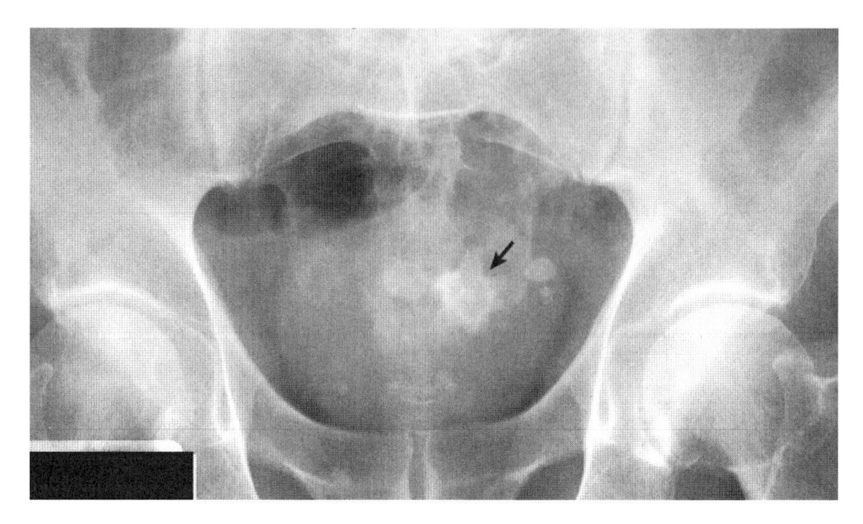

Figure 10.25.1.

Findings. Scout film from an intravenous urography demonstrates multiple calcifications projected over the true bony pelvis and a prominent "jackstone" calcification projected over the upper left margin of the bladder (Fig. 10.25.1, *arrow*).

Diagnosis. Calcium oxalate bladder stone among other bladder calculi

Discussion. Lower urinary tract calculi are much less frequent than stones in the kidneys and upper collecting systems, and most lower tract stones reside in the bladder lumen. Except for ureteral stones that may have been temporarily passed into the bladder (also known as migrant calculi), bladder calculi can be classified by their etiology as primary or secondary, depending on the presence of preexisting calculogenic factors (e.g., obstruction, stasis, infection, or foreign body). Primary or endemic calculi are most frequently seen in young men from the Middle East and Far East and likely are related to certain dietary deficiencies of milk and other proteins. These poorly opaque or radiolucent stones are composed of ammonium hydrogen urate. Most secondary calculi are seen in older patients with underlying urinary stasis, as occurs with bladder-outlet obstruction in men, bladder diverticula, or stasis associated with lower urinary tract infection. Secondary bladder calculi can vary in chemical composition, size, shape, or number. The characteristic peripheral spiculations defining the "jackstone" appearance in the current case indicate a calcium oxalate composition (55).

Aunt Minnie's Pearls

- *Bladder calculi are less common than upper tract stones.*
- *"Jackstone" appearance is associated with calcium oxalate.*
- *Secondary calculi are seen with underlying stasis, infection, obstruction, or foreign bodies.*

Case 26

History. 82-year-old man with a 1-week history of left flank pain

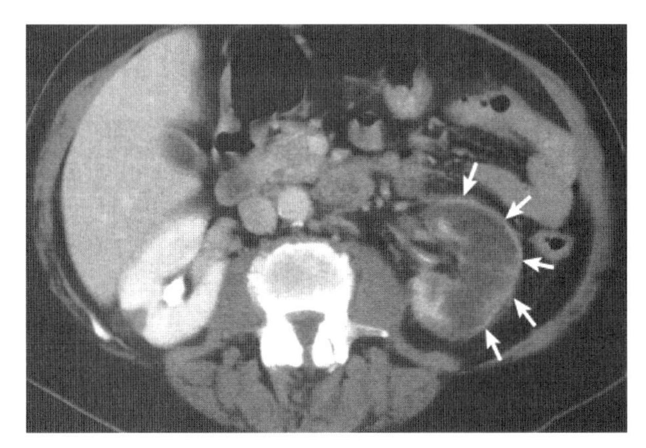

Figure 10.26.1.

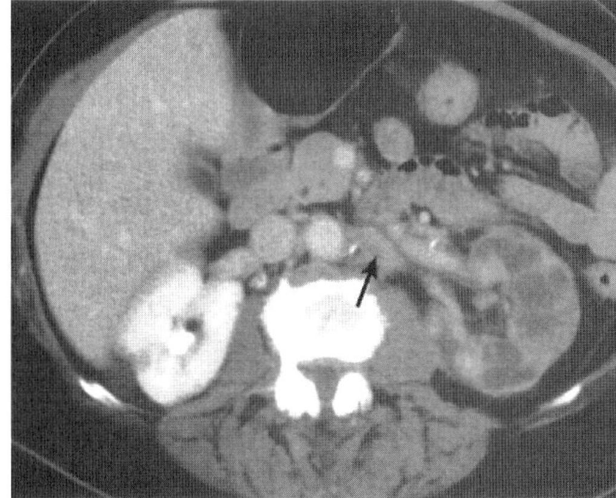

Figure 10.26.2.

Findings. Axial contrast-enhanced CT images through the kidneys reveal large areas of nonperfusion involving the parenchyma of the left kidney surrounded by a thin rim of contrast enhancement (Fig. 10.26.1, *arrows*). Focal clot is demonstrated on a CT image within the left renal artery as low attenuation at the origin of this vessel (Fig. 10.26.2, *arrow*).

Diagnosis. Embolic occlusion of the left renal artery and nearly total infarction of the left kidney

Discussion. Segmental absence of the CT nephrogram can be due to space-occupying lesions such as cysts or tumors but can also be seen with local physiologic or hemodynamic alterations affecting parenchymal blood flow. Because contrast material is prevented from reaching tissue beyond sites of vascular occlusion, areas of underperfusion are depicted as focal or multifocal peripheral wedge-shaped areas of decreased attenuation against a background of normally enhancing parenchyma. Results in most clinical series suggest that embolic phenomena are the leading cause of multifocal segmental renal infarcts, with emboli arising either from a cardiac source or from diseased peripheral vessels. The rim nephrogram surrounding unopacified tissue seen in this case is believed to represent preserved subcapsular perfusion via collateral flow through capsular, peripelvic, and periureteric vessels. This characteristic rim sign is demonstrated in approximately 50% of patients with renal infarction and provides strong evidence to support this diagnosis. Although rarely seen in other disorders such as acute tubular necrosis or renal vein thrombosis, this rim pattern of subcapsular enhancement serves as a crucial point of differential diagnosis between infarction and pyelonephritis (another abnormality with a similar CT appearance) (56).

Aunt Minnie's Pearls

- *Rim pattern of enhancement is highly suggestive of renal infarction.*
- *Emboli are the leading cause of segmental or multifocal renal infarcts.*
- *The rim pattern of enhancement has not been described with pyelonephritis.*

CASE 27

History. 50-year-old man with right flank pain

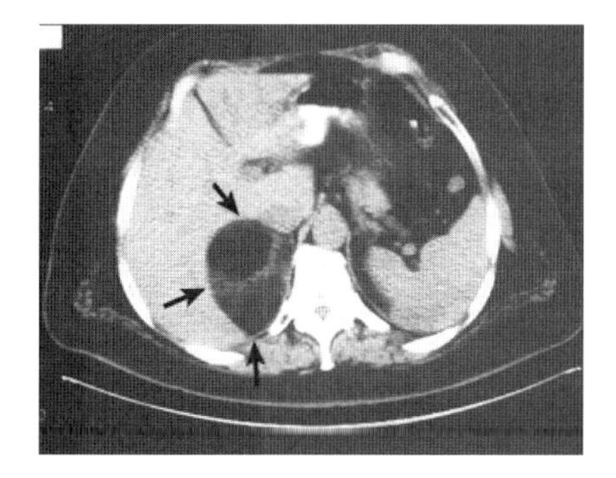

Figure 10.27.1.

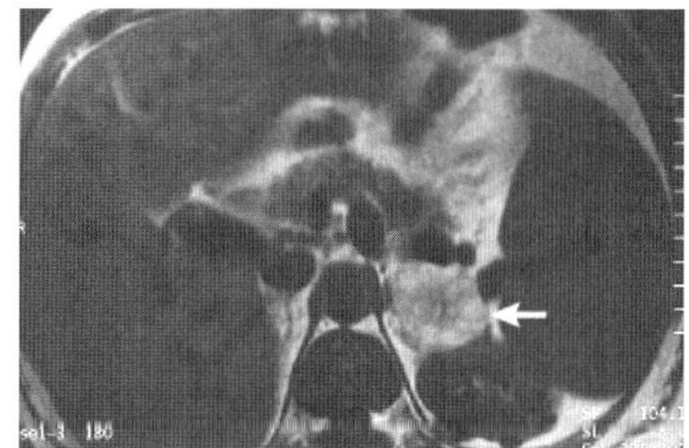

Figure 10.27.2. SE 888/12.

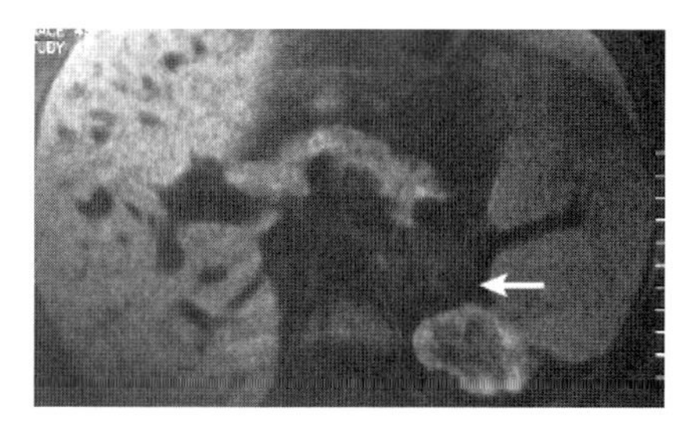

Figure 10.27.3. SE 800/12 with fat saturation.

Findings. An unenhanced axial CT image of the abdomen shows a large right adrenal mass with obvious low-attenuation fatty elements (Fig. 10.27.1, *arrows*). Axial T1-weighted MR images (Fig. 10.27.2) in a different patient reveal a left adrenal mass that has the same signal intensity as subcutaneous fat (*arrow*). Fat saturation MR image of the same lesion (Fig. 10.27.3) reveals that the mass completely loses signal (*arrow*), confirming the large quantity of fat within it.

Diagnosis. Adrenal myelolipoma

Discussion. Adrenal myelolipomas are benign tumors composed of variable amounts of mature adipose cells and hematopoietic tissue. Considered a rare lesion, this neoplasm is functionally inactive and is usually discovered incidentally during abdominal imaging or autopsy (57). Although most myelolipomas are asymptomatic, hemorrhage or necrosis can occur within the tumor, and adjacent structures may be compressed, especially with the larger lesions. The demonstration of well-defined macroscopic fat within an adrenal mass on CT examination virtually confirms the diagnosis of adrenal myelolipoma. Other considerations in the differential diagnosis of a suprarenal fatty mass would include an exophytic renal or extrarenal angiomyolipoma, a retroperitoneal lipoma, or possibly a liposarcoma. Careful analysis of the lesion for exact location, margination, internal consistency, and CT attenuation values should allow a correct diagnosis. Tumors with irregular margins, internal heterogeneity, significant contrast enhancement, and attenuation values greater than that of normal fat should be considered suggestive of malignancy (57, 58).

Aunt Minnie's Pearls

- *Myelolipomas are benign, nonfunctioning tumors containing fat and marrow elements.*
- *Precontrast CT scans or MR images are most useful to identify fat within adrenal lesions.*

Case 28

History. 62-year-old woman with recurrent symptoms of lower urinary tract infection

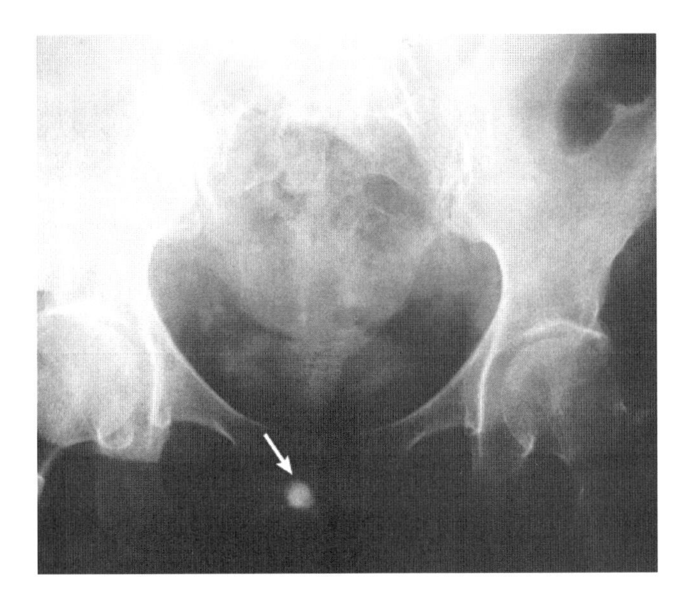

Figure 10.28.1.

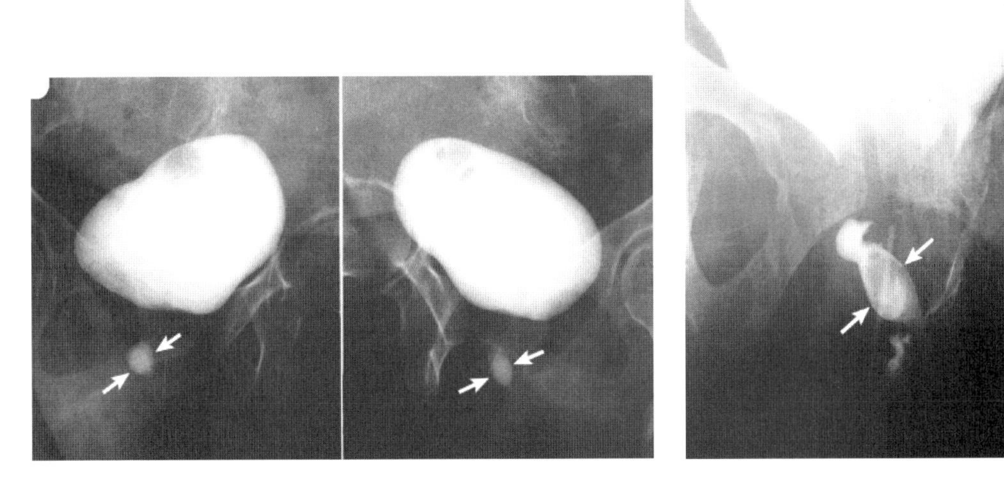

Figure 10.28.2. **Figure 10.28.3.**

Findings. Plain film of the pelvis reveals a 19 × 14 mm ovoid calcification projected over the pubis on the right (Fig. 10.28.1, *arrow*). Bilateral oblique views obtained from a VCUG study demonstrate a persistent collection of contrast material in the region of the urethra (Fig. 10.28.2, *arrows*). Subsequent positive-pressure urethrography was performed with a double-balloon catheter demonstrating a bilobed urethral diverticulum (Fig. 10.28.3, *arrows*) containing a large stone.

Diagnosis. Large urethral diverticulum containing a calculus

Discussion. The clinical diagnosis of a urethral diverticulum can be elusive, but the diagnosis should be considered in women with unexplained recurrent urinary tract infections. One common historical clue is posturinary dribbling, which occurs because the diverticulum fills during voiding and slowly empties after voiding is complete. The traditional urologic evaluation for these patients, including physical examination and cystoscopy, is often unrevealing. Careful radiographic workup with both voiding cystourethrography and a positive-pressure urethral study is considered the most sensitive means of making this diagnosis. VCUG often demonstrates the exact number and position of urethral diverticula, whereas the double-balloon study provides higher pressure and better contrast opacification of occult diverticula. Previous studies have shown that most diverticula in women occur posteriorly in the midurethra, corresponding to the anatomic location of the periurethral or Skene's glands. One theory proposes that infection and obstruction of the orifices of these glands leads to a small abscess, which later ruptures into the urethral lumen, thus forming the diverticulum (59).

Aunt Minnie's Pearls

- *Clinicians should suspect a urethral diverticulum in any female patient with recurrent lower urinary tract symptoms and posturinary dribbling.*
- *VCUG and double-balloon urethral studies are the diagnostic tests of choice.*
- *If a diverticulum is detected, it should be analyzed for lucent filling defects that could represent stones, debris, or even a neoplasm.*

Case 29

History. 43-year-old man with known chronic renal insufficiency presents with subacute left flank pain

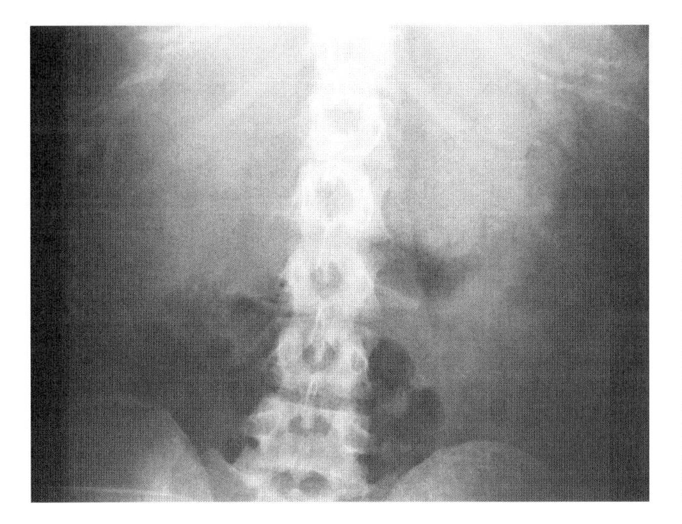

Figure 10.29.1.

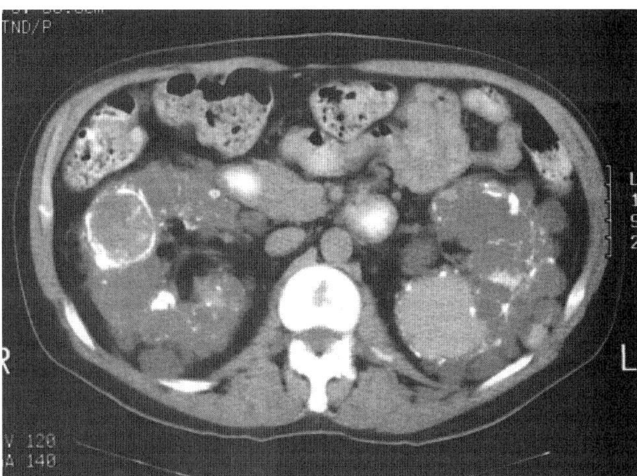

Figure 10.29.2.

Findings. An abdominal plain film (Fig. 10.29.1) reveals numerous bilateral calcifications over the renal fossae. The kidneys are quite large (left kidney extends over a length of at least five lumbar vertebral bodies), and the renal outlines are difficult to define. Note the nearly complete peripheral curvilinear calcification in the lesion in the lower pole of the right kidney. Unenhanced CT scan (Fig. 10.29.2) shows innumerable cysts within both kidneys, and innumerable calcifications within the walls of the cysts. High density cysts are seen in the dorsal aspect of the left kidney and at the periphery of the left kidney.

Diagnosis. Autosomal dominant polycystic kidney disease (ADPKD) with extensive cyst wall calcification bilaterally and cysts complicated by hemorrhage

Discussion. The discovery of enlarged kidneys with irregular or poorly defined renal outlines should always prompt consideration of the diagnosis of ADPKD. With increasing numbers of cysts, the kidneys progressively increase in size, with most patients becoming symptomatic in the fourth or fifth decade (60). On CT, renal cyst calcifications or urinary tract stones can be seen in up to 50% of patients with ADPKD (61). Cyst calcification is believed to be a consequence of cyst hemorrhage and may be more common in older patients with larger kidneys and poorer renal function. Renal stones are also more common in patients with ADPKD, as a result of urinary stasis from distortion of the renal collecting systems by the multiple cysts (61). If urography is performed, the cysts create multiple filling defects in the enlarged nephrogram giving it a Swiss cheese appearance. The collecting system is stretched by the cysts giving it a spidery or arachnoid appearance.

Aunt Minnie's Pearls

- *Enlarged kidneys with innumerable, calcified, and high density cysts = ADPKD.*

CASE 30

History. Two different patients undergoing hysterosalpingography for infertility

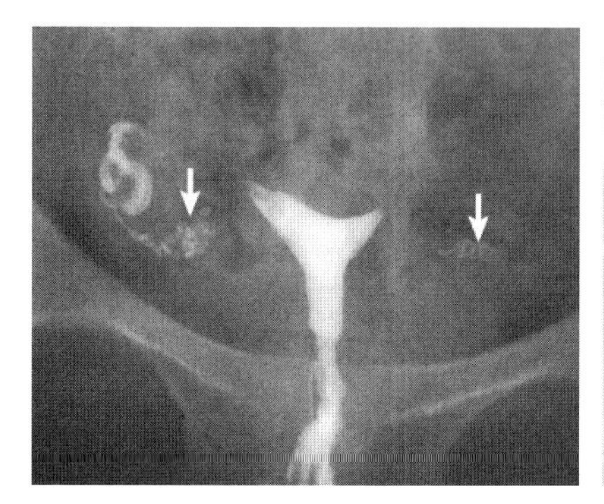

Figure 10.30.1. Patient A.

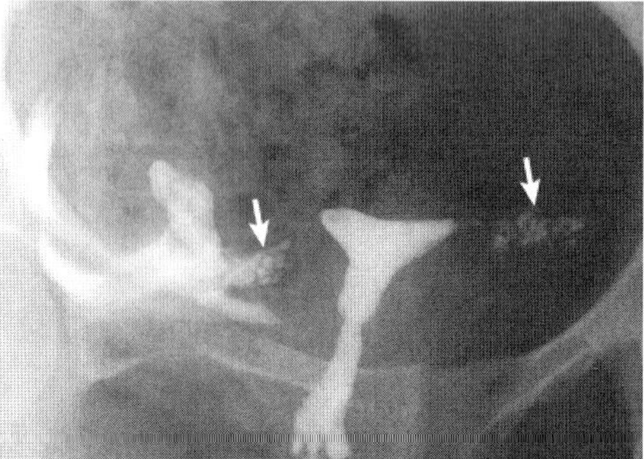

Figure 10.30.2. Patient A.

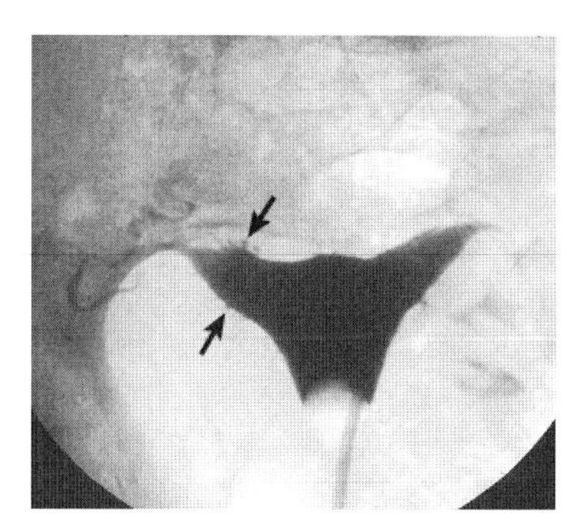

Figure 10.30.3. Patient B.

Findings. In patient A, irregular outpouchings of contrast (*arrows*) are seen in the isthmic portion of the tubes bilaterally (Figs. 10.30.1 and 10.30.2). In patient B, small collections of contrast are seen projecting into the uterine wall (Fig. 10.30.3, *arrows*).

Diagnosis. Patient A: salpingitis isthmica nodosa; patient B: adenomyosis

Discussion. Salpingitis isthmica nodosa is a distinctive abnormality of the female adnexa that affects the isthmic portion of the fallopian tubes. The disorder is diagnosed on hysterosalpingography by identifying small diverticular outpouchings that project from the lumen of the tubes. The disorder likely is a response to previous tubal inflammation, because these patients usually have a history of previous pelvic infections. Most cases are bilateral, and patients with this disorder have an increased frequency of infertility and tubal pregnancies (62).

Adenomyosis of the uterus refers to nests of endometrium that are contained in the uterine wall because of an abnormal down-growth of the basal zone of the endometrium into the myometrium. Clinically, patients with this disorder present with various signs and symptoms including uterine enlargement, dysmenorrhea, or menorrhagia. Hysterosalpingography may provide a specific diagnosis of this entity by demonstrating small diverticular outpouchings along the body or fundus of the uterus (62).

Aunt Minnie's Pearls

- *Small diverticula of the isthmic portion of the fallopian tubes = salpingitis isthmica nodosa.*
- *Small diverticula of the body or fundus of the uterus = adenomyosis.*

REFERENCES

1. McCallum RW. The adult male urethra: normal anatomy, pathology, and method of urethrography. Radiol Clin North Am 1979;17:227–244.
2. Talner LB. Specific causes of obstruction. In: Pollack HM, ed. Clinical urography: an atlas and textbook of urological imaging. Philadelphia: Saunders, 1990;2:1629–1751.
3. McCallum RW. Lower urinary tract trauma. Appl Radiol 1993;22:15–20, 25.
4. Sandler CM, Hall JT, Rodriguez MB, Corriere JN Jr. Bladder injury in blunt pelvic trauma. Radiology 1986;158:633–638.
5. Amis ES Jr, Newhouse JH. Urologic trauma. In: Essentials of uroradiology. Boston: Little, Brown, 1991:353–366.
6. Timmons JW Jr, Malek RS, Hattery RR, Deweerd JH. Caliceal diverticulum. J Urol 1975;114:6–9.
7. Middleton AW Jr, Pfister RC. Stone-containing pyelocaliceal diverticulum: embryogenic, anatomic, radiologic and clinical characteristics. J Urol 1974;11:2–6.
8. Bosniak MA. Angiomyolipoma (hamartoma) of the kidney: a preoperative diagnosis is possible in virtually every case. Urol Radiol 1981;3:135–142.
9. Hélénon O, Chrétien Y, Paraf F, Melki P, Denys A, Moreau JF. Renal cell carcinoma containing fat: demonstration with CT. Radiology 1993;188:429–430.
10. Federle MP, McAninch JW, Kaiser JA, Goodman PC, Roberts J, Mall JC. Computed tomography of urinary calculi. AJR 1981;136:255–258.
11. Lüscher TF, Lie JT, Stanson AW, Houser OW, Hollier LH, Sheps SG. Arterial fibromuscular dysplasia. Mayo Clin Proc 1987;62:931–952.
12. King BF. Diagnostic imaging evaluation of renovascular hypertension. Abdom Imaging 1995;20:395–405.
13. Ferris EJ, Bosniak MA, O'Connor JF. An angiographic sign demonstrating extension of renal carcinoma into the renal vein and vena cava. AJR 1968;102:384–391.
14. Zagoria RJ, Bechtold RE, Dyer RB. Staging of renal adenocarcinoma: role of various imaging procedures. AJR 1995;164:363–370.
15. Bergman H, Friedenberg RM, Sayegh V. New roentgenologic signs of carcinoma of the ureter. AJR 1961;86:707–717.
16. Ramchandani P, Pollack HM. Tumors of the urothelium. Semin Roentgenol 1995;30:149–167.
17. Lautin EM, Haramati N, Frager D, et al. CT diagnosis of circumcaval ureter. AJR 1988;150:591–594.
18. Pitts WR Jr, Muecke ED. Horseshoe kidneys: a 40-year experience. J Urol 1975;113:743–746.
19. Silva JM, Jafri SZH, Cacciarelli AA, Madrazo BL, Farah J, Roberts JL. Abnormalities of the kidney: embryogenesis and radiologic appearance. Appl Radiol 1995;24:19–28.
20. Lalli AF. Medullary sponge kidney disease. Radiology 1969;1992:92–96.
21. Goldman SM, Hartman DS. Medullary sponge kidney. In Hartman DS. Renal cystic disease. Philadelphia: Saunders, 1989:108–119.
22. Mayo-Smith WW, Lee MJ, McNicholas MMJ, Hahn PF, Boland GW, Saini S. Characterization of adrenal masses (<5 cm) by use of chemical shift MR imaging: observer performance versus quantitative measures. AJR 1995;165:91–95.
23. Outwater EK, Siegelman ES, Radecki PD, Piccoli CW, Mitchell DG. Distinction between benign and malignant adrenal masses: value of T1-weighted chemical-shift MR imaging. AJR 1995;165:579–583.
24. Bilbey JH, McLoughlin RF, Kurkjian PS, et al. MR imaging of adrenal masses: value of chemical-shift imaging for distinguishing adenomas from other tumors. AJR 1995;164:637–642.
25. Evanoff GV, Thompson CS, Foley R, Weinman EJ. Spectrum of gas within the kidney: emphysematous pyelonephritis and emphysematous pyelitis. Am J Med 1987;83:149–154.
26. Lautin EM, Gordon PM, Friedman AC, Dourmashkin L, Fromowitz F. Emphysematous pyelonephritis: optimal diagnosis and treatment. Urol Radiol 1979;1:93–96.
27. Michaeli J, Mogle P, Perlberg S, Heiman S, Caine M. Emphysematous pyelonephritis. J Urol 1984;131:203–208.
28. Meyers MA, Whalen JP, Evans JA, Viamonte M. Malposition and displacement of the bowel in renal agenesis and ectopia: new observations. AJR 1973;117:323–333.
29. Mascatello V, Lebowitz RL. Malposition of the colon in left renal agenesis and ectopia. Radiology 1976;120:371–376.
30. Friedland GW, Devries PA, Nino-Murciam, Cohen R, Rifkin MD. Congenital anomalies of the urinary tract. In: Pollack HM, ed. Clinical urography. Philadelphia: Saunders, 1990;1:559–787.
31. Liebeskind AL, Elkin M, Goldman SH. Herniation of the bladder. Radiology 1973;106:257–262.
32. Teasley GH. Cystitis emphysematosa: case report with a review of literature. J Urol 1949;62:48–51.
33. Ney C, Kumar M, Billah K, Doerr J. CT demonstration of cystitis emphysematosa. J Comput Assist Tomogr 1987;11:552–553.
34. Waltzer WC. The urinary tract in pregnancy. J Urol 1981;125:271–276.
35. Peake SL, Roxburgh HB, Langlois SLP. Ultrasonic assessment of hydronephrosis of pregnancy. Radiology 1983;146:167–170.
36. Dure-Smith P. Pregnancy dilatation of the urinary tract. Radiology 1970;96:545–550.
37. Harrow BR, Sloane JA, Salhanick L. Etiology of the hydronephrosis of pregnancy. Surg Gynecol Obstet 1964;119:1042–1048.
38. Eckert DE, Jonutis AJ, Davidson AJ. The incidence and manifestations of urographic papillary abnormalities in patients with S hemoglobinopathies. Radiology 1974;113:59–63.
39. Amis ES, Newhouse JH. Essentials of uroradiology. Boston: Little, Brown, 1991;12:171–188.
40. Hartman GW, Torres VE, Leago GF, Williamson Jr B, Hattery RR. Analgesic-associated nephropathy. JAMA 1984;251:1734–1738.
41. Talner LB, Gittes RF. Megacalyces. Clin Radiol 1972;23:355–361.
42. Kozakewich HPW, Lebowitz RL. Congenital megacalyces. Pediatr Radiol 1974;2:251–258.

43. Mellins HZ. Cystic dilatations of the upper urinary tract: a radiologist's developmental model. Radiology 1984;153:291–301.
44. Dunbar JS, Nogrady MB. The calyceal crescent: a roentgenographic sign of obstructive hydronephrosis. AJR 1970;110:520–528.
45. LeVine M, Allen A, Stein JL, Schwartz S. The crescent sign. Radiology 1963;81:971–973.
46. Cochran ST, Walsman J, Barbaric ZL. Radiographic and microscopic findings in multiple ureteral diverticula. Radiology 1980;137:631–636.
47. Wasserman NF, La Pointe S, Posalaky IP. Ureteral pseudodiverticulosis. Radiology 1985;155:561–566.
48. Parker MD, Rebsamen S, Clark RL. Multiple ureteral diverticula: a possible radiographically demonstrable risk factor in development of transitional cell carcinoma. Urol Radiol 1989;11:45–48.
49. Becker JA. Renal tuberculosis. Urol Radiol 1988;10:25–30.
50. Kollins SA, Hartman GW, Carr DT, Segura JW, Hattery RR. Roentgenographic findings in urinary tract tuberculosis: a 10-year review. AJR 1974:121:487–499.
51. Premkumar A, Lattimer J, Newhouse JH. CT and sonography of advanced urinary tract tuberculosis. AJR 1987;148:65–69.
52. Amis ES Jr, Newhouse JH. Congenital anomalies. In: Essentials of uroradiology. Boston: Little, Brown, 1991:57–72.
53. Mitty HA, Schapira HE. Ureterocele and pseudoureterocele: cobra versus cancer. J Urol 1977;117:557–561.
54. Thornbury JR, Silver TM, Vinson RK. Ureteroceles vs. pseudoureteroceles in adults. Radiology 1977;122:81–84.
55. Banner MP, Pollack HM. Urolithiasis in the lower urinary tract. Semin Roentgenol 1982;17:140–148.
56. Saunders HS, Dyer RB, Shifrin RY, Scharling ES, Bechtold RE, Zagoria RJ. The CT nephrogram: implications for evaluation of urinary tract disease. RadioGraphics 1995;15:1069–1085.
57. Musante F, Derchi LE, Zappasodi F, et al. Myelolipoma of the adrenal gland: sonographic and CT features. AJR 1988;151:961–964.
58. Dunnick NR. Adrenal imaging: current status. AJR 1990;154:927–936.
59. Greenberg M, Stone D, Cochran ST, et al. Female urethral diverticula: double-balloon catheter study. AJR 1981;136:259–264.
60. Goldman SM, Hartman DS. Autosomal dominant polycystic kidney disease. In: Hartman DS. Renal cystic disease. Philadelphia: Saunders, 1989:88–107.
61. Levine E, Grantham JJ. Calcified renal stones and cyst calcifications in autosomal dominant polycystic kidney disease: clinical and CT study in 84 patients. AJR 1992;159:77–81.
62. Yoder IC, Hall DA. Hysterosalpingography in the 1990s. AJR 1991;157:675–683.

FIGURE CREDITS

Figure 3.2.2. From Gutiérrez FR, Canter CE, Mirowitz SA. MR appearance of congenital heart defects. In: Gutiérrez FR, Brown JJ, Mirowitz SA, eds. Cardiovascular magnetic resonance imaging. St. Louis: Mosby, 1992:79.

Figure 3.7.2. From Gutiérrez FR, Canter CE, Mirowitz SA. MR appearance of congenital heart defects. In: Gutiérrez FR, Brown JJ, Mirowitz SA, eds. Cardiovascular magnetic resonance imaging. St. Louis: Mosby, 1992:82.

Figure 4.4.3. From Benedetti (14), with permission.

Figures 5.19.1 and 5.19.2. Courtesy of J. Philip Moyers and Scott L. Kaltman, Mallinckrodt Institute of Radiology, St. Louis, MO.

Figure 6.24.1. Reprinted by permission from Southern Med J 1994;87:1278–1279.

Figure 6.31.1. Courtesy of Thomas E. Underhill, Diagnostic Radiology Resident, Bowman Gray School of Medicine, Winston-Salem, NC.

Figures 7.2.1–7.2.4. Courtesy of Harold Bennett, Mallinckrodt Institute of Radiology, St. Louis, MO.

Figures 7.4.1–7.4.3. Courtesy of Stuart Sagel and Scott L. Kaltman, Mallinckrodt Institute of Radiology, St. Louis, MO.

Figures 7.5.1–7.5.3. Reprinted with permission from Chiles C, Choplin RH. Radiology of the chest. In: Chen MYM, Pope TL Jr, Ott DJ, eds. Basic radiology. New York: McGraw-Hill, 1995:125–127.

Figures 7.8.1–7.8.2. Reprinted with permission from Chiles C, Choplin RH. Radiology of the chest. In: Chen MYM, Pope TL Jr, Ott DJ, eds. Basic radiology. New York: McGraw-Hill, 1995:91.

Figure 7.10.1. From Chen MYM, Pope TL Jr, Ott DJ. Basic radiology. New York: McGraw-Hill, 1995.

Figure 8.2.1. Reprinted with permission from Freimanis R. Radiology of the breast. In: Chen MYM, Pope TL Jr, Ott DJ, eds., Basic radiology. New York: McGraw-Hill, 1995:169.

Figure 8.14.2. Reprinted with permission from Freimanis R. Radiology of the breast. In: Chen MYM, Pope TL Jr, Ott DJ, eds. Basic radiology. New York: McGraw-Hill, 1995:158.

Figure 8.16.2. Courtesy of John W. Gilpin, Greenville Radiology, Greenville, SC.

Figure 8.17.1. Courtesy of Barbara Monsees, Mallinckrodt Institute of Radiology, St. Louis, MO.

Figure 9.10.1. From Ott DJ, Katz PO, Wu WC. Antireflux barrier. In: Castell DO, Wu WC, Ott DJ, eds. Gastrointestinal reflux disease: pathogenesis, diagnosis, therapy. Mt. Kisco, NY: Futura, 1985:43.

Figure 9.11.1. From Ott DJ. The esophagus: diaphragmatic hernias. In: Taveras JM, Ferruci JT, eds. Radiology: diagnosis—imaging—intervention. Philadelphia: Lippincott, 1993;4:7.

Figure 9.21.1. Courtesy of Jeff Brody, Davis Community Hospital, Statesville, NC.

Figures 9.22–9.22.3. Courtesy of Jeff Brody, Davis Community Hospital, Statesville, NC.

Figures 10.30.1–10.30.3. Courtesy of Cary Lynn Siegel, Mallinckrodt Institute of Radiology, St. Louis, MO.

INDEX